Essentials of
BIOCHEMISTRY
(For Medical Students)

Essentials of
BIOCHEMISTRY
(For Medical Students)

FOURTH EDITION

Shivananda Nayak B
MSc PhD FAGE NRCC-CC (USA) FACB (USA)

Professor of Biochemistry
Department of Preclinical Sciences
Faculty of Medical Sciences
University of the West Indies
Trinidad and Tobago, West Indies

Visiting Professor
Sri Ramachandra University
Chennai, Tamil Nadu, India
Subbaiah Institute of Medical Science
Shivamogga, Karnataka, India

Foreword
Ramdas M Pai

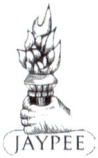

JAYPEE BROTHERS MEDICAL PUBLISHERS
The Health Sciences Publisher
New Delhi | London

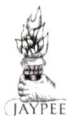 **Jaypee Brothers Medical Publishers (P) Ltd**

Headquarters

Jaypee Brothers Medical Publishers (P) Ltd
EMCA House, 23/23-B
Ansari Road, Daryaganj
New Delhi - 110 002, INDIA
Landline: +91-11-23272143,+91-11-23272703,
+91-11-23282021,+91-11-23245672
Email: jaypee@jaypeebrothers.com

Corporate Office

Jaypee Brothers Medical Publishers (P) Ltd
4838/24, Ansari Road, Daryaganj
New Delhi 110 002, India
Phone: +91-11-43574357
Fax: +91-11-43574314
Email: jaypee@jaypeebrothers.com

Overseas Office

J.P. Medical Ltd
83 Victoria Street, London
SW1H 0HW (UK)
Phone: +44 20 3170 8910
Fax: +44 (0)20 3008 6180
Email: info@jpmedpub.com

Website: www.jaypeebrothers.com
Website: www.jaypeedigital.com

© 2022, Jaypee Brothers Medical Publishers

The views and opinions expressed in this book are solely those of the original contributor(s)/author(s) and do not necessarily represent those of editor(s) of the book.

All rights reserved. No part of this publication may be reproduced, stored or transmitted in any form or by any means, electronic, mechanical, photocopying, recording or otherwise, without the prior permission in writing of the publishers/ editors.

All brand names and product names used in this book are trade names, service marks, trademarks or registered trademarks of their respective owners. The publisher is not associated with any product or vendor mentioned in this book.

Medical knowledge and practice change constantly. This book is designed to provide accurate, authoritative information about the subject matter in question. However, readers are advised to check the most current information available on procedures included and check information from the manufacturer of each product to be administered, to verify the recommended dose, formula, method and duration of administration, adverse effects and contraindications. It is the responsibility of the practitioner to take all appropriate safety precautions. Neither the publisher nor the author(s)/editor(s) assume any liability for any injury and/or damage to persons or property arising from or related to use of material in this book.

This book is sold on the understanding that the publisher is not engaged in providing professional medical services. If such advice or services are required, the services of a competent medical professional should be sought.

Every effort has been made where necessary to contact holders of copyright to obtain permission to reproduce copyright material. If any have been inadvertently overlooked, the publisher will be pleased to make the necessary arrangements at the first opportunity. The **CD/DVD-ROM** (if any) provided in the sealed envelope with this book is complimentary and free of cost. **Not meant for sale.**

Inquiries for bulk sales may be solicited at: jaypee@jaypeebrothers.com

Essentials of Biochemistry (For Medical Students)

First Edition: 2010

Second Edition: 2013

Third Edition: 2016

Fourth Edition: **2022**

ISBN: 978-93-89188-68-4

Dedicated to

My Parents and Family

Foreword

Biochemistry is such a vast branch of medical science that it has been the backbone of many studies aimed at raising the standard and effectiveness of medical procedures. It encompasses a host of subspecialties relevant to a thorough study of the subject. For medical students in particular, an in-depth knowledge of the subject is essential to ensure a successful medical career.

I am glad that Dr Shivananda Nayak B has come out with yet another book on biochemistry to enable the medical students to understand the subject thoroughly and with ease. As an author of three earlier books on biochemistry, he has dealt with the subject with lucidity and clarity in this book. His meticulous presentation of the subject with illustrations in the chapters will certainly add to the relevance of the book for medical students. The MCQs and case studies of each chapter will certainly help the medical graduates to prepare for postgraduate entrance tests. Having worked as a teacher of biochemistry for the last over 30 years, he knows the pulse of the students and the book is sure to demonstrate the wealth of his knowledge about the subject.

I am happy to write the Foreword for this book—*Essentials of Biochemistry (For Medical Students)*, and I hope the book will receive appreciation from both the medical students and their teachers.

Ramdas M Pai MBBS
President and Chancellor
Manipal University
Manipal, Karnataka, India

Message

It gives me the greatest pleasure to write this message to commemorate the publication of this fine textbook, *Essentials of Biochemistry (For Medical Students)*, authored by my colleague Dr Shivananda Nayak B.

As the Faculty of Medical Sciences in the University of the West Indies, Dr Nayak is very highly respected by all levels of staff and it is my observation that he is extremely well-liked by the student body. The reason is plain—he is totally committed to them and can be confidently described as student-centered.

He believes in making learning easy as he has been systematic in his approach so that ideas and information can be readily infused within the vast knowledge base that is required in the curriculum, which serves the future health professional.

Dr Nayak has had a meteoric rise to this position of author having already produced three successful books each of which is focused on a special audience.

He is really a visionary and truly an asset to the Department of Preclinical Sciences and the Faculty of Medical Sciences. His aim is to help and that is being accomplished admirably in the way that he has touched the lives of the many who have been able to gain from his own teaching, learning and research experience.

As a person, Dr Nayak is humble, patient and honest in his work. In a project such as this, he was ably supported by his wife who would have endured many hours without his immediate attention, as he was engrossed in this vision. I thank her for this level of devotion to him.

I am sure that this book will be one that students will read now for their initial exposure, but they will be happy to keep this for their continuing education in the years to come, when they will be looking for information, which is easy to read and assimilate.

My heartiest congratulations to him on this milestone achievement!

Samuel Ramsewak FRCOG FACOG
Professor
Faculty of Medical Sciences
University of the West Indies
Trinidad and Tobago, West Indies

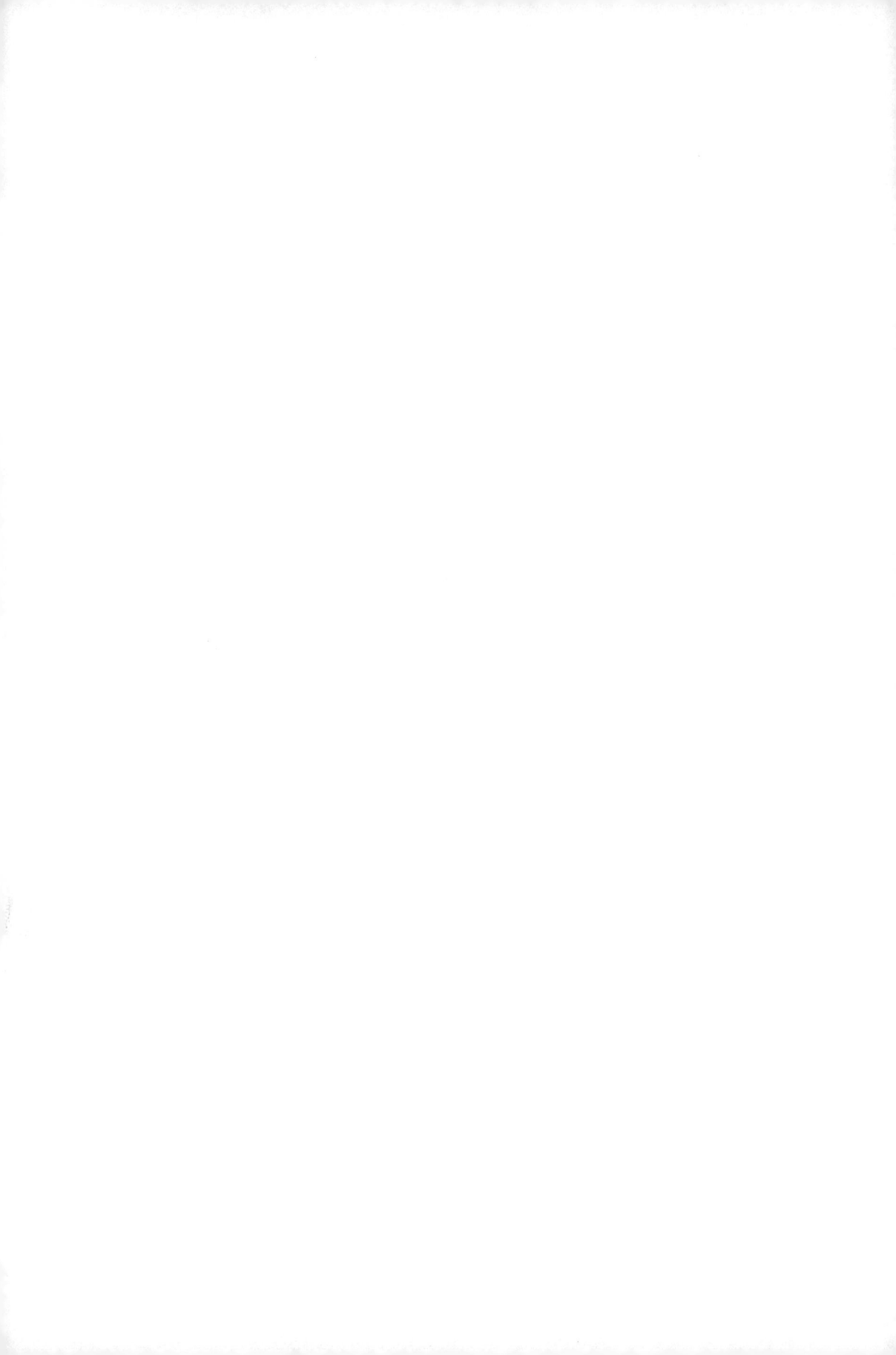

Message

I congratulate Dr Shivananda Nayak, on the upcoming publication of the fourth edition of the *Essentials of Biochemistry (For Medical Students)*. The book is concise, precise, with easy presentation of biochemistry. The illustrations are very good and informative which make theory easier to understand as well as retain the subject. I appreciate Dr Shivananda Nayak for putting all the work in this book and it deserves recognition by all. The success will keep you going well beyond this edition. I am sure that this book will most sought after by both faculty and student communities.

Santhi Silambanan MD DNB MBA
Professor of Biochemistry
Sri Ramachandra University of Higher Education and Research
Porur, Chennai, India

Message

I am glad that Dr Shivananda Nayak B has come out with fourth edition of *Essentials of Biochemistry (For Medical Students)*. The book includes the biochemical aspects that are essential for medical students. Presentation is simple, lucid, concise and easily reproducible. All chapters have been thoroughly revised and updated. New chapters have been incorporated. Diagram-based explanations and self-assessment questions given in each chapter are useful for examination preparation. I am confident that the students will be benefitted from this book.

Wilma Delphine Silvia MD DNB MNAMS FAGE
NABL Assessor, Executive Editor of IJCDR
Professor and Head
Department of Biochemistry
Bowring Institute of Medical Sciences
and Research Centre
Bengaluru, Karnataka, India

Message

I am immensely pleased to compliment Dr Shivananda Nayak B, who has authored this textbook *Essentials of Biochemistry (For Medical Students)*, which has now entered in its fourth edition.

Professor Shivananda Nayak is a meticulous scientist, an alumnus of Kasturba Medical College, Manipal, Karnataka, India, and also former Associate Professor. Throughout his career, he received several fellowships and authored numerous textbooks on biochemistry. He is an enthusiastic and fanatical teacher I have ever come across. His publications stand a key index of his knowledge in the subject.

I am sure that this book makes biochemistry comprehensible and will be chosen by thousands of medical students and graduates in biochemistry. The line drawings and diagrams help students remember the important structures and processes, while the multiple choice questions and case studies applied enable the students to test their skills. This much-awaited textbook being published will be a boon for the students.

I extend my congratulations to Dr Nayak for his achievement and also wish him many more fruitful endeavors.

Anuradha CV MSc PhD
Professor
Department of Biochemistry and Biotechnology
Faculty of Science
Annamalai University
Cuddalore, Tamil Nadu, India

Message

I am very happy that Dr Shivananda Nayak B is bringing the fourth edition of his book *Essentials of Biochemistry (for Medical Students)*. I know him as my teacher as well as my mentor throughout my studies in Manipal University. I have gone through this book, which has been presented in a simple way that anyone can understand easily. The presentation is simple, lucid, concise and easily reproducible with all chapters thoroughly revised and updated. Diagram-based explanation and self-assessment questions given in each chapter are useful for easy understanding as well as for examination preparation. Students will be benefitted from this book. I congratulate him on his achievement and for bringing out this fourth edition expediously.

Surapaneni Krishna Mohan PhD MHPE CSCI MRSC
Associate Professor
Department of Biochemistry
Faculty of Medicine
Saveetha University
Chennai, Tamil Nadu, India

Preface to the Fourth Edition

I am happy to present the fourth edition of *Essentials of Biochemistry (For Medical Students)*. My experience of more than 30 years in teaching Biochemistry to Medical, Dental and Allied health, Pharmacy and Nursing students in India as well as abroad made me to present this fourth edition in a simple way that can be easily understood by the student community. I tried my best to incorporate diagram-based explanations and self-assessment questions in each chapter. The encouragement, support and suggestions from lecturers, professors and the students inspired me to reveal this fourth edition with interesting flowcharts and case studies. I have tried to edit some of the contents as per the suggestions made by lecturers and some of my colleagues.

As per my promise, I am bringing this fourth edition. The comments, suggestions and constructive criticisms from faculty and students are always welcome. Please feel free to communicate at my e-mail address **shiv25@gmail.com**, if you have any suggestion.

Shivananda Nayak B

Preface to the First Edition

I am glad to present this edition entitled *Essentials of Biochemistry (for Medical Students)*. There are many textbooks, which deal with the theory aspects of Biochemistry in a simple way. My experience of more than 18 years in teaching Biochemistry to medical students both in India and abroad has motivated me to write this title in a simple way that can be easily grasped by the student community. I tried my best to incorporate diagram-based explanations wherever necessary that may help the readers. Also, I made an attempt to present self-assessment questions and case studies at the end of each chapter. The encouragement and support both from the teacher and the student community inspired me to present this title with interesting diagram-based explanations.

It is my duty to thank all those who warmly received my other titles like *Manipal Manual of Clinical Biochemistry* and *Handbook of Biochemistry* published by M/s Jaypee Brothers Medical Publishers (P) Ltd, New Delhi, India. I sincerely thank Dr Ramdas M Pai, President, Manipal University, Manipal, Karnataka, India, and Dr Sudhakar Nayak, Head, Department of Biochemistry, who encouraged me to offer my 15 years of service to the Kasturba Medical College, Manipal. I am always grateful to Dr Shivaraj, Professor (Biochemistry) for his inspirations throughout my service. I am indebted to Dr Bhoendradatt Tewarie, Director (PVC planning), University of the West Indies, for his support when I joined the university. It is my pleasure to thank Professor Samuel Ramsewak, Faculty of Medical Sciences, University of the West Indies, for his support. Last but not least, I thank each and every one who encouraged me to write this title at the right time. I extend my thanks to Miss Geetha Bhaktha for editing the contents.

I am immensely grateful to Dr Geetha Samanth (DVS College of Arts and Science, Shivamogga), Dr (Mrs) Vinutha Bhat and Dr Krishnananda Prabhu (Kasturba Medical College, Manipal, Karnataka, India) for contributing the following chapters—Cell, Biochemistry of Cancer and Radioisotopes in Medicine, respectively.

A textbook will be improved only by successive revisions. I will try to revise this book every two years. The comments, suggestions and constructive criticisms from faculty and students are always welcome. Please feel free to communicate at my e-mail address shiv25@gmail.com, if you have any suggestion. The success of the book was due to the active participation of the publisher. This is to record my appreciation for the support extended by Shri Jitendar P Vij (Group Chairman), Mr Ankit Vij (Managing Director), Mr Tarun Duneja (Director-Publishing), Mr Venugopal (Bengaluru Branch) and the associates of M/s Jaypee Brothers Medical Publishers (P) Ltd, New Delhi, India, for readily conceding my request to publish the book in color and taking all pains to bring out the book to my utmost satisfaction.

Shivananda Nayak B

Acknowledgments

I sincerely thank all those who warmly received the third editions, and other titles such as *Manipal Manual of Clinical Biochemistry* and *Handbook of Biochemistry* published by M/s Jaypee Brothers Medical Publishers (P) Ltd, New Delhi. It is my pleasure to thank Dr Ramdas M Pai, President and Chancellor, Manipal University, Manipal, Karnataka, India, for writing Foreword to this book. I am indebted to Professor Samuel Ramsewak, Faculty of Medical Sciences, University of the West Indies, for the message and his continuous support. Also, I thank each and every one who encouraged me to bring this fourth edition.

I am immensely grateful to Dr Geetha Samanth (DVS College of Arts and Science, Shivamogga) and Dr Krishnananda Prabhu (Kasturba Medical College, Manipal, Karnataka, India) for contributing the following chapters—Cell, and Radioisotopes in Medicine, respectively.

The success of this book was due to the active participation of the publisher. This is to record my appreciation for the support extended by Shri Jitendar P Vij (Group Chairman), Mr Ankit Vij (Managing Director), Mr MS Mani (Group President), Dr Madhu Choudhary (Publishing Head–Education), Ms Pooja Bhandari (Production Head), Ms Sunita Katla (Executive Assistant to Group Chairman and Publishing Manager), Ms Samina Khan (Executive Assistant to Publishing Head–Education), Mr Rajesh Sharma (Production Coordinator), Ms Seema Dogra (Cover Visualizer), Mr Deepak Saxena (Typesetter), Mr Narsing Kumar (Proofreader), Mr Pappu Kumar (Graphic Designer), and Mr Venugopal Vishnumurthy (Associate Director-South), Bengaluru Production Unit/Bengaluru Branch and the associates of M/s Jaypee Brothers Medical Publishers (P) Ltd, New Delhi, India, for readily conceding my request to publish the book in color and taking all pains to bring this book to my utmost satisfaction.

Content

1. Cell 1
- *Structural and Functional Aspects of Cell Organelles   1*
- *Prokaryotic and Eukaryotic Cells   4*
- *Transport Across Membranes   5*
- *Fluid Mosaic Model   6*
- *Transport Mechanisms in the Membranes   6*
- *Cell Fractionation   8*

2. Bioenergetics 13
- *Free Energy   13*
- *High-energy Compounds   14*

3. Enzymes 16
- *Chemical Nature of Enzymes   16*
- *Ribozymes   17*
- *Zymogens or Proenzymes   17*
- *Coenzymes   17*
- *Energy of Activation of Catalyzed and Uncatalyzed Reactions   18*
- *List and Explain the Factors that Affect the Enzyme Activity   18*
- *Classification of Enzymes   19*
- *Mechanism of Enzyme Catalysis   20*
- *Enzyme Kinetics   21*
- *Michaelis–Menten Equation   21*
- *Enzyme Inhibition   23*
- *Therapeutic Use of Competitive Inhibition   23*
- *Allosteric Enzymes   26*
- *Isoenzymes   26*
- *Diagnostic Enzymes   26*
- *Lactate Dehydrogenase   26*

4. Chemistry of Amino Acids and Proteins 35
- *Essential and Nonessential Amino Acids   37*
- *Glucogenic and Ketogenic Amino Acids   38*
- *Ninhydrin Reaction   38*
- *Peptides and Peptide Bond   39*
- *Classification of Proteins   40*
- *Important Functions of Proteins   41*
- *Structure of Proteins   41*
- *Denaturation of Proteins   44*
- *Plasma Proteins   44*
- *Multiple Myeloma   47*

5. Metabolism of Amino Acids 53
- Digestion and Absorption of Proteins in the Gastrointestinal Tract 53
- Metabolism of Amino Acids 55
- Urea Cycle (Krebs–Henseleit Cycle) 56
- Metabolism of Important Amino Acids 59
- One-carbon Metabolism with Examples 61
- Metabolism of Glycine Including the Products Formed from It 61
- Importance of Specialized Products Formed from Glycine 62
- Metabolism of Phenylalanine and Tyrosine 65
- Metabolism of Tyrosine 65
- Specialized Products Formed from Tyrosine 66
- Synthesis of Catecholamines 67
- Metabolism of Tryptophan 68
- Metabolic Fate of Tryptophan 68
- Disorders 69
- Histidine Metabolism 69
- Metabolism of Branched-chain Amino Acid 71
- Metabolic Disorders 72
- Inborn Errors of Metabolism 74

6. Chemistry of Carbohydrates 80
- Classification of Carbohydrates 80
- Homopolysaccharides 81
- Heteropolysaccharides with Examples and their Biomedical Importance 82
- Isomerism in Carbohydrates 83
- Optical Activity of Carbohydrates, Including Stereoisomerism with Specific Examples 83
- Invert Sugar with Example 84
- Chemical Properties of Monosaccharides 85
- Glycosidic Bond 86
- Tests for Carbohydrates 87
- Special Carbohydrates of Clinical Importance 87

7. Metabolism of Carbohydrates 91
- Digestion and Absorption of Carbohydrates 91
- Metabolism of Carbohydrate 94
- Glycolysis 96
- Compounds Formed from Pyruvate 101
- Compounds Formed from Acetyl-CoA 102
- TCA Cycle 103
- Gluconeogenesis and Its Importance in Regulating the Blood Glucose 106
- Cori Cycle and its Clinical Importance 108
- Metabolism of Glycogen 110
- Synthesis of Glycogen from Glucose 110
- Oxidative and Nonoxidative Phases of Hexose Monophosphate Pathway and its Importance 114
- Galactose Metabolism 117
- Fructose Metabolism 118
- Sorbitol Pathway and its Clinical Significance 118
- Lactose Intolerance 120
- Regulation of Blood Glucose 121

- Role of Hormones in Regulating the Blood Glucose 121
- Insulin 122
- Mechanism of Action of Insulin in Regulating the Blood Glucose 123
- Hyperglycemic Hormones and their Role in Regulating the Blood Glucose 124
- Diabetes Mellitus 124
- Criteria Used to Diagnose the Diabetes Mellitus 126
- Clinical Complications of Diabetes Mellitus 126
- Glucose Tolerance Test and Its Clinical Significance 127
- Case Study 138

8. Chemistry of Lipids 140
- Functions of Lipids 140
- Classification of Lipids with Specific Examples 140
- Simple Lipids 141
- Compound Lipids 141
- Apoproteins 144
- Derived Lipids 145
- Properties of Lipids 148

9. Metabolism of Lipids 153
- Digestion and Absorption of Lipids 153
- Metabolism of Lipids 157
- Compounds Formed from Acetyl-CoA 161
- Regulation of Cholesterol Biosynthesis and Significance of Biochemical Basis of Use of Hypolipidemic Drugs 166
- Ketone Body Metabolism 167
- Conditions in Which Ketone Body Formation Occurs 168
- Phospholipid Metabolism 169
- Lipoprotein Metabolism 171
- Fatty Liver 175
- Regulation of Lipid Metabolism 177
- Alcohol Metabolism 177
- Synthesis of Prostaglandins 179
- Biochemical Actions of Prostaglandins 181
- Leukotrienes 182
- Lipid Storage Disorders 182
- Risk Factors for Cardiovascular Disease 185

10. Integration of Metabolism 194
- Pathways of Metabolism 194
- Adipose Tissue Hormones 200
- Diabetes Mellitus: Types, Metabolic Changes, and Complications 202
- Atherosclerosis 203
- Laboratory Tests in Myocardial Infarction 204

11. Hemoglobin 209
- Structure of Hemoglobin 209
- Comparison of Myoglobin with Hemoglobin 210
- Cooperative Binding of Oxygen by Hemoglobin 212
- Clinical Aspects of Heme Metabolism 215

- Disorders of Hemoglobin Catabolism   217
- Role of Hemoglobin in Disease   219
- Abnormal Hemoglobin   220
- Hemoglobinopathy   220
- Thalassemia and its Important Types   221
- Sickle Cell Hemoglobin and its Causes and Symptoms   221
- Test for the Detection of Abnormal Hemoglobin   222
- Derived Hemoglobin Compounds   223
- Case Study   226

12. Hormones 227
- Mechanism of Hormonal Action   228
- Pituitary Hormones   228
- Thyroid Hormones   232
- Parathyroid Hormones   233
- Adrenal Gland Hormones   233
- Pancreatic Hormones   238
- Female Sex Hormones   238
- Case Studies   243

13. Acid-base Balance 246
- Regulation of Acid-base Balance   247
- Blood Buffer System   247
- Role of Respiratory and Renal Mechanism in Regulating the Blood pH   250
- Acid-base Disorders   251
- Assessment of Acid-base Analysis   254
- Case Studies   257

14. Biological Oxidation 259
- Electron Transport Chain, its Organization and Components   260
- Uncouplers   264

15. Mineral Metabolism 267
- Macrominerals or Bulk Elements   267
- Microminerals or Trace Elements   276

16. Vitamins 286
- Fat-Soluble Vitamins   286
- Water-soluble Vitamins   291
- B-complex Vitamins   292

17. Nutrition 305
- Caloric Values of Macronutrients   306
- Respiratory Quotient of Food Stuffs   306
- Nutritional Importance of Carbohydrates, Proteins, and Fats   307
- Dietary Fiber   309
- Metabolic Rate/Energy Expenditure   311
- Calculation of Basal Metabolic Rate   313
- Methods of Determining Caloric Needs   313
- Nitrogen Balance   315

- Balanced Diet   315
- Assessing Nutritional Status   316
- Methods Available to Measure the Nutritional Status   318
- Nutrition-related Diseases   321
- Causes, Signs, and Symptoms of Different Types of Protein–Energy Malnutrition   323

18. Chemistry of Nucleic Acid 328
- Nucleosides and Nucleotides   328
- Synthetic Analogs of Nucleotides or Antimetabolites   332
- The Structure of DNA   335
- Types of RNA   336

19. Nucleic Acid Metabolism 340
- Purine Metabolism   340
- Pyrimidine Metabolism   344

20. Molecular Biology 349
- Deoxyribonucleic Acid   349
- Genomics   350
- Proteomics and its Applications   350
- Difference between Genomics and Proteomics   351
- Metabolomics   351
- Replication   351
- Telomere and Telomerase   353
- Deoxyribonucleic Acid Repair   354
- Mutation   356
- Ribonucleic Acid   359
- Transcription   360
- Genetic Code   362
- Translation   362
- Recombinant DNA   372
- Polymerase Chain Reaction   374
- Southern, Northern, and Western Blotting and their Applications   376
- Restriction Enzymes   379
- Plasmid   379
- Restriction Fragment Length Polymorphism   380
- Deoxyribonucleic Acid Libraries   381

21. Organ Function Tests 387
- Liver Function Tests   387
- Renal Function Tests   391
- Thyroid Function Tests   394
- Adrenal Gland   399
- Pathophysiology   400
- Case Studies   404

22. Extracellular Matrix 407
- Biomolecules in Extracellular Matrix   407
- Collagen   407
- Elastin   409

- *Fibrillin   409*
- *Fibronectin   410*
- *Laminin   410*
- *Glycosaminoglycans   410*
- *Proteoglycans   411*

23. Biochemistry of Muscle Structure and Function 416
- *Types of Muscles   416*
- *Activation of Skeletal Muscle   418*
- *Type I versus Type II Fibers   421*
- *Cardiac Muscle   422*
- *Smooth Muscle   424*
- *Adenosine Triphosphate Hydrolysis for Muscle Contraction   425*
- *Muscle Diseases   426*

24. Water and Electrolyte Balance 432
- *Water Balance   432*
- *Causes and Symptoms of Hypovolemia and Hypervolemia   435*
- *Electrolyte Balance   436*
- *Causes and Symptoms of Different Types of Hyponatremia and Hypernatremia   438*

25. Biochemistry of AIDS 444
- *Factors Influencing Transmission of AIDS   444*
- *Symptoms of HIV Infection   444*
- *Routes of Transmission   446*
- *Pathophysiology   447*
- *Molecular Basis of HIV   448*
- *Diagnosis of AIDS   449*
- *Prevention of AIDS   449*
- *Treatment of AIDS   450*

26. Biochemistry of Cancer 452
- *Cell Cycle   454*
- *Tumor Markers   465*
- *Oncofetal Antigens   469*
- *Biochemical Basis of Cancer Therapy   470*

27. Radioisotopes in Medicine 475
- *Types of Radiation   476*
- *Handling Radioactive Material   477*
- *Applications of Radioactive Isotopes   478*
- *Radiation Effects   480*

28. Metabolism of Xenobiotics (Detoxification) 481
- *Phase I Detoxification   481*
- *Phase II Detoxification (Conjugation)   483*

29. Biochemistry of Free Radicals and Antioxidants 486
- *Reactive Oxygen Species   486*
- *Antioxidants   488*
- *Oxidative Stress in Disease   491*

30. Immunology 493
- Immunoglobulins   494
- Hypergammaglobulinemia   498

31. Biochemistry of Vision 502
- Structure of the Eye   503
- Phototransduction   504
- Visual Cycle   506
- Color Vision   506
- Human Disorders of Phototransduction   506
- Sorbitol Pathway and Diabetes Mellitus   506

32. Clinical Chemistry 509
- Purpose of the Laboratory Medicine   509
- Critical Alerts   513
- Legal and Ethical Regulations   513
- Laboratory Values   514

33. Instrumentation and Techniques 519
- Spectrophotometry/Colorimetry   519
- Centrifugation   521
- Electrophoresis   523
- Chromatography   524
- Radioimmunoassay   526
- Enzyme-linked Immunosorbent Assay   527

34. Buffers and Biochemical Tests 530
- Buffer   530
- Acids and Bases   531
- Chemical Components of Normal Urine   532
- Urine Analysis: Abnormal Constituents of Urine   534
- Determination of Creatinine Content in Urine, Calculation of Creatinine Clearance   535
- Estimation of Plasma Proteins   536

Index   *539*

Competency Table

BIOCHEMISTRY (CODE: BI)

No	Description of Competency	Core (Y/N)	Teaching/Learning Method	Chapter No.	Page No.
Topic: Basic Biochemistry				**Number of Competencies: (01)**	
BI 1.1	Describe the molecular and functional organization of a cell and its sub-cellular components	Y	Lecture, small group discussion	1	1
Topic: Enzyme				**Number of Competencies: (07)**	
BI 2.1	Explain fundamental concepts of enzyme, isoenzyme, alloenzyme, coenzyme and co-factors. Enumerate the main classes of IUBMB nomenclature	Y	Lecture, case discussion	3	17
BI 2.2	Observe the estimation of SGOT and SGPT	Y	Demonstration	3	
BI 2.3	Describe and explain the basic principles of enzyme activity	Y	Lecture, case discussion	3	21
BI 2.4	Describe and discuss enzyme inhibitors as poisons and drugs and as therapeutic enzymes	Y	Lecture, small group discussion	3	23
BI 2.5	Describe and discuss the clinical utility of various serum enzymes as markers of pathological conditions	Y	Lecture, small group discussion	3	26–30
BI 2.6	Discuss use enzymes in laboratory investigations (Enzyme-based assays)	Y	Lecture, small group discussion	3	26–30
BI 2.7	Interpret laboratory results of enzyme activities and describe the clinical utility of various enzymes as markers of pathological conditions	Y	Lecture, small group discussion, DOAP sessions	3	26–30
Topic: Chemistry and Metabolism of Carbohydrates				**Number of Competencies: (10)**	
BI 3.1	Discuss and differentiate monosaccharides, disaccharides and polysaccharides giving examples of main carbohydrates as energy fuel, structural element and storage in the human body	Y	Lecture, small group discussion	6	80–82
BI 3.2	Describe the processes involved in digestion and assimilation of carbohydrates and storage	Y	Lecture, small group discussion	7	91–93
BI 3.3	Describe and discuss the digestion and assimilation of carbohydrates from food	Y	Lecture, small group discussion	7	91–93

No	Description of Competency	Core (Y/N)	Teaching/Learning Method	Chapter No.	Page No.
BI 3.4	Define and differentiate the pathways of carbohydrate metabolism, (glycolysis, gluconeogenesis, glycogen metabolism, HMP shunt)	Y	Lecture, small group discussion	7	95
BI 3.5	Describe and discuss the regulation, functions and integration of carbohydrate along with associated diseases/disorders	Y	Lecture, small group discussion	10	195–201
BI 3.6	Describe and discuss the concept of TCA cycle as an amphibolic pathway and its regulation	Y	Lecture, small group discussion	7	102–105
BI 3.7	Describe the common poisons that inhibit crucial enzymes of carbohydrate metabolism (eg; fluoride, arsenate)	Y	Lecture, small group discussion, DOAP sessions	7	98 and 104
BI 3.8	Discuss and interpret laboratory results of analyte associated with metabolism of carbohydrates	Y	Lecture, small group discussion	7	
BI 3.9	Discuss the mechanism and significance of blood glucose regulation in health and disease	Y	Lecture, small group discussion	7	121–124
BI 3.10	Interpret the results of blood glucose levels and other laboratory investigations related to disorders of carbohydrate metabolism	Y	Lecture, small group discussion	7	126
Topic: Chemistry and Metabolism of Lipids				**Number of Competencies: (07)**	
BI 4.1	Describe and discuss main classes of lipids (Essential/non-essential fatty acids, cholesterol and hormonal steroids, triglycerides, major phospholipids and sphingolipids) relevant to human system and their major functions	Y	Lecture, small group discussion	8	140–142
BI 4.2	Describe the process involved in digestion and absorption of dietary lipids and also the key features of their metabolism	Y	Lecture, small group discussion	9	153
BI 4.3	Explain the regulation of lipoprotein metabolism and associated disorders	Y	Lecture, small group discussion	9	174
BI 4.4	Describe the structure and functions of lipoproteins, their functions, interrelations and relations with atherosclerosis	Y	Lecture, small group discussion	9	171
BI 4.5	Interpret laboratory results of analytes associated with metabolism of lipids	Y	Lecture, small group discussion	9	186
BI 4.6	Describe the therapeutic uses of prostaglandins and inhibitors of eicosanoid synthesis	Y	Lecture, small group discussion	9	179–181

Competency Table

No	Description of Competency	Core (Y/N)	Teaching/Learning Method	Chapter No.	Page No.
BI 4.7	Interpret laboratory results of analytes associated with metabolism of lipids	Y	Lecture, small group discussion,	9	186
Topic: Chemistry and Metabolism of Proteins				**Number of Competencies: (05)**	
BI 5.1	Describe and discuss structural organisation of proteins	Y	Lecture, small group discussion	4	42
BI 5.2	Describe and discuss functions of proteins and structure-function relationships in relevant areas, e.g., haemoglobin and selected hemoglobinopathies	Y	Lecture, small group discussion	4 and 11	43, 210, 221
BI 5.3	Describe the digestion and absorption of proteins	Y	Lecture, small group discussion	5	53
BI 5.4	Describe common disorders associated with protein metabolism	Y	Lecture, small group discussion	5	57–68
BI 5.5	Interpret laboratory results of analytes associated with metabolism of proteins	Y	Lecture, small group discussion	5	57–68
Topic: Metabolism and Homeostasis				**Number of Competencies: (15)**	
BI 6.1	Discuss the metabolic processes that take place in specific organs in the body in the fed and fasting stages	Y	Lecture, small group discussion	10	95
BI 6.2	Describe and discuss the metabolic processes in which nucleotides are involved	Y	Lecture, small group discussion	5, 7, 9	56, 98, 157
BI 6.3	Describe the common disorders associated with nucleotide metabolism	Y	Lecture, small group discussion	19	343, 346
BI 6.4	Discuss the laboratory results of analytes associated with gout and Lesch-Nyhan syndrome	Y	Lecture, small group discussion	19	343
BI 6.5	Describe the biochemical role of vitamins in the body and explain the manifestations of their deficiency	Y	Lecture, small group discussion	16	287
BI 6.6	Describe the biochemical processes involved in generation of energy in cells	Y	Lecture, small group discussion	5, 7, 9	56, 98, 157
BI 6.7	Describe the processes involved in maintenance of normal pH, water and electrolyte balance of body fluids and the derangements associated with these disorders	Y	Lecture, small group discussion	13 and 24	248, 433, 437
BI 6.8	Discuss and interpret results of Arterial Blood Gas (ABG) analysis in various disorders	Y	Lecture, small group discussion	13	252
BI 6.9	Describe the functions of various minerals in the body, their metabolism and homeostasis	Y	Lecture, small group discussion	15	269

No	Description of Competency	Core (Y/N)	Teaching/Learning Method	Chapter No.	Page No.
BI 6.10	Enumerate and describe the disorders associated with mineral metabolism	Y	Lecture, small group discussion	15	269
BI 6.11	Describe the functions of the haem in the body and describe the processes involved in its metabolism and describe porphyrin metabolism	Y	Lecture, small group discussion	11	214
BI 6.12	Describe the major types of haemoglobin and its derivatives found in the body and their physiological/pathological relevance	Y	Lecture, small group discussion	11	221
BI 6.13	Describe the functions of the kidney, liver, thyroid and adrenal glands	Y	Lecture, small group discussion	21	388
BI 6.14	Describe the tests that are commonly done in clinical practice to assess the functions these organs (kidney, liver, thyroid and adrenal glands)	Y	Lecture, small group discussion	21	388
BI 6.15	Describe the abnormalities of kidney, liver, thyroid and adrenal glands	Y	Lecture, small group discussion	21	388
Topic: Molecular Biology				**Number of Competencies: (07)**	
BI 7.1	Describe the structure and functions of DNA and RNA and outline the cell cycle	Y	Lecture, small group discussion	18 and 20	335–337, 350–351
BI 7.2	Describe the processes involved in replication and repair DNA and the transcription and translation mechanisms	Y	Lecture, small group discussion	20	351
BI 7.3	Describe gene mutation and basic mechanism of regulation of gene expression	Y	Lecture, small group discussion	20	356
BI 7.4	Describe applications of molecular technologies like recombinant technology, PCR in the diagnosis and treatment of diseases with genetic basis	Y	Lecture, small group discussion	20	372, 376
BI 7.5	Describe the role of xenobiotics in disease	Y	Lecture, small group discussion	28	482
BI 7.6	Describe the anti-oxidant defence systems in the body	Y	Lecture, small group discussion	29	487
BI 7.7	Describe the role of oxidative stress in the pathogenesis of conditions such as cancer, complications of diabetes mellitus and atherosclerosis	Y	Lecture, small group discussion	29	491
Topic: Nutrition				**Number of Competencies: (05)**	
BI 8.1	Discuss the importance of various dietary components and explain importance of dietary fibre	Y	Lecture, small group discussion	17	309

Competency Table

No	Description of Competency	Core (Y/N)	Teaching/Learning Method	Chapter No.	Page No.
BI 8.2	Describe the types and causes of protein energy malnutrition and its effects	Y	Lecture, small group discussion	17	323–324
BI 8.3	Provide dietary advice for optimal health in childhood and adult, in disease conditions like diabetes mellitus, coronary artery disease and in pregnancy	Y	Lecture, small group discussion	17	315 and 322
BI 8.4	Describe the causes (including dietary habits), effects and health risks associated with being overweight/obesity	Y	Lecture, small group discussion	17	324
BI 8.5	Summarize the nutritional importance of commonly used items of food including fruits and vegetables (macro-molecules and their importance)	Y	Lecture, small group discussion	17	306–311
Topic: Extracellular Matrix				**Number of Competencies: (03)**	
BI 9.1	List the functions and components of extracellular matrix (ECM)	Y	Lecture, small group discussion	22	408
BI 9.2	Discuss the involvement of ECM components in health and disease	Y	Lecture, small group discussion	22	408–413
BI 9.3	Describe protein targeting and sorting along with its associated disorders	Y	Lecture, small group discussion	22	411–412
Topic: Oncogenesis and Immunity				**Number of Competencies: (05)**	
BI 10.1	Describe the cancer initiation, promotion oncogenes and oncogene activation. Also focus on p53 and apoptosis	Y	Lecture, small group discussion	26	453, 464
BI 10.2	Describe various biochemical tumour markers and the biochemical basis of cancer therapy	Y	Lecture, small group discussion	26	466–473
BI 10.3	Describe the cellular and humoral components of the immune system and describe the types and structure of antibody	Y	Lecture, small group discussion	30	494–496
BI 10.4	Describe and discuss innate and adaptive immune responses, self /non-self- recognition and the central role of T-helper cells in immune responses	Y	Lecture, small group discussion	30	497
BI 10.5	Describe antigens and concepts involved in vaccine development	Y	Lecture, small group discussion	30	497
Topic: Biochemistry Laboratory Tests				**Number of Competencies: (24)**	
BI 11.1	Describe commonly used laboratory apparatus and equipment, good safe laboratory practice and waste disposal	Y	Lecture, small group discussion	33	520

No	Description of Competency	Core (Y/N)	Teaching/Learning Method	Chapter No.	Page No.
BI 11.2	Describe the preparation of buffers and estimation of pH	Y	Lecture, small group discussion	34	530
BI 11.3	Describe the chemical components of normal urine	Y	Lecture, small group discussion	34	532
BI 11.4	Perform urine analysis to estimate and determine normal and abnormal constituents	Y	DOAP session	34	535
BI 11.5	Describe screening of urine for inborn errors and describe the use of paper chromatography	Y	Lecture, small group discussion	33	525
BI 11.6	Describe the principles of colorimetry	Y	Lecture, small group discussion	33	520
BI 11.7	Demonstrate the estimation of serum creatinine and creatinine clearance	Y	Practical	34	535
BI 11.8	Demonstrate estimation of serum proteins, albumin and A:G ratio	Y	Practical	34	536
BI 11.17	Explain the basis and rationale of biochemical tests done in the following conditions: diabetes mellitus, dyslipidemia, myocardial infarction, renal failure, proteinuria, nephrotic syndrome, edema, jaundice liver disease, pancreatitis, disorders of acid-base balance, thyroid disorders	Y	Lecture, Small group discussion	21	388–402
BI 11.18	Discuss the principles of spectrophotometry	Y	Lecture, Small group discussion	33	520–521
BI 11.19	Outline the basic principles involved in the functioning of instruments commonly used in a biochemistry laboratory and their applications	Y	Lecture, Small group discussion	33	521–524
BI 11.20	Identify abnormal constituents in urine, interpret the findings and correlate these with pathological states	Y	DOAP sessions	34	535
BI 11.22	Calculate albumin: globulin ratio (AG) ratio and creatinine clearance	Y	Lecture, Small group discussion	34	536–537

Competency Table

No	Description of Competency	Core (Y/N)	Teaching/Learning Method	Chapter No.	Page No.
BI 11.23	Calculate energy content of different food items, identify food items with high and low glycemic index and explain the importance of these in the diet	Y	Lecture, Small group discussion	17	310–311
BI 11.24	Enumerate advantages and/or disadvantages of use of unsaturated, saturated and trans fat in food	Y	Lecture, Small group discussion	8	147

CHAPTER

1

Cell

OBJECTIVES

At the end of this chapter, students should be able to:
- Know about the ultrastructure of the cell
- State the different organelles of the cell and their individual functions
- Know the marker enzymes to identify the cell organelles.

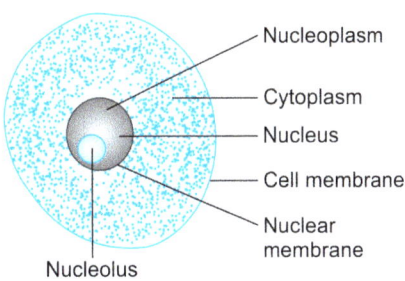

Fig. 1.1: Structure of the cell as seen with light microscope.

INTRODUCTION

Cells are the structural and functional units of all living organisms. Humans are multicellular organisms and contain at least 10^{14} cells. These cells differ considerably in shape, structure and function as a result of specialization. Tissues are an aggregation of cells that are similar in origin, structure and function. Most of the metabolic activities occur at the cellular level.

A typical cell, as seen by the light microscope, is illustrated in **Figure 1.1**. It contains two compartments such as inner nucleus and outer cytoplasm. Nucleus contains nucleoplasm suspended with genetic material. Nuclear envelope separates the nucleus from the cytoplasm. Cytoplasm is composed of aqueous cytosol, which is suspended with particles and membrane-bound organelles. Externally the cytoplasm is limited by the plasma membrane.

Normal cell ranges between 10 µm and 30 µm in diameter. **Figure 1.2** shows the ultrastructure or finer details of a typical cell as revealed under the electron microscope.

STRUCTURAL AND FUNCTIONAL ASPECTS OF CELL ORGANELLES

Plasma Membrane

- The cell membrane, which completely envelops the cell, is a thin (75-100 Å), living, dynamic and selectively permeable membrane.
- It has specialized surface structures for attachment and communication, which include (i) the tight junctions that seal the adjacent cells and (ii) the gap junctions that allow movement of the ions and electric currents between the adjacent cells. They may also possess certain modifications to carry out the physiological functions such as microvilli for absorption, invagination or infolding to carry out transportation.
- All the biological membranes including the plasma membrane and internal membranes that form the subcellular structures such as endoplasmic reticulum

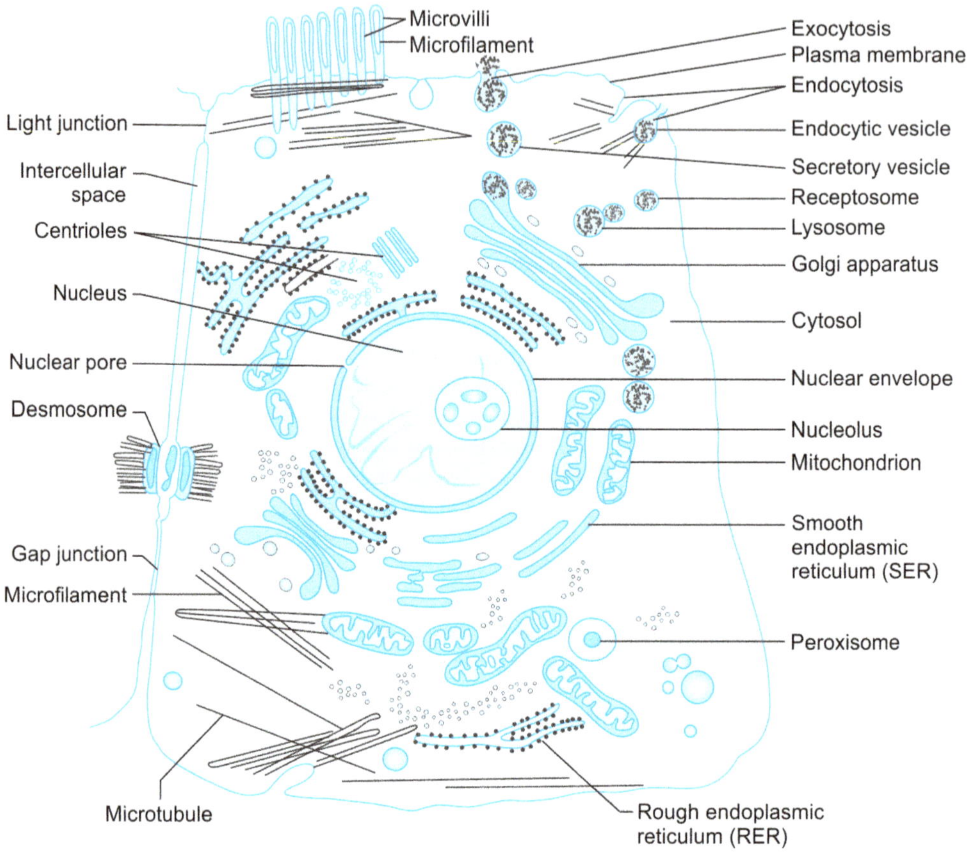

Cell

Fig. 1.2: Ultrastructure of a typical cell showing all cell organelles as seen under the electron microscope.

(ER), mitochondria, lysosomes nuclear envelope, peroxisomes, and Golgi complex are similar in structure and are made of lipoproteins, i.e. lipids (60–40%), proteins (40–60%) and carbohydrates (1–10%).

- The membranes separate the cell from the external environment and also separate different parts of the cell from one another, so that the cellular activities are compartmentalized.

Endoplasmic Reticulum

- Cytoplasm is traversed by an extensive network of interconnecting membrane-bound channels or cisternae (diameter of 40–50 µm), vesicles (diameter of 25–500 µm) and tubules (diameter of 50–190 µm), which form the ER **(Fig. 1.3).**

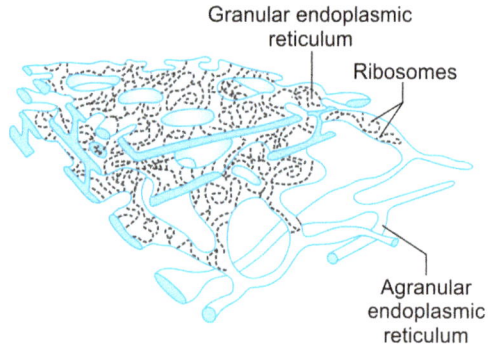

Fig. 1.3: Endoplasmic reticulum.

- Membranes of ER are continuous, with a plasma membrane and an outer nuclear envelope.
- The two basic morphological types of ER are as follows: (i) The rough ER (RER),

which possesses rough surface due to the attachment of ribosomes. The RER occurs mainly in the form of cisternae and is concerned with protein synthesis. (ii) The smooth ER (SER) that lacks ribosomes on their surface and is mainly in the form of tubules. The SER is concerned with lipid synthesis.
- Endoplasmic reticulum provides skeletal framework to cells and gives mechanical support to the colloidal cytoplasm. It also plays a role in detoxifying the xenobiotics.

Golgi Complex

- Golgi complex is a membrane-bound structure similar to ER and was discovered in 1873 by Camillo Golgi.
- It consists of a stack of flattened membrane vesicles (cisternae) surrounded by a network of tubules of 300–500 Å diameters.
- Cisternae are gently curved, and its convex part of the cis side faces the ER and the concave part of the trans side can be located near the plasma membrane **(Fig. 1.4)**.
- Golgi complex functions in association with ER and is a center of reception, finishing, packaging, and transportation of a variety of materials.
- Proteins synthesized in the ER added with sulfates, carbohydrates, lipid moieties, etc. and are dispatched in the form of secretory vesicles.
- Golgi complex also gives rise to lipoprotein of plasma membrane and lysosomes.

Lysosomes

- Lysosomes are packets of hydrolases.
- They are spherical in shape and are 1 μm in diameter surrounded by tough carbohydrate-rich lipoprotein membranes enclosing about 50 types of hydrolases such as protease, lipase, nuclease, transferase and sulfatase.
- Lysosomes provide an intracellular digestive system through which macromolecules, foreign bodies and worn-out unwanted structures are digested.

Peroxisomes

- Circular membrane-bound organelles measuring about 0.25 μm diameters and contain peroxidase and catalase enzymes.
- Peroxisomes detoxify various toxic substances and metabolites through peroxidative reactions catalyzed by peroxidases. Catalase degrades H_2O_2 obtained from the breakdown of fatty acids and amino acids.

Mitochondria

- They are spherical, oval or rod-like bodies measuring about 0.5–1 μm in diameter and up to 7 μm in length. Mitochondria consist

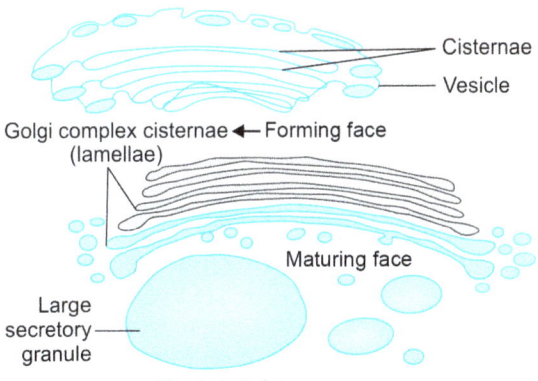

Fig. 1.4: Golgi apparatus.

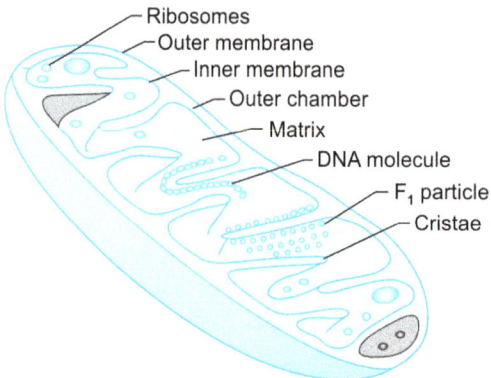

Fig. 1.5: Longitudinal section of mitochondrion.

of DNA molecules that encode information for certain mitochondrial proteins **(Fig. 1.5)**.
- Mitochondria are considered to be the powerhouse of the cell, where energy released from the oxidation of foodstuffs is trapped as chemical energy in the form of adenosine triphosphate (ATP).
- Mitochondria are the respiratory center of the cell where pyruvate oxidation, citric acid cycle, electron transport chain and ATP generation occur. Moreover, β-oxidation of fatty acid and ketone body synthesis also take place.

Centrioles

- Two cylindrical rod-shaped structures of 0.3–0.7 µm length and 0.1–0.25 µm diameters, which lie right angle to one another near nucleus, are called centrioles.
- Centriole is an array of nine triplet microtubules equally spaced from the central axis and is made of structural protein tubulin. They form mitotic poles during cell division.
- They also give rise to cilia and tail of sperm.

Nucleus

- Nucleus is the command center of cells and is spherical in shape. All the genetic materials are confined in nucleus.
- All cells in the human body contain nucleus, except the matured red blood cells (RBCs) and the upper dead skin cells.
- Generally nucleus is spherical or oval in shape and measures 3–25 µm in diameter. However, squamous epithelial cells contain discoidal and multilobed nucleus as in polymorphonuclear leukocytes.
- Nuclear envelope, which encircles the nucleus, consists of outer and inner nuclear membranes, which is a typical lipoprotein membrane. Outer nuclear membrane is continuous with the membranes of ER and is found attached to the ribosomes on its outer surface. Nuclear envelope contains numerous nuclear pores of 100–1,000 Å diameter, which regulates nucleocytoplasmic trafficking of ions, nucleotides, proteins, messenger RNA (mRNA), transfer RNA (tRNA) and ribosomal subunits.
- Nucleoplasm is the gelatinous substance within the nuclear envelope, which is also called as karyoplasm, and it consists of genetic material (chromosomes) and nucleolus. It regulates the passage of molecules between the nucleoplasm and the cytoplasm.
- Nucleolus is made up of proteins and RNAs and is the site for the formation of ribosomal subunits. The main components are nucleoproteins, proteins, enzymes, minerals and organic and inorganic substances.

PROKARYOTIC AND EUKARYOTIC CELLS

Cells are of two types, namely prokaryotes and eukaryotes. "*Karyose*" is a Greek word, meaning "kernel" as the kernel of a grain. In biology, we use this word root to refer to the nucleus of a cell. "*Pro*" means "before," and "*Eu*" means "true" or "good." Hence "prokaryotic" means "before a nucleus" and "eukaryotic" means "possessing a true nucleus." Prokaryotic cells have no nuclei,

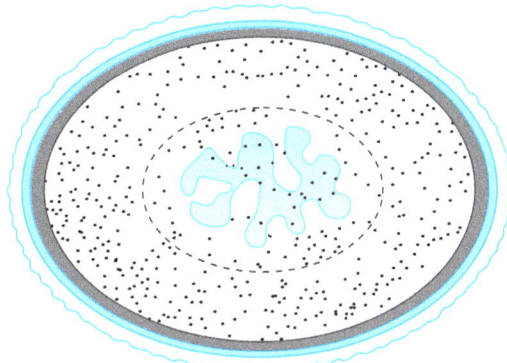

Fig. 1.6: Prokaryotic cell.

whereas eukaryotic cells have true nuclei (**Fig. 1.6**).

Differences between Eukaryotic and Prokaryotic Cells

1. Eukaryotic cells have a true nucleus bound by a double membrane (**Fig. 1.7**). Prokaryotic cells have no nucleus. The purpose of the nucleus is to sequester the DNA-related functions of the big eukaryotic cells into a smaller chamber to attain increased efficiency. This function is unnecessary in the prokaryotic cells, due to their much smaller size and closer location of all materials. Prokaryotic cells also have DNA and DNA functions.
2. Eukaryotic DNA is linear, but prokaryotic DNA is circular.
3. Eukaryotic DNA is complexed with proteins called "histones" and is organized into chromosomes. Prokaryotic DNA is "naked" (no histones) and does not have chromosomes. A eukaryotic cell contains a number of chromosomes; a prokaryotic cell contains only one circular DNA molecule and a varied assortment of much smaller circlets of DNA called "plasmids."
4. Both cell types have many ribosomes, but the ribosomes of the eukaryotic cells are larger and more complex than those of the prokaryotic cell. A eukaryotic ribosome is composed of 5 kinds of ribosomal RNA (rRNA) and about 80 kinds of proteins. Prokaryotic ribosomes are composed of only 3 kinds of rRNA and about 50 kinds of proteins.
5. The cytoplasm of eukaryotic cells is filled with a large, complex collection of organelles; many of these are enclosed in their own membranes. However, the prokaryotic cell does not have membrane-bound organelles, which are independent of the plasma membrane.

TRANSPORT ACROSS MEMBRANES

Biological membranes are lipoprotein viscous barriers, which are around all living cells and form the structural and functional components of all cell organelles. The membrane contains mainly lipids, proteins and very little amount of carbohydrates. The contents of these vary according to the nature of the membrane. Lipids are mainly amphipathic phospholipids, glycolipids and cholesterol. Proteins are of two types, namely (i) peripheral or extrinsic proteins and (ii) integral or intrinsic proteins.

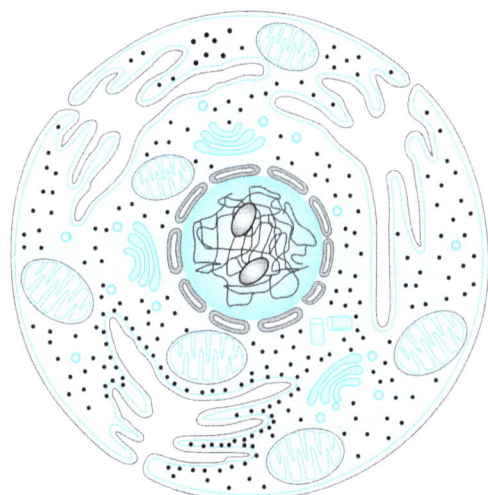

Fig. 1.7: Eukaryotic cell.

FLUID MOSAIC MODEL

Organization of biological membranes and the arrangement of lipids and proteins can be explained using the fluid mosaic model of Singer and Nicolson (1972) **(Fig. 1.8)**. According to this model, membrane is a viscous fluid with a phospholipid bilayer in which the globular proteins are inserted in a mosaic pattern. Amphipathic phospholipid consists of polar phosphate head, glycerol neck and two nonpolar fatty acid tails. The hydrophobic tails or fatty acids form the middle core of the lipid bilayer. The hydrophilic heads line both the sides. Both phospholipids and proteins are amphipathic and form permeability barrier. Degree of saturation and unsaturation of fatty acids and presence of cholesterol and carbohydrates regulate the fluidity and movement of molecules. Hydrophilic heads of inner and outer surfaces maintain constant water circulation. However, hydrophobic fatty acid core acts as a selective permeable barrier and saves the cells and cell organelles from osmotic shocks.

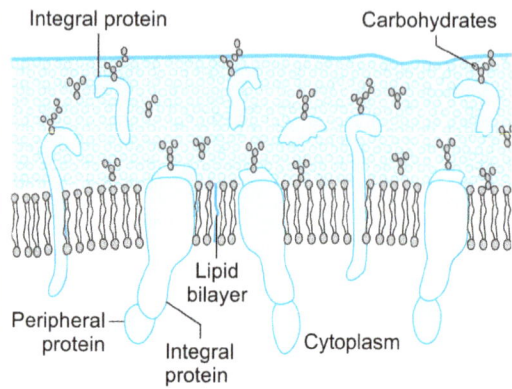

Fig. 1.8: Fluid mosaic model of plasma membrane.

TRANSPORT MECHANISMS IN THE MEMBRANES

An important function of a membrane is to withhold unwanted molecules but permits the entry of molecules necessary for cellular metabolism. Transport across the membranes occurs in the following ways:
1. Passive transport
2. Active transport
3. Exocytosis
4. Endocytosis.

Passive Transport

Passive transport of molecules across the membrane is achieved along the concentration gradient, without the use of energy. Movement of molecules from higher to lower concentration takes place without using energy. Solutes and gases passively enter into the cells. They are driven by the concentration gradient. The rate of transport is directly proportional to the concentration gradient of that solute across the membrane. Passive transport of molecules across the biomembranes can be achieved in two ways:
1. Simple diffusion
2. Facilitated diffusion.

Simple diffusion: Small uncharged molecules such as H_2O_2, O_2, CO_2, CH_4, other gases, urea and ethanol cross the lipid bilayer by simple diffusion.

Facilitated diffusion or carrier-mediated passive transport: Diffusion of molecules across the membrane happens along the concentration gradient through carrier proteins or permeases. It differs from simple diffusion in the following aspects:
- The process is stereospecific, i.e. only one of the two possible isomers, L and D, is transported.
- It shows saturation kinetics.
- A carrier is required for transport across the membranes **(Fig. 1.9)**.

The carrier proteins or permeases are specific for integral membrane proteins and highly specific for molecules that they transport. Carrier proteins are specific for individual sugars, amino acids, phosphates, etc. Based on a concentration gradient across the membrane, the solute molecules from the hypertonic side bind to specific permease of

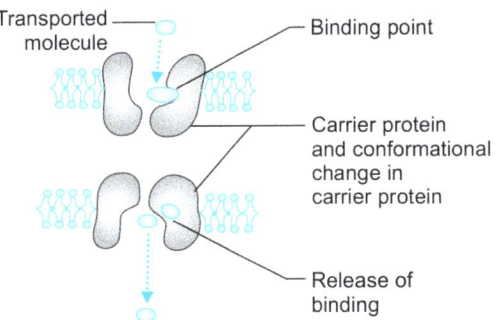

Fig. 1.9: Mechanism of facilitated diffusion.

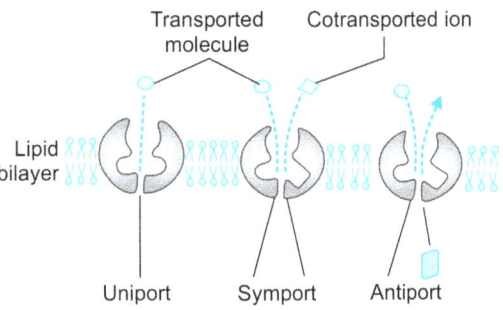

Fig. 1.10: Carrier proteins of membrane functioning as uniports, symports and antiports.

the membrane. This binding triggers certain conformational changes, producing a pore or tunnel in carrier protein through which ions, glucose, etc. may cross. Following this, the permease regains its original structure.

Uniport, Symport and Antiport

Carrier proteins, which simply transport a single solute from one side of the membrane to the other, are called uniports. Transport of one solute depends on the simultaneous transfer of a second solute, either in the same direction (symport) or in the opposite direction (antiport). Both symport and antiport are collectively called cotransport **(Fig. 1.10)**.

Symport: Examples: Glucose-Na^+ symport protein in intestinal epithelial cells.

Antiport: Examples: Na^+-K^+ ATPase pump, Cl^-/HCO_3^- anion exchange permease in erythrocytes.

Active Transport

The transport of molecules across the membrane against the concentration gradient using energy is referred to as active transport. Molecules are transported from lower concentration (hypotonic) to higher concentration (hypertonic) using energy **(Fig. 1.11)**. In all cells, a significant portion of energy is used for maintaining the concentration gradient of ions across plasma membrane and intracellular membranes. In human RBCs,

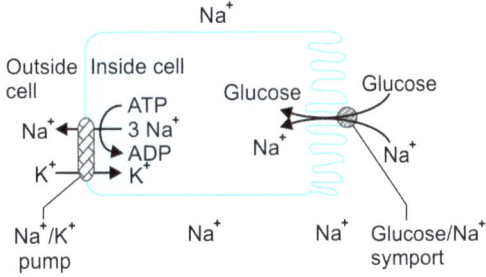

Fig. 1.11: Active transport.

50% of the energy (cellular metabolism) is used for the purpose mentioned above. Active transport is mainly of two types:

1. *ATP-driven active transport or primary active transport*: Transmembrane proteins or carrier proteins form channels to transport the molecules and ions across biological membranes using energy from ATP. The most important active transport in cells is the Na^+-K^+ ATPase pump. All cells maintain high internal concentration of K^+ and low concentration of Na^+. This Na^+-K^+ gradient across the membrane is maintained using energy from ATP hydrolysis. ATPase is a large carrier protein, and ATP hydrolysis enables the binding of 3Na^+ to ATPase, leading to some conformational changes in ATPase and resulting in pumping of 3 Na^+ outside, in exchange of 2K^+ pumped in the opposite direction.

2. *Ion-driven active transport or secondary active transport*: Secondary active transport

takes place in the presence of ionic gradient maintained across the membrane by primary active transport. For example, glucose absorption in intestinal epithelial cells. Concentration gradient maintained by Na⁺-K⁺ ATPase pump across the cell enables the symport of Na⁺ and glucose molecules into the cell.

Exocytosis

Proteins, lipids and carbohydrate secretions of cell are released out of the cell through a process called exocytosis. These secretions are packed in the form of secretory vesicles. Per the necessary stimulation, these vesicles move toward and fuse with plasma membrane. In this way, materials inside the vesicles are externalized. Examples are release of acetyl choline from synaptic vesicles in presynaptic cholinergic nerves, release of trypsinogen by pancreatic cells, and release of insulin by β cells of Langerhans, etc.

Endocytosis

Endocytosis is the mechanism by which cells uptake macromolecules in the form endocytic vesicles. Plasma membrane invaginates and encloses the materials, resulting in the formation of vesicles. Endocytosis is of two types **(Fig. 1.12)**:
1. Phagocytosis: Ingestion of large particles such as bacteria and cell debris, and plasma membrane invaginates in the form of pseudopodia and encloses the particles in the form of phagosome. Materials of phagosomes will be digested by lysosomes, for example, engulfment of bacteria by macrophages and granulocytes.
2. Pinocytosis: Uptake of nonspecific or specific extracellular molecules in the form of endocytic vesicles, which is termed as receptor-mediated endocytosis. Plasma membranes internalize these receptor-attached molecules in the form of vesicles, for example, uptake of chylomicrons by liver cells and internalization of low-density lipoprotein (LDL) through LDL receptors of plasma membrane.

CELL FRACTIONATION

To study the biochemical properties of individual organelles, it is necessary to understand subcellular fractionation. In subcellular fractionation, cells are broken down by means of mechanical force to purify the organelles.

The steps involved are as follows **(Figs. 1.13 and 1.14)**:
- Mince the tissues using a buffer.
- The minced tissues are then carefully broken up in a homogenizer using isotonic 0.25 M sucrose solution (sucrose solution is preferred because it is not metabolized, does not readily pass through the membranes and does not cause interorganelles to swell.
- The gentle homogenization with an isotonic sucrose solution ruptures the cell membrane and keeps most of the organelles intact. But ER is broken into small pieces to form microsomes.
- Homogenate is drained to remove connective tissues and fragments of blood vessels by stainless steel sieve.
- The homogenate thus obtained is centrifuged using a series of increasing centrifugal force.

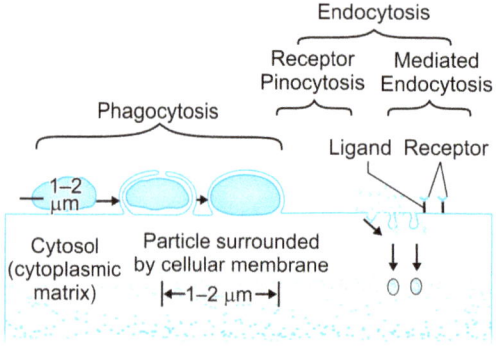

Fig. 1.12: Process of phagocytosis and endocytosis.

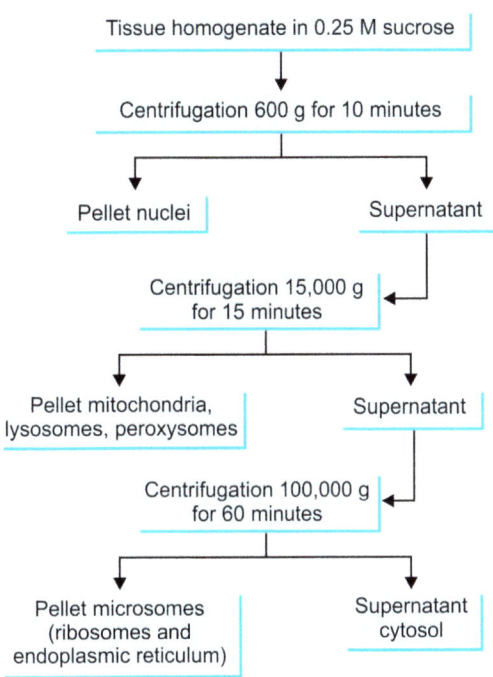

Fig. 1.13: Subcellular fractionation of cell by differential centrifugation.

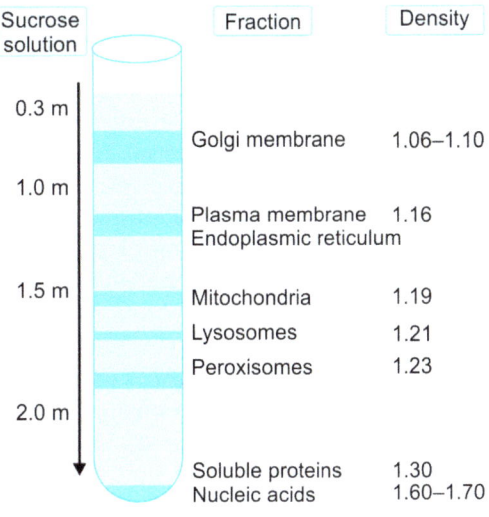

Fig. 1.14: Organelle separation by isopycnic centrifugation.

The nuclei and mitochondria differ in size and specific gravity and, therefore, sediment at different rates in a centrifugal field. This can be isolated from the homogenate by differential centrifugation. The dense nuclei are sedimented first, followed by the mitochondria and finally by the microsomal fraction. The soluble remnant is the cytosolic portion.

The mitochondria isolated in this way are contaminated with lysosomes and peroxisomes. These may be separated by isopycnic centrifugation technique. In this technique, a density gradient is setup in a centrifuge tube (the density of the solution in the tube increases from top to the bottom). Sucrose is used as the medium, and the colloidal materials such as percoll, which form density gradients with a low osmotic pressure, are often used. Particles are sedimented to an equilibrium position, i.e. the point at which their density equals that of the medium in the tube. Different organelles are separated according to their density.

The purity of the isolated subcellular fraction is assessed by analyzing the marker enzymes, which are located exclusively in a particular fraction and are specific to that fraction. Analysis of the marker enzymes confirms the degree of purity and contamination (**Table 1.1**).

Enzymes Used to Identify the Cell Organelles

Table 1.1: Marker enzymes of subcellular fractions.

Fraction	Enzyme
Plasma membrane	5′-nucleotidase and Na$^+$–K$^+$ ATPase
Golgi membrane	Galactosyl transferase and mannosidase
Endoplasmic reticulum	Glucose 6-phosphatase and cytochrome b reductase
Mitochondria	Succinate dehydrogenase and cytochrome c oxidase
Cytosol	Lactate dehydrogenase and glucose 6-phosphate dehydrogenase
Lysosomes	Acid phosphatase
Peroxisomes	Catalase
Nucleus	DNA polymerase and RNA polymerase

SUMMARY

Humans are multicellular organisms and contain at least 10^{14} cells. Cell contains two compartments such as inner nucleus and outer cytoplasm. Nucleus contains nucleoplasm suspended with genetic material. The nuclear envelope separates nucleus from the cytoplasm. Cytoplasm is composed of aqueous cytosol suspended with particles and membrane-bound organelles. The diameter of normal cell ranges between 10 μm and 30 μm. The various cell organelles are ER, Golgi complex, lysosomes, peroxisomes, mitochondria, nucleus, and centrioles. Biological membranes (lipoprotein viscous barriers) exist around all the living cells and also form structural and functional components of all the cell organelles. A membrane contains mainly lipids, proteins and very little amount of carbohydrates. Important function of the membrane is to withhold unwanted molecules and to permit the entry of molecules necessary for cellular metabolism. Transport across the membrane occurs through passive transport, active transport, exocytosis and endocytosis. Subcellular fraction of individual organelles of a cell allows to study their biochemical properties individually.

SELF-ASSESSMENT QUESTIONS

1. Briefly discuss the ultrastructure of a typical cell.
2. Add a note on the structural aspects of mitochondria and mention the metabolism that takes place in mitochondria.
3. Explain the fluid mosaic model of plasma membrane.
4. Write the features and importance of active transport mechanism.
5. How do you explain the ATP-driven and ion-driven active transport?
6. Mention the significance of endocytosis and exocytosis.
7. What is ion-driven active transport? Explain with an example.
8. Explain uniport and antiport transport mechanisms with examples.
9. Why do we call mitochondrion as a powerhouse of the cell?

MULTIPLE-CHOICE QUESTIONS

1. Concerning plasma membrane, one of the following statements is *not true*:
   a. Plasma membrane consists of specialized surface structures for attachment and for communication
   b. Tight junctions seal the adjacent cells
   c. Gap junctions allow ions and electric current between adjacent cells
   d. Consists of proteins, lipids and carbohydrates
2. Cytoplasm is traversed by extensive network of interconnecting membrane-bound channels or cisternae, vesicles and tubules to form ...
   a. Endoplasmic reticulum
   b. Golgi complex
   c. Ribosomes
   d. Microsomes
3. Concerning the Golgi complex, all of the following statements are true, *except*:
   a. It is a membrane-bound structure
   b. It is a stack of flattened membrane vesicles
   c. It does not give rise to lipoprotein of plasma membrane
   d. It helps in packaging and transportation of a variety of materials
4. Concerning mitochondria, one of the following statements is *incorrect*:
   a. It is considered to be the powerhouse of the cell
   b. They are respiratory center of the cell where pyruvate oxidation takes place
   c. It accommodates glycolysis
   d. It has electron transport chain
5. Nucleus:
   a. Presents in all cells of the body
   b. Does not have nuclear envelope
   c. Is absent in RBCs
   d. Exists in different shapes
6. Concerning passive transport, one of the following statements is *incorrect*:
   a. It requires ATP
   b. It requires carrier protein

c. It occurs along the concentration gradient
d. Its process is stereospecific

7. **Concerning active transport, one of the following statements is *incorrect*:**
   a. Transport of molecules across the membrane is against the concentration gradient
   b. It is energy dependent
   c. Most important active transport in cells is Na$^+$-K$^+$ ATPase pump
   d. 2Na$^+$ pumped outside and in exchange 3K$^+$ pumped in the opposite direction

8. **Glucose absorption in intestinal epithelial cells:**
   a. Is ion-driven active transport
   b. Is facilitated diffusion
   c. Is passive transport
   d. Does not depend on the concentration gradient

9. **Transport of macromolecules takes place through the following mechanisms, *except*:**
   a. Diffusion   b. Phagocytosis
   c. Pinocytosis   d. Exocytosis

10. **All of the following are the examples for endocytosis, *except*:**
    a. Uptake of chylomicrons by liver cells
    b. Internalization of LDL through LDL receptors of plasma membrane
    c. Uptake of glucose by intestinal cells
    d. Engulfment of bacteria by macrophages

11. **The main function of mitochondria is:**
    a. DNA synthesis
    b. Protein processing and packaging
    c. ATP production
    d. RNA synthesis

12. **The main function of the Golgi apparatus is:**
    a. DNA synthesis
    b. Protein processing and packaging
    c. ATP synthesis
    d. RNA synthesis

13. **The following are true of plasma membranes, *except*:**
    a. They are made up of a double layer of lipid molecules in which the proteins are embedded
    b. The lipid membranes include phospholipids and cholesterol
    c. The plasma membrane has RNA-binding sites on the inside surface of the membrane resembling the rough endoplasmic reticulum
    d. The plasma membrane has both integral membrane proteins and peripheral membrane proteins

14. **The function of smooth endoplasmic reticulum is:**
    a. Protein synthesis
    b. Regulation of intracellular calcium distribution
    c. Excretion
    d. Maintaining the skeleton of the cell

15. **All of the following are the functions of lysosomes, *except*:**
    a. Phagocytosis
    b. Pinocytosis
    c. Exocytosis
    d. Breakdown of some intracellular materials

16. **Hydrolytic enzymes are found in:**
    a. Golgi apparatus   b. RER
    c. Lysosomes   d. Ribosomes

17. **The site of lysosomes can be seen using a specific histochemical reaction called:**
    a. Alkaline phosphatase
    b. Acid phosphatase
    c. Peroxidase
    d. Succinic dehydrogenase

18. **Organelles most notable for producing and degrading hydrogen peroxide are:**
    a. Lysosomes
    b. Mitochondria
    c. Golgi bodies
    d. Peroxisomes

19. **The function of attached ribosomes to RER is to synthesize:**
    a. Lipids
    b. Carbohydrates
    c. Proteins that will be secreted by the cell
    d. Glycogen

20. **Ribosomal RNA is formed in:**
    a. The euchromatin
    b. The nucleolus
    c. The RER
    d. The heterochromatin

21. **Glycogen can be demonstrated using:**
    a. Best's carmine
    b. H and E
    c. Sudan black
    d. Silver

22. **Euchromatin is predominant in:**
    a. The nuclei of metabolically active cells
    b. The nuclei of metabolically inactive cells
    c. The special type of stain
    d. The type of cell organoids

23. **The nucleolus is formed of:**
    a. Proteins and DNA
    b. Proteins only
    c. Chromatin
    d. Proteins and RNA
24. **The nuclear pore:**
    a. Is hexagonal in shape
    b. Is bridged by a unit membrane
    c. Is a transient structure
    d. Allows for communication between the nucleus and the cytoplasm
25. **The feature of phospholipids that is essential for their role in biological membranes is:**
    a. Strong rigid membranes
    b. Extremely hydrophobic
    c. Hydrophilic and hydrophobic
    d. Extremely hydrophilic

Answers

1. c	2. a	3. c	4. c	5. c
6. a	7. d	8. a	9. b	10. c
11. c	12. b	13. c	14. b	15. c
16. c	17. b	18. d	19. c	20. b
21. a	22. a	23. d	24. d	25. c

CHAPTER 2

Bioenergetics

OBJECTIVES

At the end of this chapter, the learner should be able to:
- Know about the high-energy compounds and their classification
- Understand the structure of adenosine triphosphate (ATP).

INTRODUCTION

The bioenergetics mainly deals with the study of energy changes during biochemical reactions that take place inside the body. The reactions are of two types, and they are as follows:
1. Exergonic (energy releasing)
2. Endergonic (energy consumption).

FREE ENERGY

Free energy is the energy available to work:
- Changes in the free energy (ΔG) predict feasibility of chemical reactions, change in heat (ΔH) and randomness of reactants and products (ΔS).
- ΔH is enthalpy and ΔS is entropy.
- Enthalpy is a measure of the change in heat content of the reactants compared with products.
- Entropy represents a change in the randomness or disorder of reactants and products.
- Decrease in the free energy leads to spontaneous reactions to occur.
- During a chemical reaction, heat may be released or absorbed.
- $\Delta G = \Delta H - T\Delta S$, T is absolute temperature.
- More randomness (ΔS), more conversion of reactants to products or vice versa.
- Increase in ΔS increases the negative charge to ΔG, thus the loss of free energy.
- $-\Delta G$, release of energy, exergonic reaction, proceeds spontaneously, e.g. ATP hydrolysis:
$$ATP + H_2O \rightarrow ADP + Pi$$
($\Delta G° = -7.3$ kcal/mol).
$+\Delta G$, consumption of energy, endergonic reaction, cannot proceed spontaneously, e.g. ATP formation:
ADP + Pi → ATP (needs supply of 7.3 kcal/mol for reaction).
- $\Delta G = 0$, when reaction is at equilibrium.
- $\Delta G = \Delta G° + RT \ln [B]/[A]$
- $\Delta G = \Delta G° + RT \ln [A]$
ΔG = Standard free energy change
R = Gas constant (91.987 cal/mol)
T = Absolute temperature (273°C)
ln = Natural logarithm
[B] = Concentration of product
[A] = Concentration of reactant
$\Delta G°$ = Standard free energy change
- When $A \leftrightarrow B$, the reaction is at equilibrium: $G = 0$.
Then, the equation becomes:
- $\Delta G = 0 = \Delta G° + RT \ln [B]/[A]$
- $\Delta G° = -RT \ln [B] eq/[A] eq$
- $\Delta G° = -RT \ln K_{eq}$.

- In biochemical pathways involving several reactions, the sum of ΔG is important in determining the reaction.

HIGH-ENERGY COMPOUNDS

The relation between the changes of ΔG, ΔH and ΔS is expressed as follows:
- ATP on hydrolysis release –7.3 kcal/mol energy.
- Substances that release energy higher than ATP, including ATP, are called high-energy compounds.
- Substances that release energy lower than ATP are called low-energy compounds.

Free energy hydrolysis of low-energy and high-energy compounds is given in **Table 2.1**.

Table 2.1: Energy released by hydrolysis of some compounds.

Compound	kcal/mol
Phosphoenolpyruvate	–14.8
Carbamoyl phosphate	–12.3
1,3-Bisphosphoglycerate	–11.8
Creatine phosphate	–10.3
ATP* to ADP† + Pi‡	–7.3
ADP to AMP§ + Pi	–6.6
Pyrophosphate	–6.6
Glucose-1-phosphate	–5.0

*ATP, adenosine triphosphate; †ADP, adenosine diphosphate; ‡Pi, inorganic phosphate; §AMP, adenosine monophosphate.

Classification

High-energy compounds are classified into five groups:
1. Pyrophosphates—ATP
2. Acyl phosphates—1,3-bisphosphoglycerate
3. Enol phosphates—phosphoenolpyruvate
4. Thioesters—acetyl-coenzyme A (acetyl-CoA)
5. Phosphoguanidines—phosphocreatine.

High-energy phosphates act as energy currency of the cell. The following list shows the features of ATP:

- It is the most important high-energy molecule.
- It consists of adenine, ribose and triphosphate moiety linked by phosphoanhydride bond.
- It serves as an energy currency of the cell.

Biochemical pathways often involve a series of reactions. For such reactions, free energy change is an additive value. The sum of ΔG is crucial in determining whether a particular pathway will proceed or not. As long as the sum of ΔGs of individual reactions is negative, the pathway can operate. This happens despite the fact that some of the individual reactions may have positive ΔG. It should be remembered that the actual rates of biochemical reactions are determined by the activities of enzymes.

Structure of ATP

The structure of ATP is given in **Figure 2.1**:

ATP/ADP Cycle

ATP/ADP cycle and the energy transfer metabolism are shown in **Figure 2.2**.

The chapter mainly deals with the study of energy changes during biochemical reactions, which take place inside the body. The reactions are of exergonic (energy releasing) and endergonic (energy consumption). Free energy

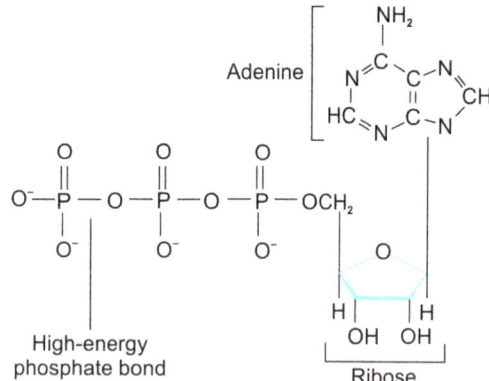

Fig. 2.1: Structure of adenosine triphosphate.

Bioenergetics

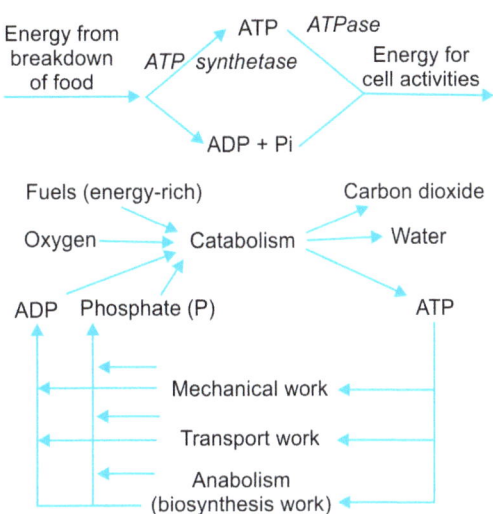

Fig. 2.2: ATP/ADP cycle and energy transfer metabolism. (ADP, adenosine diphosphate; ATP, adenosine triphosphate).

is the energy available to work. Decrease in the free energy leads to spontaneous reactions to occur. During a chemical reaction, heat may be released or absorbed. The relation between the changes of ΔG, ΔH and ΔS is expressed as ATP on hydrolysis release –7.3 kcal/mol energy. Substances that release energy higher than ATP, including ATP, are called high-energy compounds, and they are classified into five groups.

MULTIPLE-CHOICE QUESTIONS

1. A pathway has two steps: A → B → C, where $\Delta G°_{A \to B}$ = +60 kJ/mol with a K_{eq} of 6×10^{-1} and $\Delta G°_{B \to C}$ = –32.5 kJ/mol with a K_{eq} of 3×10^6. The $\Delta G°$ for the pathway of C → A is:
   a. +27.5 kJ/mol
   b. –27.5 kJ/mol
   c. +92.5 kJ/mol
   d. –92.5 kJ/mol
2. Calculate the $\Delta G°$ for the following redox reaction, given that $\Delta E°$ = –0.40 V and F = 96.5 kJ/V/mol:
   Acetaldehyde + 2H$^+$ + 2e$^-$ → Ethanol
   a. –19.3 kJ/mol
   b. +38.6 kJ/mol
   c. –57.9 kJ/mol
   d. +77.2 kJ/mol
3. The second law of thermodynamics states that for a system:
   a. Energy cannot be gained or lost
   b. Free energy exists only as heat
   c. The total entropy must increase for a process to become spontaneous
   d. Energy must be converted from one form to another to be used in a process
4. Adenosine triphosphate is considered the currency of energy in cells because:
   a. It has an energy-rich adenine base
   b. It has a $\Delta G°$ > 0, when hydrolyzed to ADP + Pi
   c. Its intermediate $\Delta G°$ allows it to couple many reactions
   d. It provides three phosphates, which are used to create energy in glycolysis
5. The following illustrates the hydrolysis of ATP:
   ATP → ADP + Pi
   It is an example of:
   a. An endothermic reaction
   b. A reaction where $\Delta G°$ < zero
   c. A reaction where $\Delta G°$ = zero
   d. A reaction where $\Delta G°$ > zero

Answers

1. b   2. d   3. c   4. c   5. b

CHAPTER 3

Enzymes

OBJECTIVES

At the end of this chapter, the learner should be able to:
- Understand the classification and function of enzymes
- Know about the active site and mechanism of enzyme action
- Explain the factors affecting enzyme activity
- Describe the different types of inhibition and use of competitive inhibition technique in the drug therapy
- Know about the diagnostic importance of enzymes.

INTRODUCTION

- Enzymes are biological catalysts produced by the living cells, and they catalyze several reactions in the body.
- They are proteins in nature.
- They are specific in action, i.e. each enzyme can catalyze only one type of reaction.
- They are required in very small quantities.
- The loss of catalytic activity was observed when they are subjected to heat or strong acids or bases or organic solvents.
- The enzymes mainly catalyze the metabolic pathways in the human body.
- The deficiency of the enzyme leads to inborn errors of metabolism.
- Most of the enzymes are produced by the cells of a particular tissue and function within that cell. Such enzymes are called as *intracellular enzymes, for example,* enzymes of glycolysis, TCA cycle and fatty acid synthesis.
- However, there are certain enzymes, which are produced by the cells of a particular tissue from where these are liberated for use in the other tissues. Such enzymes are called as *extracellular enzymes, for example,* various proteolytic enzymes of gastrointestinal tract (trypsin, chymotrypsin).

The enzyme binds with its specific substrate and forms an enzyme–substrate (ES) complex. At the end of the reaction, the substrate is converted into the product, and the enzyme remains unchanged.

$$E + S - ES \rightarrow E + Product$$

CHEMICAL NATURE OF ENZYMES

Following lists the chemical nature of enzymes:
- Enzymes with two or more subunits (polypeptides) are called as oligomeric enzymes.
- Several enzymes occur in the form of multienzyme complex. In this case, several enzymes occur in a single complex form, for example, pyruvate dehydrogenase and fatty acid synthase complex.
- Some enzymes require the presence of certain additional organic or inorganic substances and are *conjugated proteins*. Such enzymes are called as **holoenzymes**. The protein part is called as *apoenzymes*. The nonprotein part is *prosthetic group*.
- Apoenzyme + Prosthetic group [coenzyme] → Holoenzyme.

- Several apoenzymes require the presence of metal ions such as Mg^{2+} (for hexokinase) and Zn^{2+} (for the activity of carboxypeptidase). Such inorganic ions are called as **cofactors**. If the metal ion is the integral part of the enzyme, such enzymes are called as **metalloenzymes**.

RIBOZYMES

These are RNA molecules that can act as catalysts.

These ribozymes break RNA phosphodiester bonds at certain specific location in the RNA molecules, serving as ribonucleases and as peptidyl transferase (catalyzes the formation of peptide body).

These ribozymes are being considered as possible therapeutic agents for disorders caused by the inappropriate expression of RNA or the expression of a mutated RNA. However, further research is required for this to consider.

ZYMOGENS OR PROENZYMES

The protein-digesting enzymes (proteolytic enzymes) of gastrointestinal tract are produced in the form of precursor. This is to prevent unwanted degradation of body self-protein. These inactive precursor forms of enzymes (zymogen) are converted into active form by HCl and trypsin.

For example,
- Pepsinogen → pepsin (HCl activates the pepsinogen)
- Trypsinogen → trypsin (trypsin and enteropeptidase activate the enzymes), procarboxypeptidase, chymotrypsinogen.

COENZYMES

Coenzymes are dialyzable, thermostable and low molecular weight organic substances (also considered as cosubstrate or second substrate) **(Table 3.1)**.

Coenzymes are small organic molecules that transport chemical groups from one enzyme to another.

Coenzymes are usually regenerated, and their concentrations are maintained at a steady level inside the cell, for example, NADPH is regenerated through the pentose phosphate pathway and S-adenosylmethionine by methionine adenosyltransferase.

Table 3.1: Common coenzymes and their functions

Vitamin	Coenzyme	Function
Thiamine (B_1)	Thiamine pyrophosphate (TPP)	Oxidative decarboxylation and transketolase reaction
Riboflavin (B_2)	Flavin adenine dinucleotide (FAD) Flavin mononucleotide (FMN)	Oxidative and reductive reaction
Niacin	Nicotinamide adenine dinucleotide (NAD) Nicotinamide adenine dinucleotide phosphate (NADP)	Oxidative and reductive reaction
Pyridoxine (B_6)	Pyridoxal phosphate (PLP)	Transamination, deamination and decarboxylation reactions
Biotin	Biocytin	Carboxylation reactions
Folic acid	Tetrahydrofolate (THF)	Carrier of one carbon
Pantothenic acid	Coenzyme A	Acyl carrier
Cyanocobalamin (B_{12})	Methylcobalamin, deoxyadenosylcobalamin	Transfer of CH_3 group and isomerizations

ENERGY OF ACTIVATION OF CATALYZED AND UNCATALYZED REACTIONS

All chemical reactions have an energy barrier, separating the reactants and the products. This barrier, called the free energy of activation, is the energy difference between the energy of the reactant and high-energy intermediates that occur during the formation of a product **(Fig. 3.1)**.

$$S \rightleftharpoons S^* \rightleftharpoons P$$
(Reactant)   (Product)

The peak of free energy activation represents the transition state, in which the high-energy intermediates (S^*) are formed during the conversion of a reactant to a product.

Due to the effect of activation energy, the rates of unanalyzed chemical reactions are slow.

An enzyme lowers the energy required for activation to the transition state.

With an enzyme as a catalyst, the reaction may easily proceed at the normal physiological temperature; otherwise addition of heat energy is required for the reaction to occur.

Active Site of an Enzyme

The active site of an enzyme is the region where substrate binds.

This active site contains the specific amino acid residues (binding and catalytic residues) and possesses three-dimensional structure.

The amino acid residues at the active site of an enzyme have two functions:
- The binding amino acid residues recognize and bind the correct substrate to form ES complex.
- The catalytic residues create a chemical environment that enhances the rate of reaction and ES complex is converted to an enzyme (E) and a product (p).

A change in the primary, secondary, tertiary or quaternary structure may alter the three-dimensional shape of the active site to reduce its binding and catalytic activity.

LIST AND EXPLAIN THE FACTORS THAT AFFECT THE ENZYME ACTIVITY

1. pH
2. Temperature
3. Concentration of substrate
4. Concentration of enzyme.

Effect of pH

Each enzyme has an optimum pH at which the activity of the enzyme is maximum **(Fig. 3.2)**. Either decreased or increased pH causes a decrease in enzyme activity.

For example,
1. Pepsin has an optimum pH at 1.2 (its activity is maximum at this pH)
2. Optimum pH for amylase is 6.8.
3. Optimum pH for alkaline phosphatase [ALP] is 9.0.

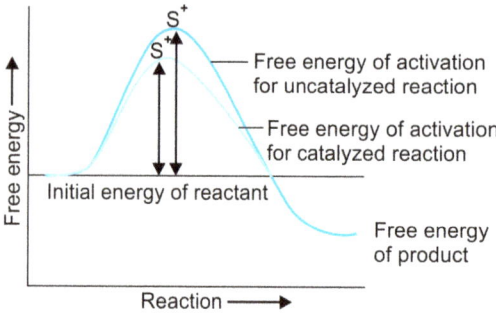

Fig. 3.1: Free energy of activation of a catalyzed and uncatalyzed reaction.

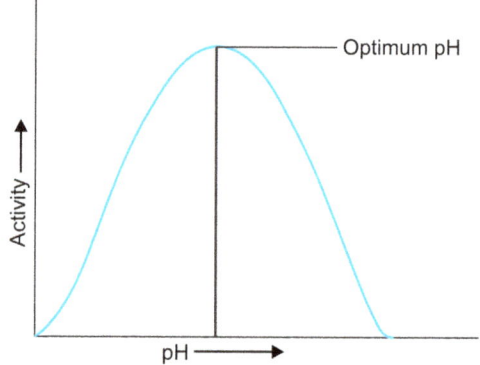

Fig. 3.2: Effect of pH on enzyme activity.

4. Optimum pH for acid phosphatase [ACP] is 5.0.

Effect of Temperature

The temperature at which the enzyme activity is more is called the optimum temperature **(Fig. 3.3)**. Any strong change in the optimum temperature results in the loss of enzyme activity. Optimum temperature of enzymes in the human body is 37°C.

Effect of Substrate Concentration

At low substrate concentration, enzyme molecules are free initially, and the ES complex formation is proportional to the substrate concentration. This means the rate of velocity is directly proportional to the [S] and follows first-order kinetics. At higher concentration, all the enzyme molecules are saturated with substrate. There will be no change in the activity further **(Fig. 3.4)** and followed by hyperbolic curve; this is zero-order kinetics.

Effect of Enzyme Concentration

The velocity of the enzyme reaction is directly proportional to the enzyme concentration **(Fig. 3.5)**.

CLASSIFICATION OF ENZYMES

Enzymes are classified into six groups according to the International Union of Biochemistry (IUB). They are as follows:
1. **Oxidoreductases:** Enzymes involved in oxidation–reduction reactions, for example, lactate dehydrogenase (LDH) and glyceraldehyde-3-phosphate dehydrogenase.
2. **Transferases:** Transfer a specific group from one substrate to another, for example, alanine transaminase and hexokinase.
3. **Hydrolases:** Hydrolyze the substrate with the addition of water molecule, for example, glucose-6-phosphatase amylase and pepsin.
4. **Lyases:** Catalyze the removal of a small molecule from a large substrate without the addition of water, for example, fumarase and enolase.
5. **Isomerases:** They isomerize substrates, for example, racemases and isomerase, etc.
6. **Ligases:** Synthesize substance by joining two substrates with the utilization of energy, for example, glutamine synthetase.

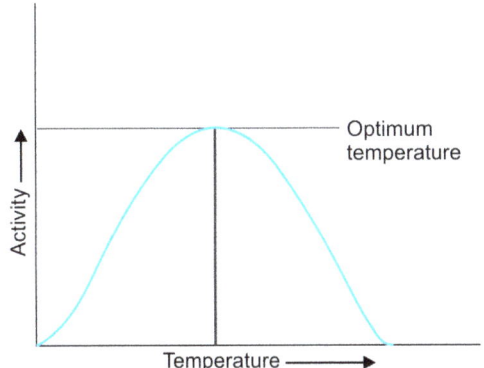

Fig. 3.3: Effect of temperature on enzyme activity.

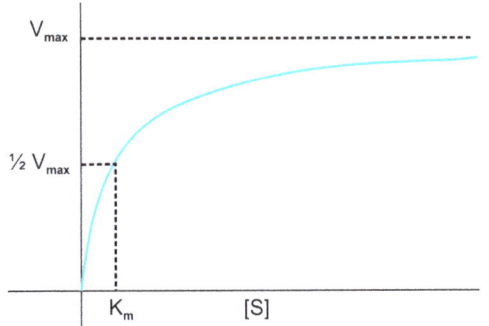

Fig. 3.4: Effect of substrate concentration.

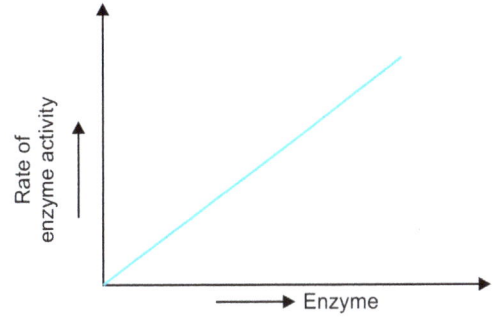

Fig. 3.5: Effect of enzyme concentration.

Enzyme Specificity

The most important property of enzyme is its specificity. They exhibit several types of specificity:
1. Stereospecificity: The group of enzyme catalyzes either L or D isomer.
2. Reaction specificity: One enzyme catalyzes only one type of reaction.
3. Substrate specificity: Pepsin hydrolyzes residues of only aromatic amino acids, while trypsin hydrolyzes residues of the basic amino acids only.
    – A. Absolute specificity: Glucokinase acts on glucose only.
    – B. Group specificity: Hexokinase catalyzes hexoses.
4. Bond specificity: Refers to the action of proteolytic enzymes. Peptidase and glycosidase act on peptide bonds of proteins and glycosidic bonds of carbohydrates, respectively. Lipases act on ester bonds of lipids.

MECHANISM OF ENZYME CATALYSIS

The substrate binds noncovalently at the active site of the enzyme and forms ES complex. This is the first step in enzyme catalysis. This complex is subsequently converted to product and free enzyme.

Two models have been proposed to explain the binding mechanism of substrate to the active site of the enzyme.
- Lock-and-key model.
- Induced fit model or hand-in-glove model of Koshland.

Lock-and-key Model (Proposed by Emil Fischer)

In this model, the enzyme is preshaped, and the active site has a rigid structure that is complementary to the substrate.

This model is called lock-and-key model, because in this model the substrate fits into the active site in the same way as a key fits into a lock (**Fig. 3.6**).

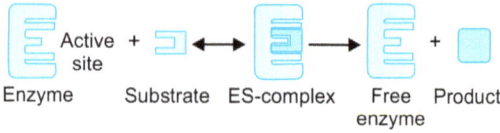

Fig. 3.6: Lock-and-key model.

This model gives the idea about the specificity of the enzymes, which bind only a specific substrate not another compound with an almost identical structure.

For example, the enzymes of glycolysis can bind D-isomer rather than L-isomer (which differs only in the configuration around a single carbon atom).

Induced-fit Model

This model explains the specificity of the enzyme as well as the changes taking place during catalysis.

Koshland explained that the enzymes are flexible and shapes of the active site can be modified by the binding of the substrate.

In the induced-fit model, the substrate induces a conformational change in the enzyme, in the same way in which placing a hand (substrate) into a glove (enzyme) induces changes in the glove's shape. Therefore, this model is also called a hand-in glove model (**Fig. 3.7**).

This arranges catalytic residues that participate in catalysis. The enzyme in turn induces reciprocal changes in its bound substrate that changes their orientation and configuration and strains the structure of the bound substrate. Such changes help to bring the ES complex into its transition state.

The intrinsic binding energy due to the ES interaction is made available for the transformation of the substrate into product.

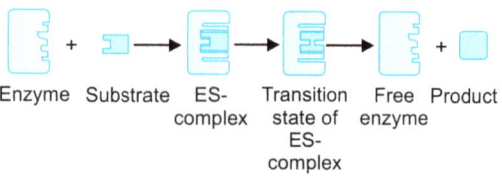

Fig. 3.7: Induced-fit model.

ENZYME KINETICS

Study of the impact made on the rate of an enzyme-catalyzed reaction by changes in experimental conditions is known as enzyme kinetics.

Knowledge of kinetics can be a very useful tool in understanding the mechanism by which an enzyme carries out its catalytic activity.

The effect of substrate concentration on the initial rate of an enzyme-catalyzed reaction is a main concept in enzyme kinetics. The substrate concentration is the important factor affecting rate of a reaction catalyzed by enzyme.

The effect on initial velocity (V_i) of varying substrate concentrations [S], when the enzyme concentration is held constant, is shown below **(Fig. 3.8)**:

- V_i = Initial velocity
- [S] = Substrate concentration
- V_{max} = Maximum velocity
- K_m = Substrate concentration when V_i is one-half V_{max} (Michaelis–Menten constant).

Observations of this type set Leonor Michaelis and Maud Menten thinking about the underlying reasons why a curve should follow this shape and led them to derive an algebraic equation that now bears their names.

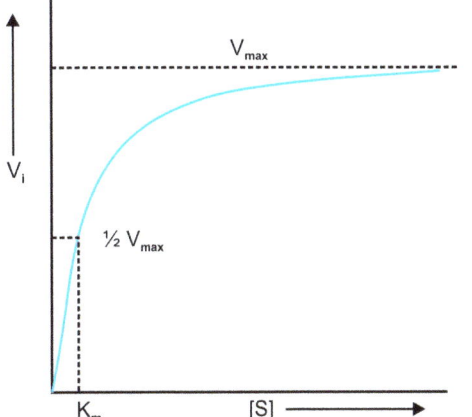

Fig. 3.8: Initial reaction velocity versus substrate concentration for Michaelis–Menten equation.

There are several modern ways to explain the way in which the Michaelis–Menten equation is derived, and the one is mentioned below.

For most enzymes, the initial velocities or reaction rates (V_i) by increasing the substrate concentration [S] with constant enzyme concentration [E] results in a hyperbolic curve. In other words, V_i increases rapidly at first as we increase the substrate concentration [S]. This is the first-order kinetics.

At higher substrate concentrations, V_i increases by smaller amounts in response to increase in [S].

Then, the rate of increase in V_i decreases, and V_i approaches a limit of the reaction rate, called V_{max}. No further increases in [S] will increase velocity. This condition is known as zero-order kinetics.

We already learned that in an enzyme-catalyzed reaction, the enzyme exists into two forms, that is, free [E] and the combined form [ES].

At low substrate concentration, most of the enzymes will be in free form E. In this condition, the rate is proportional to [S].

The maximum velocity of the catalyzed reaction is observed when the entire enzyme is present as the ES complex and concentration of E is vanishingly low. Therefore, at this condition, all the enzymes will be saturated with its substrate, and all the free enzymes will be converted into ES form. So that any increase in the [S] has no effect on the rate and the reaction immediately reaches a steady state, in which [ES] remains approximately constant. The ES complex breaks down to yield the product and the enzyme is free to bind another substrate molecule.

MICHAELIS–MENTEN EQUATION

With some assumptions, the Michaelis–Menten equation describes the relationship between [S] and reaction rate (V_i), as follows:

$$V_i = \frac{V_{max}[S]}{K_m + [S]}$$

K_m is Michaelis-Menten constant and is equal to the [S],
where

$$V_i = \frac{V_{max}}{2}$$

K_m is also an indicator of the enzyme's affinity for the substrate. The lower the K_m value, the higher the affinity, so it takes less substrate to reach half of V_{max} and the enzyme is a better catalyst for the reaction.

Begin by considering a simple reaction in which one substrate, S, in the presence of an enzyme, E, converts to one product, P. Michaelis and Menten hypothesized that the enzyme catalyzes the reaction by reacting with the substrate to form an intermediate ES complex. This complex experiences a catalytic reaction to form the enzyme, E, and the product, P. The following diagram represents the situation where K1, K2, K3 and K4 are rate constants:

$$E + S \underset{K_2}{\overset{K_1}{\rightleftarrows}} ES \underset{K_4}{\overset{K_3}{\rightleftarrows}} E + P$$

To derive their model, Michaelis and Menten made the following simplifying assumptions:

Moreover, considering $x = 1/[S]$ to be an independent variable and $y = 1/V_i$ to be a dependent variable, the equation has the form of a line, $y = mx + b$. Thus, in the graph **(Fig. 3.9)** of $1/V_i$ versus $1/[S]$, the slope is $\frac{K_m}{V_{max}}$

- The reaction rate is determined before much product is formed. Consequently, the reverse reaction from E + P to ES is negligible.
- K3 is small in comparison to K1 and K2; that is, the rate of product formation is slow in comparison with the rate of ES formation and the rate of ES dissociation to E + S.
- [S] is much greater than [E], so that [S] is virtually constant.
- [E] + [ES] is constant.

Under these assumptions, the Michaelis-Menten equation models the reaction as follows:

$$V_i = \frac{K_m[S]}{V_{max}[S]}$$

Although the Michaelis-Menten equation captures the relationship of reaction velocity to substrate concentration, K_m and V_{max} are difficult to ascertain from its graph. Hans Lineweaver and Dean Burk reorganized the equation into a form that is more helpful for determination of these constants. Taking the reciprocal of both sides, they solved for $1/V_i$ in terms of $1/[S]$, as follows:

$$\frac{1}{V_i} = \frac{K_m[S]}{V_{max}[S]}$$

$$\frac{1}{V_i} = \frac{K_m[S]}{V_{max}[S]} + \frac{[S]}{V_{max}[S]}$$

$$\frac{1}{V_i} = \left(\frac{K_m}{V_{max}}\right) + \frac{1}{[S]} + \frac{1}{V_{max}}$$

$\frac{K_m}{V_{max}}$ and $\frac{1}{V_{max}}$ are constants

Moreover, considering $x = 1/[S]$ to be an independent variable and $y = 1/V_i$ to be a dependent variable, the equation has the form of a line, $y = mx + b$. Thus, in the graph **(Fig. 3.9)** of $1/V_i$ versus $1/[S]$, the slope is $\frac{K_m}{V_{max}}$ and the vertical intercept is $\frac{1}{V_{max}}$

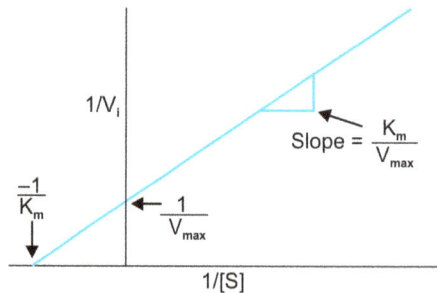

Fig. 3.9: Double reciprocal or Lineweaver–Burk plot.

Setting $1/V_i$ equal to zero, we find that the horizontal intercept is $-\dfrac{1}{K_m}$. Such a plot is called double reciprocal or Lineweaver–Burk plot.

ENZYME INHIBITION

The phenomenon of the decrease in the rate of enzymatic reaction brought about by the addition of a chemical substance is called enzyme inhibition. The substances, which inhibit the enzyme, are called as inhibitors.

1. *Competitive inhibition*: The competitive inhibitor (reversible inhibitor) closely resembles with that of substrate. Hence the inhibitor competes with the substrate for substrate-binding sites of the enzyme. This type of inhibition can be overcome by sufficiently high concentrations of substrate, i.e. by out-competing the inhibitor **(Fig. 3.10)**.

Competitive inhibitors can bind to E, but not to ES. Competitive inhibition increases K_m (i.e. the inhibitor interferes with substrate binding) but does not affect V_{max} (the inhibitor does not hamper catalysis in ES because it cannot bind to ES), *for example*, inhibition of succinate dehydrogenase by malonate.

The Michaelis–Menten equation for competitive inhibition is:

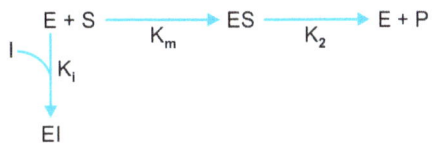

Here K_i is the dissociation constant for the enzyme-inhibitor (EI) complex. EI does not react to form E+ P, and the enzyme is unable to bind both S and I at the same time.

The Michaelis–Menten equation for competitive inhibition is:

$$V = \dfrac{V_{max}[S]}{[S] + K_m\left(1 + \dfrac{[I]}{K_i}\right)}$$

The Lineweaver–Burk equation for competitive inhibition is:

$$\dfrac{1}{V} = \dfrac{K_m}{V_{max}}\dfrac{1}{[S]}\left(1 + \dfrac{[I]}{K_i}\right) + \dfrac{1}{V_{max}}$$

For example, succinate dehydrogenase is the enzyme catalyzing the conversion of succinate to fumarate.

The malonate has the close structural resemblance to succinate.

That is why the malonate tries to occupy the active site of the enzyme.

Some of the competitive inhibitors are used in the treatment of disorders, which are explained later.

THERAPEUTIC USE OF COMPETITIVE INHIBITION

Competitive Inhibition Technique in Drug Therapy

The competitive inhibitors available are mostly synthetic compounds that are designed in such a way that it should have similarities with the substances present in the human body. So this similarity helps that compound to inhibit the enzymes that act on the particular substrates and finally block the reaction. Such type of inhibitors or drugs inhibit the important enzyme reactions in a

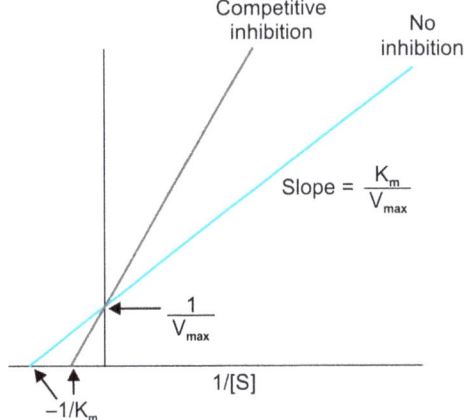

Fig. 3.10: Competitive inhibition.

bacteria or virus to control the infection. This type of treatment with chemicals or drugs to control infection is called chemotherapy.

To understand this, we should go through some of the examples **(Table 3.2)**.

a. *Treatment with sulfa drugs*: Bacteria can synthesize folic acid from para-amino-benzoic acid (PABA).
   - Sulfa drugs like sulfonamide have a structure similar to PABA.
   - When a person is treated with sulfa drugs, it inhibits the synthesis of folic acid in bacteria.
   - The folic acid is an important vitamin required for bacterial multiplication.
   - When sulfa drugs block the synthesis of folic acid, the bacterial multiplication is inhibited and infection is controlled.

b. *Treatment for gout by allopurinol*:
   - Allopurinol is the drug of choice for the treatment of gout.
   - It has a structure similar to hypoxanthine.
   - So allopurinol competitively inhibits xanthine oxidase, the enzyme that converts hypoxanthine to xanthine and then to uric acid.

c. *Control of cancer by amethopterin and aminopterin*:
   - Amethopterin and aminopterin are antifolic compounds having structural similarity with folic acid **(Fig. 3.11)**.
   - Coenzyme (tetrahydrofolic acid) of this folic acid helps in the transfer of one carbon unit (in the reactions like the synthesis of purines and pyrimidines).

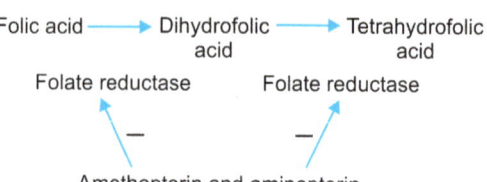

Fig. 3.11: Action of amethopterin and aminopterin.

   - Purines and pyrimidines are required for the synthesis of nucleic acids for growth and cell multiplication.
   - Aminopterin or amethopterin competitively inhibits folate reductase and interferes with the synthesis of tetrahydrofolate.
   - Thus these compounds are used in the treatment of blood cancer wherein there is excessive production of WBC.
   - Because of the coenzyme deficiency, the multiplication of WBC is inhibited.

d. *Dicumarol to thromboembolic condition*:
   - Vitamin K is involved in the γ-carboxylation (see details in Vitamin K) of glutamic acid residues of the clotting factors such as prothrombin, proconvertin factor, Christmas factor and Stuart–Prower factor.
   - There are various anticoagulants to treat the thromboembolic conditions.
   - Important and clinically useful are coumarins and heparins. Dicumarol and warfarin are the coumarins to treat the thromboembolic condition.

Table 3.2: Commonly used drugs that are competitive inhibitors.

Drug	Enzyme	Substrate	Therapeutic use
Methotrexate	Dihydrofolate reductase	FH_2	Treatment of cancer
Allopurinol	Xanthine oxidase	Hypoxanthine	Treatment of gout
Acetazolamide	Carbonic anhydrase	H_2CO_3	To treat hypertension
Mevinolin and Lovastatin	β-hydroxy-β-methylglutaryl CoA reductase (HMG CoA)	HMG CoA	To treat hypercholesterolemia
Captopril and enalapril	Angiotensin-converting enzyme (ACE)	Angiotensin	To treat high blood pressure

- When the patient is treated with dicumarol, it competes with vitamin K and decreases the formation of prothrombin by liver.
e. *Isonicotinic acid hydrazide (INH) treatment for tuberculosis*:
    - The INH drug has structural similarity with pyridoxine.
    - This drug interferes with the formation of pyridoxal phosphate (PLP), a coenzyme of pyridoxine used by TB bacillus.
    - That is the reason why patients treated with INH always supplemented with vitamin B_6.

Noncompetitive Inhibition

In this type, the inhibitor does not resemble the substrate and does not bind to the substrate-binding site of the enzyme. It binds to the enzyme other than the active site **(Fig. 3.12)**, for example, inhibition of enzymes by heavy metals such as Hg^{2+}, iodoacetamide and diisopropylphosphofluoride (DIPF).

Iodoacetamide reacts with sulfhydryl groups of cysteine residues or with the imidazole group of histidine residues of the enzyme.

Di-isopropylphosphofluoride can inhibit acetylcholine esterase by covalently reacting with the hydroxyl group of a serine residues present at the active site of an enzyme.

A noncompetitive inhibitor lowers the V_{max} with no change in the K_m value.

Noncompetitive inhibitors have identical affinities for E and ES ($K_i = K_i'$). Noncompetitive inhibition does not change K_m (i.e. it does not affect substrate binding) but decreases V_{max} (i.e. inhibitor binding affects catalysis).

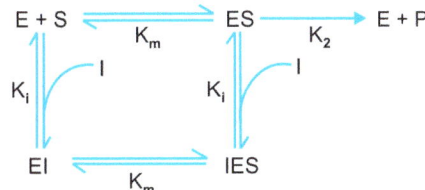

Here K_i is the dissociation constant for either the EI complex or the inhibitor enzyme substrate (IES) complex. Neither of these complexes can react to form E + P.

The Michaelis–Menten equation for noncompetitive inhibition is:

$$V = \frac{V_{max}[S]}{([S]+K_m)\left(1+\frac{[I]}{K_i}\right)}$$

The Lineweaver–Burk equation for noncompetitive inhibition is:

$$\frac{1}{V} = \frac{K_m}{V_{max}}\frac{1}{[S]}\left(1+\frac{[I]}{K_i}\right) + \frac{1}{V_{max}}\left(1+\frac{[I]}{K_i}\right)$$

Uncompetitive Inhibition

Occurs when the inhibitor binds only to the ES complex, not to the free enzyme; the EIS complex is catalytically inactive. Inhibitor binds to ES complex at locations other than the catalytic site. This mode of inhibition is rare and causes a decrease in both V_{max} and the K_m value **(Fig. 3.13)**.

Substrate and Product Inhibition

These are where either the substrate or product of an enzyme reaction inhibits the enzyme's activity. This inhibition may follow the competitive, uncompetitive, or mixed patterns. In substrate inhibition, there is

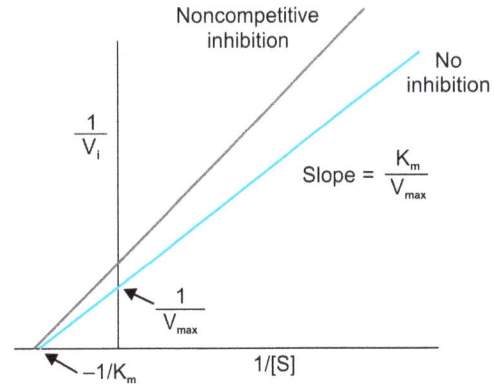

Fig. 3.12: Noncompetitive inhibition.

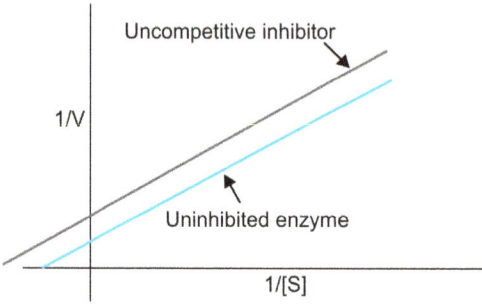

Fig. 3.13: Uncompetitive inhibition.

a progressive decrease in activity at high substrate concentrations. This may indicate the existence of two substrate-binding sites in the enzyme. At low substrate, the high-affinity site is occupied, and normal kinetics is followed. However, at higher concentrations, the second inhibitory site becomes occupied, inhibiting the enzyme. Product inhibition is often a regulatory feature in metabolism and can be a form of negative feedback, *for example*, hexokinase inhibition by glucose-6-phosphate and inhibition of β-hydroxy-β-methylglutaryl CoA reductase (HMG CoA) reductase by cholesterol.

ALLOSTERIC ENZYMES

These enzymes have more than one subunit with a catalytic and regulatory site. Allosteric activator or inhibitor binds to the regulatory site and regulates the activity of the enzyme. For example, HMG CoA reductase enzyme is a regulatory enzyme of cholesterol biosynthesis.

ADP and glucose-6-phosphate are the allosteric activator and inhibitor of hexokinase, respectively.

ISOENZYMES

Isoenzymes are defined as the different forms of a single enzyme and exist in the same species, which have same catalytic activity but differ structurally, physically, electrophoretically and chemically, for example, LDH (has five different forms) and creatine phosphokinase (CK; has three different forms).

LDH: Each of five forms consists of four subunits (polypeptide chains). It is made up of two types of subunits (H and M) and contains four of them in different proportions as LDH_1, LDH_2, LDH_3, LDH_4 and LDH_5.

CK: It is a dimeric enzyme having two types of subunits (B and M). There are three isoenzyme forms of CK (CK_1 [BB], CK_2 [MB] and CK_3 [MM]).

DIAGNOSTIC ENZYMES

The cells produce enzymes, and they remain within the cells. Very small amount of the enzymes is released into the bloodstream, due to the normal breakdown of the cells. Hence the enzymes are present even in the blood in very small amounts under normal conditions. The levels of these enzymes are significantly increased in blood under certain diseased conditions, which leads to breakdown of cells. Estimation of these enzyme levels in blood or plasma is useful in the diagnosis of various diseases. These enzymes indicate the organ from which they are released, and based on this, it is easy to find out which organ is affected **(Table 3.3)**.

The diagnostic enzymes are grouped according to the organ they belong. Important groups are as follows:
1. Liver enzymes: [Aspartate aminotransferase (AST), alanine aminotransferase (ALT), alkaline phosphatase (ALP) and gamma glutamyl transferase (GGT)]
2. Cardiac enzymes: (LDH, LD_1, CK, CKMB, AST)
3. Muscle enzymes: (CK, LDH, AST)
4. Pancreatic enzymes: (amylase, lipase)
5. Bone enzymes: (ALP and ACP).

LACTATE DEHYDROGENASE

LDH is present in almost all the tissues of the body. There are different forms of LDH, which

Table 3.3: Diagnostic importance of certain serum enzymes.

Serum enzymes	Diagnostic significance
1. Acid phosphatase	Increases in carcinoma of prostate
2. Alkaline phosphatase	Increases in obstructive jaundice and bone disorders such as rickets, Paget's disease, hyperthyroidism
3. Amylase	Increases in acute pancreatitis, intestinal obstruction, decreases in acute liver disease
4. Creatine phosphokinase	
CPK 1 (BB)	Brain disorder
CPK 2 (MB)	Myocardial infarction (within 4 hours of onset)
CPK 3 (MM)	Muscular dystrophy
5. Ceruloplasmin	Increases in liver cirrhosis, decreases in Wilson's disease
6. Choline esterase	Increases in nephrotic syndrome and decreases in acute liver disease and organophosphorus poisoning
7. Aspartate aminotransferase (AST) or serum glutamate oxaloacetate transaminase (SGOT)	Increases in myocardial infarction and toxic liver cell necrosis
8. Alanine aminotransferase (ALT) or serum glutamate pyruvaye transaminase (SGPT)	Increases in viral hepatitis and other liver diseases
9. Lactate dehydrogenase	
LDH_1, LDH_2	Myocardial infarction
LDH_4, LDH_5	Acute viral hepatitis
10. Lipase	Increases in acute pancreatitis
11. 5′ nucleotidase	Increases in liver disease, obstructive jaundice
12. γ-glutamyl transpeptidase	Alcoholic liver disease

are known as isoenzymes; it is one of the best examples for isoenzymes.

Isoenzyme	Subunits	Source
LD_1	HHHH	Heart, RBC
LD_2	HHHM	RBC, heart
LD_3	HHMM	Liver, lung and spleen
LD_4	HMMM	Liver, lung and spleen
LD_5	MMMM	Skeletal muscle

Since LDH presents in almost all the tissues, its increase in the serum is nonspecific. LDH level mainly increases in the following conditions:

- Myocardial infarction (LD_1 and LD_2 increased)
- Skeletal muscle diseases (LD_5 increased)
- Liver diseases (LD_3 and LD_4 increased)
- Cancer of lung, liver and many other organ diseases (LD_3 and LD_4 increased).

Cardiac Enzymes in Myocardial Infarction

The enzymes such as CKMB, LDH, LDH_1 and AST are included under cardiac enzymes. Estimation of these may help in the diagnosis, assessment and prognosis of the heart diseases **(Fig. 3.14)**.

The increase and decrease in the levels of cardiac enzymes follow a particular pattern in myocardial infarction. It is as follows:

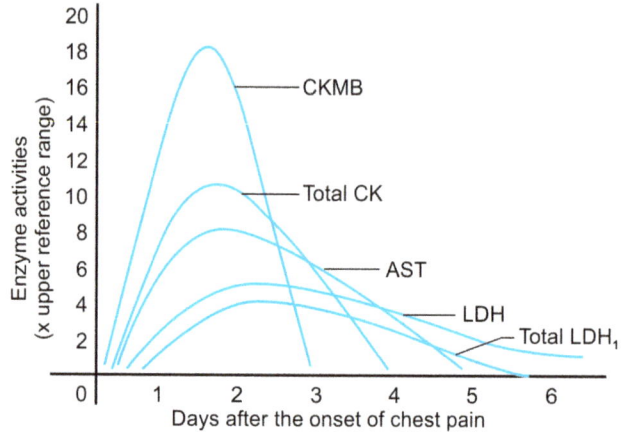

Fig. 3.14: Pattern of cardiac enzymes following myocardial infarction.

CK and CKMB

Following myocardial infarction (MI), the first enzyme to increase is CKMB. Immediately after the heart attack, the CKMB levels start increasing in the serum. It goes on increasing and reaches a maximum level by the end of first day. After reaching the peak level, CKMB decreases and reaches the normal level by third day. Total CK also follows the same pattern (normally CKMB is about 6% of the total CK value). In myocardial infarction, CKMB form may go up to 10–30% of the total CK.

AST

AST levels in plasma increase after 6–8 hours of chest pain, and it reaches the peak value by second day but comes to normal by fourth or fifth day.

LDH_1 and LDH

Total LDH and LDH_1 begin to increase 8–12 hours after the chest pain. It goes on increasing and reaches the maximum value by third day and slowly comes to normal by about seventh day.

The level of these enzymes in serum is related to the severe damage to heart muscle. So, in severe MI, these enzymes are elevated. CKMB and LD_1 are the most sensitive and specific markers for the diagnosis of MI.

Phosphatases

These are enzymes, which catalyze the removal of PO^{2-} group from organic monophosphoric esters. Two types of phosphatases are present: normally alkaline phosphatase, which has maximum activity at pH 10, and acid phosphatase, with maximum activity at acidic pH 5.0.

Alkaline Phosphatase

The alkaline phosphatase is present in all tissues of the body.

Its level is high in liver, bone, intestine, kidney and placenta. Each of these organs contains a specific isoenzyme of alkaline phosphatase.

There are totally five isoenzyme forms of ALP. Normal adult serum contains ALP, which is mainly from liver and bile duct.

The source of serum ALP is mainly from bone in children.

Placenta ALP is found in pregnancy only.

The functions of ALP in the body are the transport of phosphate across the

cell membranes and the addition of phosphates during mineralization of the bone.
Normal range: 40–200 U/L (35–140 U/L).

Acid Phosphatases

The prostate gland is the richest source for ACP. Other sources are red blood cells, platelets, bone, etc.
1. Serum ACP is increased in prostate gland enlargement (BPH—benign prostate hypertrophy) and carcinoma of the prostate gland.
2. The elevation of ACP is also seen in bone diseases.

Gamma-glutamyl Transferase

Source: Liver and bile ducts are the main sources of plasma GGT. Pancreas, prostate gland and kidneys also contain this enzyme.

Clinical Significance

GGT levels in serum are increased in:
1. Obstructive jaundice
2. Hepatitis
3. Alcoholic cirrhosis.
   Plasma GGT level is a very sensitive indicator to diagnose alcoholic cirrhosis.
Normal value: 5–40 U/L.

Amylase

Amylase helps in the digestion of starch in the small intestine. Amylase breaks down α-1,4-glucoside linkages of starch into maltose. Serum amylase originates from pancreas and salivary gland.

Clinical Significance

Amylase level in serum is increased in acute pancreatitis, pancreas injury and carcinoma of pancreas, tumors of lung, mumps and other salivary lesions.
Normal range: 80–240 U/L.

Lipase

The enzyme presents in the intestine, which hydrolyzes triglycerides (FAT) of the diet and finally helps to digest the fat. Bile salts are essential for the action of lipase.

Source: Pancreas is the major source for lipase in the serum.

Serum lipase is increased in chronic pancreatitis.

Serum amylase is increased in mumps, pancreatic diseases or due to some other cause, whereas lipase is increased only in pancreatitis. Therefore, the determination of both amylase and lipase together help in the diagnosis of acute pancreatitis.
Normal range: 40–200 U/L.

Cholinesterase

Two types have been distinguished: true cholinesterase (acetylcholine hydrolase, acetylcholine esterase) presents in the nerve tissue and RBC and is responsible for the hydrolysis of acetylcholine at synapses and the neuromuscular junction.

Serum cholinesterase level is an important indicator of insecticide poisoning. Its level is markedly decreased in persons who have consumed insecticides, which are organophosphorus compounds.
Normal level: 4,000–12,000 U/L.

Glucose-6-phosphate Dehydrogenase (G6PD)

Glucose-6-phosphate dehydrogenase (G6PD) is present within the RBC. Deficiency of G6PD is inborn, and it is prevalent throughout the world. The deficiency is of the mild type in most people. Deficiency is also observed in some rare cases and it is observed in the childhood itself.

G6PD is the enzyme required in hexose monophosphate (HMP) pathway of carbohydrate metabolism. The enzyme catalyzes the reaction, with the production of NADPH.

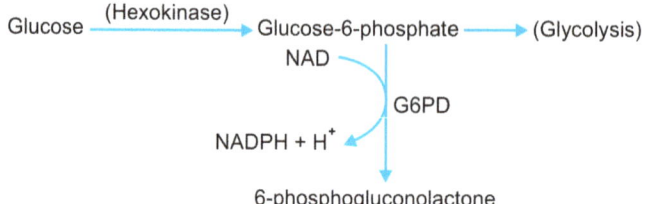

NADPH is essential for the stability of RBC membranes (NADPH is required to maintain reduced glutathione range, which maintains the stability of RBCs). In case of G6PD deficiency, NADPH production will be decreased leading to the breakdown of RBC and anemia. In the case of mild deficiency, a person will be healthy when he or she is treated with certain drugs like primaquine, and sulfonamides cause severe hemolysis. The NADPH supply is not sufficient to maintain the stability of RBC when these drugs are given. Hence hemolysis takes place and may lead to anemia and death.

G6PD estimation in blood is required in the following conditions:

1. When the patient is suffering from severe hemolytic anemia.
2. While treating a patient with malarial drugs.

Reference: 8–18 U/g Hb.

SUMMARY

Enzymes are biological catalysts produced by the living cells, and they catalyze several reactions in the body. All enzymes are proteins in nature and specific in action. The enzymes mainly catalyze the metabolic pathways in the human body. The deficiency of the enzyme results in metabolic errors. Most of the enzymes are of intracellular enzymes and few are extracellular enzymes. During the reactions, they catalyze the enzyme binds with its specific substrate to form ES complex and then generate the product. The active site of an enzyme is the region where the substrate binds to. Enzymes require coenzymes, which are small organic molecules that transport chemical groups from one enzyme to another. The factors that affect enzyme activity are pH, temperature, concentration of substrate, concentration of enzyme and activators. Enzymes are classified into six classes depending on their specific functions. The phenomenon of the decrease in the rate of enzymatic reaction brought about by the addition of a chemical substance is called enzyme inhibition. The substances that inhibit the enzyme are called inhibitors. The inhibition is of competitive and noncompetitive in nature. The competitive inhibition technique is utilized in the drug therapy to synthesize many drugs to treat various disorders. Most of the enzymes are regulated by allosteric regulation to control the metabolic reactions. The enzymes are produced by the cells and remain within the cells. Very small amount of the enzymes is released into the blood stream, due to the normal breakdown of the cells. Hence, the enzymes are present in the blood in very small amounts under normal conditions. The levels of these enzymes are significantly increased in blood under certain diseased conditions, which is due to breakdown of the cells. Estimation of these enzymes in blood or plasma is useful in the diagnosis of various diseases. Alanine transaminase, aspartate transaminase, creatine kinase, LDH, lipase and gamma glutamyl transaminase are used as the diagnostic enzymes to diagnose the diseases.

SELF-ASSESSMENT QUESTIONS

1. What are enzymes?
2. What are extracellular and intracellular enzymes? Explain with examples.
3. Briefly discuss the factors affecting enzyme activity.
4. Classify enzymes with an example for each class.
5. What is inhibitor? Give three examples.
6. What are the antimetabolites? Mention any two importance of it.
7. Can competitive inhibition be reversed by increasing substrate concentration?
8. How do you explain the competitive type of inhibition? Mention some of the uses of competitive inhibitors in drug therapy.
9. How the noncompetitive inhibition differs from competitive type of inhibition?
10. What are proenzymes? Give an example.
11. How trypsinogen is converted to trypsin?
12. Briefly discuss the isoenzymes with some examples.
13. Mention the clinical importance of diagnostic enzymes.
14. Add a note on the specificity of enzymes.
15. Give the formula for Michaelis–Menten constant.
16. Give the normal serum value for LDH and alkaline phosphatase.
17. Mention the importance of G-6-P dehydrogenase and which pathway needs this enzyme?
18. How many isoenzyme forms of lactate dehydrogenase are possible?
19. Mention the five organs that release alkaline phosphatase.
20. Derive the Michaelis–Menten equation.
21. Give the clinical significance of GGT estimation.
22. Write the different forms of CK.
23. Which form of LDH increases in MI?
24. Which form of LDH moves fast on electrophoresis?
25. Give the cardiac enzyme panel.
26. What are proenzymes?
27. What are coenzymes? Explain with examples.
28. Briefly explain the mechanism of enzyme actions using different models.
29. What is enzyme inhibition and what are its types? Explain with specific examples.
30. What are allosteric enzymes? Explain with example.
31. What are isoenzymes? Briefly explain with examples.
32. What are diagnostic enzymes? List them with the clinical importance.

MULTIPLE-CHOICE QUESTIONS

1. Most of the enzymes of glycolysis are:
   a. Intracellular   b. Extracellular
   c. Intermediate   d. Neutral
2. All the following statements regarding the coenzymes are correct, *except*:
   a. Dialyzable and thermostable
   b. Organic substances
   c. NADH is the coenzyme for lactate dehydrogenase
   d. They do not bind to the enzyme
3. One of the following factors does not affect the enzyme activity:
   a. pH
   b. Temperature
   c. Isoenzyme concentration
   d. Substrate concentration
4. Amylase is a:
   a. Hydrolase class of enzyme
   b. Lyase class of enzyme
   c. Oxidoreductase class of enzyme
   d. Ligase class of enzyme
5. Optimum pH for alkaline phosphatase is:
   a. 5.0   b. 7.0
   c. 9.0   d. 2.0
6. The enzyme that inhibits xanthine oxidase is:
   a. Malonate
   b. Succinate
   c. Allopurinol
   d. Methotrexate
7. Aminopterin or amethopterin competitively inhibits:
   a. Folate reductase
   b. Glutathione reductase
   c. Lactate dehydrogenase
   d. Xanthine oxidase
8. The enzyme that elevates in prostate cancer is:
   a. Alkaline phosphatase
   b. Acid phosphatase
   c. Lactate dehydrogenase
   d. Amylase

9. The isoenzyme form of lactate dehydrogenase increases in skeletal muscle disease is:
   a. LD5
   b. LD1
   c. LD3
   d. LD4
10. Following myocardial infarction, the first enzyme to increase is:
   a. CKMB
   b. LDH
   c. AST
   d. None of the above
11. Concerning alkaline phosphates, one of the following statements is *incorrect*:
   a. It has more than five isoenzyme forms
   b. It is not present in placenta and kidney
   c. It elevates in bone disorder
   d. It elevates in obstructive jaundice
12. The enzyme that elevates in alcoholic cirrhosis is:
   a. GGT
   b. ACP
   c. CK
   d. LDH
13. Enzymes used to break down proteins in biological washing powders belong to the group:
   a. Lactases
   b. Lipases
   c. Proteases
   d. Hydrolases
14. Enzymes act as biological:
   a. Inhibitors
   b. Substrates
   c. Solvents
   d. Catalysts
15. Enzymes speed up biochemical reactions by:
   a. Increasing the activation energy of the reaction
   b. Lowering the activation energy of the reaction
   c. Increasing the temperature of the reaction
   d. Lowering the temperature of the reaction
16. The diagram shows a typical relationship between enzyme activity and:

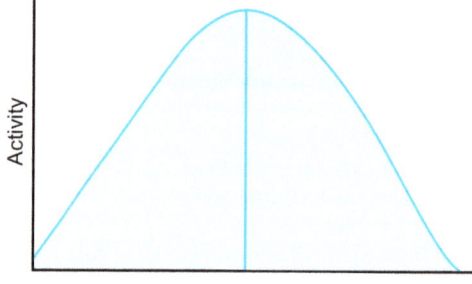

   a. pH
   b. Enzyme concentration
   c. Substrate concentration
   d. Temperature

17. Chemicals (other than the substrate) that affect enzyme activity are called:
   a. Exhibitors
   b. Activators
   c. Inhibitors
   d. Inactivators
18. Enzymes belong to which group of chemicals:
   a. Proteins
   b. Polysaccharides
   c. Lipids
   d. Phospholipids
19. The diagram shows a typical relationship between enzyme activity and:

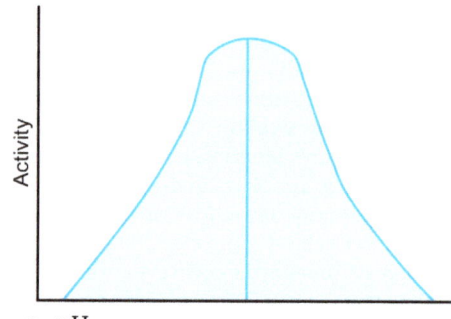

   a. pH
   b. Enzyme concentration
   c. Substrate concentration
   d. Temperature
20. Allosteric enzymes:
   a. Have a single subunit
   b. Obey Michaelis–Menten kinetics
   c. Have a catalytic and a regulatory site
   d. Have affinity toward inhibitors only
21. Concerning the allosteric enzymes, one of the following statements is *incorrect*:
   a. The inhibitor can bind to the enzyme at the same time as the enzyme's substrate
   b. Binding of inhibitor to allosteric site changes the enzyme conformation
   c. They contain many subunits and catalyze the committed step in a pathway
   d. They do not obey Michaelis–Menten kinetics
22. To confirm the Koshland mechanism, an enzyme must:
   a. Have more than one subunit
   b. Exhibit allosteric behavior
   c. Demonstrate negative cooperativity
   d. Have more than one binding site
23. All of the following about the MCW enzyme model are true, *except*:
   a. The enzyme exists in two states only
   b. The T-state has greater affinity for substrate
   c. In the absence of substrate, there is little R-state

d. This model cannot account for negative cooperativity

24. Concerning the cooperativity, all are true, *except*:
a. Positive cooperativity occurs when binding of the first substrate molecule increases the affinity of the other active sites for substrate
b. Phosphofructokinase shows negative cooperativity
c. Negative cooperativity makes enzymes insensitive to small changes in [S]
d. Hill equation is often used to describe the degree of cooperativity quantitatively in non-Michaelis-Menten kinetics

25. The disorder of a system is measured by its:
a. Activation energy   b. Heat of reaction
c. Entropy   d. Energy

26. The optimum pH of the most human enzymes is:
a. 2.0   b. 6.0
c. 8.0   d. 7.1

27. The "lock-and-key" model of enzyme action illustrates that a particular enzyme molecule:
a. Forms a permanent enzyme-substrate complex
b. Forms a denatured and renatured several time
c. Interacts with a specific type of substrate molecule
d. Reacts at identical rates under all conditions

28. An enzyme-substrate complex may result from the interaction of molecules of:
a. Fructose and lipase
b. Fat and amylase
c. Sucrose and maltase
d. Protein and protease

29. The place of the enzyme molecule into which the substrate fits is:
a. Active site
b. Coenzyme
c. Peptide
d. Key part

30. One of the following variables is least likely to affect an enzyme's rate of reaction is:
a. Temperature
b. Enzyme concentration
c. CO_2 concentration

d. Hydrogen bonds

31. Which of the following is characteristic of enzymes?
a. They lower the energy of activation of a reaction by binding the substrate
b. They raise the energy of activation of a reaction by binding the substrate
c. They lower the amount of energy present in the substrate
d. They raise the number of molecules moving quickly

32. An allosteric site on an enzyme is:
a. Similar to active site
b. Nonprotein in nature
c. Where ATP attaches and gives up its energy
d. Involved in feedback inhibition

33. In noncompetitive inhibition, the allosteric inhibitor:
a. Attaches to the active site, preventing the substrate from attaching there
b. Attaches to the substrate, preventing it from attaching to the active site
c. Changes the pH of the environment, thus preventing enzyme-substrate complex formation
d. Attaches to the enzyme at a site away from the active site, altering the shape of the enzyme

34. The minimum amount of energy needed for a process to occur is called the:
a. Minimal energy theory
b. Process energy
c. Kinetic energy
d. Activation energy

35. An inhibitor that changes the overall shape and chemistry of an enzyme is known as:
a. Allosteric inhibitor
b. Competitive inhibitor
c. Noncompetitive inhibitor
d. Active inhibitor

36. Inactive precursors of some enzymes that are activated through hydrolysis reactions are called:
a. Allosteric enzymes
b. Apoenzymes
c. Prosthetic groups
d. Zymogens

37. L-Amino acid dehydrogenase is an enzyme that can catalyze the oxidation of different L-amino acids. It cannot catalyze the oxidation of D-amino acids. Based on these

characteristics, this enzyme one can say that it shows:
   a. Allosteric regulation
   b. Absolute specificity over substrate
   c. Relative specificity over substrate
   d. Specific inhibition
38. These enzymes have different structures but the same catalytic function. Frequently they are oligomers made from different polypeptide chains. These enzymes are called:
   a. Isozymes
   b. Allosteric enzymes
   c. Proenzymes
   d. Zymogens
39. The models that explain that the active site is flexible and the catalytic group of the enzyme is brought into proper alignment by the substrate are called:
   a. Concerted model
   b. Induced-fit model
   c. Lock-and-key model
   d. Sigmoid model

Answers

1. a	2. d	3. c	4. a	5. c
6. c	7. a	8. b	9. a	10. a
11. c	12. a	13. c	14. d	15. b
16. d	17. c	18. a	19. a	20. c
21. d	22. c	23. d	24. b	25. d
26. c	27. c	28. d	29. a	30. c
31. a	32. d	33. d	34. d	35. c
36. d	37. b	38. a	39. b	

CHAPTER 4

Chemistry of Amino Acids and Proteins

OBJECTIVES

At the end of this chapter, the students should be able to:
- Understand the classification of amino acids on the basis of their properties and functions
- Know about the biologically important peptides
- Define and classify proteins on the basis of their properties
- Explain the different structural organization of proteins
- Define the process of denaturation, causes and properties of the denatured proteins.

INTRODUCTION

Proteins are a group of organic compounds of carbon, hydrogen, oxygen and nitrogen (sulfur and phosphorus may also be present). They are of prime importance to the living systems. All the biologically active proteins comprise nearly 22 different amino acids (α-L-amino acids), which are called building blocks of proteins.

α-Amino Acid

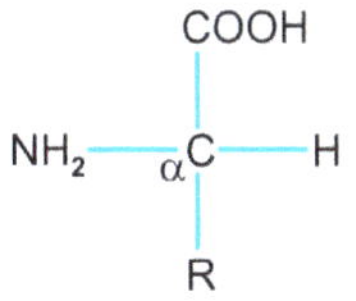

$$NH_2 - \underset{R}{\underset{|}{\overset{COOH}{\overset{|}{C_\alpha}}}} - H$$

L-amino acid

Definition of an α-amino Acid

Amino acids are organic compounds containing two functional groups: the basic NH_2 group (amino group) and the COOH group (carboxyl group).

The carbon atom attached with NH_2 and COOH group is called as α-carbon, where R- is the side chain of amino acid, which can be a hydrogen or an aliphatic, aromatic or heterocyclic group.

Following are the 20 different amino acids, which occur in the nature.

Name	Abbreviation	Symbol	Structural formula
Alanine	ala	A	$CH_3 - CH(NH_2) - COOH$ 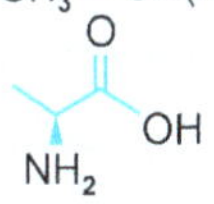 ![structure] $\underset{NH_2}{\overset{O}{\underset{\|}{C}}} - OH$
Arginine	arg	R	$HN=C(NH_2) - NH - (CH_2)_3 - CH(NH_2) - COOH$ 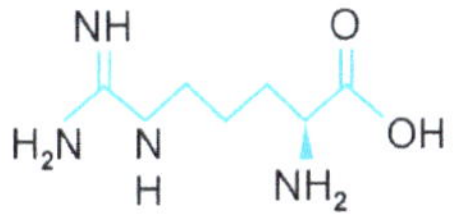 $\underset{H_2N}{\overset{NH}{\|}} \underset{H}{\overset{}{N}} \quad \underset{NH_2}{\overset{O}{\|}} OH$

Contd...

Contd...

Name	Abbreviation	Symbol	Structural formula
Asparagine	asn	N	$H_2N-CO-CH_2-CH(NH_2)-COOH$ 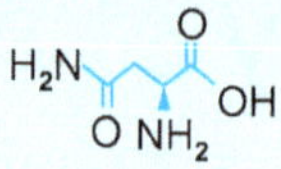
Aspartic acid	asp	D	$HOOC-CH_2-CH(NH_2)-COOH$ 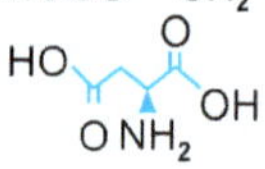
Cysteine	cys	C	$HS-CH_2-CH(NH_2)-COOH$ 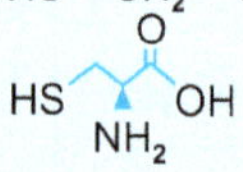
Glutamine	gln	Q	$H_2N-CO-(CH_2)_2-CH(NH_2)-COOH$ 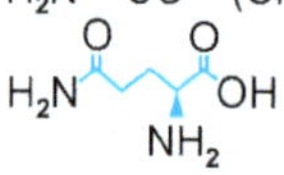
Glutamic acid	glu	E	$HOOC-(CH_2)_2-CH(NH_2)-COOH$ 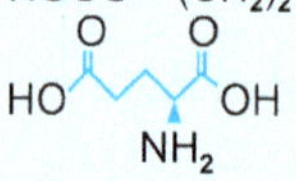
Glycine	gly	G	NH_2-CH_2-COOH 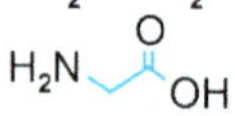
Histidine	his	H	$HNH-CH=N-CH=C-CH_2-CH(NH_2)-COOH$ 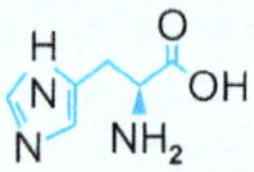
Isoleucine	ile	I	$CH_3-CH_2-CH(CH_3)-CH(NH_2)-COOH$ 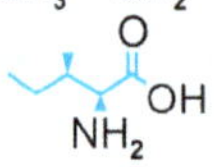
Leucine	leu	L	$(CH_3)_2-CH-CH_2-CH(NH_2)-COOH$ 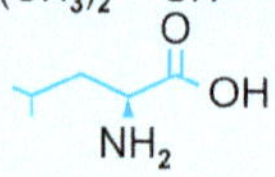
Lysine	lys	K	$H_2N-(CH_2)_4-CH(NH_2)-COOH$ 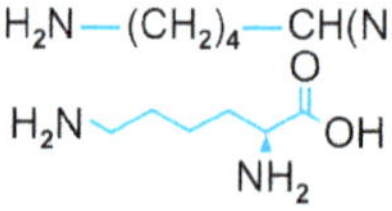
Methionine	met	M	$CH_3-S-(CH_2)_2-CH(NH_2)-COOH$ 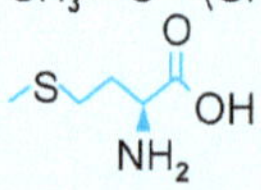

Contd...

Chemistry of Amino Acids and Proteins

Contd...

Name	Abbreviation	Symbol	Structural formula
Phenylalanine	phe	F	$Ph-CH_2-CH(NH_2)-COOH$
Proline	pro	P	$NH-(CH_2)_3-CH-COOH$
Serine	ser	S	$HO-CH_2-CH(NH_2)-COOH$
Threonine	thr	T	$CH_3-CH(OH)-CH(NH_2)-COOH$
Tryptophan	trp	W	$Ph-NH-CH=C-CH_2-CH(NH_2)-COOH$
Tyrosine	tyr	Y	$HO-Ph-CH_2-CH(NH_2)-COOH$
Valine	val	V	$(CH_3)_2-CH-CH(NH_2)-COOH$

Classification of Amino Acids

Amino acids are mainly classified into three groups depending on their reaction in solution as neutral, acidic and basic (**Fig. 4.1**).

They are also classified on the basis of charge they carry, as well as on their essentiality in the diet. Those that carry a net negative charge at pH 6.0 are called as acidic amino acid and those that carry a net positive charge are called as basic amino acid. Neutral amino acids carry no net charge at pH 6.0.

According to their chemical structure, they are also classified as aliphatic, aromatic and heterocyclic amino acids.

ESSENTIAL AND NONESSENTIAL AMINO ACIDS

Nutritionally, amino acids are classified as essential and nonessential amino acids.

Of the 20 amino acids, our body has the ability to synthesize 10 of them even if they are absent in our dietary proteins. Hence, they

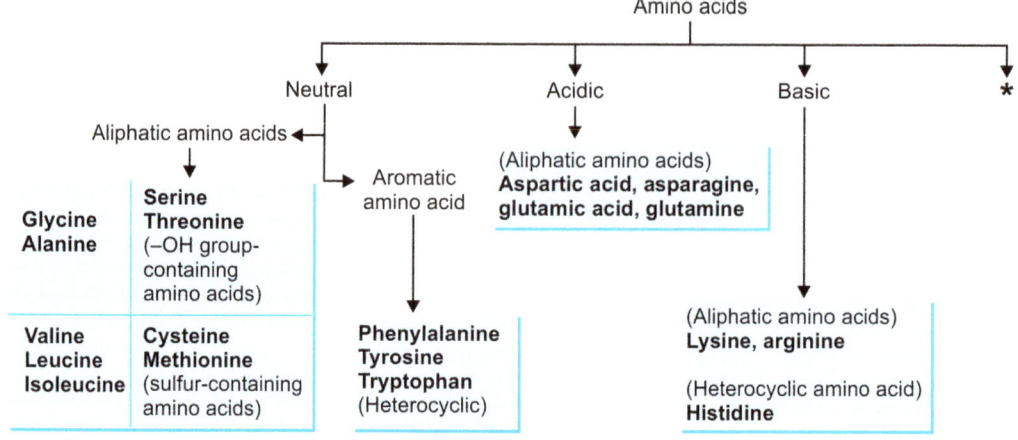

Fig. 4.1: Classification of amino acids.

are known as nonessential amino acids. They are glycine, alanine, serine, cysteine, cystine, glutamine, glutamic acid, aspartic acid and asparagine.

However, our body cannot synthesize the remaining 10 amino acids and should be supplied through diet. Hence, they are called as essential amino acids.

Essential Amino Acids

Essential amino acids are as follows:
- Methionine
- Valine
- Phenylalanine
- Arginine
- Isoleucine
- Histidine
- Threonine
- Leucine
- Lysine
- Tryptophan

The code word to remember them is *MATTVILPHLy*.

GLUCOGENIC AND KETOGENIC AMINO ACIDS

After the removal of amino group of amino acid, if the carbon skeleton of amino acid can be converted into glucose in the body, such amino acids are called as glucogenic amino acids.

Similarly, if the carbon skeleton of amino acid is converted into ketone body (acetoacetic acid), such amino acids are called as ketogenic amino acids.

If one part of the carbon skeleton is converted into glucose and other part is converted into ketone body, such amino acids are termed as both glucogenic and ketogenic amino acids **(Table 4.1)**.

Chemical Properties of Amino Acids

The chemical properties of amino acids are due to their carboxyl group, amino group and side chain R. All amino acids contain amino and carboxyl groups and undergo chemical reactions, which are characteristic for these groups.

NINHYDRIN REACTION

It is used to detect and quantify the amount of amino acid. When amino acids are heated with ninhydrin, the free α-amino groups react and give a purple-colored product.

Ninhydrin + α-amino acid $\rightarrow$ Purple pigment

Proline has imino group as α-amino group that gives yellow product.

This ninhydrin reaction is used for quantifying amino acids by colorimetric method and to stain chromatographic plates. Fluorescamine reacts rapidly with amino acids, yielding highly fluorescent derivative that permits the detection of amino acid.

Table 4.1: Glucogenic and ketogenic amino acids.

Glucogenic AA		Ketogenic AA	Glucogenic and ketogenic AA	
Glycine	Methionine	Leucine	Lysine	Phenylalanine
Alanine	Aspartic acid		Isoleucine	Tyrosine
Serine	Glutamic acid			Tryptophan
Threonine	Asparagine			
Valine	Glutamine			
Cysteine, cystine	Histidine			
Proline	Arginine			

Dansyl chloride and 1-fluoro 2-4 dinitro-benzene (Sanger's reagent) give stable derivative. These derivatives absorb light and facilitate the detection and quantification of amino acid.

1-Fluoro 2-4 dinitro-benzene + amino acid → 2, 4-dinitrophenyl amino acid.

PEPTIDES AND PEPTIDE BOND

The proteins have many amino acids, and these are joined by peptide bonds (**Fig. 4.2**).

The dipeptide formation from two amino acids occurs with a loss of a water molecule.

If amino acid 1 is glycine and 2 is alanine, then the dipeptide formed is glycylalanine. If the amino acids are interchanged, then the resulting peptide is alanylglycine. Always the amino group of the first amino acid in the peptide is free and the carboxyl group of the last amino acid is also free. The amino terminal of the peptide is always written on the left side and the carboxyl terminal will be on the right side.

Naturally Occurring Peptides

1. *Dipeptide*: It is made up of two amino acids.

   For example,
   A. Carnosine
   B. Anserine.

   The two amino acids are β-alanine and histidine. Anserine is the derivative of carnosine. Both these peptides are found in muscle.

2. *Tripeptide*: It is made up of three amino acids.

   For example,
   Glutathione (abbreviated as GSH). The three amino acids present are glutamic acid, cysteine and glycine. It contains –SH group (sulfhydryl group) from amino acid cysteine as an active group. The oxidized form of GSH is represented as GS-SG.
   - Glutathione presents in RBC in the large amount.
   - It plays a major role in the oxidation–reduction reaction.
   - It protects the SH group of various other proteins.
   - It decomposes H_2O_2 and maintains the integrity of the cells and keeps hemoglobin in reduced state (Fe^{2+} form) when it is oxidized to Fe^{3+} form.

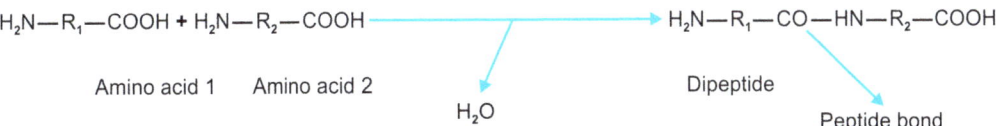

Fig. 4.2: Peptide bond formation between amino acids.

Glu—Cys—Gly (with SH on Cys)
Glutathione

Thyrotropin-releasing hormone *(TRH)*: secreted from hypothalamus.

3. *Pentapeptide*: It is made up of five amino acids, e.g. enkephalins. They influence transmission in some parts of the brain.
4. *Nonapeptide*: It is made up of nine amino acids. Oxytocin and vasopressin (ADH—antidiuretic hormone) secreted by posterior pituitary gland are the best examples for nonapeptides.
5. *Polypeptide*: They are made up of large number of amino acids, e.g. hemoglobin, myoglobin and insulin. Hemoglobin (made up of four polypeptide chains); each polypeptide chain contains several amino acids.

The insulin is the hormone secreted from cells of pancreas. It is made up of 51 amino acids. Insulin contains two polypeptide chains joined by disulfide bridge.

Charge Properties of Amino Acids and Proteins

Each amino acid has at least two ionizable groups:

$-NH_2$ and the COOH group (in addition, charged groups present in the side group of amino acid if present).

In acidic medium, the $-NH_2$ group behaves as a base and accepts a proton and becomes positively charged (cationic form).

In basic medium, the –COOH group acts as a proton donor and the amino acid becomes negatively charged (anionic form).

This property in which amino acids act as acid and base is known as amphoteric nature of amino acids.

At specific pH, the amino acids carry both the charges in equal number and thus exist as dipolar ion or zwitterions. At this point, the net charge on the amino acid is zero. The number of positive charge is equal to the number of negative charges at this condition.

The pH at which the amino acid or protein exists in zwitterionic form is called as isoelectric pH or pI.

$^+H_3N-\underset{R}{\overset{COOH}{C}}-H$ $^+H_3N-\underset{R}{\overset{COO^-}{C}}-H$ $H_2N-\underset{R}{\overset{COO^-}{C}}-H$

Cation form at acidic pH   Zwitterion form at isoelectric pH   Anionic form at basic pH

Proteins are made up of amino acids, and hence they also exhibit charged properties similar to amino acids.

For example, the isoelectric pH of:
- Albumin is 4.7
- Hemoglobin is 6.7
- Casein is 4.6.

Proteins do not move under electrical field at their isoelectric pH (pI). Hence, for the electrophoretic separation, selection of pH of the medium should be different from the pI.

Proteins tend to aggregate and precipitate at their isoelectric pH. As a result, they exhibit least solubility.

CLASSIFICATION OF PROTEINS

There are several classifications of proteins:

1. Based on solubility: Different proteins of different soluble property are listed in **Table 4.2**.
2. Based on composition: They are classified into simple, conjugated and derived proteins.
   - Simple proteins: Proteins made up of only amino acids are simple proteins, for example, serum albumin, keratin and lactalbumin.

Table 4.2: Proteins of different soluble property.

Class	Soluble in	Example
Albumins	Water	Serum albumin, egg albumin
Globulins	Dilute salt solutions	Serum globulins
Histones	Dilute acids	Nucleoproteins, histones
Basic proteins		
Scleroproteins	Insoluble in H_2O	Collagen, elastin

Chemistry of Amino Acids and Proteins

Table 4.3: Different conjugated proteins.

Example for conjugated proteins	Nonprotein part + protein
1. Hemoglobin (Hb)	Heme + globin
2. Nucleoprotein	DNA + histone
3. Lipoprotein	Lipids + apolipoprotein
4. Phosphoprotein (casein)	Phosphate + protein
5. Glycoprotein (egg albumin)	Carbohydrate + protein
6. Rhodopsin	11-cis retinal + opsin (protein)
7. Ferritin	Iron + apoferritin

- Conjugated proteins: Proteins containing amino acid and an additional nonprotein part are called as conjugated proteins. Nonprotein part is called as prosthetic part. **Table 4.3** gives the examples of conjugated proteins and their composition.
- Derived proteins: These are the proteins that are formed by partial hydrolysis of high molecular weight proteins. Peptone and gelatin are the examples. Gelatin is formed from native protein collagen.

3. Based on the shape (conformation):
   - Globular proteins: These are spherical in shape, e.g. hemoglobin and albumin.
   - Fibrous proteins: They are long and fiber like, e.g. keratin, myosin and collagen.

IMPORTANT FUNCTIONS OF PROTEINS

Biological Role of Proteins

General Functions of Proteins

The functions of proteins are as follows:
1. Proteins play a central role in cell functions and cell structure. It constitutes 17% of body weight **(Table 4.4)**.
2. Proteins form an essential part of the particular structure in the body. Membrane, muscle, connective tissues and organs are the examples.

Table 4.4: Biological importance of proteins with example.

Biological role	Proteins	Function
1. Structural proteins	Collagen, keratins	Bone and hair, respectively
2. Enzymes	Pepsin, amylase	Help in digestion of food
3. Hormones	Insulin, prolactin	Regulate the metabolism
4. Transport proteins	Hemoglobin (Hb)	Transport of oxygen
5. Protein receptor	Hormone receptor	Insulin receptor on liver cell
6. Storage proteins	Ferritin	Storage form of iron in liver
7. Immune proteins	γ-Globulins	Act against antigens
8. Contractile proteins	Actin, myosin	Muscle contraction
9. Buffering proteins	Plasma protein and Hb	Maintain the pH of blood

3. Various proteins are enzymes in nature and catalyze biological reactions.
4. Several proteins act as hormones and thus regulate various metabolic processes of the body.
5. A number of proteins serve as a carrier for the transport of various substances.
6. Some proteins act as a receptor molecule for the transport of the compounds, across the cell membrane, such as a hormone receptor.
7. Various proteins bind to certain substances and store them in different tissues, acting as storage proteins.
8. Some proteins like γ-globulins act as antibodies and provide immunity.
9. Proteins function as buffers to maintain pH of the cell.

STRUCTURE OF PROTEINS

Proteins are made up of one or more polypeptide chains. Four levels of structural organization recognized in proteins:
A. Primary structure

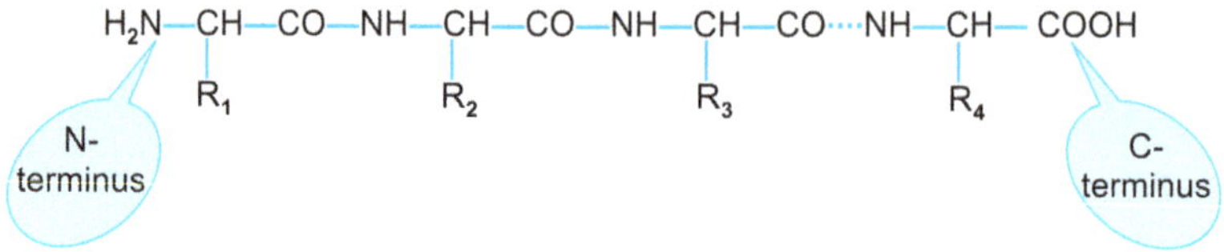

$H_2N-CH-CO-NH-CH-CO-NH-CH-CO\cdots NH-CH-COOH$
  R_1 R_2 R_3 R_4

N-terminus   C-terminus

Peptide structure: R_1, R_2, R_3 and R_4 are the side group of the amino acids

Fig. 4.3: Primary structure of protein.

B. Secondary structure
C. Tertiary structure
D. Quaternary structure.

Primary Structure

Primary structure of proteins refers to the order and sequence of α-L-amino acids in a polypeptide chain in which these different amino acids are linked through the peptide linkage. It has an N-terminus (amino terminal) and a C-terminus (carboxyl terminal) **(Fig. 4.3)**.

Secondary Structure

Folding or twisting the large polypeptide molecule possessing primary structure obtains the secondary level of structure.

For the secondary level of protein structure, hydrogen bonds and disulfide linkages are involved.

Hydrogen bonds: Weak, low energy noncovalent bond sharing single H between two electronegative atoms such as O and N. These occur between polar side chains of amino acids.

Disulfide linkages: They occur between two cysteine residues. These are strong, high-energy covalent bonds. Cystine contains the disulfide (–S–S–) bridge formed by the oxidation of two cysteine molecules.

These forces cause indefinite number of configurations in the protein structure. Hydrogen bond in secondary structure may form one or all of the following structure:
1. α-helix (this is a coiling up like a slinky or spring).

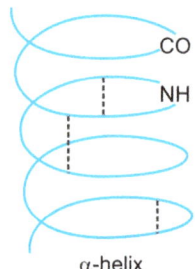

α-helix
Secondary structure of the protein

Fig. 4.4: α-Helix structure.

2. β-pleated sheets (this is a fan-shaped bending).
3. Random coils (this is when we cannot describe any real pattern to the folding).

α-helix: Hydrogen bonds may be formed between –CO and –NH groups within the same polypeptide chain (intrachain peptide linkage) resulting in its folding and forming a coil or helix **(Fig. 4.4)**.

The right-handed folding, of protein chain, results in the formation of α-helix. For example, α-helix of many globular proteins such as myoglobin and hemoglobin.

β-pleated sheets: They are formed by the formation of H bonds between –CO and –NH groups of different polypeptides (interchain peptide linkage).

Stretching, the helices of the polypeptide chains, result in β-pleated sheets **(Fig. 4.5)**.

For example, β-pleated sheets of ribonuclease and fibroin protein of silk.

Tertiary Structure

Refolding of the polypeptide chain possesses the secondary level of structure like:

Chemistry of Amino Acids and Proteins

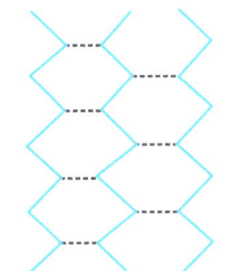

β-pleated sheets
Secondary structure of the protein

Fig. 4.5: β-Pleated sheet.

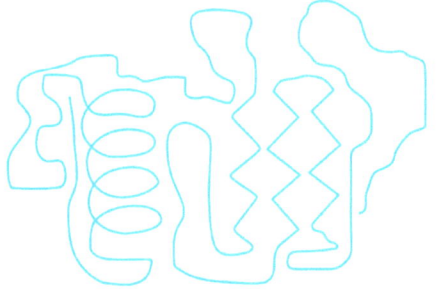

Fig. 4.6: Tertiary structure of protein.

α-helix, β-pleated sheets and random coils lead to the formation of tertiary structure **(Fig. 4.6)**.

The forces responsible for the interaction between different groups of amino acids are hydrogen bonds, hydrophobic interactions, ionic interactions and van der Waals forces.

Hydrogen bonds: It is formed between –CO and –NH groups of two different peptide bonds. It is also formed between –OH group of serine and –COOH groups of acidic amino acids.

Hydrophobic interactions: Hydrophobic interactions occur between nonpolar side chains of amino acids such as alanine and phenylalanine.

Ionic interactions: Ionic or electrostatic interactions occur between oppositely charged polar side groups of amino acids. They are lysine, arginine, histidine and acidic amino acids.

van der Waals forces: These forces occur between nonpolar side chains of amino acids.

Quaternary Structure

Some proteins contain more than one polypeptide chain. They are known as oligomeric (multisubunit) proteins. Each subunit possesses primary, secondary and tertiary level of structure as explained above.

When these subunits are held together by noncovalent interactions or by covalent crosslinks (–S–S– bridge), it is referred to as quaternary structure. Same weak bonds involved in the secondary and tertiary structure are also involved here. Disintegration of the quaternary structure leads to the loss of biologic activity of the proteins.

For example,

1. *Hemoglobin*: A tetramer having four polypeptide chains held together by noncovalent bonds. These polypeptide chains are called as α1, α2, β1 and β2 chains **(Fig. 4.7)**.
2. *Lactate dehydrogenase (LDH)*: It has four polypeptide chains.
3. *Creatine kinase (CK)*: It has two polypeptide chains.
4. *Immunoglobulin (Ig)*: They are also called as antibodies. They are made up of two heavy and two light chains.
5. Collagen is a fibrous protein containing three helical polypeptide chains bound

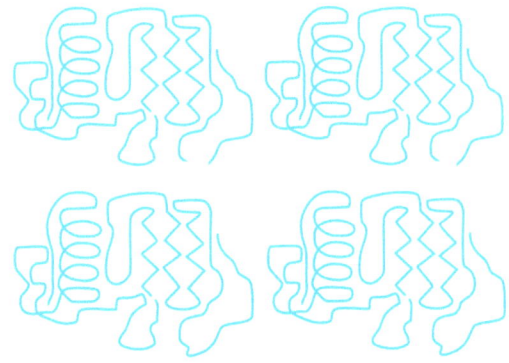

Fig. 4.7: Quaternary structure of hemoglobin.

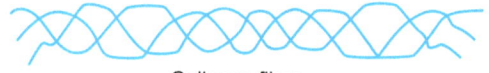

Collagen fiber
Triple helical structure of collagen

Fig. 4.8: Collagen.

together. Glycine, proline and lysine are the important amino acids present **(Fig. 4.8)**.

DENATURATION OF PROTEINS

The following lists the denaturation properties:
- Denaturation of proteins may be defined as a disruption of the secondary, tertiary and wherever applicable quaternary organization of protein molecule due to the cleavage of noncovalent bonds.
- Primary structure is not affected during this process.
- Peptide bonds are not broken.
- Various agents bring about denaturation of protein are as follows:
  - Physical agents: Heat, UV light, ultrasound, high pressure and even violent shaking can cause denaturation.
  - Chemical agents: Organic solvents, acids, alkalies, urea and various detergents cause protein denaturation.

Modification of Protein after Denaturation

Following are the changes that occur after denaturation of proteins:
1. Physical changes: Protein becomes more viscous and rate of diffusion decreases.
2. Chemical changes: Decreased solubility at pI and floccules may occur. Many chemical groups become inactive (e.g. –SH group).
3. Biological changes: Biologically enzymes and hormones become inactive.

PLASMA PROTEINS

The major six plasma proteins are as follows:
1. Albumin
2. α_1-Globulin
3. α_2-Globulin
4. β-Globulin
5. Fibrinogen
6. γ-Globulin.

They are separated using electrophoresis technique and also by precipitation methods. Fibrinogen is absent in serum.

Albumin

The name is derived from the white precipitate formed when egg is boiled (albus=white). It is present in high concentration that is about 60% of the total proteins is albumin. It has one polypeptide chain with about 585 amino acids and 17 disulfide bonds having a molecular weight of 69,000. Liver produces 12 g of albumin per day.

The decrease in serum albumin is called hypoalbuminemia. This is seen in cirrhosis, nephrotic syndrome and malnutrition. In cirrhosis, the synthesis of albumin decreases, and in nephrotic syndrome, the damaged nephrons lead to the excretion of more albumin in the urine.

Briefly Explain the Functions of Albumin

Plasma albumin performs the following functions:
- Osmotic function
- Transport function
- Nutritive function
- Buffering functions.

Osmotic function: Due to its high concentration and low molecular weight, albumin contributes to 80% of the total plasma osmotic pressure (25 mm Hg). It plays a major role in maintaining blood volume and body fluid distribution. Decrease in plasma albumin level results in a fall in the osmotic pressure. This leads to enhanced fluid retention in tissue spaces leading to edema. Edema is seen in conditions where albumin level in blood is below 2 g/dL.

Transport function: Albumin is necessary for the transport of many hydrophobic substances such as:

- Bilirubin
- Free fatty acids
- Drugs (such as sulfa drugs, aspirin, salicylates, phenytoin and dicumarol)
- Steroid hormones
- Thyroxin
- Calcium
- Copper
- Heavy metals.

Nutritive function: Albumin serves as a source of amino acids for tissue protein synthesis when it is broken down.

Buffering function: All proteins have buffering capacity. Since albumin is present in the high concentration in blood, it shows the maximum buffering capacity. The large number of histidine residues present in the albumin is responsible for the buffering action of albumin.

Globulins

The different types of globulins present in plasma are α_1, α_2, β_1, β_1 and γ-globulins. These proteins are glycoproteins with the molecular weight ranges from 90,000 to 130,000. The α and β-globulins also function as transport proteins, which transport hormones, vitamins, minerals and lipids, etc. The γ-globulins are known as Igs, and they provide mainly immunity against any infections.

Proteins belong to different globulins

α_1-Globulin

1. α_1-antitrypsin
2. α_1-acid glycoprotein
3. α_1-lipoproteins
4. Thyroxine-binding globulin (TBG).

α_1 Antitrypsin

- It is an acute-phase reactant (APR) and protease inhibitor present in the extracellular fluid throughout the body.
- The level of certain proteins in blood may increase up to 1,000 folds in several inflammatory and neoplastic conditions.

Such proteins are called as **acute-phase proteins** or **APRs**. It neutralizes the lysosomal elastase, which is released during phagocytosis of particles by polymorphonuclear leukocytes.

- Thus α_1-antitrypsin has a protective role in the body.
- α_1-antitrypsin level is increased during any infection or inflammation because of this protective role. Hence it is known as APR.
- α_1 antitrypsin inhibits activity of proteases particularly elastase, which degrades elastin.

Relationship of excessive cigarette smoking and emphysema?

Cigarette smoke inhibits the activity of α_1 antitrypsin by oxidizing a specific methionine residue of α_1 antitrypsin. Thus α_1 antitrypsin loses the capacity of inhibiting elastase activity.

Cigarette smoking increases the number of neutrophils in the lung and therefore increases the amount of elastase (elastase is released from neutrophils in lungs). Elastase then causes the tissue breakdown and loss of elasticity in the lungs, i.e. emphysema.

α_2-Globulins

Important proteins under this group are as follows:
1. α_2-macroglobulins
    - This has protective role in the body.
    - It is synthesized by hepatocytes.
    - It inactivates all the proteases; therefore, it is considered as *in vivo* anticoagulant.
2. Haptoglobins
    - The proteins that bind with hemoglobin and help in the breakdown of hemoglobin to bilirubin.
3. Ceruloplasmin
    - It is a copper-containing protein in the plasma.
    - It is known to have an antioxidant property.
    - It is an acute-phase reactive protein.
    - Its level is increased in the plasma in infections and malignant conditions, especially in Hodgkin's disease.

- Ceruloplasmin levels decreased in Wilson's disease, and it is used in the diagnosis of this disease.

Beta Globulins

C-reactive Protein (CRP) (β_2-Microglobulin)

The following lists the characteristics of C-reactive protein:
- It is an APR. It is released in response to acute injury, infection or other inflammatory stimuli.
- Recent development of a high sensitivity assay for CRP has enabled investigation of this marker of systemic inflammation.
- It consists of five identical nonglycosylated polypeptide subunits noncovalently linked to form a disk-shaped cyclic polymer.
- This consists little or no carbohydrate and migrates both on cellulose or agarose electrophoresis anywhere from γ to β region.

Clinical significance:
The clinical significance is as given below:
- Its level rises more than 6 hours after triggering stimulus.
- Peaks within 48 hours. Short half-life of 5–7 hours (rapidly declines after condition resolves).
- The plasma CRP level increases in inflammation and infections.
- The determination of CRP level is clinically useful:
    - For screening of organic disease
    - For assessing the activity of an inflammatory diseases such as rheumatoid arthritis
    - For detecting intercurrent infections in systemic lupus erythematosus, leukemia and after surgery
    - For managing neonatal septicemia and meningitis.

Reference range: 0–10 mg/L.

Fibrinogen

The fibrinogen is an acute-phase protein. It is an essential factor in blood coagulation.

Table 4.5: Concentration of various plasma proteins.

Plasma protein	g/dL	%
Total protein	6.5–8	100%
Albumin	3.5–5	60%
Globulins	1.8–3	40%
α_1		3%
α_2		11%
β		11%
γ		16%
Fibrinogen	0.2–0.4	

The conversion of fibrinogen to fibrin occurs by cleaving of Arg–Gly peptide bonds of fibrinogen. It is synthesized by the liver. The fibrin monomers aggregate and precipitate to form a clot.

Different types of plasma proteins and their concentration in the blood are shown in **Table 4.5**.

Separation of Plasma Proteins

Chemical and immunological methods are available that can quantify the concentration of a specific plasma protein with a high degree of specificity. Less commonly electrophoresis is used to provide a semiquantitative estimate of the pattern of serum proteins. Plasma proteins can be separated by different techniques, which mainly depend on certain properties of proteins:

i. Charged groups that are present in the protein.
ii. Molecular weight of the protein.
    Gel filtration: Columns that are packed with gel are used to separate the proteins. The proteins are separated depending on their molecular weight.
iii. *Precipitation of proteins by salts (salt fractionation)*: Albumin is soluble in water, whereas globulins are less soluble in water. All proteins are soluble in dilute salt solutions. As the concentration of the salt increases, proteins get precipitated

from their solution. For example, when ammonium sulfate is added to a solution of protein until it completely saturates, so the availability of water molecules for the protein is decreased causing the proteins to precipitate. This process is called salting out. Albumin is precipitated at full saturation with ammonium sulfate. Since albumin is having hydrophilic property, it requires higher concentration of salt to get precipitated. At full saturation, all the proteins are precipitated. Globulins are precipitated at half saturation with ammonium sulfate. Solutions of sodium sulfite (21-28%) are also used to precipitate globulins.

iv. *Precipitation by organic solvents*: Organic solvents such as methanol, ethanol and acetone are dehydrating agents that cause the precipitation of proteins. These solvents reduce the amount of water required to keep protein in solution; this results in precipitation. The protein may get denatured in this process. Hence, this process is usually carried out at 0°C.

Electrophoresis

Electrophoresis separates the proteins into five broad fractions—albumin, α_1 and α_2, β_1 and β_2 globulins **(Fig. 4.9)**. Each of the globulin fractions consists of a mixture of several proteins. Electrophoresis is the migration of the charged molecule in an electric field. Negatively charged particles (anions) move toward anode (positively charged electrode). Positively charged particles (cations) move toward cathode (negatively charged electrodes). Proteins in solution or plasma can be separated from one another by electrophoresis, because they are charged molecules. Proteins contain charges due to the presence of amino group (NH_3^+) and carboxyl group (COO^-). The presence of more number of negative charges depends on the number of COO^- group. If a protein has more NH_3^+ group, it will have more positive charges. At acidic pH, the proteins will have more positive charges so proteins will be positively charged and moves toward negative electrode in an electric field. At alkaline pH, the proteins have more negative charges. Hence the protein will be negatively charged and moves toward positive electrode in an electric field.

MULTIPLE MYELOMA

This is a malignant disease of the plasma cell.

In this case, one type of plasma cell multiplies abnormally and produces one type of Ig (IgG or IgA) in excess quantities.

The electrophoresis of such a serum shows a thick deeply stained protein band in the γ-globulin region. This band is called "M" band.

Biochemical Findings

The biochemical findings of multiple myeloma are increased total proteins, decreased albumin, increased globulins and Ca^{2+} levels in plasma. Some cases of multiple myeloma patients excrete light chains of Igs in the urine, which are known as Bence-Jones proteins.

Bence-Jones Proteins

The characteristics of Bence-Jones proteins are as follows:
- Bence-Jones proteins are light chain fragments of Igs, which are excreted in urine, in some cases of multiple myeloma.
- It was discovered in the urine by its characteristic behavior on heating.
- Bence-Jones proteins precipitate between 40°C and 60°C. But as the temperature increases above 60°C, the protein redissolves. Again on cooling, the protein gets precipitated.

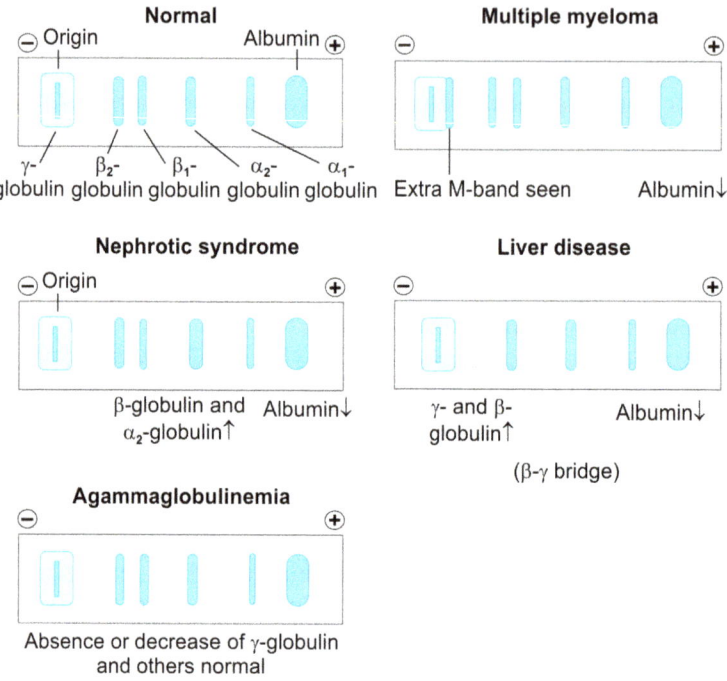

Fig. 4.9: Serum electrophoresis pattern of serum of normal and diseased conditions..

SUMMARY

Proteins are the group of organic compounds of carbon, hydrogen, oxygen and nitrogen. All the biologically active proteins comprise nearly 22 different amino acids, which are called building blocks of proteins. Amino acids contain two functional groups such as amino (NH_2) and carboxyl (COOH) groups. The carbon atom attached to $-NH_2$ and $-COOH$ group is called α-carbon and "R" is the side chain of amino acid, and it can be hydrogen or an aliphatic group and aromatic or heterocyclic group. Amino acids are classified mainly into three groups depending on their reaction in solution as neutral, acidic and basic amino acids. Nutritionally, amino acids are classified as essential and nonessential amino acids. Amino acids are of ketogenic (acetoacetic acid) and glucogenic (glucose from carbon skeleton). Amino acids joined by peptide bonds to form peptides (proteins). Proteins play a central role in cell functions and cell structure. Proteins are made up of one or more polypeptide chains. Four levels of structural organization of proteins can be recognized such as primary, secondary, tertiary and quaternary structure. Disruption of the secondary, tertiary and wherever applicable quaternary without affecting the primary organization of protein molecule is denaturation. Human plasma has albumins, globulins and fibrinogen. Albumin level falls below the range in cirrhosis of liver and nephrotic syndrome. Globulins are classified into $α_1$, $α_2$, $β_1$, $β_2$ and γ globulins. Globulin levels elevated in multiple myeloma, a plasma cell cancer. Plasma proteins can be separated by electrophoresis and which helps in the diagnosis of various diseases.

SELF-ASSESSMENT QUESTIONS

Long Questions

1. Classify proteins and give an example for each.
2. Classify amino acids and give an example for each.
3. What are essential and nonessential amino acids and list them?
4. What are glucogenic and ketogenic amino acids. List them.
5. Proteins are very important for humans. Justify this with few functions of it.
6. Explain the different levels of organization of protein structure.
7. What is denaturation of proteins? Give its consequences.
8. Name the proteins that belong to α_1-globulins and α_2-globulins.
9. What are essential and nonessential amino acids? Explain with examples.
10. What are glucogenic and ketogenic amino acids? Explain with examples.
11. Which reaction can be used to detect the amino acids with alpha-amino groups? Explain.
12. What are peptides? Explain with biologically important peptides as examples.
13. Classify proteins with examples.
14. What are the different structural organization of proteins? Explain with examples.
15. What is denaturation? List the denaturing agents and what changes will happen with structure of protein after denaturation.
16. What are the different types of plasma proteins? Explain with examples.

Short Questions

1. Which test is used as a general test for protein?
2. Which bond mainly stabilizes the primary structure of protein?
3. Give an example for a phosphoprotein.
4. Name the plasma protein that provides immunity to our body.
5. Mention the important functions of albumin.
6. How many polypeptide chains are present in the hemoglobin molecule?
7. Give an example for tertiary structure of a protein.
8. Name the sulfur-containing amino acids.
9. What is the isoelectric pH of casein?
10. Name the urine protein that helps in the diagnosis of multiple myeloma.
11. Give an example for acute-phase proteins.
12. State the causes of Wilson's disease.

MULTIPLE-CHOICE QUESTIONS

1. All the following statements are true regarding the amino acids, *except*:
   a. They contain an α-amino group and a carboxyl group
   b. Proteins are made up of α-L-amino acids
   c. They form peptide bond with each other to form a polypeptide
   d. They react in alkaline medium with copper to form violet color
2. Which of the following amino acids is an acidic amino acid?
   a. Arginine
   b. Aspartic acid
   c. Lysine
   d. Leucine
3. Which of the following amino acids is both neutral and aromatic in nature?
   a. Alanine   b. Histidine
   c. Phenylalanine   d. Proline
4. Which of the following amino acids is called essential amino acid?
   a. Glycine   b. Glutamine
   c. Phenylalanine   d. Proline
5. All the following statements are true regarding a peptide, *except*:
   a. A peptide is formed by bond between α-carboxyl group of an one amino acid and the amino group of the second amino acid
   b. Glutathione is an example of dipeptide
   c. Dipeptide reacts in biuret reaction
   d. Carboxy terminal of a peptide is written on the left side
6. Following are the properties of proteins at pI, *except*:
   a. Proteins will have the maximum solubility at pI
   b. Protein possesses equal number of positive and negative charges
   c. Proteins exist in zwitterionic form
   d. Below the isoelectric point, they possess net positive charge

7. Which one of the following proteins is *not* a conjugated protein?
   a. Egg albumin   b. Hemoglobin
   c. Serum albumin   d. Casein
8. Which of the following statements is *false* regarding the structure of a protein?
   a. Immunoglobulin (Ig) possesses quaternary structure
   b. Upon denaturation, the primary structure is broken
   c. Proteins lose their biological activity if their secondary, tertiary and quaternary structures are damaged
   d. Hydrogen bond is predominant force stabilizing the α-helix and β-pleated sheets
9. Which of the following proteins is absent in a normal person's serum:
   a. Albumin   b. γ-globulin
   c. Fibrinogen   d. γ2-globulin
10. Following are the examples of globular proteins, *except*:
    a. Hemoglobin   b. Collagen
    c. Albumin   d. Myoglobin
11. The tripeptide that plays an important role in oxidation–reduction reactions is:
    a. Glutathione   b. Oxytocin
    c. Carnosine   d. Vasopressin
12. Concerning amino acids, which one of the following statements about amino acids is false?
    a. They all have at least two ionizable groups
    b. Amino and carboxyl groups are attached to an α-carbon
    c. In an acidic medium, the amino group is positively charged
    d. In a basic medium, the amino acid exists in zwitterionic form
13. The carbon skeleton of the following amino acids can be converted to glucose as well as ketone bodies:
    i. Isoleucine   ii. Tryptophan
    iii. Lysine   iv. Leucine
    a. i only
    b. i and ii only
    c. i, ii and iii only
    d. iii and iv only
14. The conjugated protein with a quaternary structure is:
    a. Albumin   b. Insulin
    c. Hemoglobin   d. Myoglobin
15. An amino acid has pKa_1, pKa_2 and pKa_3 values of 2.0, 3.9 and 10 respectively. Which of the following symbols best represents this amino acid?
    a. K   b. M
    c. D   d. F
16. Which one of the following is *not* an essential amino acid?
    a. Valine   b. Phenylalanine
    c. Lysine   d. Glutamine
17. Which of the following bonds is *not* affected when a protein is denatured?
    a. Hydrogen bond   b. Ionic bond
    c. Disulfide bond d. Peptide bond
18. Which of the following is a basic amino acid?
    a. Lysine   b. Asparagine
    c. Glutamine   d. Alanine
19. A protein's ability to absorb ultraviolet radiation is based mainly on the presence of:
    a. Cysteine   b. Aspartic acid
    c. Tryptophan   d. Valine
20. All of the following proteins contain a quaternary structure, *except*:
    a. Ig
    b. Myoglobin
    c. Collagen
    d. Lactate dehydrogenase
21. Concerning pI of an amino acid, which one of the following statements is *false*?
    a. It is the pH at which the amino acid exists as a zwitterion.
    b. It is the same as the isoelectric pH of the amino acid.
    c. It is the pH at which the net charge on the amino acid is zero.
    d. It is the point at which amino acid has maximum solubility.
22. The alpha helix and beta sheet represent the following level of structural organization of a protein:
    a. Primary level
    b. Secondary level
    c. Tertiary level
    d. Quaternary level
23. All of the following amino acids are polar, *except*:
    a. Phenylalanine   b. Aspartic acid
    c. Tryptophan   d. Histidine

Chemistry of Amino Acids and Proteins

24. Which one of the following pairs contains only fibrous proteins?
    a. Collagen and myoglobin
    b. Albumin and keratin
    c. Hemoglobin and myosin
    d. Collagen and keratin
25. The Ig, which crosses placenta, is:
    a. IgG b. IgM
    c. IgE d. IgA
26. Concerning the structure of Ig, all of the following statements are true, *except*:
    a. Heavy chains are linked to carbohydrates
    b. Amino acid sequence of the variable regions is responsible for binding with antigen
    c. Light chains have four hypervariable regions
    d. Light chains are of two types
27. Myoglobin:
    a. Transports oxygen to the peripheral tissues
    b. Returns CO_2 to the lungs
    c. Has secondary structure similar to hemoglobin subunits
    d. Has four heme groups
28. Concerning myoglobin, which one of the following statements is *incorrect*?
    a. It is a monomeric protein of red muscle
    b. Stores and transports oxygen to the peripheral tissues
    c. Its secondary structure contains high proportion of α-helical structure.
    d. Its histidine residues are responsible for binding oxygen.
29. Concerning the binding of oxygen to hemoglobin, all of the following statements are true, *except*:
    a. Binding of first oxygen molecule results in the rupture of salt bridges between the carboxy-terminal residues
    b. T state of the hemoglobin increases the affinity for oxygen
    c. Changed structure of hemoglobin facilitates gain or loss of oxygen molecule by the heme
    d. It has cooperative interaction between binding sites
30. The binding of first oxygen molecule to deoxyhemoglobin:
    a. Shifts the heme molecule
    b. Creates the salt bridges between the carboxy-terminal residues of Hb
    c. Changes only the secondary structure of Hb
    d. Induces the transfer of Hb from the low-affinity T to R state
31. Concerning gaseous transport of hemoglobin, all of the following statements are true, *except*:
    a. It transports CO_2 from peripheral tissues to the lungs.
    b. It carries 80% of CO_2 as carbamates.
    c. It carries CO_2 also as bicarbonates.
    d. It also carries protons to the lungs.
32. Deoxyhemoglobin:
    a. Binds one proton for every two oxygen molecules released in lungs
    b. Binds one CO_2 for every two protons released in lungs
    c. Binds one proton for every two oxygen molecules released in peripheral tissues
    d. Binds two oxygen for one CO_2 released
33. 2,3-bisphosphoglycerate:
    a. Binds to oxygenated hemoglobin (R) and destabilizes it
    b. Binds weakly to fetal hemoglobin (HbF) than to adult hemoglobin (HbA)
    c. Synthesis is a spontaneous reaction
    d. Synthesis promoted by high PO_2
34. Concerning the oxygen dissociation curve of hemoglobin and myoglobin, which one of the following statements is *false*?

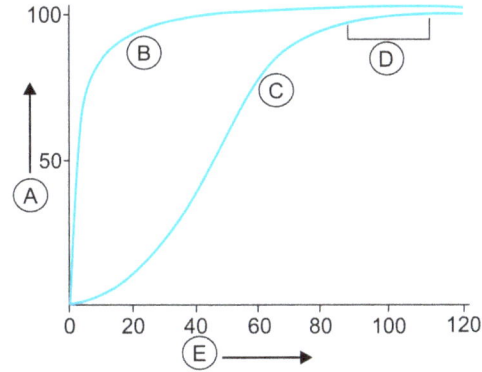

a. A represents percent of oxygen saturation
b. B represents myoglobin-oxygen dissociation curve
c. C represents hemoglobin-oxygen dissociation curve
d. D represents deoxygenated blood leaving the lungs

35. **Concerning fetal hemoglobin, all are true, *except*:**
    a. Compared to adult hemoglobin, it is less sensitive to 2,3-bisphoglycerate
    b. Its binding curve is to the right of myoglobin
    c. It consists of 2α and 2γ chains
    d. Compared to adult hemoglobin, the critical substitution involves replacement of histidine residues with tryptophan

36. **Concerning oxygen-binding proteins:**
    a. Increased pH shifts the oxygen-binding curve of hemoglobin to the right
    b. Increased 2,3-bisphosphoglycerate shifts the oxygen binding curve of myoglobin to the left
    c. CO_2 shifts the oxygen-binding curve of hemoglobin to the left
    d. Successive oxygen molecules bind with increasing affinity to myoglobin

37. **Hydrophobic interaction in protein is giving important stabilization contributions:**
    a. To protein's secondary and tertiary structure
    b. Just to the orientation of polar amino acids
    c. To the protein's primary structure
    d. After every possible hydrogen bond is formed

38. **Which amino acid is very important for optimal immune function?**
    a. Phenylalanine   b. Glutamine
    c. Isoleucine   d. Leucine

Answers

1. d	2. b	3. c	4. c	5. b
6. a	7. c	8. b	9. c	10. b
11. a	12. d	13. c	14. c	15. c
16. d	17. d	18. a	19. c	20. b
21. d	22. b	23. a	24. d	25. a
26. c	27. d	28. b	29. b	30. d
31. b	32. c	33. b	34. d	35. d
36. c	37. d	38. b		

CHAPTER 5

Metabolism of Amino Acids

OBJECTIVES

After reading this chapter, the learner should be able to:
- Explain the process of digestion and absorption of proteins through our gastrointestinal (GI) tract
- Understand the transamination, oxidative deamination and urea cycle
- Know the synthesis, catabolic products formed and inborn errors of different amino acids.

INTRODUCTION

Digestion is the breakdown of large polypeptide protein molecules into dipeptides and amino acids so that they can be absorbed into the blood. In certain organisms, these smaller substances are absorbed through the small intestine into the blood stream.

The proteolytic enzymes act on proteins to convert them finally into amino acids. The amino acids are absorbed by active transport into the intestinal epithelial tissue **(Fig. 5.1)**.

Amino acids undergo the process of catabolism to generate several products that are essential for the body.

DIGESTION AND ABSORPTION OF PROTEINS IN THE GASTROINTESTINAL TRACT

Digestion in the Stomach

The following list shows the process of digestion in the stomach:

- The protein does not undergo any digestion in the mouth. When it enters the stomach, it stimulates the secretion of the hormone gastrin from gastric mucosal cells.
- The gastrin stimulates the release of gastric juice-containing hydrochloric acid (HCl) and pepsinogen (rennin in infants).
- The HCl secreted by parietal cells unfolds the proteins and activates the proteolytic enzyme pepsin. This type of activation is called zymogen activation.
- Pepsin secreted by chief cells as pepsinogen and later converted to pepsin by HCl. Pepsin converts protein polypeptides into tripeptides, dipeptides and amino acids.
- Rennin in infants is also called chymosin or rennet.
- Rennin clots milk and then milk casein undergoes slight hydrolysis to produce paracasein, which coagulates in the presence of calcium ions, resulting in an insoluble calcium paracaseinate (curd). Then this calcium paracaseinate is acted upon by pepsin. This is required to convert milk into solid form, which prevents rapid passage of milk from the stomach.

Digestion in the Intestine

The following list shows the process of digestion in the intestine:
- When the acidic contents from the stomach pass into the small intestine, the low pH triggers the secretion of hormones such as **cholecystokinin** and **secretin**.

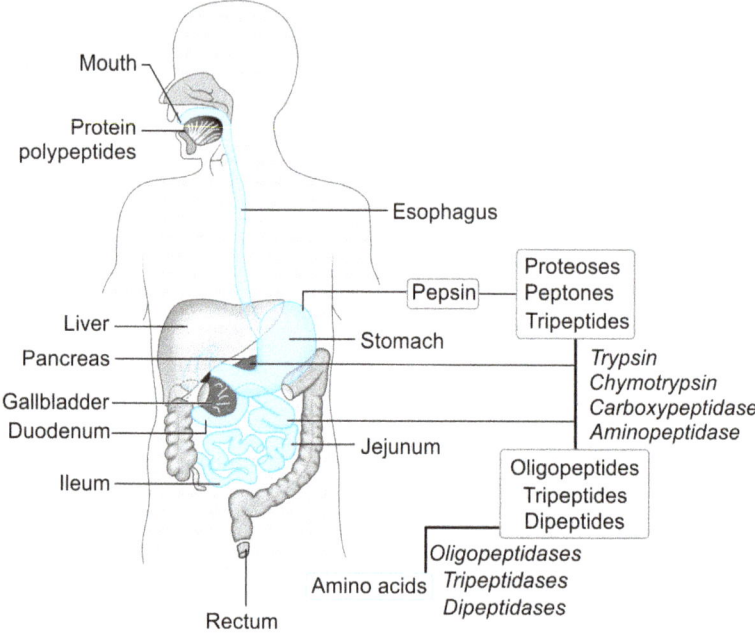

Fig. 5.1: Digestion of proteins.

- Secretin stimulates the release of bicarbonate and pancreatic juice from pancreas into the small intestine.
- Bicarbonate neutralized the contents from the stomach entered.
- Cholecystokinin stimulates the secretion of pancreatic endo- and exopeptidases.
- Endopeptidases cleave internal peptide bonds of proteins to convert into smaller peptides. The endopeptidases are trypsin, chymotrypsin, elastase and carboxypeptidase, which are secreted in the proenzyme forms and are converted to active forms by enteropeptidase or enterokinase is an exopeptidase.
- Trypsin hydrolyzes peptide bonds of proteins, whose carboxyl groups are contributed by lysine and arginine residues.
- Chymotrypsin cleaves peptide bonds involving carboxyl group of aromatic amino acids and peptide linkages of leucine, methionine, asparagine and histidine.
- Elastase hydrolyzes peptide bonds involving nonpolar amino acids such as alanine, serine and glycine.
- Carboxypeptidase removes amino acids from the carboxyterminal end.
- The oligopeptidase acts on the oligopeptides and converts them into tri- and dipeptides. The enzymes such as aminopeptidase, tripeptidase and dipeptidase finally convert these peptides into amino acids.

Absorption

The absorption of amino acids includes Na^+-dependent active transport mechanism, which requires adenosine triphosphate (ATP) as energy source. After the absorption, amino acids are utilized for the synthesis of protein and the remaining will go for catabolism **(Fig. 5.2)**.

Importance of amino acid in human body: Once the amino acids are released by the

Metabolism of Amino Acids

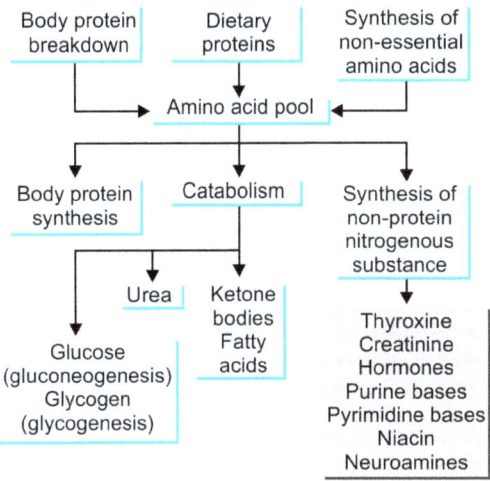

Fig. 5.2: Amino acid pool.

hydrolysis of dietary proteins, it forms an amino acid pool **(Fig. 5.2)**. Amino acids are used for the synthesis of proteins and nitrogen-containing substances.

Protein Degradation/Nitrogen Balance

The following list shows the process of protein degradation/nitrogen balance:
- Cells constantly turn over proteins
- It is a normal process, balanced by protein intake
- Proteins can be degraded if:
  - Damaged by free radicals
  - Oxidative damage
  - Misfolded
  - No longer needed.

Nitrogen Balance Expresses the Balance between Anabolism and Catabolism

Nitrogen balance is measured by assessing dietary nitrogen intake versus urinary nitrogen output (as urea).

Positive nitrogen balance: It is the net storage of nitrogenous compounds, which is seen during:

- Childhood growth
- Pregnancy
- Muscle building
- Healing.

Negative nitrogen balance: It is the net breakdown of stored nitrogenous compounds and excreted in urine, which is observed during:
- Illness
- Uterine resorption
- Starvation
- Amino acid deficiency
- Wounding.

METABOLISM OF AMINO ACIDS

Removal of Amino Groups

The **α-amino** group of amino acids is removed as ammonia (NH_3). The conversion of amino group to NH_3 takes place in several tissues, but liver is the major site of removal of NH_3 from amino acid. There are two major processes, which can remove the amino groups. These are transamination and deamination.

Transamination

Transamination is the process of transfer of α-amino group ($-NH_2$) of an amino acid to α-keto acid forming a new amino acid and ketoacid. Enzymes, which catalyze the reversible set of reaction, are called transaminases or aminotransferases, and they require pyridoxal phosphate (PLP), a coenzyme form of vitamin B_6.

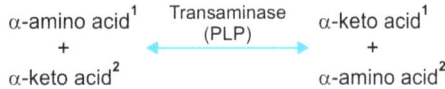

Liver contains two most important transaminases; they are serum glutamate pyruvate transaminase (SGPT) or alanine transaminase (ALT):

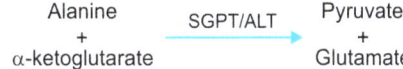

Serum glutamate oxaloacetate transaminase (SGOT) or aspartate transaminase (AST):

$$\text{Aspartate} + \alpha\text{-ketoglutarate} \xrightarrow{\text{SGOT/AST}} \text{Oxaloacetate} + \text{Glutamate}$$

Transamination is very important for the redistribution of amino groups and production of nonessential amino acids per requirement of the cell.

As shown, the amino acids undergo transamination to finally concentrate nitrogen in glutamate. Glutamate is the amino acid that undergoes oxidative deamination to a significant amount to generate free NH_3 for the urea production.

Diagnostic significance: The level of these enzymes increases in cardiac disorders (myocardial infarction) as well as in liver diseases.

Deamination

Since transamination involves only the transfer of a α-amino group from amino acid to α-keto acid and as such there is no net loss of the amino group, deamination is the actual process resulting in the removal of the α-amino group of an amino acid, which is released in the form of NH_3. Liver and kidney are the main organs involved in the deamination of an amino acid. There are two types of deamination reactions:
1. Oxidative deamination
2. Nonoxidative deamination.

Oxidative deamination
Oxidative deamination is the generation of free NH_3 from the amino group of amino acids coupled with oxidation. This mainly takes place in liver and kidney. The importance of oxidative deamination is to provide NH_3 for urea synthesis and α-keto acids for a variety of reactions.

L-amino acid oxidase, D-amino acid oxidase and glutamate dehydrogenase are the main enzymes involved in the deamination of amino acids. These enzymes remove electrons from the amino acids:

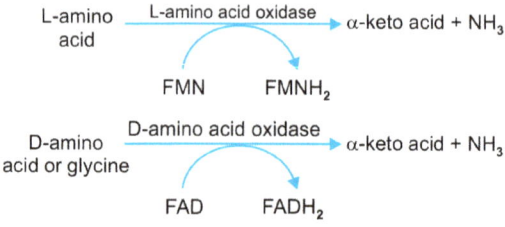

Nonoxidative deamination
Deamination of some of the amino acids such as serine, cysteine and histidine is catalyzed by dehydratases, desulfhydrases and histidase enzyme, respectively. Transdeamination using transaminase and glutamate dehydrogenase is as follows:

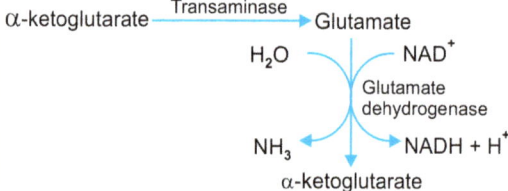

Metabolic Fate of NH_3

In human beings and primates, the NH_3 is converted to urea in the liver mainly through the urea cycle and it is excreted as such. Therefore, human beings and primates are called ureotelic.

UREA CYCLE (KREBS–HENSELEIT CYCLE)

The process where the highly toxic substance NH_3 is converted to a less toxic excretory waste product urea (NH_2-CO-NH_2) in liver **(Fig. 5.3)**. Human beings are known as ureotelic, whereas birds are uricotelic (excrete uric acid):
- In the first step, ATP activates NH_3, and it combines with CO_2 to form carbamoyl phosphate. This reaction is catalyzed by carbamoyl phosphate synthetase I enzyme, which requires *N*-acetyl glutamate as an activator.

Metabolism of Amino Acids

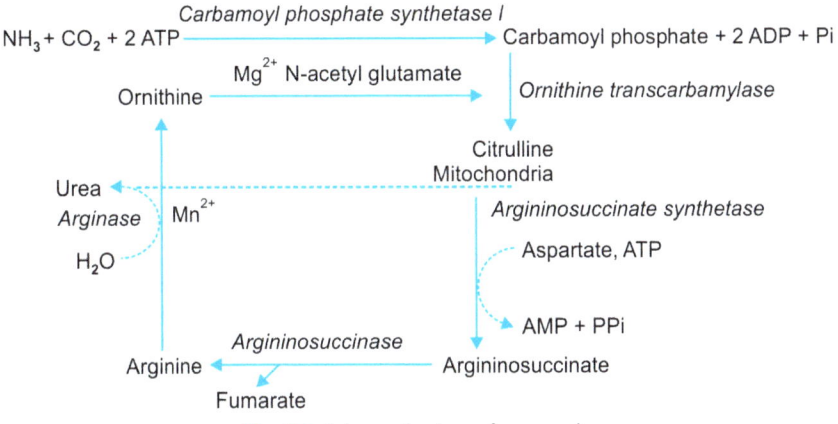

Fig. 5.3: Schematic view of urea cycle.

- Ornithine transcarbamylase transfers carbamyl group from carbamoyl phosphate to ornithine and produces citrulline.

  These first two reactions occur in the mitochondria.

  Other reactions proceed in cytosol:
- Citrulline combines with L-aspartate in the presence of argininosuccinate synthetase enzyme and ATP to form argininosuccinic acid.
- Argininosuccinic acid is hydrolyzed by argininosuccinase to form arginine and fumaric acid.
- In the last step, arginine is hydrolyzed by arginase to form ornithine and urea. Ornithine again enters the urea cycle.

Inborn Errors of Urea Cycle

The decreased or absence of urea cycle enzymes results in urea cycle disorder (**Table 5.1**), and this turn leads to many clinical symptoms such as vomiting, lethargy, irritability, rejection of high-protein diet and mental retardation.

Case
A newborn becomes lethargic and drowsy 48 hours after birth. The doctor requested blood investigations and the results showed the elevated level of NH_3 and urinary orotic acid (orotic aciduria). This baby has deficiency of an enzyme that leads to an inability to directly produce:
a. Ornithine
b. Citrulline
c. Arginine
d. Argininosuccinate

Answer is B. This is a disorder of pyrimidine biosynthesis pathway. There is no direct link between urea cycle and pyrimidine biosynthesis, but the channeling of metabolites of urea cycle to pyrimidine biosynthetic pathway can occur due to block at the level of ornithine transcarbamoylase (enzyme helps in the condensation of transcarbamoylase with ornithine to form ornithine).

Table 5.1: Inborn errors of urea cycle.

Defective enzyme	Disorder
Carbamoyl phosphate synthetase I	Hyperammonemia type I
Ornithine transcarbamylase	Hyperammonemia type II
Argininosuccinic acid synthetase	Citrullinemia
Argininosuccinase	Argininosuccinic aciduria
Arginase	Hyperargininemia

What are the Signs and Symptoms of NH₃ Intoxication?

NH₃ Intoxication

Increased blood NH$_3$ level may be genetic or acquired. Any impairment in urea synthesis due to a defect in the enzymes of urea cycle leads to disorders, and all these disorders result in hyperammonemia, which causes mental retardation. Accumulated NH$_3$ results in the following symptoms:
- Impaired brain function
- Ataxia
- Convulsions
- Lethargy
- Nausea
- Vomiting
- Slurred speech
- Blurred vision.

Why is NH₃ Toxic?

Glutamate level is disturbed, and since it is a neurotransmitter, its levels may be critical to proper neural function. Glutamate is recycled from postsynaptic neuron to presynaptic neuron as glutamine and that step is probably disturbed by high-NH$_3$ levels.

Glutamate is also the precursor of another neurotransmitter, gamma-aminobutyric acid (GABA), which thus may be affected by hyperammonemia. Alterations in glutamate levels may influence energetics. Moreover, removing NH$_3$ uses ATP also with potentially detrimental effects on energetics.

Treatment: Low-protein diet and substitution of α-keto analogs for essential amino acids (carbon skeletons of essential amino acids are important and not their amino groups).

Other Fates of NH₃

1. Biosynthesis of nonessential amino acid: NH3 is used in the amination of α-keto acids derived from the carbohydrates:

$$\alpha\text{-ketoglutarate} + NH_3 \xrightarrow[\text{dehydrogenase}]{\text{Glutamate}} \text{L-glutamate}$$
$$NADH + H^+ \quad \quad NAD^+$$

2. Formation of glutamine: This is the main route for the disposal of NH$_3$ from brain. NH$_3$ is converted to glutamine by glutamine synthetase. Glutamine is an important form for the transport of NH$_3$ to kidney where glutaminase enzyme hydrolyses glutamine to glutamic acid and NH$_3$:

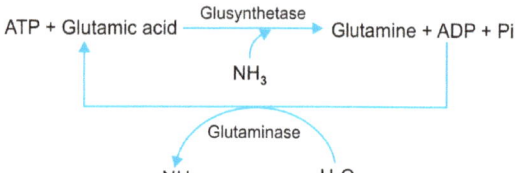

Urea and Its Clinical Significance
- Normal serum/plasma urea is:
  - 8.0–40 mg/dL
  - 2.49–7.47 mmol/L.
- Normal blood urea nitrogen (BUN) is: 7–21 mg/dL.
- Greater than normal levels may indicate:
  - Pre-renal causes:
    - Congestive heart failure
    - Myocardial infarction
    - Hypovolemia due to burns, shock or dehydration
    - Excessive protein catabolism
    - Gastrointestinal bleeding.
  - Renal causes:
    - Acute glomerulonephritis
    - Chronic nephritis
    - Pyelonephritis
    - Acute tubular necrosis.
  - Post-renal causes: Urinary tract obstruction to urine flow (stone, tumor and enlarged prostate).
- Lower than normal levels may indicate:
  - Liver failure
  - Low-protein diet
  - Malnutrition
  - Over hydration.

Urea is a non-protein nitrogen-containing substance. The molecular weight of urea is 60 and about half is contributed by the two nitrogen atoms. In some places, estimations of BUN are used instead of blood urea. BUN = ½ NPN (non-protein nitrogen).

METABOLISM OF IMPORTANT AMINO ACIDS

Catabolism of Carbon Skeleton of Amino Acids

After the removal of α-amino group as NH_3, the carbon skeletons of the amino acids form amphibolic intermediates, which are either converted into glucose or to fats and ketone bodies (Fig. 5.4):

- Transamination of alanine, glutamate and valine forms pyruvate, α-ketoglutarate and succinyl-CoA, respectively. These can be converted into glucose by gluconeogenesis. Such amino acids are called glucogenic amino acids.
- Catabolism of phenylalanine forms acetyl-CoA or acetoacetyl-CoA, which are the precursors of ketone bodies. Phenylalanine also forms fumaric acid, which is glucogenic. Hence, phenylalanine is grouped under both glucogenic and ketogenic amino acids (Table 5.2).

Table 5.2: Catabolic products of different amino acid.

Amino acids	End products
Glucogenic amino acids	
Glycine, alanine, serine, threonine, cysteine and hydroxyl-proline	Pyruvate
Glutamic acid, glutamine, proline, arginine and histidine	α-ketoglutarate
Valine and methionine	Succinyl-CoA
Both glucogenic and ketogenic amino acids	
Isoleucine	Succinyl-CoA + Acetyl-CoA
Phenylalanine and tyrosine	Fumarate + Acetoacetyl-CoA
Tryptophan	Pyruvate
Ketogenic amino acid	
Leucine and lysine	Acetyl-CoA + Acetoacetyl-CoA

- Leucine is the only amino acid whose end product of catabolism is acetoacetyl-CoA. Hence leucine is called ketogenic amino acid.

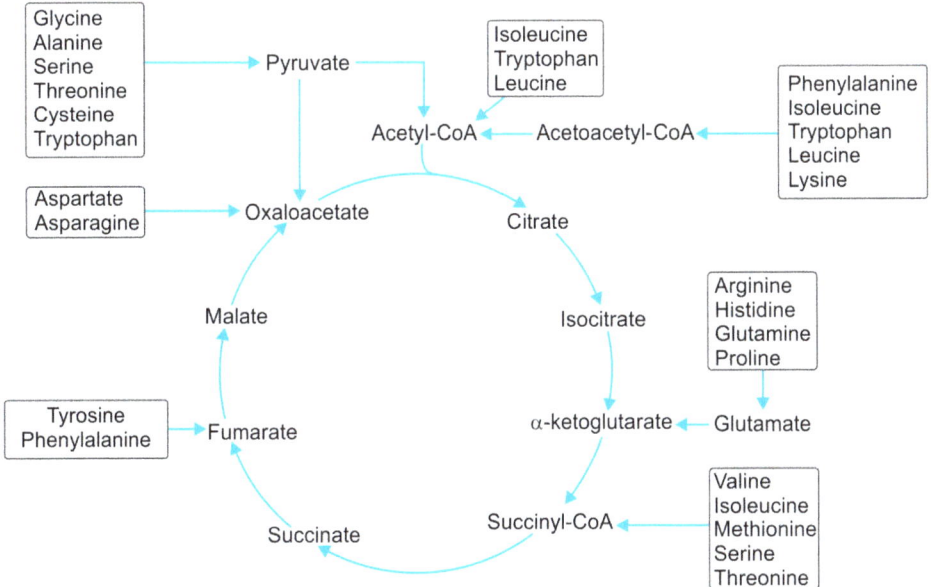

Fig. 5.4: Metabolic fates of carbon skeletons of amino acids.

Important Reactions Involved in Amino Acid Metabolism

There are some important reactions in the amino acid metabolism, which are responsible for generating many clinically important compounds. The reactions are as follows:
- Decarboxylation
- Transmethylation
- Transcarboxylation.

Decarboxylation

What are Biogenic Amines and List Them

The decarboxylation of amino acids or their derivatives results in the formation of amines:
- Amino acid decarboxylases (with PLP as the coenzyme) catalyze the removal of carboxyl group as CO_2 to form amines.
- Decarboxylases catalyze the formation of GABA and histamine from glutamate and histidine, respectively.
- Most of the biogenic amino acids are synthesized from basic amino acids through decarboxylation reactions.

Summary of Biogenic Amines
- Serine → Ethanolamine (forms choline)
- Glutamate → Gamma-aminobutyric acid → Inhibitory neurotransmitter
- Histidine → Histamine → Vasodilator promotes gastric HCl and pepsin synthesis
- Phenylalanine → Dopamine → Synthesis of norepinephrine and epinephrine
- Tyrosine → Tyramine → Vasoconstrictor
- Tryptophan → Tryptamine → Elevates blood pressure
- Tryptophan → Serotonin → Stimulates cerebral activity
- Tryptophan → Melatonin → Circadian rhythms
- Cysteine → Taurine → Taurocholic acid (constituent of bile acid).

Polyamines and their clinical significance
- Polyamines possess multiple amino groups.
- Putrescine, spermidine and spermine are the biologically important polyamines. These are derived from ornithine and methionine. These are positively charged at physiological pH and combine with negatively charged nuclear deoxyribonucleic acid (DNA). These are the constituents of semen.
- Polyamines have a role in transcription and translation.
- They act as a growth factor and help in proliferation and growth of cell.
- Ornithine and *S*-adenosylmethionine (SAM) are the precursors for polyamine synthesis.
- Putrescine is converted to spermidine and then spermine with the involvement of SAM.
- Degradation: Polyamine oxidase present in peroxisome oxidizes spermine to spermidine and spermidine to putrescine. This putrescine is then oxidized by a copper-containing diamine oxidase to CO_2 and NH_3. Major portions of putrescine and spermidine are excreted in urine after conjugation with acetyl-CoA as acetylated derivatives.

Clinical importance of polyamines:
- Polyamines are essential for the growth, maintenance and functioning of normal cells.
- Polyamines and their derivatives have application in diagnosis and treatment of cancer.
- Many researchers have shown the increased level in response to cell growth and differentiation.
- Putrescine and spermidine are found to be abnormally high in kidney, bladder and prostate cancer.
- Urinary and blood polyamines have been used to detect cancer and to determine the success of therapy.
- Ornithine decarboxylase, which catalyzes the rate-limiting step in polyamine synthesis, can serve as a marker of proliferation.

Metabolism of Amino Acids

Transmethylation

Transfer of methyl group to acceptor is termed as transmethylation. These reactions are responsible for generating methylated derivatives, such as choline, creatine, carnitine, epinephrine and melatonin. The active form of methionine and SAM, where the methyl group of methionine is available for transmethylation.

Transcarboxylation

Transcarboxylation is a transfer of carboxy groups through biotin.

ONE-CARBON METABOLISM WITH EXAMPLES

One-carbon Metabolism

Groups containing single carbon atoms are called one-carbon groups. One-carbon groups are formed from several amino acids during metabolic reactions. The amino acids such as serine, glycine, histidine and tryptophan generate one-carbon groups **(Fig. 5.5)**.
- Methyl (CH_3)
- Methylene (CH_2)

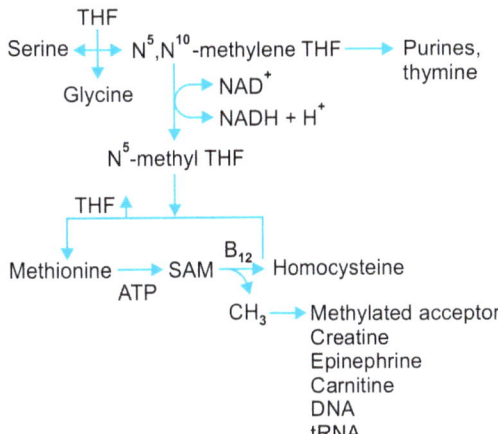

Glycine → Formate → N^{10}-formyl THF → Purines

Tryptophan → Formate → N^{10}-formyl THF → Purines

Glycine → Formate ⎤
Tryptophan → Formate ⎦ → N^{10}-formyl THF
↕
N^5,N^{10}-methylene THF
↓ THF
Purines, thymine

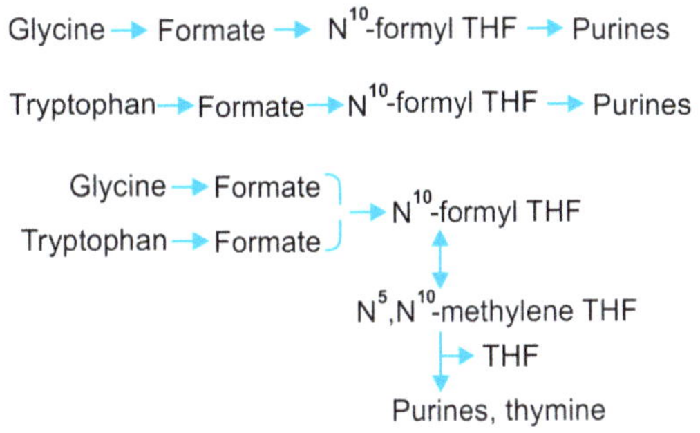

Fig. 5.6: Source of one-carbon group.

- Methenyl (CH)
- Formyl (CHO).

The above one-carbon groups are transferred by way of tetrahydrofolate (THF). The N5- and N10-nitrogen atoms participate in the transfer of one-carbon group **(Fig. 5.6)**. There are six one-carbon derivatives of THF such as:
1. N5-methyl THF
2. N5, N10-methylene THF
3. N5, N10-methenyl THF
4. N5-formyl THF
5. N10-formyl THF
6. N5-formimino THF.

The sources of one-carbon groups are serine, glycine, tryptophan, formaldehyde and formate.

METABOLISM OF GLYCINE INCLUDING THE PRODUCTS FORMED FROM IT

Metabolism of Glycine

- Simplest amino acid
- Nonessential in the diet.

Synthesis

The synthesis of glycine is shown below:

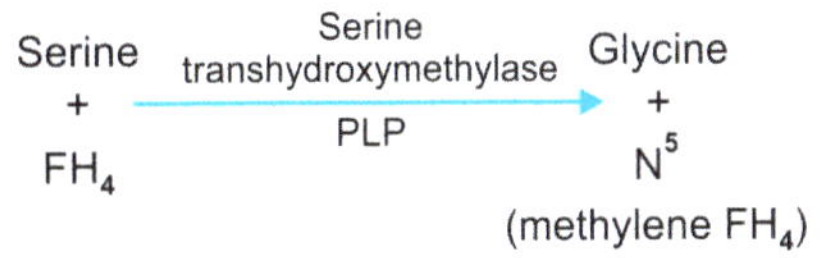

Serine + FH_4 →[Serine transhydroxymethylase / PLP]→ Glycine + N^5 (methylene FH_4)

Fig. 5.5: Schematic diagram showing one-carbon metabolism.
(SAM, S-adenosylmethionine; THF, tetrahydrofolate)

IMPORTANCE OF SPECIALIZED PRODUCTS FORMED FROM GLYCINE

Metabolic Fate of Glycine

Biologically important compounds synthesized from glycine are as follows (**Fig. 5.7**):

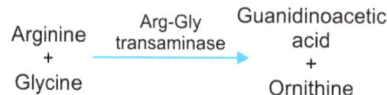

- C^4, C^5 and N^7 of purine base present in adenine guanine are contributed by glycine.
- Six glycine molecules combined with succinyl-CoA totally form heme group of the heme proteins (namely, hemoglobin).
- Bile acids (namely, cholic acid) get conjugated with glycine and form glycocholic acid.
- Glycine detoxifies benzoic acid in liver and forms hippuric acid.
- Creatine constitutes about 0.5% of total muscle weight. It is synthesized from three amino acids such as glycine, arginine and methionine.
- Creatine phosphate is the phosphorylated derivative of creatine found in muscle, which is a high-energy compound that can reversibly donate a phosphate group to ADP to form ATP. This can be used to maintain the intracellular level of ATP during the first few minutes of intense muscular contraction.

In kidney, the guanidinoacetic acid is methylated by SAM:

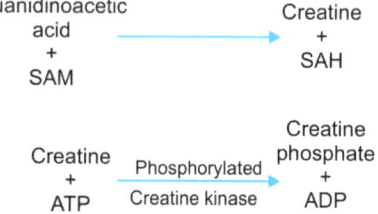

Metabolic Disorder

1. **Primary hyperoxaluria:** It is an inborn error characterized by high-urinary excretion of oxalate. This is an endogenous origin from glycine. Metabolic defect involves a failure to catabolize glyoxylate, which therefore gets oxidized to oxalate and results in urolithiasis, and nephrocalcinosis (presence of calcium deposits in kidneys).
2. **Glycinuria:** It is an inborn error characterized by increased excretion of glycine in urine.

Glutamic Acid

- Nonessential amino acid
- It is synthesized by action of glutamate dehydrogenase using α-ketoglutarate and NH_3.

Synthesis

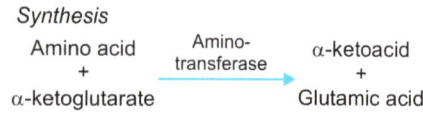

List the Compounds Formed From Glutamate

Metabolic Fate of Glutamate

Glutamine is formed by glutamate through the glutamine synthetase activity, which adds NH_4^+ to the carboxyl side chain. Glutamine is reconverted to glutamate by glutaminase. Glutamine is the major transport form of NH_3 (**Fig. 5.8**).

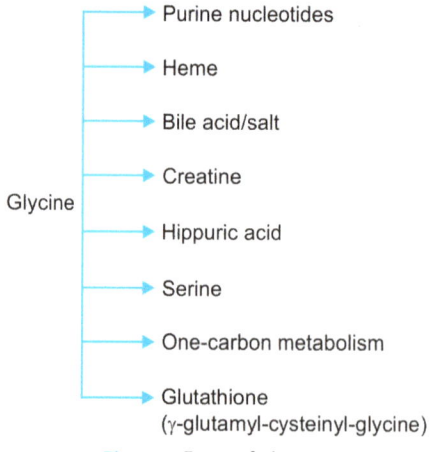

Fig. 5.7: Fates of glycine.

Metabolism of Amino Acids

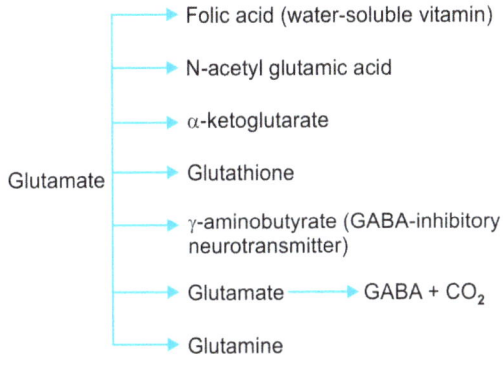

Fig. 5.8: Fates of glutamate.

Metabolism of Aspartic Acid and Asparagine

- Aspartic acid is synthesized from tricarboxylic acid (TCA) cycle intermediate by transamination process.
- It can be converted back to oxaloacetate.
- Asparagine is formed from aspartate.
- Asparaginase hydrolyzes the asparagine and releases NH_3, and aspartate.
- Certain types of tumor cells like leukemic cells require asparagine. Therefore, asparagine has been used as an antitumor agent.
- This acts on asparagine and converting asparagine to aspartate, decreasing the amount of asparagine available for tumor cell proliferation.

Glutamate and aspartate are important in collecting and eliminating amino nitrogen via glutamine synthetase and the urea cycle, respectively. The catabolic path of the carbon skeletons involves simple one-step aminotransferase reaction that directly produces net quantities of a TCA cycle intermediate. The glutamate dehydrogenase reaction operating in the direction of α-ketoglutarate production provides a second avenue leading from glutamate to gluconeogenesis.

Metabolism of Threonine

Threonine is an essential amino acid. There are at least three pathways for threonine catabolism that have been identified in yeasts, insects and vertebrates including mammals. The principal threonine catabolism pathway in humans involves glycine-independent serine/threonine dehydratase yielding α-ketobutyrate, which is further catabolized to propionyl-CoA and finally the TCA cycle intermediate, succinyl-CoA. Serine/threonine dehydratase is expressed at high levels only in the liver. It appears that in newborn infant's catabolism of threonine occurs exclusively via the action of the serine/threonine dehydratase. Therefore, it is presumed that this is the predominant threonine-catabolizing pathway in humans (**Fig. 5.9**).

Metabolism of Lysine

- It is an essential amino acid.
- Both are glucogenic and ketogenic, and it has two amino groups.
- Lysine generates acetyl-CoA as the end product of its catabolism.
- It is involved in the synthesis of carnitine, which is required to transfer acyl groups across mitochondrial membrane.
- There are two metabolic disorders of lysine metabolism:
  - Periodic hyperlysinemia
  - Persistent hyperlysinemia.

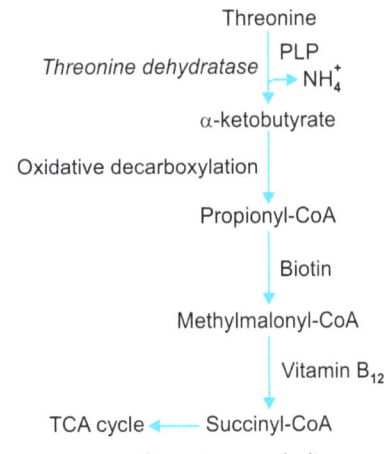

Fig. 5.9: Threonine metabolism.

Metabolism of Arginine

Arginine is a semi-essential amino acid and can be synthesized from glutamate, but it is not sufficient to meet the requirement of the body for growth **(Fig. 5.10)**.

Fates of Arginine

The fate of arginine is shown schematically in **Figure 5.11**.

Proline Metabolism

Synthesis

Synthesis of proline is illustrated in **Figure 5.12**.

Catabolism

Catabolism of proline is depicted in **Figure 5.13**.

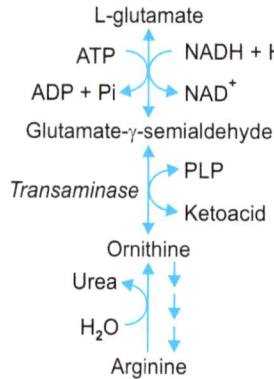

Fig. 5.10: Synthesis and catabolism of arginine.

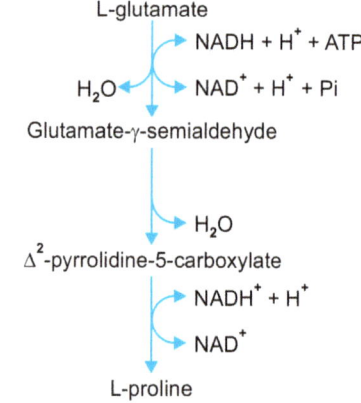

Fig. 5.12: Synthesis of proline.

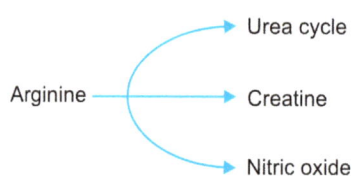

Fig. 5.11: Fates of arginine.

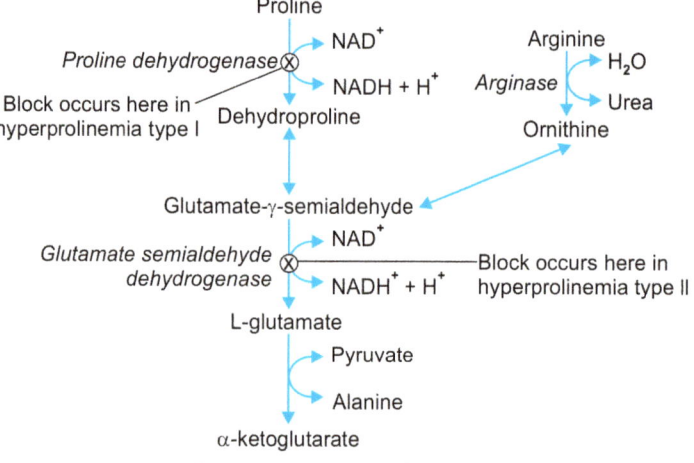

Fig. 5.13: Catabolism of proline.

METABOLISM OF PHENYLALANINE AND TYROSINE

Phenylalanine and tyrosine are not synthesized in human body (essential amino acids) **(Fig. 5.14)**.

Normal Condition

Proteins and tyrosine are formed from phenylalanine. Formation of tyrosine from phenylalanine requires phenylalanine hydroxylase enzyme.

Disorders

Defect in phenylalanine hydroxylase leads to phenylketonuria (PKU). Mental retardation and convulsions are the signs. The metabolites of phenylalanine such as phenylpyruvate, phenyl lactate and acetate are excreted in urine. The detection of these compounds helps in the diagnosis of PKU.

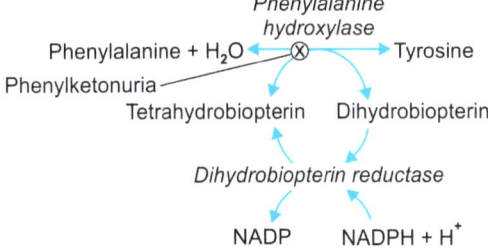

Fig. 5.14: Synthesis of tyrosine from phenylalanine.

METABOLISM OF TYROSINE

A newborn infant was diagnosed with PKU, and this was confirmed by the presence of phenylpyruvic acid, phenyl acetate and phenyllactate in the urine sample. Which of the following enzymes is absent in this infant?
a. Homogentisate oxidase
b. **Phenylalanine hydroxylase**
c. Fumarase
d. Ketoacyl dehydrogenase
Answer is B

What is PKU? Explain Briefly.

Phenylketonuria
- Phenylketonuria is an inborn error of phenylalanine metabolism associated with the defect in converting phenylalanine to tyrosine.
- Cause: This occurs due to deficiency of phenylalanine hydroxylase.
- Because of the block due to enzyme deficiency, the phenylalanine accumulates in the body.
- The accumulation leads to the high level of phenylalanine in blood.
- The accumulated phenylalanine is metabolized further by other route, which normally does not take place in the body.
- Transamination of phenylalanine produces phenylpyruvate.
- The phenylpyruvate gives phenyllactate and phenylacetate by reduction and oxidative decarboxylation reactions, respectively **(Fig. 5.15)**.
- The phenylacetate may conjugate with glutamine and excreted as phenylacetylglutamine.
- So finally urine contains phenyllactate, and phenylacetylglutamine along with phenylalanine.
- Symptoms are mental retardation, failure to talk, seizures, fair hair and blue eyes due to the deficiency of melanin pigment (hydroxylation of tyrosine by tyrosinase is inhibited by high levels of phenylalanine in PKU) **(Fig. 5.16)**.
- The PKU may be classified into three groups:
   a. Classic PKU: Due to defect in phenylalanine hydroxylase. This is most common error.
   b. Atypical PKU or hyperphenylalaninemia types II and III: Defect in dihydrobiopterin reductase.

c. Hyperphenylalaninemia types IV and V: Defect in dihydrobiopterin synthesis.
• Treatment: Low-phenylalanine diet.

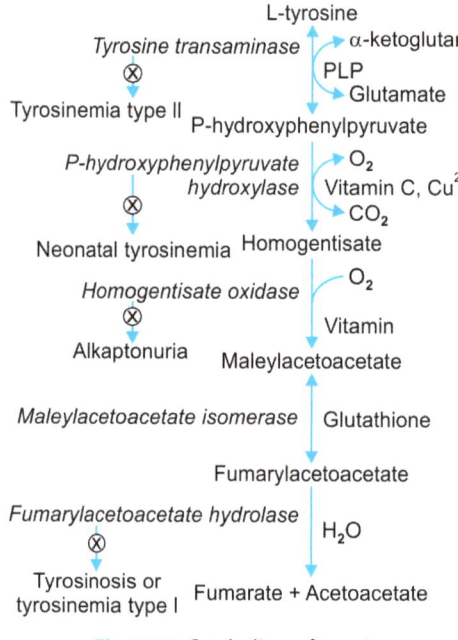

Fig. 5.15: Catabolism of tyrosine.

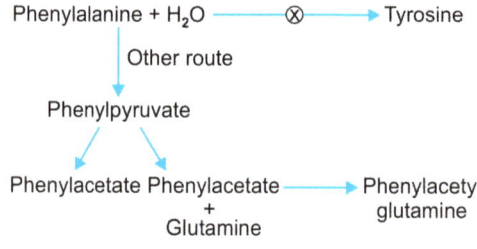

Fig. 5.16: Phenylalanine catabolism in PKU.

Case

A 40-year-old Mathew presented with complaints of severe back ache, pain in the hip joint, and inability to walk without support since last 2–3 years in orthopedic department. History revealed that patient noticed dark-colored pigmentation over face, eyes and hands since last 8–10 years. He had noticed that his urine used to turn dark on standing since childhood. There was no systemic complaint. On examination, bluish-black pigmentation was seen on the sclera bilaterally, between limbus and lateral canthus. Dark discoloration was observed over both palms, along thenar, hypothenar eminence, and sides of fingers along with pits with relative sparing of center. Nails and dorsum of hands were also showing bluish-colored discoloration mainly along the extensor tendons. Which of the following diagnosis is made?

A. A case of alkaptonuria
B. A case of PKU
C. A case of Maple syrup urine disease (MSUD)
D. A case of gouty arthritis

Answer is A. Alkaptonuria is due to deficiency of homogentisic acid oxidase in kidney and liver. This leads to accumulation of homogentisic acid, an immediate metabolite of phenylalanine and tyrosine metabolism. As homogentisic acid accumulates both intracellularly and extracellularly, it is oxidized to benzoquinone acetate, which polymerizes to form melanin-like polymer, resulting in deposition of polymer, a dark yellow pigment or "ochre" occurs in the cartilage and other connective tissue. One of the first symptoms of alkaptonuria is darkening of the urine upon standing (due to the oxidation and polymerization of homogentisic acid). Dark urine stains on the diaper are sometimes the first telltale sign of the disease in infants. Darkening of urine is the only feature suggestive of alkaptonuria in the pediatric age group in most patients.

SPECIALIZED PRODUCTS FORMED FROM TYROSINE

Metabolic Fates of Tyrosine

Metabolic fates of tyrosine is shown in **Figure 5.17**.

Metabolism of Amino Acids

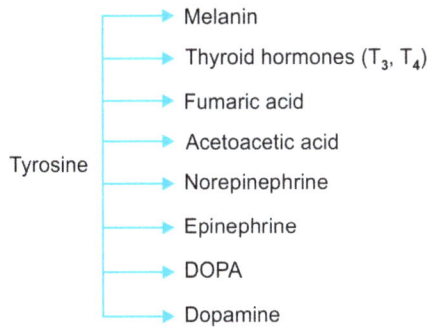

Fig. 5.17: Metabolic fates of tyrosine.

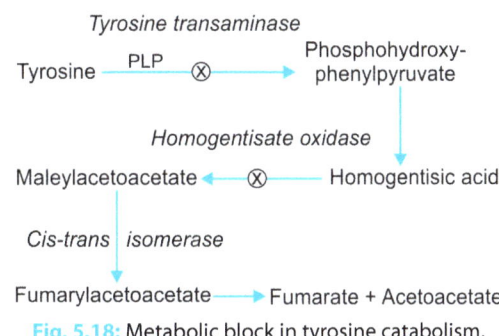

Fig. 5.18: Metabolic block in tyrosine catabolism.

Tyrosinemia

Tyrosinemia is a hereditary disease due to the lack of hepatic *tyrosine transaminase* enzyme **(Fig. 5.18)**. There are three types of tyrosinemia:
1. Tyrosinemia I (tyrosinosis).
2. Tyrosinemia II (Richner–Hanhart syndrome).
3. Benign transient neonatal tyrosinemia.

Tyrosinemia I
Cause: The deficiency of fumarylacetoacetate hydroxylase causes tyrosinemia.
Clinical features: Increased tyrosine level in blood and urine. Increased methionine in the blood. Excretion of large amounts of 3,4-dihydroxyphenylalanine (DOPA).

Tyrosinemia II (Richner–Hanhart syndrome)
Cause: It causes due to the genetic deficiency of tyrosine transaminase.
Clinical features: Increased tyrosine level in blood and urine. Increased levels of *p*-hydroxyphenylacetate, *N*-acetyl tyrosine and *p*-hydroxyphenylpyruvate. Eye lesions and skin lesions of palm.

Benign transient neonatal tyrosinemia
Cause: Defect in the synthesis of *p*-hydroxyphenylpyruvate hydroxylase in the infants due to immature liver. But as age advances, the accumulated tyrosine is metabolized, and serum levels come to normal within 4–8 weeks of age.
Treatment: Low-phenylalanine diet.

State the Causes and Clinical Symptoms of Alkaptonuria

Alkaptonuria
Cause: The deficiency of *homogentisate oxidase*. It is an inherited metabolic disorder. Homogentisic acid is excreted in urine. Urine turns black upon exposure to light. In the later stages, the black pigment is deposited in sclera, ear, nose and cartilages. This is called **ochronosis**, and it may lead to tissue damage and may develop arthritis.
Symptoms: Mental retardation, children have low IQ and low-serotonin levels in brain.

Melanin

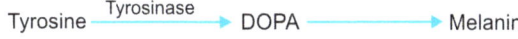

Tyrosinase deficiency leads to albinism. Melanin is a pigment that occurs in the eye, hair and skin. In the epidermis, the pigment-forming cells are called melanocytes. Here the melanin is synthesized to protect the underlying cells from the harmful effects of sunlight.

SYNTHESIS OF CATECHOLAMINES

Synthesis of Dopamine, Epinephrine and Norepinephrine (Catecholamines)

- **Epinephrine is produced in** the adrenal medulla.

- Norepinephrine is a neurotransmitter produced in central nervous system (CNS) and postganglionic sympathetic nerves.
- Dopamine is present in localized regions of the brain and also functions in the peripheral organs.
- Both dopamine and norepinephrine are primary amines, whereas epinephrine is a secondary amine.
- Dopamine and norepinephrine functions as transmitters of nerve signals in the CNS.
- Epinephrine influences carbohydrate metabolism.
- These catecholamines have their characteristic physiological and pharmacological actions through the interaction with adrenergic or dopaminergic receptors (α or β) that are located on the surface of target cells throughout the body.
- The overproduction of these catecholamines produces disorders.
- The α-receptors interact with epinephrine and norepinephrine; β-receptors interact with only epinephrine **(Fig. 5.19)**.
- Excess or reduced production of catecholamines is associated with many diseases such as thyroid hormone deficiency, congestive heart failure and stress.
- Low levels of catecholamines are seen in idiopathic postural hypotension.
- Measurements of catecholamines are helpful in the diagnosis of catecholamine secreting tumors such as pheochromocytomas, paraganglions or neuroblastomas.
- In Parkinson disease, dopamine levels in the CNS are decreased due to a deficiency of cells that produce dopamine and depression is associated with low levels of serotonin.

The diphenyl is used to treat this disease because this drug inhibits the action of mono-amine oxidase:

- Tyrosine + $I^+ \rightarrow$ Monoiodotyrosine (MIT)
- MIT + $I^+ \rightarrow$ Diiodotyrosine (DIT)
- MIT + DIT $\rightarrow$ Triiodothyronine (T3)
- DIT + DIT $\rightarrow$ Tetraiodothyronine (T4 or thyroxine).

METABOLISM OF TRYPTOPHAN

- It is an essential amino acid **(Fig. 5.20)**.
- It is mainly required for the synthesis of proteins, niacin, serotonin and melatonin.

METABOLIC FATE OF TRYPTOPHAN

- Nicotinamide adenine dinucleotide (NAD^+) and nicotinamide adenine dinucleotide

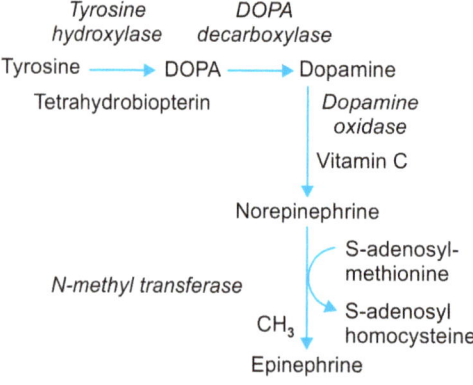

Fig. 5.19: Formation of catecholamines.

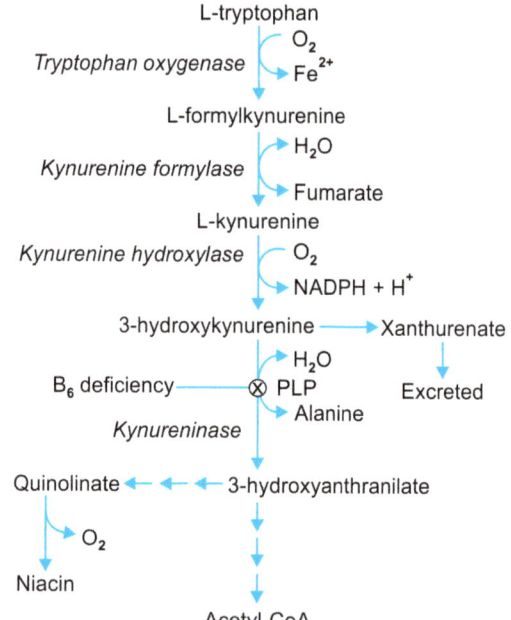

Fig. 5.20: Metabolism of tryptophan.

Metabolism of Amino Acids

phosphate (NADP⁺) are the acceptor of reducing equivalents (H⁺) provided by various metabolic intermediates. 60 mg of tryptophan forms 1 mg of niacin, which is required for the formation of its coenzyme form NAD⁺ and NADP⁺ **(Fig. 5.21)**.

- *Synthesis of serotonin* **(Fig. 5.22)**:
  - Serotonin is a neurotransmitter and vasoconstrictor stimulator of smooth muscle contraction.
  - It is synthesized by neurons, pineal gland and argentaffin tissue.
  - The degradation product of serotonin is 5-hydroxyindoleacetic acid (5-HIAA).

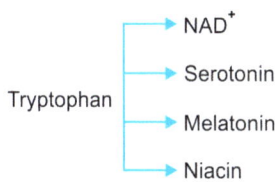

Fig. 5.21: Fate of tryptophan.

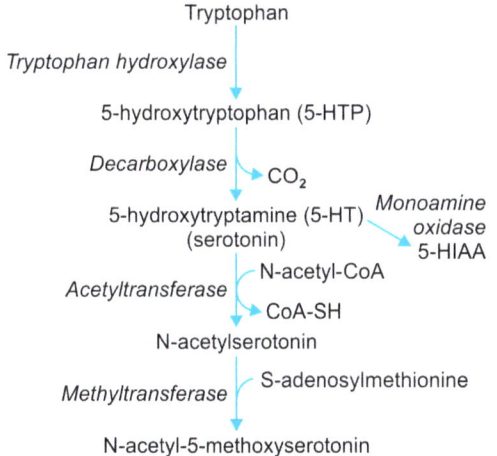

Fig. 5.22: Synthesis of serotonin.

DISORDERS

Physiological Role of Serotonin

The important physiological role of serotonin is transmitter in serotonergic neurons within the brain. In humans, it has a role in sleep, perception of pain, schizophrenia and mental depression (low level of serotonin).

Hartnup's disease

Hartnup's disease is an autosomal-recessive trait caused by a defect in the intestinal absorption and renal reabsorption of tryptophan. Tryptophan and its catabolic products, indole acetic acid, excreted in large amounts in the urine. Indole acetic acid being excreted as indole-acetyl glutamine after conjugation with glutamine. Pellagra-like symptoms may be seen.

Signs and symptoms: Photosensitive red scaly rash resembling rash of pellagra, reversible cerebellar ataxia.

Diagnosis: It can be made on the level of indole acetic acid and other indole derivatives in urine.

Treatment: Oral administration of nicotinic acid.

Malignant carcinoid (argentaffinoma)

Malignant carcinoid is characterized by serotonin producing tumor cells in the argentaffin tissue of the abdominal cavity. Instead of 1%, the 60% of tryptophan is diverted to form serotonin resulting in pellagra-like symptoms. Urine also contains large amount of 5-HIAA.

HISTIDINE METABOLISM

- Histidine is a basic essential genetically coded amino acid.
- Histidine is also a precursor of histamine, a compound released by immune system cells during an allergic reaction.
- It is needed for growth and for the repair of tissue, as well as in the maintenance of the myelin sheaths that act as protector for nerve cells.
- It is further required for the formation of both red and white blood cells and helps to protect the body from damage caused by radiation and in removing heavy metals from the body.

- In the stomach, histidine is also helpful in producing gastric juices, and people with a less secretion of gastric juices or suffering from indigestion may also benefit from this nutrient:

$$\text{Histidine} \xrightarrow[\text{PLP}]{\text{Decarboxylase}} \text{Histamine} + CO_2$$

- Histamine strongly stimulates the secretion of HCl by the parietal cells of the stomach.

Catabolism/Disorders

Catabolism of histidine is shown in **Figure 5.23**.

Histidinemia

Histidinemia is a rare autosomal-recessive metabolic disorder caused by a deficiency of the enzyme histidase. Histidase is needed for the metabolism of the amino acid histidine. Histidinemia is characterized by increased levels of histidine in blood, urine and cerebrospinal fluid and decreased levels of the metabolite urocanic acid in blood, urine and skin cells.

> **FIGLU Excretion**
> *Cause:* Folic acid deficiency leads to decreased concentration of FH_4, which is required for the conversion of N-formimino-glutamate to glutamic acid. Accumulation of FIGLU results in excretion in urine.

> *Diagnostic importance:* Megaloblastic anemia occurs in both folic acid and vitamin B_{12} deficiency. To differentiate the anemia due to folic acid deficiency from that of vitamin B_{12} deficiency, FIGLU excretion test can be conducted.

> *Case*
> Mr Raju, a 12-year-old boy was brought to the pediatric outpatient department with a complaint of tiredness and abdominal pain. His mother explained to the doctor that Raju gets tired very often. The doctor noticed the Raju as anemic and requested for complete blood count and renal function test (RFT). The RFT report came normal and CBC showed reduced hemoglobins. The doctor requested for formiminoglutamic acid (FIGLU) and methyl malonic acid excretion test. The FIGLU excretion test showed positive and the doctor diagnosed it as megaloblastic anemia and suggested Raju's mother to give folic acid every day. Which of the following metabolisms requires folic acid as coenzyme to convert N-formiminoglutamate to glutamic acid?
> a. Histidine
> b. Tryptophan
> c. Phenylalanine
> d. Glycine
> **Answer is A**

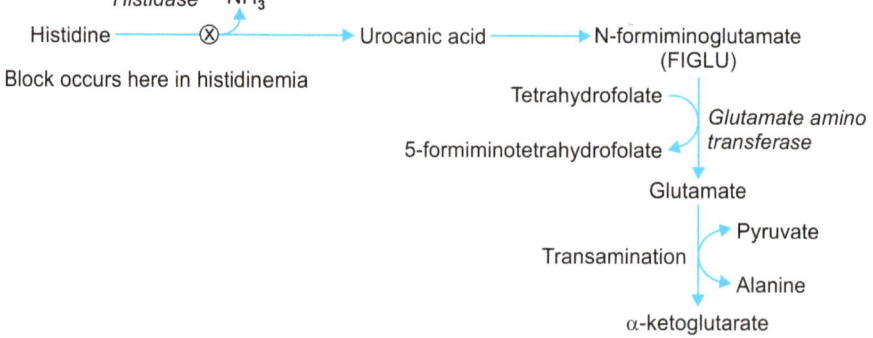

Fig. 5.23: Catabolism of histidine.

METABOLISM OF BRANCHED-CHAIN AMINO ACID

Valine, leucine and isoleucine are branched-chain amino acids **(Fig. 5.24)**.

Maple Syrup Urine Disease (MSUD)
The MSUD is an inborn error of branched-chain amino acid metabolism.

Cause: Deficiency or complete absence of α-ketoacid dehydrogenase. Accumulated α-ketoacids are excreted in the urine. These ketoacids give a characteristic smell to the urine. It is similar to that of maple syrup. Seizures, coma and mental retardation are the common symptoms.

Diagnosis: Antenatal diagnosis may be done by measuring decarboxylase activity in cultured cells from amniotic fluid. Analysis of urine with dinitrophenylhydrazine (DNPH) and measurement of plasma amino acid levels.

Treatment: Replacing dietary protein by mixture of amino acids that excludes leucine, isoleucine and valine.

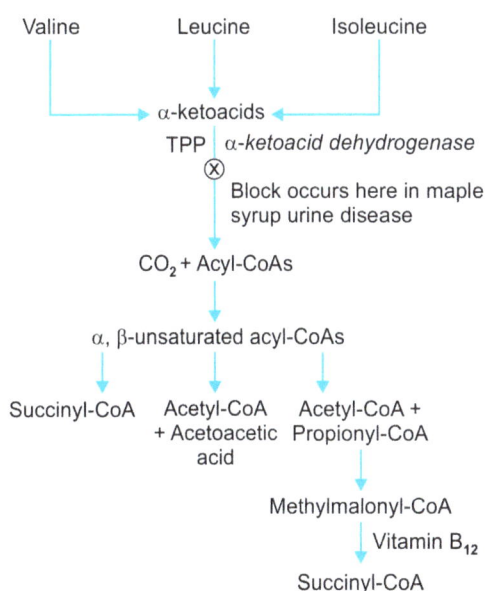

Fig. 5.24: Metabolism of branched-chain amino acids.

Methionine

Methionine is one of the essential amino acids (building blocks of protein), i.e. it cannot be produced by the body and must be provided by the diet. It supplies sulfur and other compounds required by the body for normal metabolism and growth. Methionine also belongs to a group of compounds called lipotropics, or chemicals that help the liver to process fats (lipids) **(Fig. 5.25)**.

Methionine and cysteine are the only sulfur-containing proteinogenic amino acids.

The methionine derivative SAM serves as a methyl donor. Methionine plays a role in cysteine, carnitine and taurine synthesis by the transsulfuration pathway, lecithin production, the synthesis of phosphatidylcholine, and other phospholipids. Improper conversion of methionine can lead to atherosclerosis.

Methionine is one of only two amino acids encoded by a single codon (AUG) in the standard genetic code (tryptophan, encoded by UGG is the other).

S-adenosylmethionine

The SAM is an enzymatic cofactor involved in methyl group transfers. It methylates targets, many of which are in the brain. It deactivates dopamine by methylating a hydroxy group on the catechol:

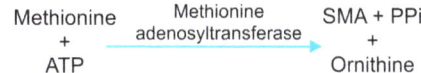

Formylmethionine

Formylmethionine (fMet) is a modified form of methionine in which a formyl group has been added to methionine amino group. fMet is a starting residue in the synthesis of proteins in prokaryotes and consequently is located at the N-terminal end of the polypeptide. fMet is delivered to the ribosome (30S) mRNA complex by a specialized tRNA (tRNA^fMet), which has a 5'-CAU-3' anticodon that is capable of binding with the AUG start codon located on the mRNA.

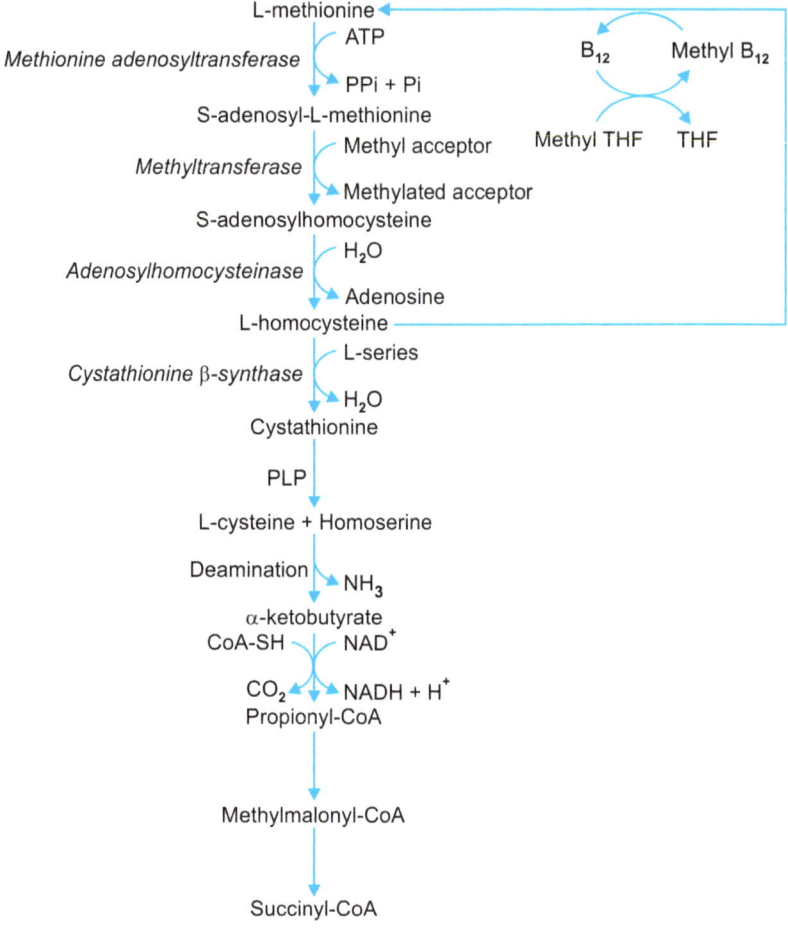

Fig. 5.25: Metabolism of methionine.

The addition of the formyl group to methionine is catalyzed by the enzyme transformylase. Transformylase will catalyze the addition of the formyl group to methionine, only if methionine has been loaded onto tRNA^{fMet} and not onto tRNA^{Met}.

METABOLIC DISORDERS

Cystinuria
It is the most common inborn error of amino acid transport. In this disorder, the renal tubules fail to absorb basic amino acids such as cysteine, ornithine, arginine and lysine. Therefore, these amino acids are excreted in the urine in a large way.

Cause: Defect in the carrier protein, which carries these amino acids once reabsorbed from the proximal renal tubules.

Clinical findings: Cystine is least soluble and its over-excretion results in the formation of cystine calculi in the renal tubules and leads to obstruction, infection and renal insufficiency in cystinuric patients.

Treatment: Reduction of the concentration of cystine in urine by taking large amounts

Metabolism of Amino Acids

of water, which increases cystine solubility through maintenance of alkaline urine.

Homocysteinemia

Normally, it does not occur because the homocysteine is unstable and, when present in excess, undergoes oxidation to homocysteine. The blood level of homocysteine is 15 µmol/L. Increased level is associated with cardiovascular disease.

Homocystinuria

Homocystinuria is an inherited disorder of methionine metabolism.

Cause: Deficiency or complete absence of cystathionine-α-synthase in the liver, which converts homocysteine and serine to cystathionine. Another cause is deficiency of methyltetrahydrofolate or methyl B_{12} due to inadequate intake of folic acid or vitamin B_{12} (or due to defective enzyme that joins methyl groups to THF, transferring methyl from methyl B_{12} to homocysteine to form methionine).

Types: There are four types of homocystinuria (Fig. 5.26):

1. Homocystinuria I (deficiency in cystathionine-β-synthase).
2. Homocystinuria II (defect in N^5, N^{10}-methylene THF reductase).
3. Homocystinuria III (defect in homocysteine transmethylase).
4. Homocystinuria IV (defect in absorption from intestine).

Signs and symptoms: Myopia, glaucoma, retinal detachment, osteoporosis, thinning and lengthening of the long bones and knock knee. The serious symptoms are caused by arterial and venous thrombosis.

Treatment: Therapy with pyridoxine to activate the enzyme cystathionine-α-synthase is helpful. Those with complete enzyme deficiency should be treated with a diet low in methionine and supplemented with cystine. Vitamin B_{12} can be given in its deficiency. Silver nitroprusside test is helpful in the diagnosis.

Cystathioninuria

Cystathioninuria is a genetic disorder due to cystathionase deficiency.

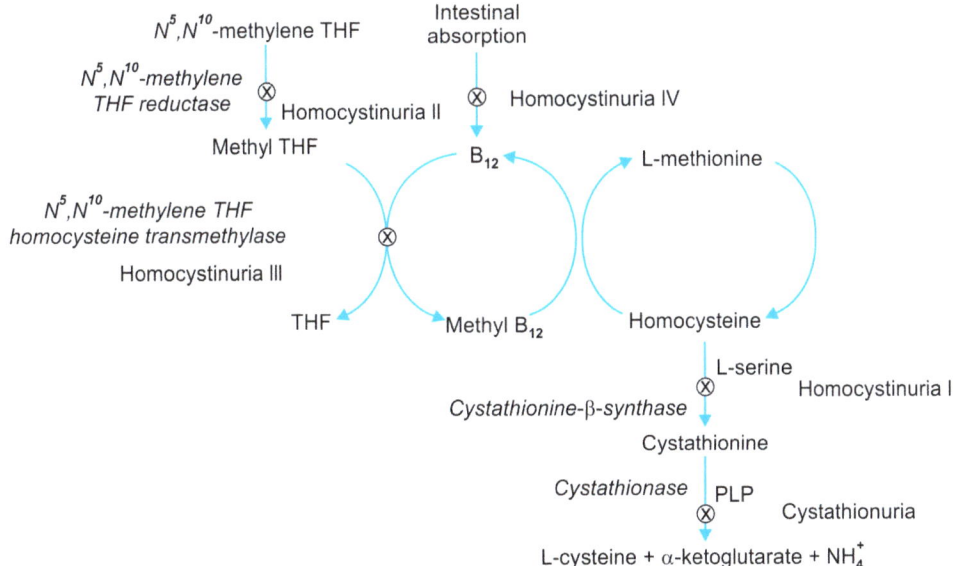

Fig. 5.26: Metabolic blocks in different types of homocystinuria.

Metabolism of Serine

- It is a nonessential amino acid.
- It is a constituent of phospholipid and phosphatidylserine of brain.
- It is also required for the synthesis of cysteine.
- It is synthesized from glycine (refer glycine catabolism).
- Glycine + N^5, N^{10}-methylene THF + H_2O hydroxymethyltransferase serine.

Catabolism of Serine

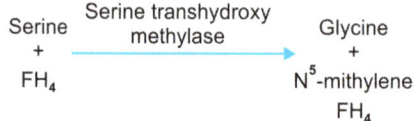

Synthesis of Creatine

The synthesis of creatine is shown in **Figure 5.27**.

Creatine is present in muscle, liver and kidney. Synthesis takes place in kidney and liver using three amino acids glycine, arginine and SAM (methyl donor).

Creatinine excretion in urine is always constant in normal person (1–1.5 g/day). It varies in kidney disease and muscle diseases.

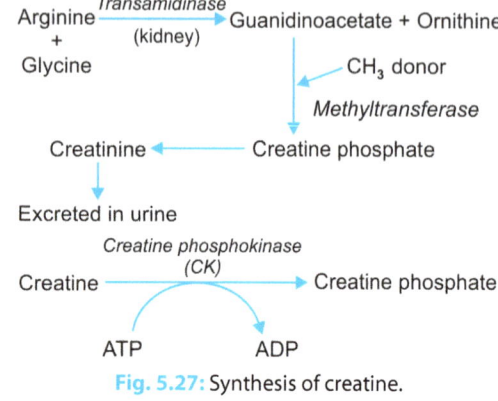

Fig. 5.27: Synthesis of creatine.

Special Compounds Formed from Other Amino Acids

See **Table 5.3**.

Table 5.3: Amino acids and the special compounds formed.

Amino acids	Special compounds
Histidine	Histamine, carnosine, anserine and formiminoglutamic acid (FIGLU)
Cysteine	Taurine and glutathione
Methionine	Cysteine, S-adenosylmethionine (SAM) and one-carbon donor

INBORN ERRORS OF METABOLISM

See **Table 5.4**.

Table 5.4: Summary of inborn errors of metabolism.

Metabolic disorder	Defect	Signs and symptoms
Primary hyperoxaluria	Failure to catabolize glyoxylate	High urinary excretion of oxalate
Glycinuria		Increased excretion of glycine in urine
Phenylketonuria	Deficiency of phenylalanine hydroxylase	Accumulation of phenylalanine converted to phenylpyruvate, phenyllactate and phenylacetate; excretion of phenyllactate, and phenylacetylglutamine along with phenylalanine Mental retardation, failure to talk, seizures
Tyrosinemia I	Fumaryl acetoacetate hydroxylase	Increased tyrosine levels in blood and urine. Increased methionine in the blood Excretion of large amounts of 3,4-dihydroxyphenylalanine (DOPA)

Contd...

Metabolic disorder	Defect	Signs and symptoms
Tyrosinemia II (Richner–Hanhart syndrome)	Deficiency of tyrosine transaminase	Increased tyrosine levels in blood and urine Increased levels of P-OH phenylacetate, N-acetyl tyrosine, P-OH phenylpyruvate, eye lesions and skin lesions of palm
Alkaptonuria	Deficiency of homogentisate oxidase	Homogentisic acid is excreted in urine. Urine turns black upon exposure to light In the later stages, black pigment is deposited in sclera, ear, nose and cartilages
Albinism	Tyrosinase deficiency	Mental retardation Children have low intelligence quotient (IQ) Low serotonin levels in brain Fair hair and blue eyes due to deficiency of pigment melanin
Hartnup's disease	Defect in the intestinal absorption renal reabsorption of tryptophan	Tryptophan and its catabolic products, indoleacetic acid excreted in large amounts in the urine Symptoms include photosensitive red scaly rash resembling rash of pellagra and reversible cerebellar ataxia
Formiminoglutamic acid (FIGLU) excretion	Folic acid deficiency	Excretion of formiminoglutamate
Maple syrup urine disease	Deficiency or complete absence of α-ketoacid dehydrogenase	Accumulated α-ketoacids excreted in the urine; these ketoacids give a characteristic smell to the urine; it is similar to that of maple syrup; seizures, coma and mental retardation are the common symptoms
Homocystinuria	Deficiency of cystathionine-α-synthase, deficiency of methyl-tetrahydrofolate or methyl B_{12}. There are four type of homocystinuria: i. Homocystinuria I (deficiency in cystathionine-β-synthase). ii. Homocystinuria II (defect in N_5, N_{10}-methylene THF reductase). iii. Homocystinuria III (defect in homocysteine transmethylase). iv. Homocystinuria IV (defect in absorption from intestine).	Myopia, glaucoma, retinal detachment, osteoporosis, thinning and lengthening of the long bones and knock knee

SUMMARY

Digestion of dietary proteins starts in the stomach. Secretion of HCl activates formation of pepsin from pepsinogen, which hydrolyzes peptide bonds of dietary proteins to release aromatic amino acids. Similarly, in the small intestine, digestion continues. Zymogens are activated for the breakdown of peptide bonds to release amino acids, which are absorbed into the small intestine through active transport mechanism. The absorbed amino acids are utilized to synthesize protein and undergo catabolism to generate nonprotein nitrogenous substances, urea, fatty acids, ketone bodies and so on. The catabolism of amino acids results in the formation of NH_3, which is toxic to human body and will convert to urea for excretion. Any defect with the urea cycle enzymes results in the accumulation of NH_3 or intermediates of urea cycle. This causes several neurological problems including mental retardation. Glycine is the simplest amino acid and responsible for the production of heme, glutathione and purine nucleotides. Glutamate catabolism results in GABA and glutathione. Tyrosine can be synthesized by phenylalanine with the help of phenylalanine hydroxylase. The deficiency of this enzyme results in PKU. The tyrosine is responsible for the generation of DOPA, dopamine, melanin, epinephrine and norepinephrine. Homogentisate oxidase deficiency results in alkaptonuria with symptoms of dark urine and mental retardation. Serotonin, melatonin and niacin are the metabolic intermediates of tryptophan. The MSUD is the clinical condition arises due to the deficiency of α-ketoacid dehydrogenase enzyme of branched-chain amino acid metabolism. Homocystinuria is an inherited disorder of methionine metabolism.

SELF-ASSESSMENT QUESTIONS

1. Outline the urea cycle and note the site of synthesis.
2. What is the need for urea synthesis in our body?
3. Describe the process of removal of ammonia from amino acids.
4. Explain the specialized compounds formed from glycine, phenyl and trypsin.
5. Name the enzymes required for the following enzymes:
   a. $NH_3 + ATP + CO_2 \rightarrow$ Carbamoyl phosphate
   b. Phenylalanine $\rightarrow$ Tyrosine
   c. Creatine $\rightarrow$ Creatine phosphate
   d. Tyrosine $\rightarrow$ DOPA
6. Describe the synthesis of creatine in the body.
7. Write a note on inborn errors of amino acid metabolism.
8. What are glucogenic amino acids? List both glucogenic and ketogenic amino acids.
9. Write the metabolic fate of tryptophan.
10. What are the compounds formed from tyrosine?
11. How tyrosine is formed from phenylalanine?
12. Write the cause for the following inborn errors of metabolism:
    a. Alkaptonuria
    b. PKU
    c. Maple syrup urine disease (MSUD)
    d. Albinism
13. Write the flowchart to show the synthesis of serotonin from tryptophan.
14. Which amino acid is responsible for the synthesis of niacin in the body?
15. What is FIGLU excretion test and what is its significance?
16. Write the importance of glycine.
17. Name the compounds formed from glutamate.
18. Briefly discuss the transamination and oxidative deamination process.
19. What is the fate of ammonia?
20. Add a note on the inborn errors of urea cycle.
21. Write a note on transamination and oxidative deamination.
22. Explain with a flow diagram showing the synthesis of tyrosine from phenylalanine.
23. Briefly discuss the metabolism of tryptophan including its metabolic fate.
24. Discuss the metabolism of branched-chain amino acids including the maple syrup urine disease.

MULTIPLE-CHOICE QUESTIONS

1. **Pepsin is secreted in:**
   a. Intestine   b. Liver
   c. Stomach   d. Pancreas
2. **The coenzyme required for the catalytic activity of transaminase is:**
   a. Thiamine pyrophosphate (TPP)
   b. PLP
   c. NAD
   d. Flavin adenine dinucleotide (FAD)
3. **Toxic ammonia produced in the body converted to:**
   a. Uric acid   b. Citrulline
   c. Purine   d. Urea

4. **Hyperammonemia type I is due to the deficiency of:**
   a. Carbamoyl phosphate synthetase 1
   b. Arginase
   c. Argininosuccinase
   d. Argininosuccinic acid synthetase

5. **Which one of the following compounds is not synthesized from glycine?**
   a. Heme
   b. Creatine
   c. Serine
   d. Tyrosine

6. **Concerning glutamic acid, one of the following is *not* true:**
   a. It is required for folic acid synthesis
   b. It is a nonessential amino acid
   c. Aspartate transaminase catalyzes its synthesis
   d. It is a component of glutathione

7. **Phenylalanine:**
   a. Is synthesized in the human body
   b. Synthesis depends on phenylalanine hydroxylase
   c. Synthesis defect results in the alkaptonuria
   d. Can synthesize tyrosine

8. **Concerning tyrosine metabolism, one of the following statements is *incorrect*:**
   a. It is essential for thyroid hormone synthesis
   b. It is required to synthesize DOPA and dopamine
   c. Tyrosine transaminase deficiency results in PKU
   d. Tyrosine deficient children will have low IQ

9. **Concerning tryptophan, all of the following statements are true, *except*:**
   a. It is required to synthesize serotonin
   b. It is an essential amino acid
   c. It can form niacin
   d. It is essential to synthesize melanin

10. **Malignant carcinoid is a metabolic disorder of:**
    a. Tyrosine
    b. Tryptophan
    c. Histidine
    d. Glycine

11. **Concerning histidine, one of the following statements is *incorrect*:**
    a. It is an acidic essential amino acid
    b. It is required for the formation of both red and white blood cells
    c. It is also helpful in producing gastric juices
    d. It is a precursor of histamine

12. **Maple syrup urine disease:**
    a. Is an inborn error of glycine metabolism
    b. Is the result of deficiency of α-ketoacid dehydrogenase
    c. Results in increased levels of amino acids in the urine
    d. Does not result in mental retardation

13. **Concerning methionine, one of the following statements is *incorrect*:**
    a. Methionine is the only sulfur-containing proteinogenic amino acid
    b. It supplies sulfur and other compounds for metabolism and growth
    c. Its derivative SAM serves as a methyl donor
    d. It is coded by AUG

14. **Methionine without methyl group is:**
    a. Homocysteine
    b. Cysteine
    c. Cystine
    d. Formylmethionine

15. **All of the following are the steps in creatine metabolism, *except*:**
    a. Arginine + Glycine → Guanidinoacetate
    b. Creatine phosphate → Creatine
    c. Creatine → Creatine phosphate
    d. Ornithine → Creatine phosphate

16. **All of the special compounds are formed from histidine, *except*:**
    a. Histamine
    b. Carnosine
    c. Taurine
    d. Anserine

17. **Which of the following statements is correct?**
    a. Urea is produced directly by the hydrolysis of ornithine
    b. ATP is required for the reaction in which argininosuccinate is cleaved to form arginine
    c. The urea cycle occurs exclusively in the cytosol
    d. In humans, the major route of nitrogen metabolism from amino acids to urea is catalyzed by the combined actions of transaminase (aminotransferase) and glutamate dehydrogenase

18. **Which of the following statements about the synthesis of carbamoyl phosphate by carbamoyl phosphate synthetase I is incorrect?**
    a. The enzyme catalyzes the rate-limiting reaction in the urea cycle
    b. The reaction is allosterically activated by N-acetylglutamate
    c. The reaction is reversible
    d. The reaction requires two high-energy phosphates for each carbamoyl phosphate molecule synthesized

19. **Tyrosine would be an essential amino acid in the diet of a child with:**

a. Lesch–Nyhan syndrome
b. Defective tyrosine aminotransferase
c. Deficiency of thiamine
d. Classical PKU

20. One of the following amino acids gives rise to α-ketoacids that accumulate in the urine in maple syrup urine disease is:
a. Phenylalanine   b. Valine
c. Lysine   d. Tyrosine

21. The collagen defect present in scurvy is:
a. Decreased protein stability due to decreased hydroxylation of proline and lysine residues
b. Substitution of valine for proline and lysine residues in the collagen sequence
c. Increased formation of Schiff-base crosslinks
d. Decreased protein stability due to increased glycosylation

22. Smokers tend to develop emphysema more readily than nonsmokers. This is due to oxidation of a methionine residue in:
a. Elastin
b. Pulmonary collagen
c. Neutrophil elastase
d. α-1-antitrypsin

23. Which amino acid serves as a carrier of ammonia from skeletal muscle to liver?
a. Alanine   b. Methionine
c. Arginine   d. Glutamine

24. Type of covalent bonds linking the amino acid in a protein is:
a. Peptide bonds   b. Hydrogen bonds
c. Glycosidic bonds d. Ester bonds

25. Which of the following statements is false?
a. After a resistance training session, the rate of protein synthesis in the exercised muscles is increased
b. After a resistance training session, the rate of protein breakdown in the exercised muscles is increased
c. Exercise increases the rate of secretion of growth
d. Protein cannot be used as a fuel for exercise

26. Which of the following is true?
a. Increasing the protein intake above 5 g/kg body mass per day will stimulate muscle growth and increase strength
b. Creatine supplements can increase muscle strength and power
c. Amino acid supplements can increase muscle strength and power
d. Muscle damage is induced by shortening contractions

27. When branched-chain amino acids are deaminated in muscle, the ammonia produced is mostly:
a. Converted into glucose and released from the muscle
b. Converted into alanine and glutamine and released from the muscle
c. Converted into urea and released from the muscle
d. Used to synthesize purines and pyrimidines in the muscle

28. One of the following promotes glucose and amino acid uptake by muscle is:
a. Adrenaline   b. Insulin
c. Glucagon   d. Cortisol

29. Which amino acid is very important for optimal immune function and exhibits a reduced plasma concentration during heavy training?
a. Arginine   b. Glutamine
c. Phenylalanine   d. Isoleucine

30. Absorption of which one of the following amino acids is defective in Hartnup's disease:
a. Lysine   b. Leucine
c. Tyrosine   d. Tryptophan

31. Which one of the following deficiencies results in homocystinuria?
a. Cystathionine-β-synthase
b. Phenylalanine hydroxylase
c. Methyltransferase
d. Creatine phosphokinase

32. The cofactors involved in the regeneration of methionine from homocysteine are:
a. Retinoic acid
b. Tetrahydrofolic acid and vitamin B_{12}
c. TPP
d. Biotin and vitamin K

33. Amino acid, which is both glucogenic and ketogenic, is:
a. Phenylalanine   b. Alanine
c. Leucine   d. Lysine

34. The precursor for the synthesis of dopamine is:
a. Phenylalanine   b. Tryptophan
c. Lysine   d. Isoleucine

35. The rate-limiting step of urea cycle is:
a. Carbamoyl phosphate synthetase
b. Ornithine transcarbamylase

c. Arginase
d. Argininosuccinase
36. **Which of the following is not an essential amino acid?**
   a. Serine
   b. Tyrosine
   c. Isoleucine
   d. Histidine
37. **The PKU results from the deficiency of:**
   a. Ketoacid decarboxylase
   b. Arginase
   c. Homogentisate oxidase
   d. Phenylalanine hydroxylase
38. **Excess lysine in the diet may impair the absorption of:**
   a. Arginine
   b. Phenylalanine
   c. Tyrosine
   d. Tryptophan
39. **The intermediate that links urea cycle directly with TCA cycle is:**
   a. Arginine
   b. Fumarate
   c. Glutamate
   d. Pyruvate
40. **The coenzyme involved in transamination reactions is:**
   a. Niacin
   b. Pyridoxine
   c. Niacin
   d. Thiamine pyrophosphate
41. **The major nonprotein nitrogen substance present in urine is:**
   a. Creatinine
   b. Uric acid
   c. Urea
   d. Amino acids
42. **Catabolism of serine and alanine produces:**
   a. Pyruvate
   b. Fumarate
   c. Lactate
   d. Succinate
43. **All of the following are formed from amino acid precursors, *except*:**
   a. Parathyroid hormone
   b. Thyroid hormone
   c. Glucocorticoid hormone
   d. Follicular-stimulating hormone
44. **The site of urea synthesis is:**
   a. Liver
   b. Kidney
   c. Brain
   d. Adrenal gland
45. **The oxidative deamination of the amino acid alanine in muscle produces:**
   a. One molecule of pyruvic acid and a molecule of ammonia
   b. One molecule of pyruvic acid and a molecule of carbon dioxide
   c. One molecule of glutamic acid and another amino acid
   d. One molecule of pyruvic acid and a molecule of urea
46. **David, an 8-month-old male infant, emigrated with his parents from India to the Trinidad and Tobago a month ago. He was normal at birth, but in the past several days, a tremor in his extremities has appeared. Last night, he presented gross switching movements in his crib. When examined, the physician noted a musty odor to the baby's wet diaper.**
   Immediately requested for a screening test for PKU and it showed positive.
   Which of the following compounds can you expect that is elevated in this patient urine?
   a. Phenyl lactate
   b. Histidine
   c. Methylmalonic acid
   d. Homogentisate
47. **Multiple myeloma:**
   a. Results from a polyclonal proliferation of lymph node plasma cells
   b. Often presents with eye pain
   c. Hypercalcemia develops in 50% of patients
   d. Most patients have a serum alpha proteinemia

Answers

1. c	2. b	3. d	4. a	5. d
6. c	7. b	8. c	9. d	10. b
11. a	12. b	13. a	14. a	15. c
16. c	17. d	18. c	19. d	20. b
21. a	22. d	23. a	24. a	25. d
26. b	27. b	28. b	29. b	30. d
31. a	32. b	33. a	34. a	35. a
36. a	37. d	38. a	39. b	40. b
41. c	42. a	43. d	44. a	45. a
46. a	47. c			

CHAPTER 6

Chemistry of Carbohydrates

OBJECTIVES

At the end of this chapter, students should be able to:
- Classify the carbohydrates with examples
- Explain the structure and function of starch and glycogen
- Understand the isomerism property of carbohydrates.

INTRODUCTION

Carbohydrates are organic substances containing carbon (C), hydrogen (H), and oxygen (O) atoms usually in the ratio of 1:2:1. They are polyhydroxy aldehyde or ketone derivatives.

CLASSIFICATION OF CARBOHYDRATES

Carbohydrates are classified into four major groups, as follows:

1. Monosaccharides

Monosaccharides are simple sugars that cannot be hydrolyzed further into simpler forms (**Table 6.1**).

Monosaccharides are further classified on the basis of number of carbon atoms present as well as on the presence of functional groups.

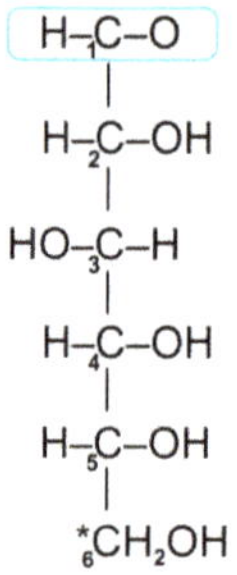

D-glucose:
$$_1H-C-O$$
$$_2H-C-OH$$
$$HO-_3C-H$$
$$_4H-C-OH$$
$$_5H-C-OH$$
$$_6^*CH_2OH$$

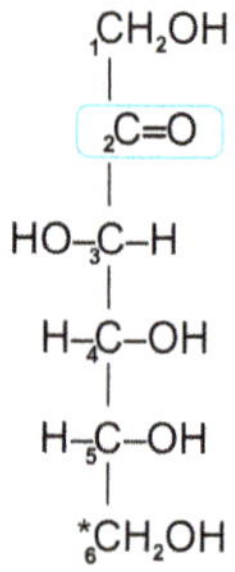

D-fructose:
$$_1CH_2OH$$
$$_2C=O$$
$$HO-_3C-H$$
$$_4H-C-OH$$
$$_5H-C-OH$$
$$_6^*CH_2OH$$

Table 6.1: Monosaccharides.

Number of carbon atoms	Examples	Functional groups present
Trioses (three carbons)	Glyceraldehyde	Aldehyde (aldotriose)
	Dihydroxy-acetone	Ketone (ketotriose)
Tetroses (four carbons)	Erythrose	Aldehyde (aldotetrose)
Pentoses (five carbons)	Ribose	Aldehyde (aldopentose)
	Xylose	Aldehyde (aldopentose)
	Xylulose	Ketone (ketopentose)
Hexoses (six carbons)	Glucose	Aldehyde (aldohexose)
	Galactose	Aldehyde (aldohexose)
	Fructose	Ketone (ketohexose)

Chemistry of Carbohydrates

Table 6.2: Examples of disaccharides.

Examples	Product formed upon hydrolysis	Glycosidic linkage	Sources
Maltose	Glucose+glucose	α-1,4	Malt
Lactose	Galactose+glucose	β-1,4	Milk
Sucrose	Glucose+fructose	β-1,2	Sugarcane
Isomaltose	Glucose+glucose	α-1,6	Digestion of amylopectin

2. Disaccharides

Disaccharides contain two molecules of the same or different monosaccharide units that get separated on hydrolysis. These units are joined by glycosidic bond **(Table 6.2)**.

3. Oligosaccharides

Oligosaccharides contain 3–10 molecules of monosaccharide units, e.g. maltotriose (glucose+glucose+glucose).

4. Polysaccharides

Polysaccharides contain more than 10 molecules of monosaccharide units. They are further classified into homopolysaccharides and heteropolysaccharides.

HOMOPOLYSACCHARIDES

Homopolysaccharides are polymer of same monosaccharide units **(Table 6.3)**.

Starch: It is a mixture of two polysaccharides—amylose and amylopectin **(Fig. 6.1)**. The

Table 6.3: Examples of homopolysaccharides.

Examples	Monosaccharide unit	Sources
Starch	Glucose	Plants, rice
Dextrin	Glucose	From starch hydrolysis
Glycogen	Glucose	Liver, muscle
Cellulose	Glucose	Plant fibers
Inulin	Fructose	Dahlia roots
Chitin	N-acetyl glucosamine	Arthropod

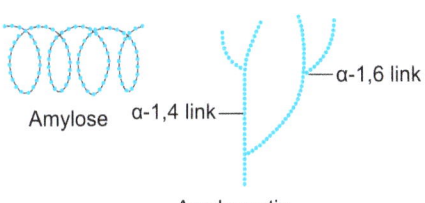

Fig. 6.1: Structure of starch.

major differences between amylose and amylopectin are shown in **Table 6.4**.

Glycogen: It is stored in liver and muscle. It is a polymer of glucose units. It is also called animal starch. It is similar to the amylopectin component of starch. But it has more branches than starch. There are 11–18 glucose residues between any branch points.

Dextrin: These are partially hydrolyzed product of starch.

Cellulose: It is made up of β-D-glucose joined by β-1,4-glycosidic bonds. Cellulose is digested by *cellulase* enzyme, which is not present in human body. However, cellulose acts as dietary fiber, adds bulk to the food, and helps in peristalsis.

Inulin: It consists of a small number of β-D-fructose joined by β-2,1-glycosidic linkages. It is used to measure glomerular filtration rate, a test to assess the function of kidney.

Difference between Amylose and Amylopectin

Differences between amylose and amylopectin are shown in **Table 6.4**.

Table 6.4: Differences between amylose and amylopectin.

Characteristics	Amylose	Amylopectin
Amount present in starch	15–20%	80–85%
Structure	Unbranched, linear	Highly branched; branch point appears after every 24–30 glucose in straight chain form
Molecular weight	60 kDa	500 kDa
Linkage	250–300 glucose residues are joined by α-1,4-glycosidic linkage	Mainly formed by α-1,4 linkages between glucose residues; branch point occurs by forming α-1,6-glycosidic linkage
Reaction with iodine solution	Blue color forms because the iodine molecules are trapped inside the helical structure. Color disappears upon heating and reappears upon cooling	Reddish-violet color

HETEROPOLYSACCHARIDES WITH EXAMPLES AND THEIR BIOMEDICAL IMPORTANCE

Heteropolysaccharides are polymer of different monosaccharide units or their derivatives, e.g. mucopolysaccharides (MPS) and blood group substances.

Mucopolysaccharides

Hyaluronic acid, chondroitin sulfate, heparin, keratan sulfate, heparan sulfate, and dermatan sulfate are the examples for mucopolysaccharides **(Table 6.5)**. Mucopolysaccharides are heteropolysaccharides, which remain when protein is removed from proteoglycan. Mucopolysaccharides are also known as glycosaminoglycans.

Biomedical importance of mucopolysaccharides

1. Mucopolysaccharides are acidic in nature because of their polyanionic property. They are the components of ground substances throughout the extracellular space. They are attached to proteins and form proteoglycans.
2. Hyaluronic acid acts as a barrier in tissues against the penetration of bacteria. Hyaluronidase present in

Table 6.5: Mucopolysaccharides.

Mucopolysaccharide	Composition	Occurrence
Chondroitin sulfate	Glucuronic acid and N-acetyl galactosamine	Cartilage
Dermatan sulfate	Glucuronic acid or iduronic acid and N-acetylgalactosamine	Animal tissue
Keratan sulfate	Galactose and N-acetyl glucosamine	Cornea and helps in corneal transparency
Heparin (highly sulfate)	Glucuronic acid and N-acetyl glucosamine	Liver, lungs, arterial wall, and blood anticoagulant
Hyaluronic acid (sulfate free)	Glucuronic acid and N-acetylgalactosamine	Synovial fluid of joint, vitreous humor of eye, umbilical cord, cell membrane, and skin

bacteria can digest hyaluronic acid and acts as "spreading factor." Hyaluronidase present in testicular secretions helps in fertilization by favoring the entry of spermatozoa into the ovum.
3. Heparin acts as anticoagulant in vitro as well as in vivo. It inhibits thrombin.

ISOMERISM IN CARBOHYDRATES

The presence of asymmetric carbon atoms (a carbon atom to which four different atoms or groups attached is known as asymmetric carbon) in a compound produces the following effects:
- Formation of the stereoisomerism of the compound
- Confers optical activity to the compound.

OPTICAL ACTIVITY OF CARBOHYDRATES, INCLUDING STEREOISOMERISM WITH SPECIFIC EXAMPLES

Optical Activity

The compounds having asymmetric carbon atoms can rotate the beam of plane-polarized light and are said to be optically active.
1. An isomer, which rotate the plane of polarized light to the right is called dextrorotatory and is designated as (*d*) or +, for example, D-(*d*)-glucose or it is also known as dextrose.
2. While the isomer, which rotates the plane of polarized light to the left is known as levorotatory and is identified as (*l*) or (-), for example, D-(*l*)-fructose.
3. A compound with D-configuration can be dextrorotatory (D+) or levorotatory (D-), for example, D+ glucose and D- fructose.

Mutarotation

Ordinary crystalline glucose (a form of glucose) is dissolved in water. Then, the plane of polarized light is passed through this solution. The optical rotation of plane-polarized light gradually changes to a constant fixed rotation. This change in rotation is called mutarotation. The mechanism behind this is a slow change α form of sugar to its β form to an equilibrium mixture.

Sugar:

α-D-glucose→Equilibrium→β-D-glucose
 mixture

Optical rotation:

+112→+52.2→+19

Stereoisomerism

Compounds, which are identical in composition and structural formula but differ in spatial configuration, are called stereo-isomers. These include the following:

Enantiomers

Dextrose (D)- and levo (L)-sugars are referred to as enantiomers. Their structures are the mirror images of each other. Only D-glucose or D-sugars are utilized by humans. The D- and L-glucose are termed D, and L form depending on the arrangement of –H and –OH on the penultimate carbon atom. When the sugar has –OH group on the right side, then it is D-isomer. If the OH group is on left side, then it is L-isomer.

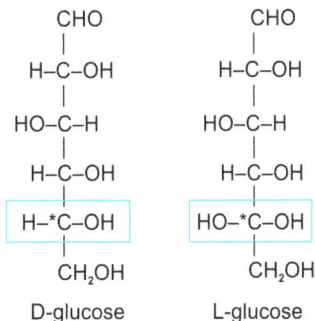

Anomerism

Sugars in a solution exist in a ring form and not in a straight chain form. Aldo sugar forms mainly pyranose ring and keto-sugar form furanose ring structure. Carbon 1, after ring formation, becomes asymmetric, and it is called anomeric carbon atom. The two sugars, which differ in the configuration at only C1 in case of aldoses and C2 in ketoses, are known as anomers and represented as α- and β-sugars. For example:

- α-D-glucose and β-D-glucose
- α-D-fructose and β-D-fructose.

α-D-glucose

β-D-glucose

α-D-fructose

β-D-fructose

Epimerism

The isomers formed due to variations in the configuration of –H and –OH around a single-carbon atom in a sugar molecule is called epimers. For example:

- Mannose is an epimer of glucose because these two have different configurations only around C2.
- Similarly, galactose is an epimer of glucose because these two have different configurations only around at C4.

D-galactose   D-glucose   D-mannose

- Ribose and xylose are epimers differing in configuration of groups around carbon:

D-ribose   D-xylose

INVERT SUGAR WITH EXAMPLE

Inversion

- Sucrose shows this phenomenon.
- Sucrose is dextrorotatory in nature.
- After hydrolysis, it gives the mixture of glucose and fructose.
- The hydrolyzed mixture shows levorotatory activity. This phenomenon is called inversion. This is because optical activity of fructose is −92° and glucose is 52.5°. The sum is negative.
- The enzyme that digests sucrose is sucrase, it is also known as invertase.
- Sucrose is the example for invert sugar.

CHEMICAL PROPERTIES OF MONOSACCHARIDES

Action of Strong Acids

When monosaccharide reacts with strong acids such as sulfuric acid or hydrochloric acid, it loses a water molecule and forms furfural derivatives. These derivatives may combine with α-naphthol or resorcinol to form colored complex:

```
    CHO                              CHO
    |                                |
  H–C–OH                             C—
    |                                |  
 HO–C–H                             H–C
    |          H₂SO₄ or HCl          |    O + 3 H₂OH
  H–C–OH       ─────────────►       H–C
    |                                |
  H–C–OH                             C—
    |                                |
   CH₂OH                            CH₂OH
  D-glucose                   Hydroxymethyl furfural
```

Action of Alkali

Monosaccharides when reacted with alkali are converted to enediols (involves either free aldehyde or keto group in the molecule). This enediol is the enol form of sugar because two hydroxyl groups (-OH) are attached to the double-bonded carbon. Enediols are the good reducing agents and which form on the basis of the Benedict's test. The alkali enolizes the sugar and causes them to be a strong reducing agent:

```
           Dilute alkali        Dilute alkali
D-glucose ◄──────────► 1,2-enediol ◄──────────► D-fructose
                            ↕
                         Mannose
```

Oxidation of Monosaccharides

1. Glucose undergoes oxidation in the presence of hypobromous acid to form gluconic acid. Similarly, mannose and galactose form mannonic and galactonic acid, respectively.
2. Oxidation of aldoses with nitric acid under proper conditions converts both aldehyde and terminal primary alcohol groups, forming dibasic saccharic or aldaric acids.
3. Uronic acid (D-glucuronic acid) is formed when aldose (D-glucose) is oxidized.
4. This glucuronic acid is involved in the process of detoxification of benzoic acid, bilirubin, and certain drugs. It is also a component of heteropolysaccharides and glycoproteins.

```
    CHO                        CHO
    |                          |
  H–C–OH                     H–C–OH
    |                          |
 HO–C–H                     HO–C–H
    |         Oxidation        |
  H–C–OH     ─────────►      H–C–OH
    |                          |
  H–C–OH                     H–C–OH
    |                          |
   CH₂OH                      COOH
  D-glucose              D-glucuronic acid
```

Reduction Reaction

Aldoses and ketoses may be reduced (enzymatically or nonenzymatically) to corresponding polyhydroxy alcohols:

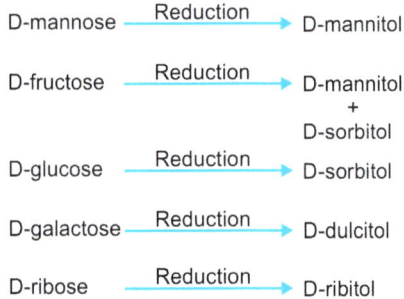

Sorbitol concentration increases in the lens in diabetic cataract.

Action of Phenylhydrazine

1. The presence of a free aldehyde or ketone group in the molecule is essential for the osazone formation (**Fig. 6.2**).

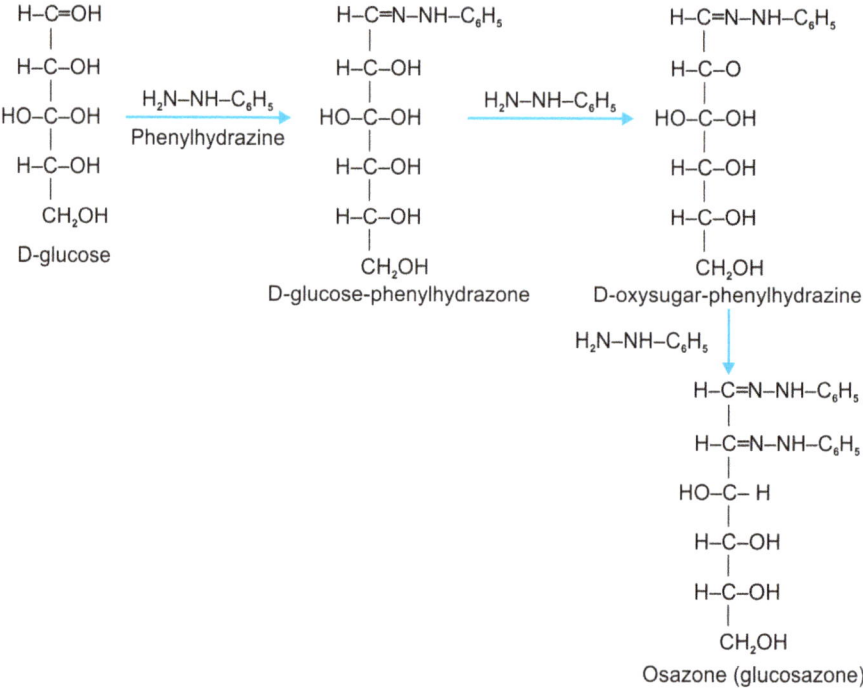

Fig. 6.2: Action of phenylhydrazine and osazone formation.

2. This osazone formation is helpful in the characterization and identification of different sugars having closely related properties.
3. Osazones are yellow or orange crystalline derivatives of reducing sugars with phenylhydrazine.
4. Phenylhydrazine in acetic acid on heating to 100°C reacts with the carbonyl carbon of reducing sugar and forms glucose phenylhydrazine with the elimination of a water molecule.
5. Then, the second molecule of phenylhydrazine reacts with the second carbon of D-glucose-phenylhydrazine and creates carbonyl carbon group on it.
6. The third molecule of the phenylhydrazine reagent reacts with the newly formed carbonyl carbon with the elimination of water molecule.
7. The osazone formed from glucose (glucosazone), mannose (mannosazone), and fructose (fructosazone) are identical because they are similar in the carbon 3-6:
    a. Maltose forms maltosazone crystals, which are sunflower shaped.
    b. Lactose forms lactosazone crystals, which are powder puff or tennis ball shaped.
    c. Glucosazone is needle shaped.
    d. Therefore the osazone crystal formation helps to identify glucose, lactose, and maltose.
8. Sucrose will not form osazone due to the absence of a free carbonyl (aldehyde or keto) group.

GLYCOSIDIC BOND

Glycosidic bond is the linkage formed between –OH group of anomeric carbon of one sugar with any –OH group of another sugar (or alcohol), which results in the loss of a water molecule. This linkage is involved in the formation of disaccharide and polysaccharides.

TESTS FOR CARBOHYDRATES

Reduction Tests

Due to the presence of a free aldehyde or ketone group, carbohydrates are readily oxidized and behave as the reducing agents. These sugars have the capacity to reduce cupric ion (Cu^{2+}) to cuprous ion (Cu^+). Therefore only the reducing sugars such as glucose will give positive reactions. Nonreducing sugars, i.e. sucrose will respond to these tests provided it is first hydrolyzed into its reducing components—glucose and fructose.

Benedict's Test

When 0.5-mL solution containing reducing sugar is boiled with 5.0-mL Benedict's reagent (blue color) for 5 minutes, brick red-, green-, or yellow-colored precipitate appears. This indicates the presence of reducing sugar in the given sample. This test is applied for the detection of reducing sugars in urine in the case of diabetes and galactosemia. (Benedict's reagent contains sodium citrate, sodium carbonate, and copper sulfate.)

SPECIAL CARBOHYDRATES OF CLINICAL IMPORTANCE

Amino Sugars

Sugars containing an amino (NH_2) group in their structure are called amino sugars, e.g. D-glucosamine. N-acetyl derivative of D-glucosamine and D-galactosamine occurs as a constituent of mucopolysaccharides. It is also present in some antibiotics.

Glycosides

Glycosides are compounds containing a carbohydrate and a noncarbohydrate residue in a same molecule linked together by a glycosidic bond.

Cardiac glycosides:
- Digitoxin or digoxin—stimulates muscular contraction (cardiac stimulant)
- Streptomycin—antibiotic used in treatment of tuberculosis
- Cardiac glycosides—used in cardiac insufficiency
- Ouabain—a sodium pump inhibitor.

Sialic Acid

Sialic acid is N-acetylneuraminic acid (NANA). It is present in mucopolysaccharide, glycolipid, and ganglioside.

Sugar Alcohols

D-Sorbitol and D-dulcitol, when accumulated in large amounts, cause strong osmotic effects leading to swelling of cells, including cataract, peripheral neuropathy, and nephropathy.

D-Mannitol: Is useful in reducing intracranial tension by forced diuresis.

Xylitol—sweetener.

Deoxy Sugar

Deoxy sugar lacks one oxygen atom in carbon and two or three of a carbohydrate.
For example:
- Deoxyribose: It is present in nucleic acid DNA.
- 6-deoxy-L-galactose or fructose: It is present on cell membrane.

Glycoproteins

Glycoproteins are proteins to which carbohydrates are covalently attached, e.g. immunoglobulin and egg albumin.

Proteoglycans

Proteoglycans are also proteins to which carbohydrates are covalently attached, but the carbohydrates differ chemically from those attached to glycoproteins. The carbohydrates may be glucosamine or galactosamine and/or their acetyl derivatives, uronic acids, and sulfate groups.

SUMMARY

Carbohydrates are organic substances of polyhydroxy aldehyde or ketone derivatives. They are classified into monosaccharides (glucose), disaccharides (sucrose), oligosaccharides (maltotriose), and polysaccharides. Polysaccharides are of two types—homo (starch, glycogen, cellulose, and inulin) and heteropolysaccharides (hyaluronic acid, dermatan sulfate, keratan sulfate, and heparin). Carbohydrates form stereoisomers, such as D- and L-sugars, and they are referred to as enantiomers (mirror images of each other). Carbon 1 of sugars is anomeric carbon atom (α-D-glucose and β-D-glucose). The isomers formed due to variations in the configuration of –H and –OH around a single carbon atom in a sugar molecule is called epimers (mannose and galactose are two and four epimers of glucose, respectively). Sucrose, also called invert sugar, is nonreducing.

SELF-ASSESSMENT QUESTIONS

1. Define carbohydrates.
2. Classify the carbohydrates with a suitable example for each class.
3. Explain the stereoisomerism of carbohydrates.
4. How monosaccharides are further classified?
5. What are the two types of polysaccharides?
6. Define the asymmetric carbon atom.
7. Explain the term "mutarotation."
8. What are disaccharides? Give example and composition.
9. What are proteoglycans and mucopolysaccharides?
10. Write briefly on mucopolysaccharide. Write their biomedical importance.
11. Discuss on the structure of starch and glycogen.
12. Differentiate between amylose and amylopectin.
13. If the two monosaccharides differ in the configuration around a single carbon atom, then what are they called as?
14. Name the nonreducing disaccharide.
15. Name the α- and β-cyclic forms of D-glucose?
16. Name the noncarbohydrate moiety present in glycoside.
17. Give an example for a glycoside.
18. Name the polysaccharide employed for the assessment of kidney function tests.
19. Name the glycosaminoglycan that serves as a lubricant and shock absorbent of joints.

MULTIPLE-CHOICE QUESTIONS

1. Which of the following is not an aldose sugar?
   a. Glucose b. Galactose
   c. Mannose d. Fructose
2. One of the following serves as an anticoagulant:
   a. Heparin
   b. Hyaluronic acid
   c. Chondroitin sulfate
   d. Keratan sulfate
3. The polysaccharide containing β-glycosidic linkage is:
   a. Starch b. Glycogen
   c. Dextrin d. Cellulose
4. In general, the carbon atoms involved in reducing action are:
   a. 1 and 2 b. 2 and 3
   c. 3 and 4 d. 5 and 6
5. Concerning glucose, all of the following statements are true, *except*:
   a. It is an aldohexose
   b. It is a reducing sugar
   c. It is present in starch and cellulose
   d. It is an epimer of fructose
6. The glycosaminoglycan, which does not contain uronic acid, is:
   a. Heparin
   b. Hyaluronic acid
   c. Chondroitin sulfate
   d. Keratan sulfate
7. Which of the following is a deoxy sugar?
   a. Ribose b. Fucose
   c. Glucosamine d. Xylulose
8. _____ is not found in glycosaminoglycan.
   a. L-Iduronic acid
   b. D-glucuronic acid
   c. Ribose
   d. *N*-Acetylgalactosamine
9. _____ is a heteropolysaccharide.
   a. Dextrin b. Chitin
   c. Inulin d. Heparin

Chemistry of Carbohydrates

10. Concerning starch, one of the following statements is incorrect:
    a. Starch is made of both linear and branched polysaccharide
    b. Starch gives red color with I_2 reactions
    c. Starch can be hydrolyzed to glucose in the body
    d. Glycogen is known as animal starch

11. One of the following is an example of invert sugar:
    a. Glucose   b. Fructose
    c. Sucrose   d. Maltose

12. All the following are the examples of monosaccharide, *except*:
    a. Glucose   b. Fructose
    c. Sucrose   d. Galactose

13. The bond, which links the monosaccharide units, is:
    a. Ester bond   b. Phosphate bond
    c. Disulfide bond   d. Glycosidic bond

14. All of the following polysaccharides contain glucose as the monosaccharide units *except*:
    a. Starch   b. Inulin
    c. Glycogen   d. Dextrin

15. Regarding amylopectin component of starch, the following statements are true, *except*:
    a. It is highly branched
    b. It is unbranched
    c. It gives reddish-violet color with iodine
    d. Its amount present in starch is 80–85%

16. Concerning glycogen, one of the following statements is incorrect:
    a. A polymer of glucose
    b. Stored in liver and muscle
    c. Stored in liver and brain
    d. Having 11–18 glucose residues between any branching points

17. Concerning cellulose, one of the following statements is incorrect:
    a. Contains β-D-glucose and β-1,4-glycosidic bonds
    b. Digested by sucrase enzyme
    c. Acts as a dietary fiber
    d. Digested by cellulase enzyme

18. Regarding the heteropolysaccharides, the following statements are correct, *except*:
    a. Polymer of different monosaccharide units
    b. Heparin and chondroitin sulfate are the examples
    c. Components of ground substances throughout the extracellular space
    d. Glycogen and starch are the examples

19. All the following are the functions of heteropolysaccharides, *except*:
    a. Hyaluronic acid acts as a barrier in tissues against the penetration of bacteria
    b. Hyaluronidase present in testicular secretions helps in fertilization by favoring the entry of spermatozoa into the ovum
    c. Chondroitin sulfate acts as anticoagulant
    d. Heparin acts as anticoagulant in vitro as well as in vivo. It inhibits thrombin

20. Concerning stereoisomerism of carbohydrates, all the following statements are true, *except*:
    a. D- and L-sugars are referred to as enantiomers
    b. D-Sugars are utilized by humans
    c. When the sugar has –OH group on right, it is D-isomer
    d. When the sugar has –OH group on left, it is D-isomer

21. Anomerism means:
    a. Carbon 1, after ring formation becomes asymmetric and it is called anomeric carbon atom
    b. Carbon 6, after ring formation becomes asymmetric and it is called anomeric carbon atom
    c. Carbon 2, after ring formation becomes asymmetric and it is called anomeric carbon atom
    d. Mirror images

22. Regarding epimerism, all of the following statements are true, *except*:
    a. The isomers formed due to variations in the configuration of –H and –OH around a single carbon atom in a sugar molecule is called epimers
    b. Mannose is 2-epimer of glucose
    c. Galactose is 4-epimer of glucose
    d. Fructose is α-4-epimer of glucose

23. Which of the following is not a reducing sugar?
    a. Glucose   b. Sucrose
    c. Fructose   d. Mannose

24. Concerning carbohydrates, one of the following statements is incorrect:
    a. Are most abundant dietary source of energy for all organisms

b. Are precursors for many organic compounds such as fats and amino acids
c. Participate in the structure of cell membrane and cellular functions
d. Build the muscle mass

25. The monosaccharide, which is present in DNA, is:
   a. Glucose
   b. Ribose
   c. Fructose
   d. Mannose

26. The 2-epimer of glucose is:
   a. Mannose
   b. Galactose
   c. Ribose
   d. Gibulose

27. Glucose is an:
   a. Ketohexose
   b. Aldohexose
   c. Aldotriose
   d. Aldopentose

28. Polysaccharide, which has fructose as their monosaccharide unit, is:
   a. Starch
   b. Dextrin
   c. Inulin
   d. Cellulose

29. Concerning the structure of starch, one of the following statements is false:
   a. It has 85% of amylopectin
   b. Amylose is highly branched
   c. Blue color appears when amylose reacts with iodine
   d. The glucose units in amylose held by α-1,4-glycosidic linkage

30. Concerning cellulose, all the following statements are true, *except*:
   a. It has β-D-glucose joined by β-1,4-glycosidic bonds
   b. It is digested by cellulase enzyme in the humans
   c. It acts as dietary fiber
   d. It acts as a storage form of glucose

31. Which of the following is not a heteropolysaccharide?
   a. Hyaluronic acid
   b. Heparin
   c. Dextrin
   d. Chondroitin sulfate

32. 4-Epimer of glucose is:
   a. Galactose
   b. Mannose
   c. Fructose
   d. Maltose

33. All the following include answers of Benedict's test, *except*:
   a. Glucose
   b. Ascorbic acid
   c. Sucrose
   d. Fructose

34. Concerning stereoisomerism, all the following statements are true, *except*:
   a. D- and L-sugars are referred to as enantiomers
   b. Sugars in solution exist in ring form and not in the straight chain form
   c. Carbon 1 in aldo sugars is the anomeric carbon atom.
   d. Keto sugar forms pyranose ring

35. A 16-year-old male patient complains that lately after the ingestion of dairy products, he experiences bloating, cramps, flatulence, and sometimes diarrhea. Therefore the patient is intolerant to:
   a. Lactose
   b. Mannose
   c. Sucrose
   d. Maltose

36. This heteropolysaccharide has multiple uses in medicine that include its use in blood transfusions to prevent the blood from coagulating before administration, as anticoagulant therapy in prophylaxis and treatment of venous thrombosis and its extension in pulmonary embolisms, and in other similar situations:
   a. Hyaluronic acid
   b. Chondroitin sulfate
   c. Heparin
   d. Dermatan sulfate

37. Human beings do not have the enzymes necessary for the hydrolysis of the β-1,4-O-glycosidic linkages between molecules of glucose. That is why humans cannot digest this compound and it is part of some laxatives:
   a. Glycogen
   b. Cellulose
   c. Amylopectin
   d. Sucrose

Answers

1. d	2. a	3. d	4. a	5. d
6. d	7. b	8. c	9. d	10. b
11. c	12. c	13. d	14. b	15. b
16. c	17. b	18. d	19. c	20. d
21. a	22. d	23. b	24. d	25. b
26. a	27. b	28. b	29. b	30. c
31. c	32. a	33. c	34. d	35. a
36. c	37. b			

CHAPTER 7

Metabolism of Carbohydrates

OBJECTIVES

At the end of this chapter, students should be able to:
- Understand the digestion and absorption of carbohydrates
- Explain the process of various metabolism, including their regulation and significance
- Describe the blood glucose regulation
- Explain diabetes and the criteria to diagnose
- Know about various disorders of carbohydrate metabolism, including lactose intolerance.

DIGESTION AND ABSORPTION OF CARBOHYDRATES

Introduction

Digestion is the process of hydrolysis of naturally occurring foodstuffs into simpler forms. There are many digestive enzymes and other chemicals secreted from the gastrointestinal tract **(Table 7.1)**. The saliva of mouth contains salivary amylase and its action on foodstuffs is very limited.

- The carbohydrates, fat, and proteins present in our diet are of high-molecular weight complex compounds.
- They are absorbed only when they get hydrolyzed to simpler forms.
- The major carbohydrates of our diet such as starch and glycogen are the polysaccharides.
- Sucrose and lactose are two different disaccharides.
- Glucose and fructose are the monosaccharides, which need no digestion before they are absorbed because they are simpler sugars **(Figs. 7.1A and B)**.
- The polysaccharides are hydrolyzed to maltose and glucose by the action of number of enzymes.
- The digestion of carbohydrates starts in the mouth.
  1. Salivary amylase hydrolyzes α-1,4-glycosidic linkages randomly within the polysaccharide chain and produces disaccharides and monosaccharides.
  2. The further digestion takes place in the small intestine by the intestinal enzymes, which hydrolyze terminal α-1,4-glycosidic linkage.
  3. When acidic contents of stomach reaches duodenum, they stimulate mucosal cells of the duodenum to release *secretin* and *cholecystokinin*. These are two local hormones that stimulate the exocrine pancreas to release pancreatic juice into the intestinal lumen. Secretin stimulates the release of bicarbonate to neutralize the acidic chyme from the stomach and the cholecystokinin stimulates the release of digestive enzymes, including pancreatic amylase.
  4. After the food reaches the duodenum, pancreatic amylase also helps in the digestion of polysaccharides. This results in maltose, isomaltose, and a limit dextrin. The limit dextrins are smaller oligosaccharides containing 3–5 glucose units.

Metabolism of Carbohydrates

Table 7.1: Enzymes of gastrointestinal tract.

Gastric juice	Pancreatic juice	Intestinal juice
Pepsinogen (inactive form of the enzyme pepsin, which is secreted by chief cells of stomach)	Trypsinogen → trypsin	Aminopeptidase
Hydrochloric acid (HCl) (secreted by parietal cells)	Chymotrypsinogen (inactive form) → chymotrypsin (active form)	Dipeptidase
Intrinsic factor (parietal cells)	Procarboxypeptidase (inactive) → carboxypeptidase (active)	Nucleotidase
Mucin (mucus cells)	Amylase	Maltase
	Lipase	Sucrase
	Proelastase → elastase	Lactase
	Ribonuclease	Isomaltase

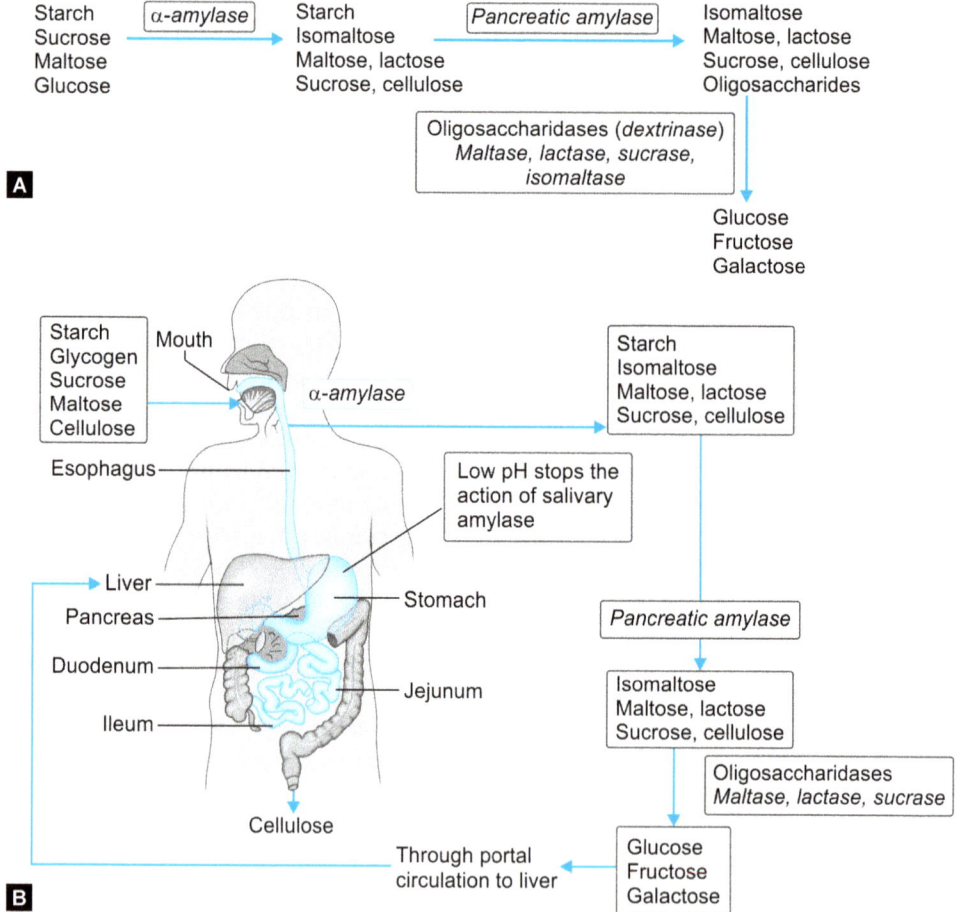

Figs. 7.1 A and B: Digestion of carbohydrates: (A) mechanism of digestion and (B) digestion in the gastrointestinal tract.

5. At the same time, disaccharidases such as maltase, lactase, and sucrase digest disaccharides, including maltose, lactose, and sucrose, respectively, into their respective monosaccharide units.
6. All the enzymes in the brush border membrane are disaccharidases except dextrinase (oligosaccharidase). These enzymes are protected from degradation by mucous known as glycocalyx present in the membrane.

Digestion of important food products
1. Cellulose is not digested further because humans do not produce and secrete 1,4-endoglycosidase in digestive juice. But this undigested cellulose helps in easy peristalsis and provides bulk to the feces.
2. Lactase deficiency results in **lactose intolerance.**

Absorption of Monosaccharides

- Monosaccharides formed are almost completely absorbed from the intestinal lumen through the mucosal epithelial cells into the bloodstream of the portal venous system **(Fig. 7.2)**.
- The galactose and glucose are absorbed very rapidly by the active process, which is linked to the transport of sodium, and require energy in the form of hydrolysis of high-energy phosphate bond adenosine triphosphate (ATP).
- Glucose cannot diffuse through lipid bilayer of the cell membrane because of its polar nature.
- Absorption from intestinal lumen into intestinal cell is by cotransport mechanism called sodium-dependent glucose transporter.
- It occurs against the concentration gradient and requires a carrier protein.
- Ouabain indirectly inhibits the glucose absorption.
- Fructose and mannose are absorbed by sodium-independent facilitated diffusion, which requires a carrier protein, but not energy. It occurs across the concentration gradient through portal circulation to liver.
- Sodium-independent transporter of glucose (GLUT-2) facilitates transport of sugars out of the mucosal cells, thereby entering the portal circulation to reach the liver.

Case 1:
A mother came to physician carrying her 2-year-old child with a complaint of history of abdominal cramps, diarrhea, and flatulence. She mentioned to physician that the symptoms appear about an hour after consuming food and disappear when she avoids dairy products.

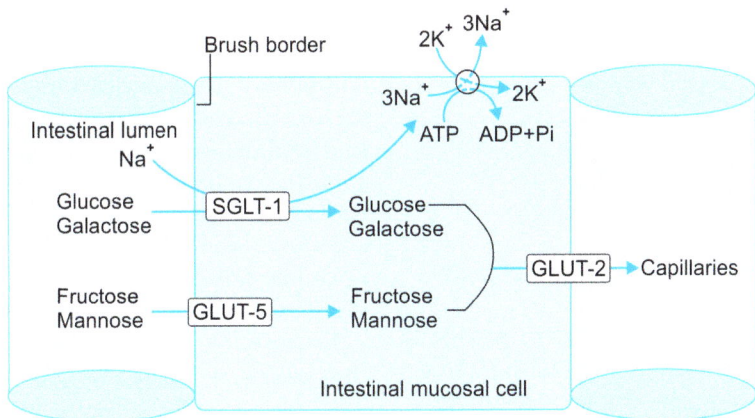

Fig. 7.2: Absorption of carbohydrates.

Laboratory investigation: Hydrogen breath test positive

Diagnosis: Lactose intolerance

Advice: Mother was advised to feed the child without dairy products

Lactose Intolerance

Cause: A deficiency of the brush border enzyme lactase found frequently in people of East Asian descent past their infant age

If lactose is not cleaved, it cannot be absorbed, so it makes its way "down the drain" from the small into the large intestine. Many of the bacteria found there have the capacity to metabolize lactose, which they convert to acids and gas. This leads to abdominal discomfort and diarrhea.

Since the environment in the large intestine lacks oxygen, hydrogen (H_2) generated in the bacterial fermentation is not oxidized but instead released as such and in part is exhaled.

An increase in exhaled hydrogen upon ingestion of lactose can be used to diagnose the condition.

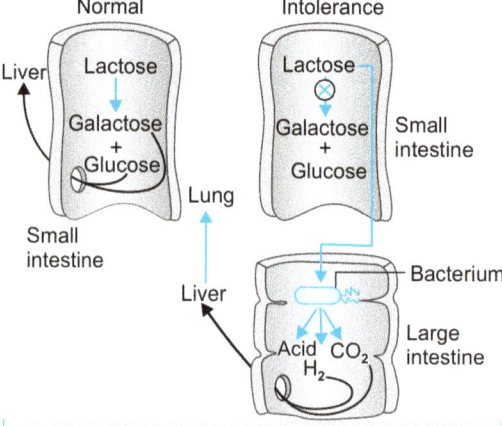

Treatment consists in omission of lactose in the diet.

Milk can be pretreated with purified bacterial α-galactosidase, rendering it suitable for consumption by lactose-intolerant individuals. Fermented milk products such as yoghurt and cheese are depleted of lactose by bacterial fermentation and therefore do not pose a problem for lactose-intolerant individuals.

Lactosuria: Second common reducing sugar found in the urine.

Observed in the urine of normal women during third trimester of pregnancy and lactation

Also seen in neonates.

METABOLISM OF CARBOHYDRATE

Introduction

Glucose is the main source of energy to our body. When glucose is oxidized, the free energy released is converted into energy in the form of ATP, which is the energy currency of our body. If the glucose is oxidized without trapping the free energy, then much of the energy will be wasted. Hence, the body preserves the energy in the form of ATP just as a battery cell.

In our body, glucose can be obtained from:
- Digestion of dietary carbohydrates **(Fig. 7.3)**.
- Glycogen breakdown.
- Gluconeogenesis (synthesis of glucose from noncarbohydrate sources). Different pathways, which involve glucose, are detailed next.

Glycolysis: It is a process of oxidation of glucose either to pyruvate or lactate.

Gluconeogenesis: Synthesis of glucose in liver and kidney using noncarbohydrate sources such as pyruvate, lactate, glycerol, propionic acid or from the carbon skeleton of glucogenic amino acids such as alanine and aspartic acid. Other pathways, which involve glucose, are:
- Hexose monophosphate (HMP) shunt
- Uronic acid pathway
- Interconversion of glucose, galactose, and fructose.

Glycogenesis: Synthesis of glycogen from glucose in liver or muscle for the purpose of storing glucose for energy is called glycogenesis.

Metabolism of Carbohydrates

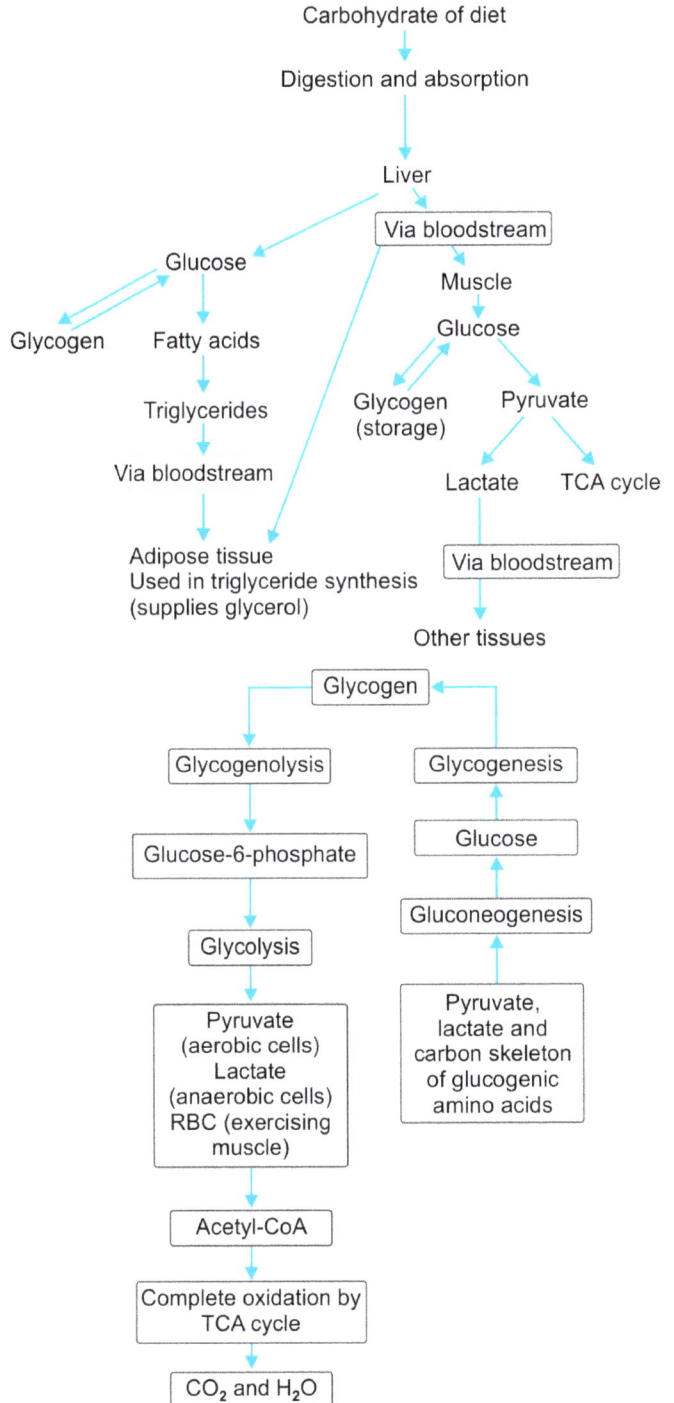

Fig. 7.3: Different pathways involving glucose.

Glycogenolysis: The formations of glucose or glucose-1-phosphate by breaking down glycogen in liver or muscle respectively are called glycogenolysis.

GLYCOLYSIS

Glycolysis involves the following steps:
- The pathway of breakdown or oxidation of glucose to yield energy is called glycolysis.
- This pathway is also called Embden–Meyerhof–Parnas pathway.
- This occurs in all types of living cells.
- It takes place in all the cells of the body.
- This is the source of energy in erythrocytes.
- Anaerobic glycolysis forms the major source of energy for muscle during exercise.
- This provides carbon skeletons for the synthesis of nonessential amino acids.
- Most of the reactions are reversible.
- The entry of glucose from extracellular fluid to cell is under the control of insulin.
- Glycolysis occurrence is prerequisite for the aerobic oxidation of carbohydrates.
- Aerobic oxidation takes place in cells possessing mitochondria.
- This is the major pathway for ATP synthesis in tissues lacking mitochondria, e.g. erythrocytes, cornea, and lens.

Aerobic Glycolysis

This occurs in cells in the presence of oxygen. They are the cells containing mitochondria actively using oxygen. Here glucose is broken down to two molecules of pyruvate and net ATP formed is equal to 7.0 ATP **(Fig. 7.4)**:
Site of occurrence: Cytosol.
1. Reactions of aerobic glycolysis **(Fig. 7.5)**: In the first step, the glucose is irreversibly activated to glucose-6-phosphate in the cell. This step is catalyzed by hexokinase enzyme using Mg^{2+} and ATP. In liver, glucokinase, the specific enzyme also catalyzes this reaction at higher concentration of glucose **(Table 7.2)**. Glucose-6-phosphate: Impermeable to the cell membrane. Central molecule with a variety of metabolic fates; glycolysis, glycogenesis, gluconeogenesis, and HMP shunt.
2. In the next step, glucose-6-phosphate is isomerized to fructose-6-phosphate by phosphohexose isomerase enzyme.
3. Fructose-6-phosphate is then irreversibly phosphorylated by phosphofructokinase (PFK) enzyme to fructose-1,6-bisphosphate (F-1,6-BP). F-1,6-BP contains two phosphoric acid groups at C1 and C6 of fructose via phosphate ester bond.
4. Fructose 1,6-bisphosphate (6-carbon sugar) is cleaved by aldolase enzyme to yield glyceraldehyde-3-phosphate and dihydroxyacetone phosphate [two 3-carbon sugars (trioses)].
5. *Dihydroxyacetone phosphate formed in the above* step can be converted back to glyceraldehyde-3-phosphate by phosphotriose isomerase enzyme.
6. Now, we have two molecules of glyceraldehyde-3-phosphate, which gets oxidized to 1,3-bisphosphoglycerate with the action of glyceraldehyde-3-phosphate dehydrogenase (DH) enzyme. This step utilizes inorganic phosphate (Pi) to convert glyceraldehyde-3-phosphate into 1,3-bisphosphoglycerate. In 1,3-bisphosphoglycerate, the phosphate group at carbon atom number 1 is the high-energy group.

During oxidation of glyceraldehyde-3-phosphate, the reducing equivalents are transferred to the acceptor nicotinamide adenine dinucleotide (NAD^+). The reduced NADH under aerobic conditions enters mitochondria and produces three molecules of ATP through its passage into electron transport chain (ETC) or respiratory chain. This type of formation of energy currency ATP through respiratory chain is called oxidative phosphorylation.

Metabolism of Carbohydrates

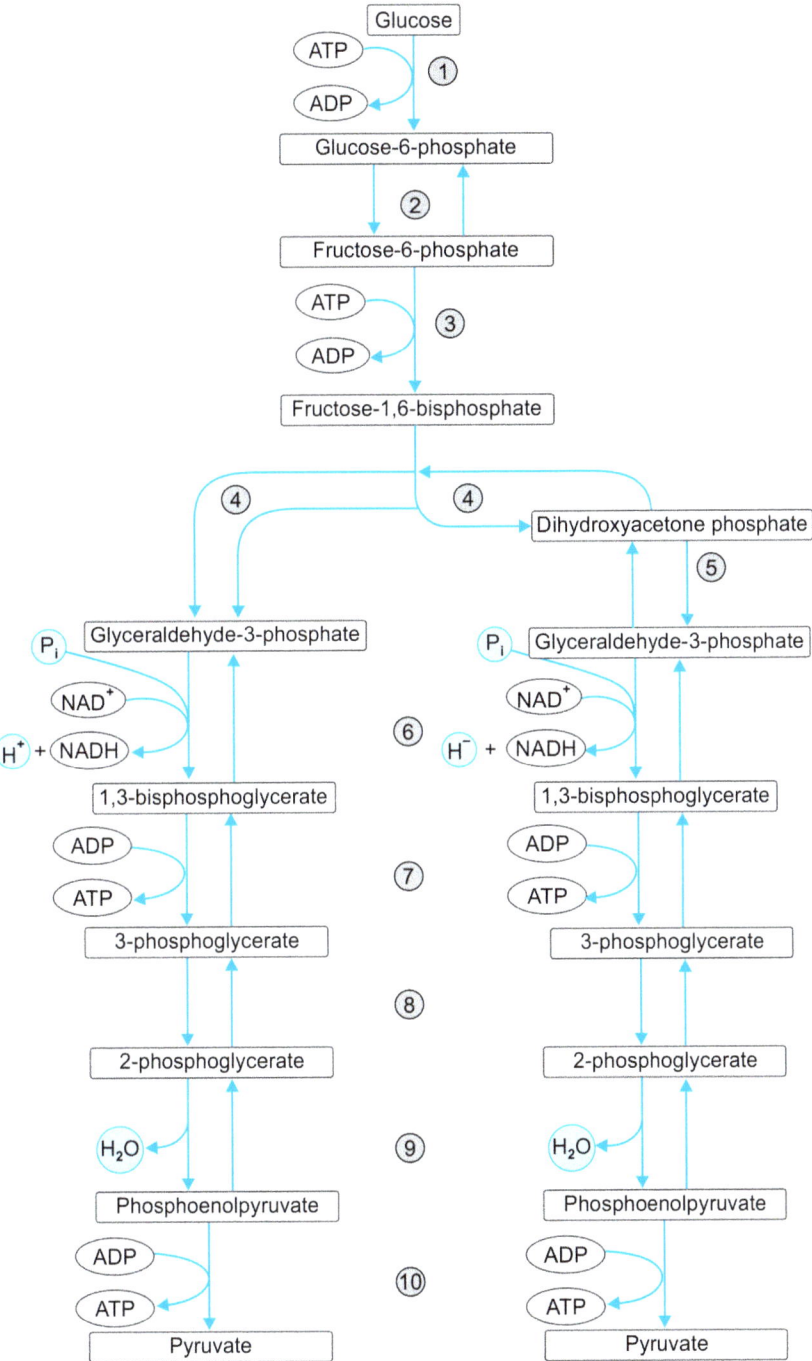

Fig. 7.4: Reactions of glycolysis (aerobic).

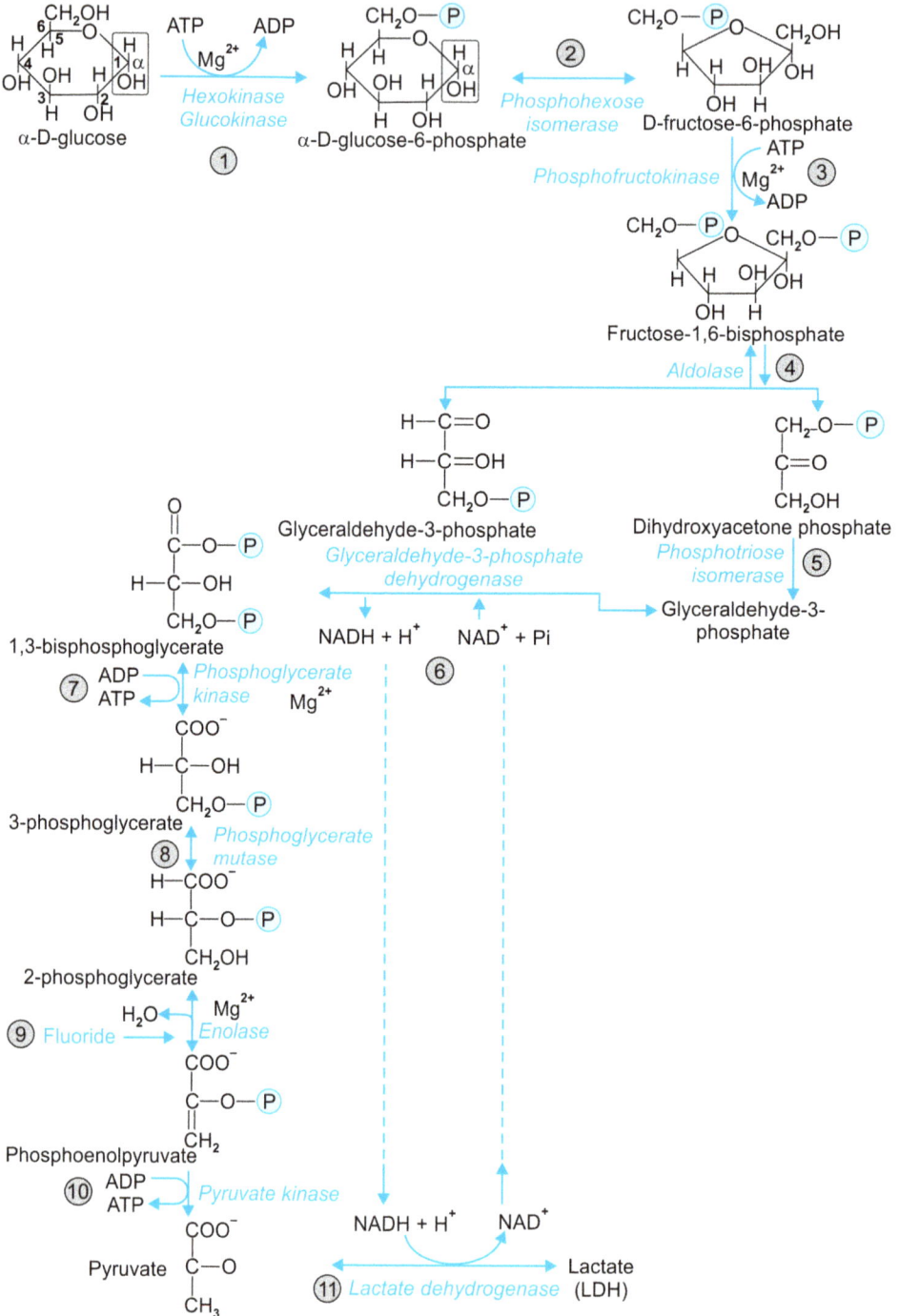

Fig. 7.5: Reactions of glycolysis (reactions showing aerobic and anaerobic steps).

Table 7.2: Features of glucokinase and hexokinase.

Glucokinase	Hexokinase
Presents in liver and pancreas	Presents in all tissues
Low affinity for glucose (high K_m)	High affinity for its substrate glucose (low K_m)
Specific for glucose	Catalyzes the phosphorylation of other hexoses
Not inhibited by glucose-6-phosphate	Inhibited by glucose-6-phosphate
Increases its synthesis in response to insulin	Not affected by insulin
It functions to remove glucose from the blood, when blood glucose increases	It functions to ensure enough supply of glucose from the blood for the tissues irrespective of the blood glucose concentration

7. In the next step, the high-energy compound 1,3-bisphosphoglycerate transfers its high energy to ADP, to form ATP resulting in the formation of 3-phosphoglycerate. This reaction is catalyzed by phosphoglycerate kinase enzyme. This type of formation of energy currency (ATP) by high-energy substrate is called substrate-level phosphorylation.
8. The 3-phosphoglycerate is then isomerized to 2-phosphoglycerate by phosphoglycerate mutase enzyme.
9. Then the 2-phosphoglycerate is converted into one more high-energy compound called phosphoenolpyruvate. This reaction is catalyzed by enolase enzyme. The activity of this enzyme is completely inhibited by fluoride. Hence, fluoride is used during blood collection for glucose estimation. This prevents the utilization of glucose by red blood cell (RBC).
10. Phosphoenolpyruvate is converted to pyruvate by pyruvate kinase enzyme. In this step, one molecule of ATP is formed through substrate-level phosphorylation. Under aerobic conditions, pyruvate is the end product of glycolysis. Hence, pyruvate is then converted into acetyl-CoA or oxaloacetate in the mitochondria. Fructose is more rapidly oxidized by the liver than glucose, because it bypasses the step in glucose oxidation catalyzed by PFK.

Anaerobic Glycolysis

This occurs in the cells under hypoxic conditions. During severe exercises, there will be depletion of oxygen in the tissues. Also RBC gets its energy by anaerobic glycolysis. Two molecules of lactate are formed as the end product. In this type, only two molecules of ATP are formed.

If anaerobic conditions prevail, the reoxidation of NADH (formed in step 6) by transfer of reducing equivalents through the respiratory chain to oxygen is prevented and gets reoxidized by conversion of pyruvate to lactate by lactate DH enzyme. Thus the number of ATP produced will be less in anaerobic condition.

Steps 6 and 11 are linked to operate the pathway in anaerobic condition **(Fig. 7.5)**:
- Glycolysis is the only major source of energy in anaerobiosis.
- For smooth operation of the pathway, NADH is to be converted to NAD^+.
- The formation of lactate allows the regeneration of NAD^+.
- NAD^+ reused by glyceraldehyde-3-phosphate DH so that glycolysis proceeds even in the absence of oxygen to supply ATP.
- Fate of pyruvate depends on the presence or absence oxygen in the cells.
- The occurrence of uninterrupted glycolysis is very important in skeletal muscle during strenuous exercise.
- Brain, retina, renal medulla, and GI tract derive energy from glycolysis.
- Glycolysis in the erythrocytes leads to the production of lactate, since the mitochondria, the centers for oxidation, are absent.

Energetics of Aerobic Glycolysis

- Energy consuming steps of glycolysis are:
  - Step 1 and step 3 → 2 ATP.
- Energy-yielding steps of glycolysis are:
  - Oxidative phosphorylation
    Step 6 → NADH × 2 → 2.5 ATP × 2 = 5.0 ATP.
  - Substrate-level phosphorylation
    Step 7 and step 10 → 2 ATP × 2 = 4 ATP.
- Total ATP produced = 9.0 ATP
- Net ATP production (9.0–2) = 7.0 ATP.

Energetics of Anaerobic Glycolysis

- Energy-consuming steps of glycolysis are:
  - Step 1 and step 2 → 2 ATP.
- Energy-yielding steps of anaerobic glycolysis are:
  - Substrate-level phosphorylation
    Step 7 and step 10 → 2 ATP × 2 = 4 ATP.
- Total ATP produced = 4 ATP
- Net ATP production (4–2) = 2 ATP.

Shuttle Pathways

If the cytosolic NADH uses malate–aspartate shuttle, 2.5 ATP are produced. If it uses glycerol phosphate shuttle, it produces 1.5 ATP.

Regulation of Glycolysis

The following list shows the regulation of glycolysis:
1. Insulin favors glycolysis by activating key glycolytic enzymes such as glucokinase, PFK-1, and pyruvate kinase **(Figs. 7.6A to C)**.
2. PFK-1 is the most important regulatory enzyme.
3. ATP, citrate, and H^+ ions are the important allosteric inhibitors.
4. F-2,6-BP, adenosine monophosphate (AMP), and Pi are the allosteric activators of PFK-1.
5. Pyruvate kinase is an inducible enzyme that increases its synthesis in response to insulin and decreases in response to glucagon.
6. Glucocorticoid inhibits glycolysis and favors gluconeogenesis.
7. Glucose-6-phosphate inhibits hexokinase and the enzyme prevents the accumulation of glucose-6-phosphate.

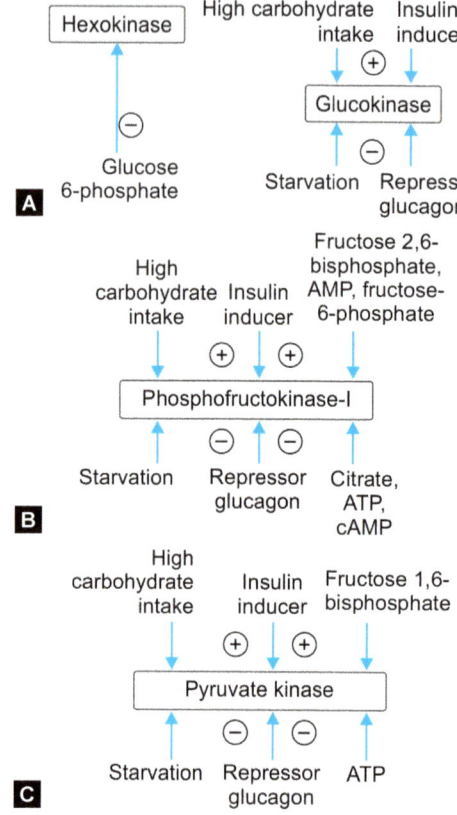

Figs. 7.6A to C: Regulation of glycolysis through various enzymes: (A) glucokinase, (B) phosphofructokinase, and (C) pyruvate kinase.

Role of Fructose-2,6-bisphosphate and Regulation by Phosphofructokinase-2 in the Regulation of Blood Glucose

1. It is the most regulatory factor for controlling PFK and ultimately glycolysis in the liver.
2. The function of synthesis and degradation of F-2,6-BP is brought out by a single enzyme (with two active sites), which is called bifunctional or "tandem enzyme."

Metabolism of Carbohydrates

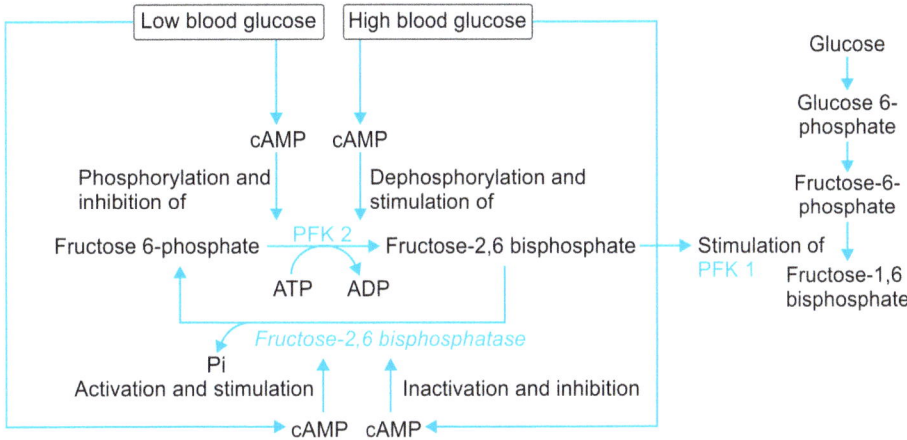

Fig. 7.7: Role of fructose-2,6-bisphosphatase and PFK-2 in regulation of blood glucose.
(PFK: phosphofructokinase.)

The activity of these enzymes is controlled by covalent modification, which in turn regulated by cyclic AMP (cAMP). The cAMP brings about the phosphorylation of the tandem enzyme, resulting in inactivation of active site of the enzyme, which is responsible for the synthesis of F-2,6-BP, but the activation of the active site of the enzyme hydrolyzes F-2,6-BP.

3. There is no stimulation, when F-2,6-BP decreases with low blood glucose, as the PFK-1 remains inactive (**Fig. 7.7**).

Rapoport–Luebering Cycle and Its Significance

Rapoport–Luebering Cycle

This cycle comprises the following steps:
- It is the side reaction of the glycolytic pathway, occurring in erythrocytes (**Fig. 7.8**).
- Kinase reaction of glycolysis is bypassed in the erythrocytes.
- No energy is trapped during the formation of 2,3-biphosphoglycerate (2,3-BPG).
- BPG, when combines with hemoglobin (Hb), reduces the affinity of Hb toward oxygen. In the presence of 2,3-BPG oxyhemoglobin will unload oxygen more easily in tissues. This is the reason

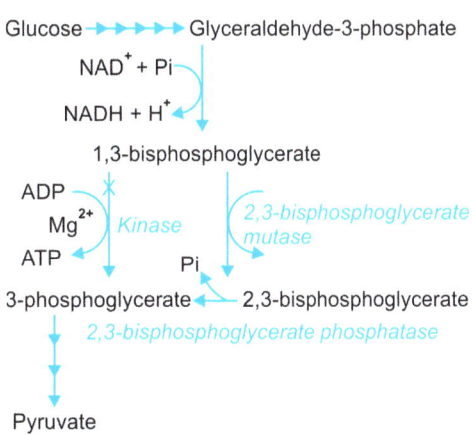

Fig. 7.8: Rapoport–Luebering cycle.

for increased 2,3-BPG during hypoxic condition.
- About 15–25% of the lactate formed goes through this pathway.
- In hexokinase deficiency, phosphorylation does not take place further. So 2,3-BPG decreases. Then affinity to Hb increases.

COMPOUNDS FORMED FROM PYRUVATE

Under aerobic conditions, pyruvate is transported into mitochondria via pyruvate transporter. Then it is dehydrogenated to acetyl-CoA by pyruvate DH complex enzyme.

Metabolism of Carbohydrates

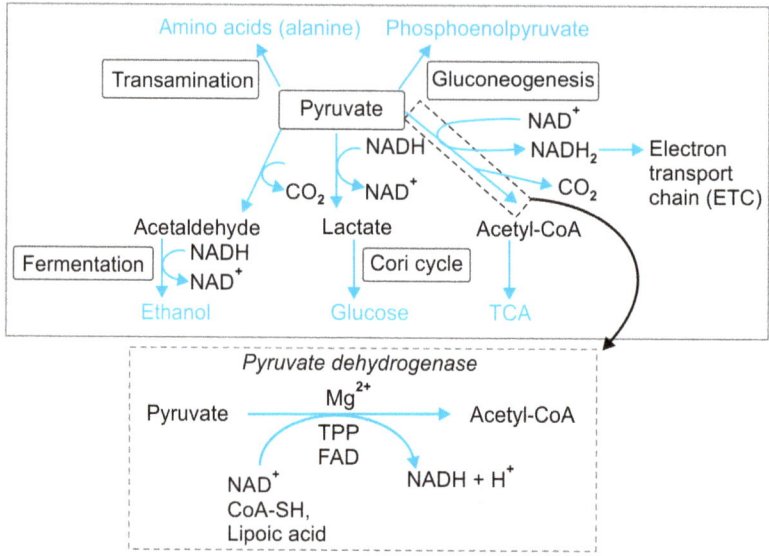

Fig. 7.9: Metabolic fates of pyruvate and the compounds formed.

This enzyme requires five coenzymes derived from water-soluble vitamin [they are thiamine pyrophosphate (TPP), coenzyme A (CoA-SH), NAD^+, flavin adenine dinucleotide (FAD)], and lipoic acid **(Fig. 7.9)**.

What happens if pyruvate dehydrogenase is inhibited and what is the significance of lactate determination? Explain why anaerobic glycolysis takes place in cancer cells?
- The arsenic and mercuric ions react with the SH groups of lipoic acid and inhibit pyruvate dehydrogenase, as does a dietary deficiency of thiamin, allowing pyruvate to accumulate. Alcoholics are thiamine deficient and may develop pyruvic and lactic acidosis. Patients with inherited pyruvate dehydrogenase deficiency develop lactic acidosis after a glucose load.
- The determination of blood lactate is very useful in assessing the presence and severity of shock and to monitor the patient recovery.
- The lactate determination also helps in the early detection of oxygen debt (excess oxygen required to recover from the anoxic episodes) in various disorders.
- In cancer, the cancer cells stimulate the glucose uptake and glycolysis. As the cancer cells grow rapidly, blood vessels are unable to supply desired oxygen. Therefore the metabolic adoption will occur for the survival of cancer cells and they continue to grow in the absence of oxygen. In this condition, the glucose is oxidized anaerobically to lactic acid to supply ATP for tumor cells.
- Alcoholics develop thiamine deficiency due to the inhibition of transport of thiamine through intestinal mucosal cells. Lack of TPP, a coenzyme form of thiamine, inhibits the pyruvate dehydrogenase, which results in the conversion of pyruvate to lactate, which leads to lactic acidosis and neurological disorders.

COMPOUNDS FORMED FROM ACETYL-COA

Metabolic Fates of Acetyl-CoA

The metabolic fates of acetyl-CoA detailed in citric acid cycle **(Fig. 7.10)**.

Metabolism of Carbohydrates

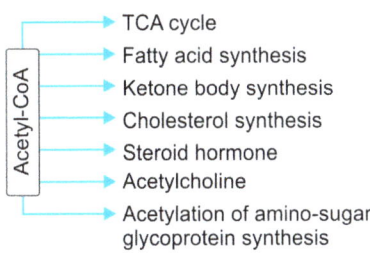

Fig. 7.10: Metabolic fates of acetyl-CoA.

TCA CYCLE

Krebs Citric Acid Cycle

Citric acid cycle is also called tricarboxylic acid (TCA) cycle because of the presence of three COOH group in citric acid.

Site of occurrence: Mitochondria.

These reactions occur in a cyclic manner and generate large amounts of ATP since the enzymes of the cycle are located in mitochondria facilitating the transfer of reducing equivalents from Krebs cycle to the respiratory chain, the enzymes of which are also located in the inner mitochondrial membrane:

1. In the first step of Krebs citric acid cycle, acetyl-CoA, which is formed from pyruvate under aerobic condition and also by fatty acid (FA) oxidation combined with oxaloacetic acid and forms citric acid (a TCA). The reaction is catalyzed by a condensing enzyme citrate synthase (Fig. 7.11).
2. Citrate is converted into isocitrate by the action of aconitase enzyme. Isocitrate undergoes dehydrogenation by the isocitrate dehydrogenase enzyme in the third step to oxalosuccinate. Molecule of NADH formed enters ETC and forms 3 ATPs.
3. Decarboxylation of oxalosuccinate to form α-ketoglutarate (α-KG) with the help of isocitrate dehydrogenase enzyme.
4. The α-KG undergoes decarboxylation to form succinyl-CoA in a manner similar to the conversion of pyruvate to acetyl-CoA, which is catalyzed by α-KG dehydrogenase enzyme. One molecule of NADH formed enters ETC and forms 3 ATPs.
5. Succinyl-CoA is then converted into succinate by the enzyme succinate thiokinase. In this step, a high-energy phosphate is produced by **substrate-level phosphorylation**.
6. Dehydrogenation of succinate is catalyzed by inner mitochondrial membrane enzyme succinate DH. This step produces 1.5 ATPs because of production of one molecule of flavin adenine dinucleotide ($FADH_2$).
7. Fumarase catalyzes the addition of water molecule to fumarate and forms malate.
8. Malate is converted into oxaloacetate by malate DH enzyme with the production of one molecule of NADH, which is equivalent to 2.5 ATPs.

Points to Note

a. Citrate → *Cis*-aconitate → Isocitrate → Oxalosuccinate.
b. *Cis*-aconitate is a transient one with very short half-life. Immediately a molecule of H_2O is added to it and forms isocitrate.
c. Isocitrate CO_2 → oxalosuccinate → α-KG. It is an oxidative decarboxylation. Oxalosuccinate is an unstable form, so it undergoes spontaneous decarboxylation to from α-KG. In each turn of TCA cycle, it yields 12 ATPs: Ten ATPs are formed per turn of TCA cycle:
Step 3,4, 8 (3 NADH+) →3 × 2.5 ATP = 7.5 ATP
Step 6 (1 FADH2) → 1.5 ATP = 1.5 ATP
Step 5 (1 ATP) → 1 ATP = 1 ATP
10 ATP

Total number of ATPs formed by the complete oxidation of glucose is = 32 ATP
From aerobic glycolysis = 9ATP
Action of pyruvate dehydrogenase (2.5 × 2) = 5 ATP
TCA cycle (2 mole pyruvate)10 ATP × 2 = 20 ATP
34 ATP
Number of ATPs utilized = 2 ATP
ATP Total = 32 ATP

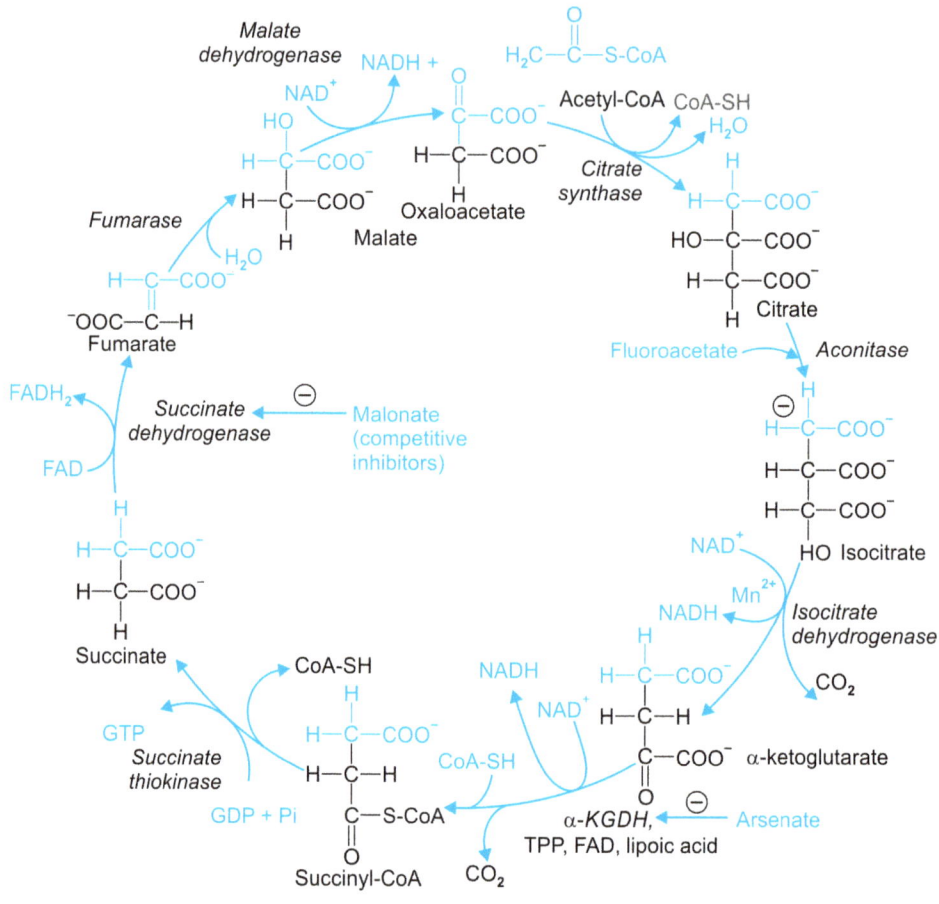

Fig. 7.11: Reactions of TCA cycle.
(TCA: tricarboxylic acid.)

Inhibitors that inhibit the enzymes of TCA cycle are:
- Fluoroacetate for aconitase
- Arsenate for α-KG DH
- Malonate for succinate DH (competitive).

Regulation of Tricarboxylic Acid Cycle

The TCA cycle is controlled by respiratory rate, which is proportional to the energy consumption. The level of NAD^+ also stimulates the TCA cycle:
1. Citrate synthase: Inhibited by ATP, NADH, acyl-CoA, and succinyl-CoA.
2. Isocitrate DH: Inhibited by ATP and NADH, and activated by ADP.
3. α-KG: Inhibited by NADH and succinyl-CoA.
4. The availability of ADP is important to proceed the TCA cycle, if not oxidation of NADH and $FADH_2$ through electron chain stops. Accumulation of NADH and $FADH_2$ inhibits the enzymes of TCA cycle.

Importance of Tricarboxylic Acid Cycle

The importance of TCA cycle is as follows:
1. The TCA cycle is the energy producing final pathway for the oxidation of glucose and

acetyl-CoA formed from FA breakdown, and from the product of breakdown of amino acids.
2. It also provides citrate for FA synthesis.
3. The intermediates of TCA cycle are used for the synthesis of amino acids and glucose by gluconeogenesis.
4. Since citric acid cycle is involved in the synthesis as well as breakdown of biological compounds, it is called amphibolic pathway (anabolic and catabolic). TCA cycle takes part in gluconeogenesis, transamination, deamination, and synthesis of FAs.

Amphibolic Role of Tricarboxylic Acid Cycle

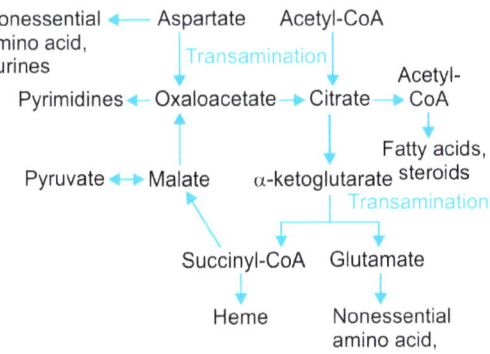

Anapleurotic Reactions of Tricarboxylic Acid Cycle

The following list shows the anapleurotic reactions of TCA cycle:
1. The reactions concerned to replenish the intermediates of TCA cycle are called anaplerotic reactions or anaplerosis (Fig. 7.12).
2. The intermediates of TCA cycle α-KG, succinate and oxaloacetate, can be removed from the TCA cycle to synthesize many compounds required by the human body.
3. For example, the acids such as succinate and α-KG are removed to synthesize heme- and gamma-aminobutyrate, respectively.

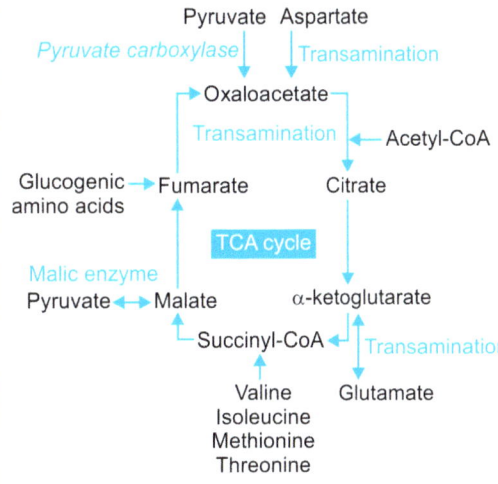

Fig. 7.12: Anaplerotic reactions.

Like this many of the intermediates of the TCA cycle are removed to synthesize the compounds. If this continues, the rate of TCA cycle may decrease. However, the intermediates of the TCA cycle can be replenished again by the action of certain enzymes by the following reaction:

Glyoxylate Cycle

This cycle comprises the following steps:
- Glyoxylate cycle is a modification of the TCA cycle, which occurs in plants and some microorganisms.
- This will not occur in animals due to absence of enzymes isocitrate lyase and malate synthase.
- In plants glyoxylate cycle occurs in cytoplasmic organelles and glyoxysomes.
- In each turn of the glyoxylate cycle, two molecules of acetate and one molecule of succinate are formed, which is used for the synthesis of glucose.
- Acetyl-CoA condenses with oxaloacetate to form citrate, which is then isomerized to isocitrate. The isocitrate is cleaved by lyase into succinate and glyoxylate. This glyoxylate combines with another molecule of acetyl-CoA to form malate by malate synthase. Malate finally oxidized to oxaloacetate.

GLUCONEOGENESIS AND ITS IMPORTANCE IN REGULATING THE BLOOD GLUCOSE

Gluconeogenesis

It is the process of formation of glucose from the various noncarbohydrate sources such as the glucogenic amino acids **(Figs. 7.13 and 7.14)** (refer Chapter 4 "Chemistry of Amino Acids and Proteins"), lactate, pyruvate, glycerol, or propionate.

Gluconeogenesis occurs in the fasting state or on a low-carbohydrate diet particularly in liver and some other tissues, which are solely dependent on glucose for their energy demand. The major metabolic significance of gluconeogenesis is to maintain the blood glucose level and to supply glucose for brain and cardiac muscle.

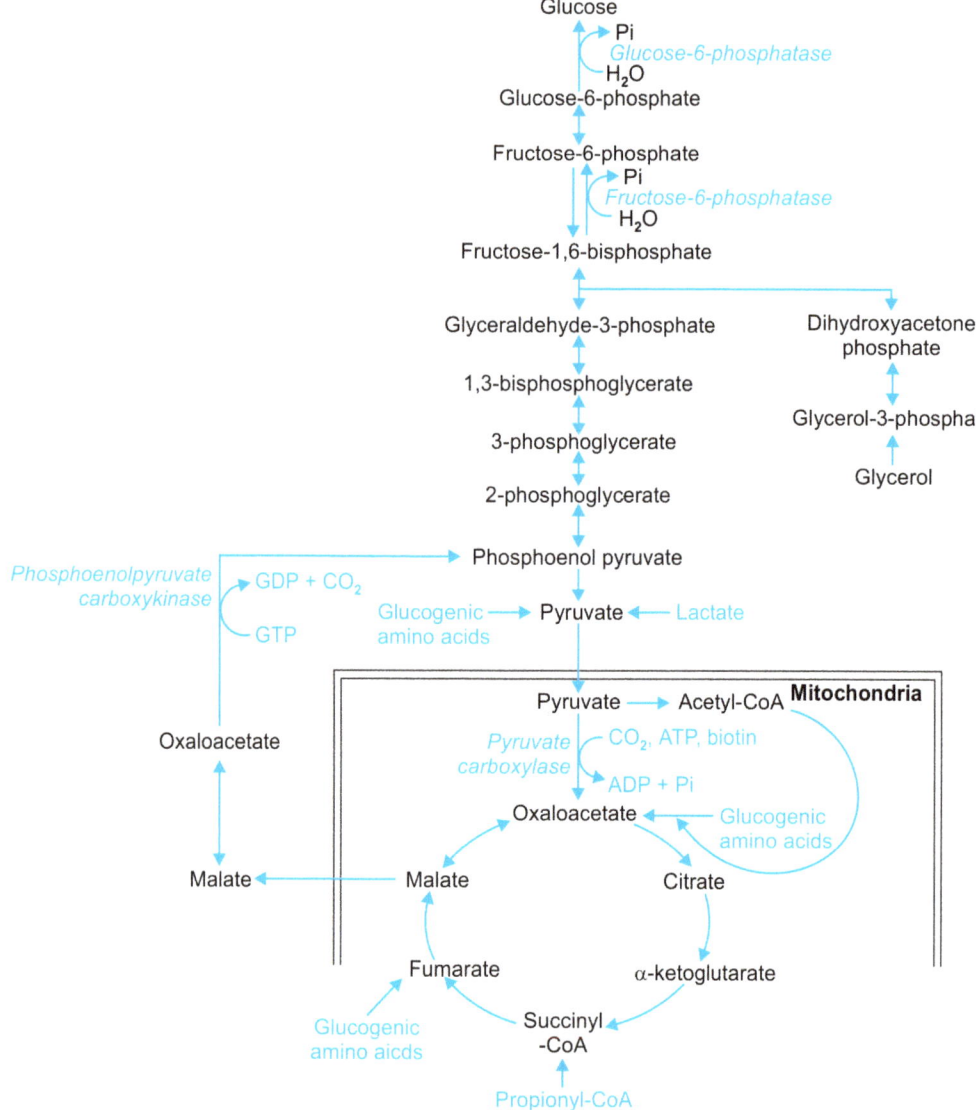

Fig. 7.13: Gluconeogenesis.

Metabolism of Carbohydrates

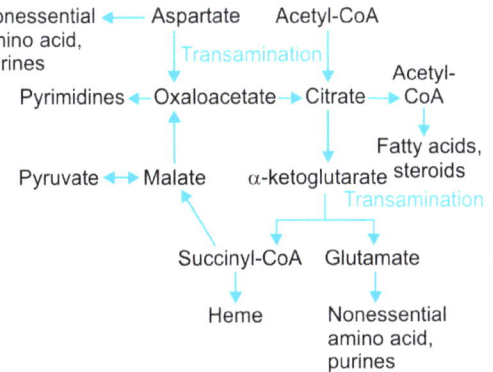

Fig. 7.14: Glucogenic amino acid.

Glycolysis is the breakdown of glucose, whereas gluconeogenesis is the synthesis of glucose from noncarbohydrate sources. But, both these process are not exactly reciprocal to each other. This is because three reactions in glycolysis are of irreversible nature:
- It mainly occurs in cytosol.
- Some precursors are produced in the mitochondria.
- It takes place in liver and kidney.
- Synthesis of glucose or glycogen from noncarbohydrates such as pyruvate, lactate, glucogenic amino acids, glycerol, and propionic acid.
- Pathway involves steps of TCA cycle and reversal of glycolysis.
- The three irreversible steps of glycolysis are catalyzed by hexokinase, PFK, and pyruvate kinase.
- These three stages are bypassed by alternate enzymes specific to gluconeogenesis and they are called key enzymes of gluconeogenesis:

- Pyruvate carboxylase
- Phosphoenolpyruvate carboxykinase (PEPCK)
- Fructose-1,6-bisphosphatase
- Glucose-6-phosphatase.
- The pathway meets the needs of the body for glucose.
- Continuous supply of glucose as a source of energy for the CNS, brain, RBC, and skeletal muscle during starvation.

Regulation of Gluconeogenesis

The following lists the regulation of gluconeogenesis (Fig. 7.15):
1. The hormone glucagon and the availability of substrates are mainly regulating gluconeogenesis.
2. Glucagon and glucocorticoid increase gluconeogenesis.
3. Insulin inhibits gluconeogenesis.
4. Glucagon inactivates pyruvate kinase (which converts phosphoenolpyruvate to pyruvate) through cAMP-dependent phosphorylation.
5. Glucagon reduces the concentration of F-2,6-BP so that PFK-1 remains inactive and activates fructose-1,6-bisphosphatase that increases gluconeogenesis.
6. Glucogenic amino acids have stimulating effect on key gluconeogenic enzymes.
7. Acetyl-CoA promotes gluconeogenesis.
8. Starvation results in excessive lipolysis in adipose tissues. The FAs released are oxidized and the acetyl-CoA accumulates in the liver. This acetyl-CoA stimulates the gluconeogenic enzymes.

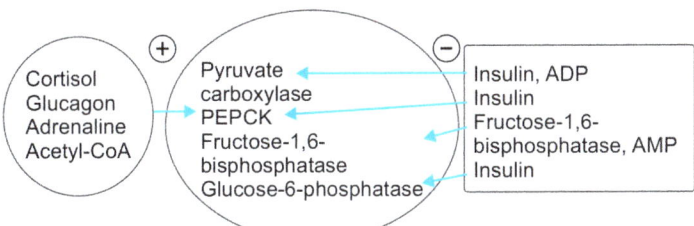

Fig. 7.15: Regulation of gluconeogenesis.

Substrates for Gluconeogenesis

Lactate and glucogenic amino acids are the most important substrates; methylmalonyl-CoA and glycerol also form glucose **(Figs. 7.16A and B)**.

Glucose Alanine Cycle

Alanine is the major amino acid released from muscle to liver during fasting by glucose alanine cycle. Some of the pyruvate resulting from glycolysis in skeletal muscle and transaminated to alanine and transported to liver, where it is converted back to pyruvate. This pyruvate in the liver is used to synthesize glucose, which is returned to muscle. This is one of the processes also used to maintain nitrogen balance **(Fig. 7.17)**.

CORI CYCLE AND ITS CLINICAL IMPORTANCE

The following lists the information about Cori cycle:

1. Glucose/glycogen is converted to lactate in the muscle and this lactate is converted back to glucose in liver **(Fig. 7.18)**.
2. During active muscle contraction, the glycogen breaks down and glucose6-phosphate formed enters anaerobic glycolysis to generate lactate, which enters the blood and then to the live. It will be converted to glucose in liver. Glucose enters the blood and back to tissues. It can be summarized as:

Muscle → Lactate → Blood → Liver → Glucose → Blood → Back to tissues.

This whole process is called Cori cycle. Acetyl-CoA is not converted to glucose in humans due to:

1. Irreversible reaction, catalyzed by pyruvate DH, prevents the direct conversion of acetyl-CoA to pyruvate.
2. There is no net conversion of acetyl-CoA to oxaloacetate via TCA cycle. Only one molecule is regenerated, which is used during TCA cycle.

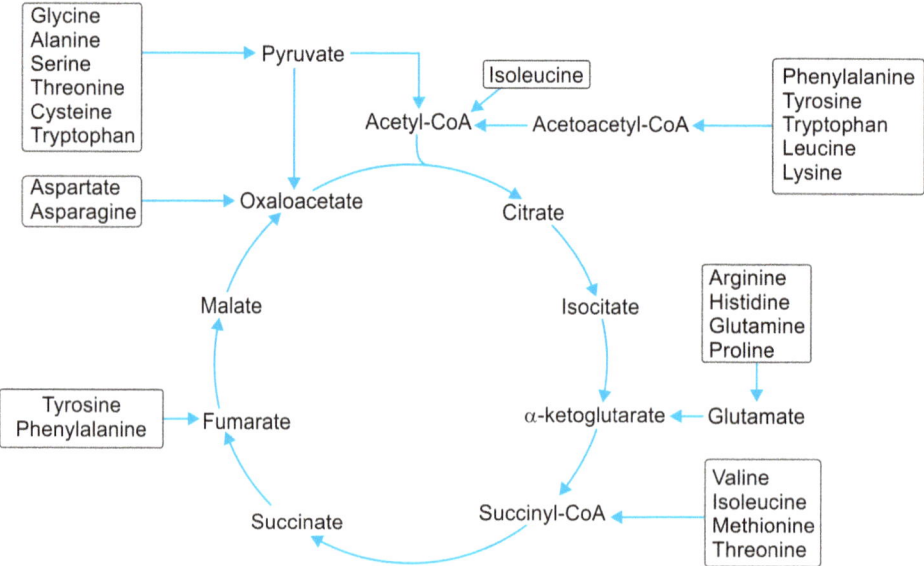

Fig. 7.16A: Substrates for gluconeogenesis.

Metabolism of Carbohydrates

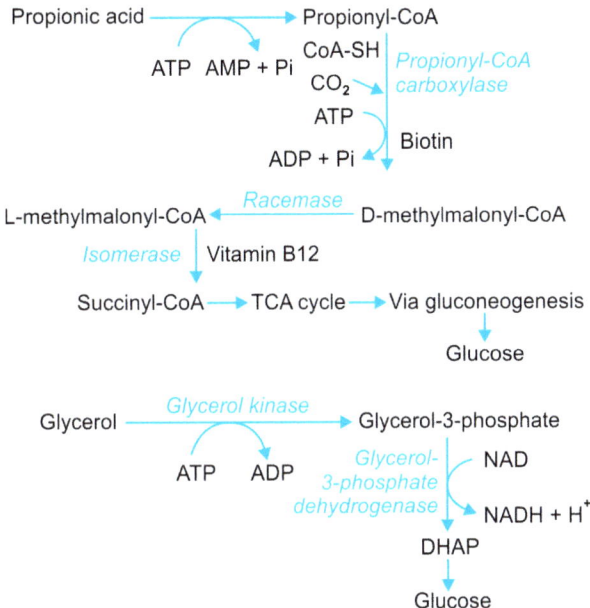

Fig. 7.16B: Formation of glucose from methylmalonyl-CoA and glycerol (glucogenic lipid).

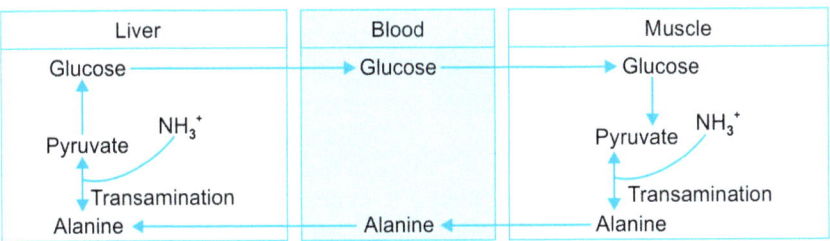

Fig. 7.17: Glucose–alanine cycle.

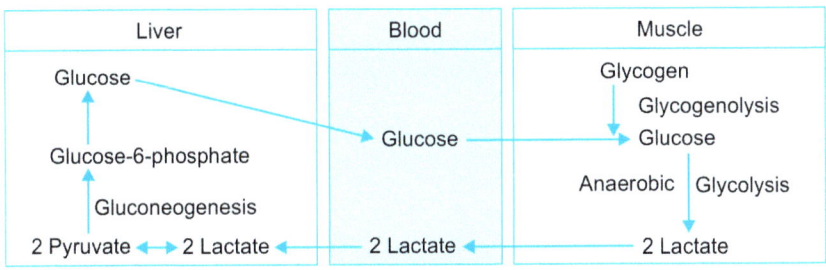

Fig. 7.18: Cori cycle.

Formation of Glucose from Lactate

See **Figure 7.19**.

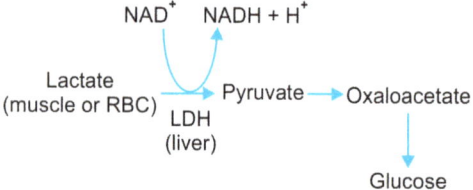

Fig. 7.19: Formation of glucose from lactate.

METABOLISM OF GLYCOGEN

The following steps show the metabolism of glycogen:
- Glycogen is the storage form of glucose in the body.
- It is mainly stored in muscle and liver.
- Stored glycogen of liver is used for maintaining blood glucose level during the period of hypoglycemia.
- The muscle glycogen is used for providing energy during exercise.

SYNTHESIS OF GLYCOGEN FROM GLUCOSE

Glycogenesis

The synthesis of glycogen from glucose is called glycogenesis. It is operative in several tissues, but liver and muscle are the main organs for the synthesis of glycogen (**Fig. 7.20**).

For its conversion to glycogen, glucose is first phosphorylated to form glucose-6-phosphate by the enzyme hexokinase, which also requires ATP and Mg^{2+}. In the fed state, another enzyme glucokinase, present in the liver, converts most of the glucose into glycogen:

1. Glucose-6-phosphate is then epimerized to form glucose-1-phosphate by phosphoglucomutase enzyme.
2. Glucose-1-phosphate reacts with uridine triphosphate (UTP) and is converted to uridine diphosphate glucose (UDP-glucose). This reaction is catalyzed by UDP-glucose pyrophosphorylase enzyme. Pyrophosphate released during this process is hydrolyzed to Pi.
3. From UDP-glucose, glucose is transferred to preexisting glycogen molecule called glycogen primer. The incoming glucose is linked to the precursor glycogen by α-1,4-glycosidic linkage resulting in the elongation of preexisting branches.
4. In the absence of glycogen primer, *glycogenin* (protein) can accept glucose from uridine diphosphate glucose (UDPG). The initial glucose is attached to the OH group of tyrosine residue of glycogenin.
5. When the chain length is increased by 10–12 glucose molecules, a minimum length of

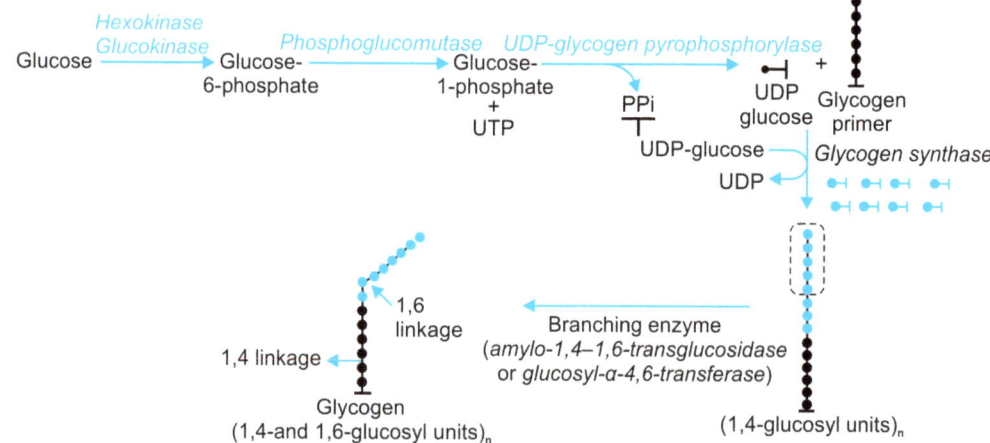

Fig. 7.20: Glycogen synthesis.

6 glucose molecules is transferred from this by the branching enzyme onto the neighboring chain in such a way that it forms a new branching point (α-1,6 linkage).
6. The branch again grows by the addition of the glucose molecules at the α-1,4 linkage. With the further branching, it results in the formation of a highly branched polymer of glucose called glycogen.
7. The UDPG is the carrier of glucose.
8. Glucose from UDPG is attached at the nonreducing end of glucose molecules of glycogen primer.
9. Branching enzyme (amylo-1,4–1,6-transglucosidase) transfers 6-glucose residue portion from one chain to a neighboring chain to form an α-1,6 linkage.

Glycogenolysis

Glycogenolysis is the process of breakdown of glycogen either to glucose-6-phosphate in muscle or to free glucose in liver:
1. In the first step, glucose molecules are sequentially removed as glucose 1-phosphate. This reaction is rate-controlling step and is catalyzed by glycogen phosphorylase enzyme. It removes glucose from the glycogen molecule until nearly four glucose residues are left on the outermost chain (**Figs. 7.21 and 7.22**).
2. Glucan transferase enzyme transfers a trisaccharide unit out of the four molecules of glucose left on the outer branch to the neighboring exposed branch point.
3. Debranching enzyme removes the glucose molecule present at the branch point as free glucose.
4. Thus with the combined action of glycogen phosphorylase, glucan transferase, and debranching enzyme, the glycogen molecule is hydrolyzed to glucose-1-phosphate and free glucose.
5. Glucose-1-phosphate formed is converted into glucose-6-phosphate by phosphoglucomutase enzyme.
6. In liver and kidney, glucose-6-phosphate further hydrolyzed to glucose by the action of glucose-6-phosphatase enzyme. This enzyme is absent in muscle. Hence, muscle

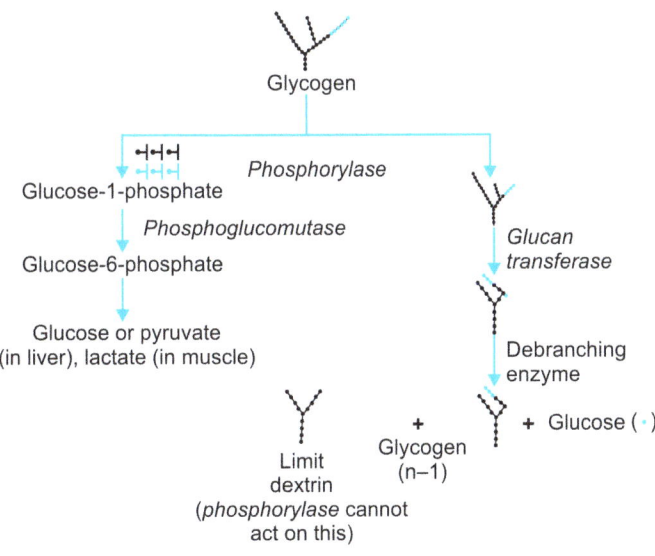

Fig. 7.21: Glycogenolysis.

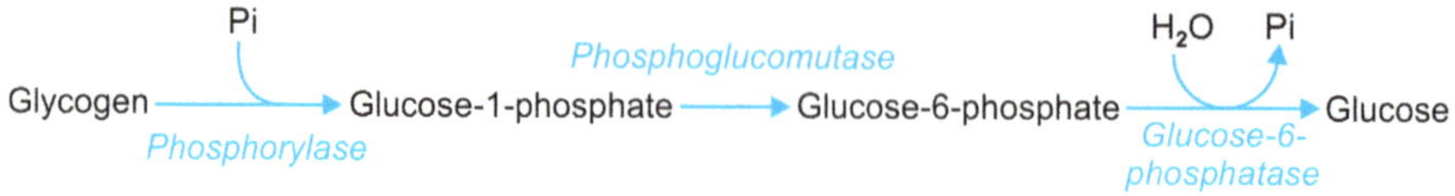

$$\text{Glycogen} \xrightarrow[\text{Phosphorylase}]{\text{Pi}} \text{Glucose-1-phosphate} \xrightarrow{\text{Phosphoglucomutase}} \text{Glucose-6-phosphate} \xrightarrow[\text{Glucose-6-phosphatase}]{\text{H}_2\text{O} \quad \text{Pi}} \text{Glucose}$$

Fig. 7.22: Glycogenolysis.

glycogen cannot be converted to glucose. Liver glycogen is mainly used to maintain the level of blood glucose.

7. Phosphorylase phosphorolytically splits α-1,4-glucoside bonds from the outermost chains of glycogen until four residues remain on either side of α_1,6 branch point (limit dextrin).
8. α_1,4-glucan transferase transfers 3-glucose residue portion from one side chain to the other exposing α-1,6 branch points.
9. Amylo-1,6-glucosidase splits the 1,6 linkages.

Muscle Glycogenolysis

Glycogen → Glucose-1-phosphate → Glucose-6-phophate → Glycolysis → Lactate.

Lysosomal Degradation of Glycogen

A small amount of glycogen is degraded by lysosomal enzyme α_1,4-glucosidase (acid maltase).

Regulation of Glycogenesis and Glycogenolysis

This list shows the regulation of glycogenesis and glycogenolysis:
- The glycogen synthase and phosphorylase exist in both active and inactive forms **(Figs. 7.23 and 7.24)**.
- The dephosphorylated form of glycogen synthase is active.
- Phosphorylated form of phosphorylase is active.
- The activation of phosphorylase depends on high cAMP level. At the same time, high cAMP level inactivates glycogen synthase.

Regulating Compounds of Glycogen Metabolism

Allosteric Regulation

- In a well-fed state, glucose-6-phosphate level is high, which activates glycogen synthase.
- On the other hand, glucose-6-phosphate and ATP allosterically inhibit phosphorylase.
- The free glucose also acts as inhibitor to phosphorylase.

Allosteric Regulation of Glycogenolysis by Calcium

Effect of Calcium

Calcium (Ca^{2+}) allosterically activates phosphorylase kinase and it is independent of cAMP and phosphorylation. When muscle contracts Ca^{2+} ions are released from the sarcoplasmic reticulum. Ca^{2+} binds allosterically to calmodulin, a subunit of phosphorylase kinase, and activates the enzyme without the need for its phosphorylation and allows glycogenolysis. When muscle relaxes Ca^{2+} returns to the sarcoplasmic reticulum and phosphorylase kinase becomes inactive.

Futile Cycle

Futile cycle is a situation wherein substrate is converted to a product through one pathway and the same product is converted back to the substrate through another pathway. The biosynthetic pathway is energy requiring and futile cycling results in a waste of high-energy phosphate bonds.

For example, in glycolysis the PFK catalyzes the phosphorylation of fructose-6-phosphate

Metabolism of Carbohydrates

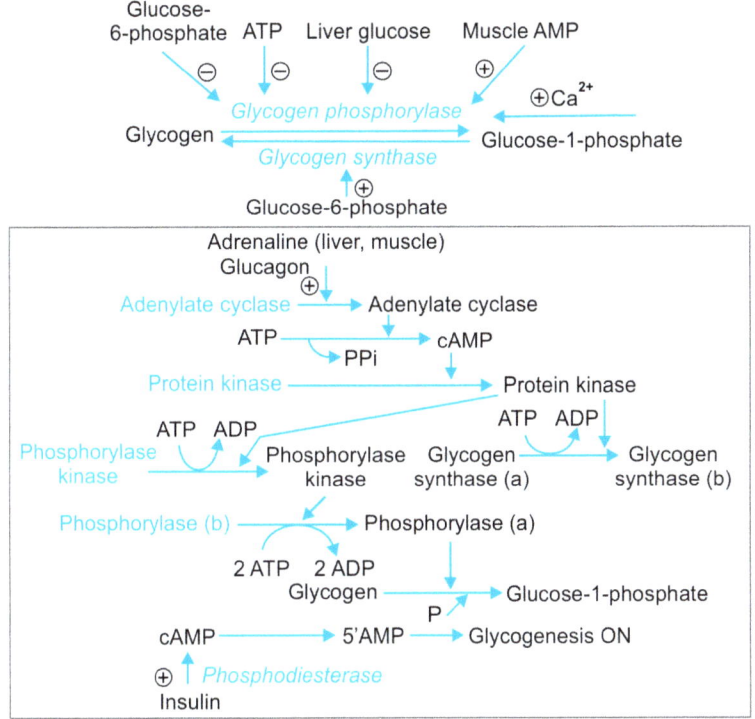

Fig. 7.23: Glycogen metabolism regulation.

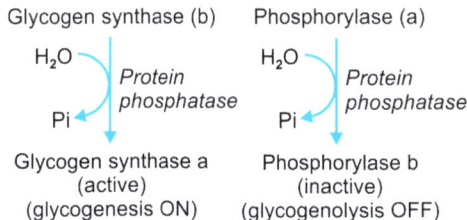

Fig. 7.24: ON and OFF mechanism of glycogenesis and glycogenolysis.

by ATP, whereas in gluconeogenesis, fructose bisphosphatase catalyzes the hydrolysis of F-1,6-BP to fructose-6-phosphate.

The sum of these two reactions is an energy-wasting reaction with a hydrolysis of ATP without any net metabolic work. If these two reactions occur simultaneously at a high rate in the same cell, it results in loss of a large amount of energy as heat. This type of ATP degrading cycle is called futile cycle.

Glycogen Storage Diseases

- Genetic diseases (may be inherited)
- Deposition of abnormal type or abnormal quantity of glycogen in the tissues is as shown in **Table 7.3**.

Case

Glycogen
Stanley, a 19-year-old male, visited his general practitioner with a complaint of experiencing early muscle fatigue and cramping muscle pain during strenuous exercise. He observed that this condition did not improve with additional exercise, with a sports drink containing electrolytes,

Table 7.3: Deposition of abnormal type or abnormal quantity of glycogen in the tissues.

Diseases	Defect and features
Type I: von Gierke's disease	• Glucose-6-phosphatase (liver), accumulation of glycogen in the liver • Fasting hypoglycemia • Lactic acidemia: Glucose is not synthesized from the lactate produced in muscle and liver. Lactate level increases and pH decreases • Hyperlipidemia: Block in gluconeogenesis leads to mobilization of fat to meet energy requirement. So, this increases plasma-free fatty acid and ketone bodies • Hyperuricemia: Accumulated glucose-6-phosphate diverted to HMP pathway, leading to increased synthesis of ribose and nucleotides, this enhances catabolism of purine nucleotides to uric acid • The massive liver enlargement leads to cirrhosis. Children fail to grow. Food should be given in small quantity at frequent intervals
Type II: Pompe disease	Lysosomal-α-1, 4-glucosidase, glycogen accumulates in lysosomes in all tissues, enlarged liver and heart
Type III: Limit dextrinosis (Cori disease)	• Debranching enzyme (amylo-α-1, 6-glucosidase) • Accumulation of polysaccharide (limit dextrin) in liver, heart, and muscle
Type IV: Amylopectinosis or Andersen's disease	• Branching enzyme (glucosyl-4,6-transferase) • Accumulation of polysaccharide with few branch points, cirrhosis of liver
Type V: McArdle's disease	• Muscle glycogen phosphorylase, glycogen accumulates in the muscle • Diminished tolerance to exercise
Type VI: Hers disease	Liver glycogen phosphorylase

or with anti-inflammatory medications. His activities associated with daily living were not affected. A blood sample taken after exercise contained a very low level of plasma lactate and increased levels of plasma creatine kinase. Further investigations showed the low level of muscle glycogen phosphorylase. Which of the following glycogen storage disorder Mr Stanley has?
A. von Gierke's disease
B. McArdle's disease
C. Anderson' disease
D. Hers disease.

Answer is B: McArdle's disease is due to the deficiency of muscle glycogen phosphorylase, which breaks down the glycogen. The energy source during strenuous exercise is through glycogen breakdown and the glucose released from this glycogen goes for anaerobic glycolysis with the production of lactate. But Stanley is not getting any energy through this due to the deficiency of phosphorylase. But muscle is able to get the energy by creatine phosphate. Therefore his blood lactate is low and creatine kinase (the enzyme helps in the formation of ATP from creatine phosphate) is high.

OXIDATIVE AND NONOXIDATIVE PHASES OF HEXOSE MONOPHOSPHATE PATHWAY AND ITS IMPORTANCE

Hexose Monophosphate Shunt, Pentose Phosphate Pathway, Phosphogluconate Pathway

It is an alternative pathway to glycolysis and TCA cycle for the oxidation of glucose (**Fig. 7.25**).

Location

The enzymes of pathway are located in cytosol. This pathway found in all cells such as liver, adipose tissue, adrenal gland, RBC,

Metabolism of Carbohydrates

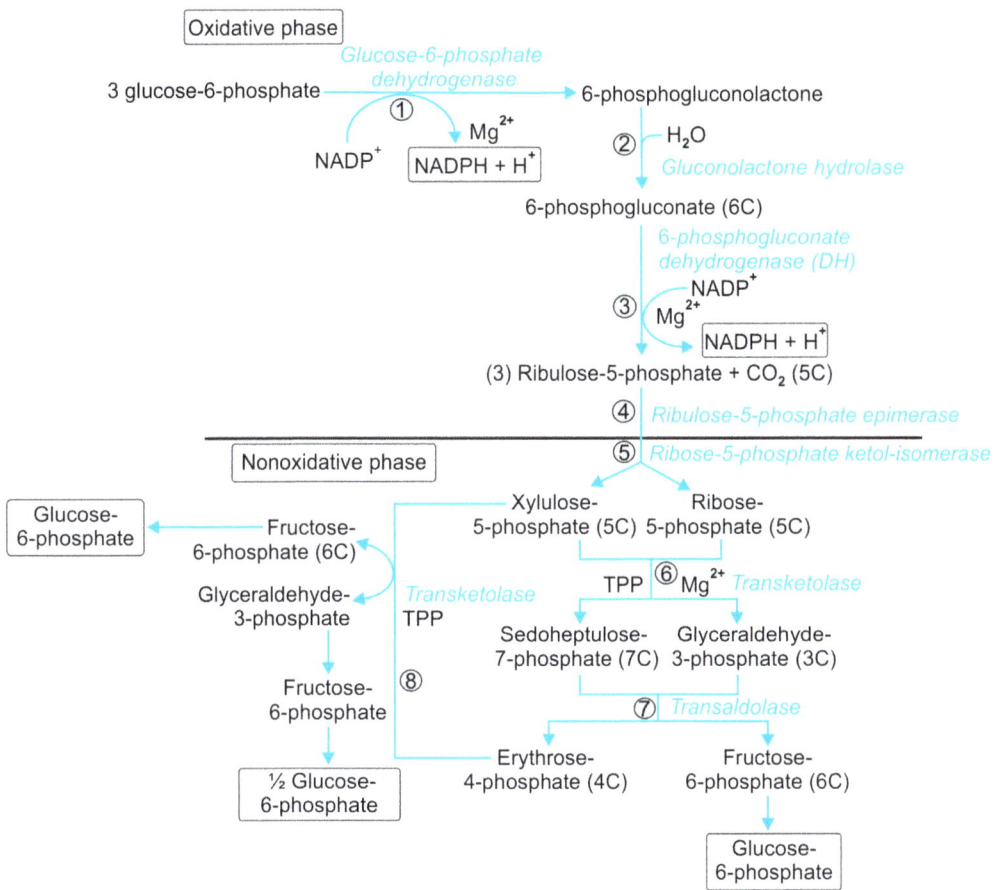

Fig. 7.25: Reactions of HMP shunt.
(HMP: hexose monophosphate.)

testes, ovaries, and lactating mammary gland, which are highly active in HMP shunt. These tissues have high amount of pentose pathway enzymes for their determined functions, which depends on NADPH:
- Adrenal gland → Steroid synthesis
- Testes → Steroid synthesis
- Ovaries → Steroid synthesis
- Adipose tissue → Fatty acid synthesis
- Mammary gland → Fatty acid synthesis
- Liver → Fatty acid, bile acids, and cholesterol synthesis
- RBCs → Maintenance of reduced glutathione (GSH).

Phases

The reactions of the pathway are divided into two phases—oxidative irreversible phase and nonoxidative reversible phase.

Oxidative Irreversible Phase

1. The reactions start with three molecules of glucose-6-phosphate.
2. Glucose-6-phosphate is converted to 6-phosphogluconolactone by glucose-6-phosphate DH, which is NADP dependent; this reaction produces first molecule of NADPH.

3. 6-phosphogluconolactone is then converted to 6-phosphogluconate by 6-phosphogluconolactone hydrolase.
4. 6-phosphogluconate undergoes decarboxylation step, which is catalyzed by 6-phosphogluconate DH. This reaction is NADP dependent and produces ribulose-5-phosphate, CO_2 and a second molecule of NADPH.

Nonoxidative Irreversible Phase

1. Ribulose-5-phosphate formed is converted back to glucose-6-phosphate by a series of reactions. Ribulose-5-phosphate serves as substrate for two different enzymes:
   1. Ribulose-5-phosphate epimerase forming two molecules of xylulose5-phosphate (ketopentose) from two molecules of ribose-5-phosphate.
   2. Ribose-5-phosphate keto-isomerase converts a molecule of xylulose-5-phosphate to ribose-5-phosphate, which is a precursor for ribose residues required for the synthesis of nucleotide and nucleic acids.
2. Transketolase transfers two carbons from a molecule of xylulose-5-phosphate (ketose) to ribose-5-phosphate (aldopentose) forming sedoheptulose-7-phosphate (with two more carbons). The xylulose-5-phosphate after losing two carbon forms glyceraldehyde-3-phosphate.
3. In the next reaction, the transaldolase transfers three-carbon dihydroxyacetone group from sedoheptulose-7-phosphate to the glyceraldehyde-3-phosphate to form fructose-6-phosphate and four carbon and erythrose-4-phosphate.
4. Transketolase transfers two carbon units from remaining molecule of xylulose-5-phosphate to erythrose-4-phosphate forming fructose-6-phosphate and glyceraldehyde-3-phosphate.
5. In order to oxidize glucose completely to CO_2 via HMP shunt, it is important to convert glyceraldehyde-3-phosphate to glucose-6-phosphate. This involves the enzymes of the glycolysis and gluconeogenesis (fructose-1,6-bisphosphatase). The reaction can be summarized as:
3 glucose-6-phosphate+H_2O + 6 $NADP^+ \rightarrow$ 3 Ribulose 5-phosphate+CO_2+6 NADPH+6 H^+.

> Significance of hexose monophosphate shunt
> 1. HMP shunt generates pentoses and NADPH.
> 2. The pentoses or its derivatives (ribose-5-phosphate) are useful for the synthesis of nucleic acids and nucleotides such as ATP, NAD^+ and FAD.
> 3. The NADPH is required for the biosynthesis of fatty acids, steroids and synthesis of glutamic acid.
> 4. The continuous production of H_2O_2 in living cells can chemically damage unsaturated lipids and proteins. This is prevented through antioxidant reactions involving NADPH, i.e. through glutathione-mediated reduction of H_2O_2. NADPH is necessary for the regeneration of reduced glutathione.
>
> In blood, RBC has a high concentration of reduced form of glutathione (GSH), which protects RBC from oxidative damage by H_2O_2. In the GSH decomposition of H_2O_2, the oxidized form of GSH (GSSG) is formed. The GSSG is reduced back to GSH by NADPH (**Fig. 7.26**) formed in HMP shunt.

Glucose-6-Phosphate Dehydrogenase Deficiency

The following list shows the information about G-6-PD deficiency:
- This is an inborn genetic disease.
- The RBC does not have active HMP shunt to provide enough NADPH to maintain high GSH concentration.
- It increased susceptibility of RBC to hemolysis.

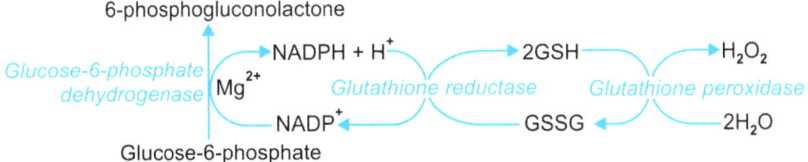

Fig. 7.26: Role of nicotinamide adenine dinucleotide phosphate (NADPH) in glutathione (GSH) concentration.

- Babies with G6PD deficiency are very sensitive to antimalarial drugs such as primaquine.
- Primaquine necessitates high GSH level and G6PD deficiency attenuates oxidation stress.
- When the drugs given, RBCs tends to get hemolyzed.
- Drugs such as aspirin and sulfa drugs also cause hemolysis of RBCs.
- The G6PD estimation is useful when:
  - The patient is suffering from severe hemolytic anemia
  - Treating the patient with antimalarial drugs.

Favism
- *Cause*: Due to ingestion of fava bean)
- The hemolytic anemia occurs due to ingestion of fava beans (broad beans) in individuals with glucose-6-phosphate dehydrogenase deficiency.
- Fava beans contain the purine glycosides, vicine and isovarmil. These compounds react with glutathione leading to decreased cellular levels of GSH.
- Favism is not observed in all individuals with G6PD deficiency, but all patients with favism have G6PD deficiency.

Regulation of the Hexose Monophosphate Shunt

The first regulatory step in the pathway is catalyzed by glucose-6-phosphate DH, the rate-limiting step. The activity of this enzyme dependent on the concentration of NADPH (it is a competitive inhibitor).

Under well-fed state, the ratio of NADPH/NADP+ decreases and the pathway is stimulated. The insulin also enhances the pathway by inducing glucose-6-phosphate DH and 6-phosphogluconolactone DH.

In starvation and diabetes, the ratio of NADPH/NADP+ is high and inhibits the pathway.

GALACTOSE METABOLISM

Galactose is required for the formation of glycolipids, glycoproteins, and lactose during lactation. In the liver, galactose is readily converted to glucose **(Fig. 7.27)**.

Galactosemia: Its Signs and Symptoms

Galactosemia

Cause: Deficiency of galactose-1-phosphate uridyltransferase
- It is a rare congenital disease in infants.
- Galactose accumulated → Galactosemia (blood)→Galactosuria (urine).
- High level of galactose in blood is reduced by aldose reductase in the eye to galactitol, which accumulated and caused cataract.
- The accumulation of galactose-1-phosphate and galactitol in tissues such as liver, nervous tissue, lens, and kidney leads to impaired functions.

Symptoms: Weight loss in infants, hepatosplenomegaly, jaundice, mental retardation, etc. In severe conditions, cataract aminoaciduria and albuminuria are observed.

Treatment: Withdrawal of the diet containing galactose and lactose.

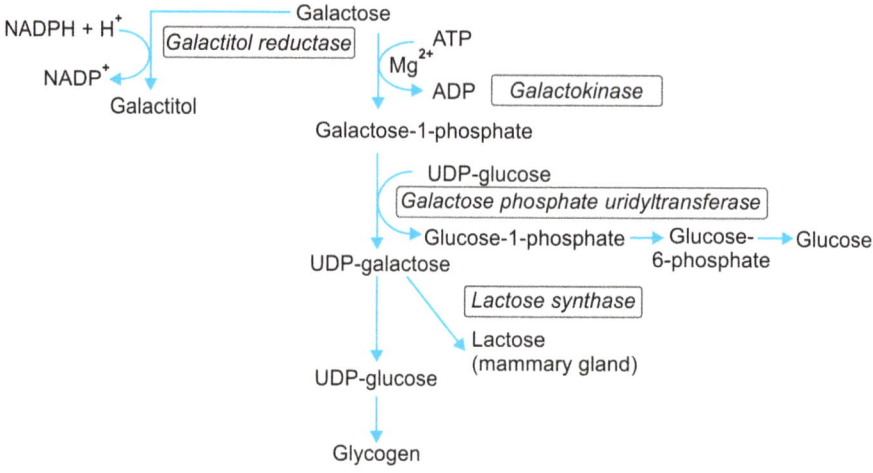

Fig. 7.27: Galactose metabolism.

Fates of Galactose

1. In liver, most of the galactose is converted into UDP-galactose and then to liver glycogen.
2. It is also used for the synthesis of glycolipid in brain and nervous tissue.
   In lactating mammary gland, galactose is converted into lactose by synthase enzyme.

FRUCTOSE METABOLISM

The following list shows the information about fructose metabolism:
- Liver is the major site of fructose metabolism **(Fig. 7.28)**
- *Fructose intolerance*: It is an inborn error of metabolism. Aldolase B is absent in this case.
- *Essential fructosuria*: Fructokinase absent in this condition.

Role of High Fructose in Atherosclerosis

High-fructose content and atherosclerosis
Fructose undergoes glycosylation more rapidly by the liver than glucose due to by passed step in the glucose metabolism catalyzed by phosphofructokinase (metabolic control is exerted at this step). This allows fructose to flood the pathways in the liver with more production of acetyl-CoA, which is deviated to synthesize fatty acid and cholesterol. In the same way, the glyceraldehyde part is reduced to glycerol and then to glycerol-3-phosphate, which forms triacylglycerol after combining with fatty acid molecules. At the end, this will lead to the increased production of very low-density lipoprotein (VLDL) and low-density lipoprotein (LDL) and risk of atherosclerosis becomes more.

SORBITOL PATHWAY AND ITS CLINICAL SIGNIFICANCE

Sorbitol Pathway (Polyol Pathway)

Mainly occurs in human lens. The enzyme aldolase reductase reduces glucose to sorbitol (glucitol) in the presence of NADPH. The enzyme sorbitol DH oxidizes sorbitol to fructose **(Fig. 7.29)**.

Aldolase

- Absents in liver

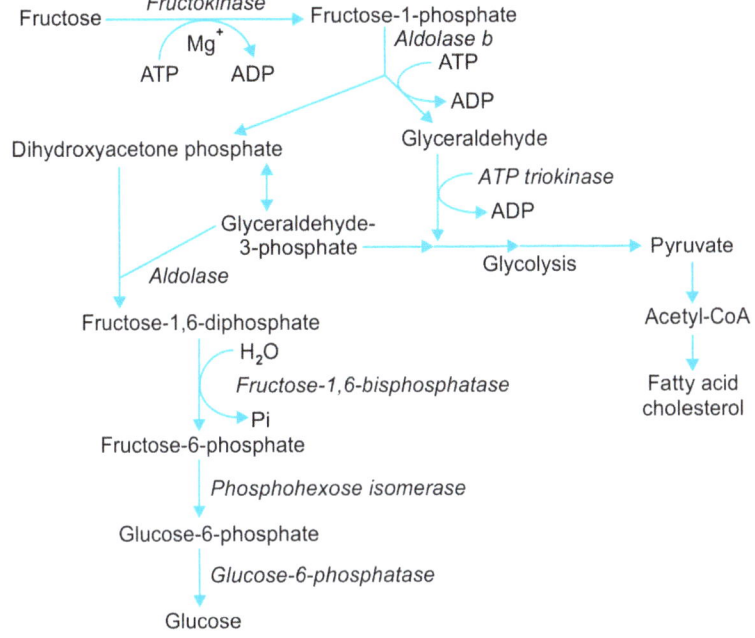

Fig. 7.28: Fructose metabolism.

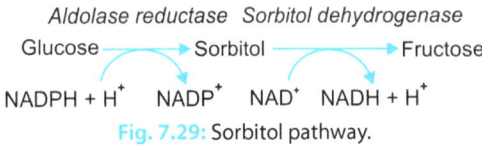

Fig. 7.29: Sorbitol pathway.

- Presents in lens, retina, kidney, nerve cells, RBC, and seminal vesicles.

Sorbitol Dehydrogenase

Sorbitol is present in liver, seminal vesicles, spleen, and ovaries. In uncontrolled diabetes, a large amount of glucose enters the cells, which are not dependent on insulin. Significant increase in intracellular glucose takes place in diabetes in cells (lens, retina, nerve cells, and kidney), which possess high activity of aldolase reductase and sufficient supply of NADPH. This results in a rapid and efficient conversion of glucose to sorbitol.

In the case of absence or decreased level of sorbitol DH, the sorbitol is not converted to fructose and gets accumulated in the cells, thus involved in pathogenesis of diabetic cataract.

Uronic Acid Pathway

Uronic acid pathway comprises the following steps:
1. It is an alternative oxidative pathway for glucose, but does not generate ATP (**Fig. 7.30**).
2. Synthesis of glucuronic acid, pentoses, and vitamin C takes place in this pathway.
3. In this pathway, free sugars or sugar acids are involved (phosphate esters in other pathways of carbohydrate).

Importance of Uridine Diphosphate Glucose-Glucuronate

1. The metabolically active UDP-glucuronate utilized for conjugation with bilirubin, steroid hormones, and some drugs.
2. It is required for the synthesis of glycosaminoglycans and proteoglycans.

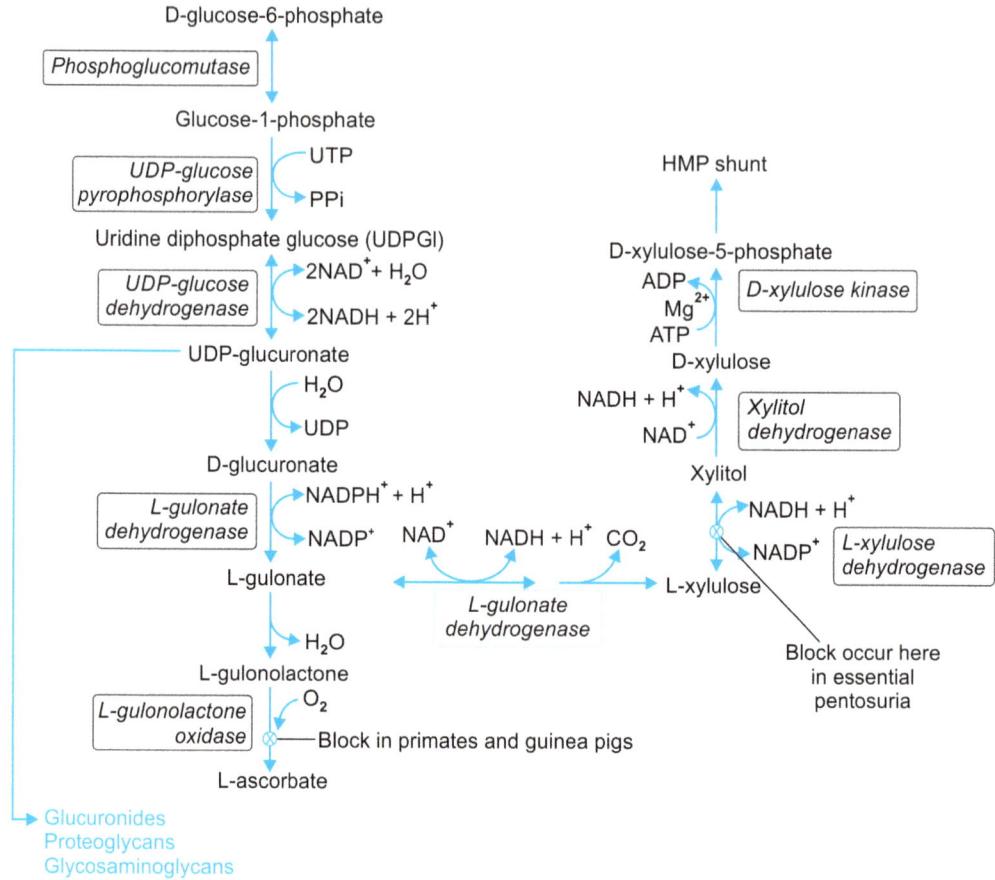

Fig. 7.30: Glucuronic acid metabolism.

3. It is required for the synthesis of vitamin C in many animals; L-gulonate, which is formed from UDP-glucuronate, is the precursor for this.
4. Essential pentosuria is a rare genetic disorder related to the deficiency of an NADP-dependent enzyme, i.e. xylulose DH.
5. L-xylulose accumulated and appears in the urine in large amounts.

LACTOSE INTOLERANCE

Cause, Signs, and Symptoms

Cause: A deficiency of the brush border enzyme lactase gives rise to a condition named lactose intolerance (**Fig. 7.31**).

- Found frequently in people of East Asian descent past their infant age. If lactose is not cleaved, it cannot be absorbed, so it makes its way "down the drain" from the small into the large intestine. Many of the bacteria found there have the capacity to metabolize lactose, which they convert to acids and gas. This leads to abdominal discomfort and diarrhea.
- Since the environment in the large intestine lacks oxygen, hydrogen (H_2) generated in the bacterial fermentation is not oxidized but instead released as such and in part is exhaled (**Fig. 7.31**).
- An increase in exhaled hydrogen upon ingestion of lactose can be used to diagnose the condition.

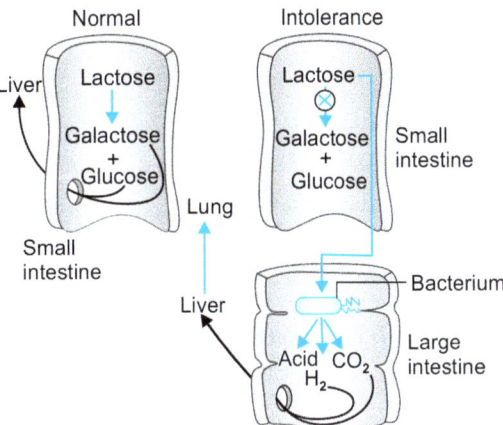

Fig. 7.31: Lactose intolerance.

- Treatment consists in omission of lactose in the diet.
- Milk can be pretreated with purified bacterial α-galactosidase, rendering it suitable for consumption by lactose-intolerant individuals. Fermented milk products such as yoghurt and cheese are depleted of lactose by bacterial fermentation and therefore do not pose a problem for lactose-intolerant individuals. *Lactosuria*: Second common reducing sugar found in the urine
- Observed in the urine of normal women during 3rd trimester of pregnancy and lactation
- Also seen in neonates.

REGULATION OF BLOOD GLUCOSE

The concentration of glucose in the blood is regulated by several metabolic pathways, which are mainly modulated by several hormones. The major metabolic pathways are glycogenesis, glycogenolysis, gluconeogenesis, glycolysis, TCA cycle, HMP shunt, lipogenesis, lipolysis, and protein synthesis.

During a brief fast, the decrease in the blood glucose level is avoided by breakdown of glycogen stored in the liver. After a meal, the absorbed glucose is converted to glycogen or fat.

Postprandial Blood Sugar Regulation

After the meal, absorption of glucose from the intestine increases the glucose level in the blood. The increased blood glucose stimulates the cells of pancreas to secrete insulin.

Fasting Blood Sugar Regulation

In normal conditions after 4–5 hours, of a meal, blood glucose level decreases near to fasting levels. Further decrease in the blood glucose is prevented by the hyperglycemic hormones.

Normal Levels

Fasting: After 12 hours of fasting, the sugar estimated 70–100 mg/100 mL.

Postprandial blood sugar (PPBS): After 2 hours of normal breakfast or lunch, the sugar estimated 90–140 mg/100 mL.

Random blood sugar: At any time sugar estimated to 90–150 mg/100 mL.

ROLE OF HORMONES IN REGULATING THE BLOOD GLUCOSE

Regulation by Hormones

Insulin (Hypoglycemic Hormone)
- Lowers blood glucose (**Fig. 7.32**)
- Favors glycogen synthesis
- Promotes glycolysis
- Inhibits gluconeogenesis.

Glucagon
- Promotes gluconeogenesis
- Enhances glycogenolysis
- Decreases glycogen synthesis
- Inhibits glycolysis
- Promotes FA oxidation, energy production, and ketone body synthesis.

Cortisol
- Increases glycogenolysis
- Enhances release of amino acids by the muscle

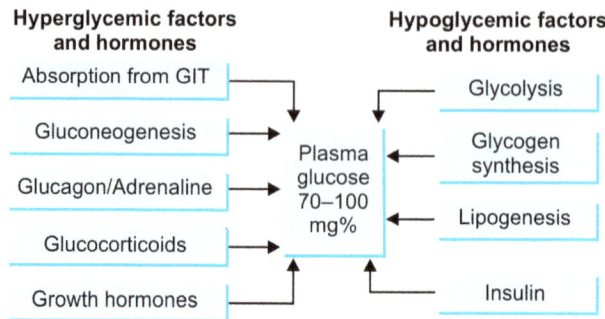

Fig. 7.32: Role of hormones and other factors in regulation of blood.

- Induces the enzymes PEPCK, fructose-1,6-bisphosphatase, glucose-6-phosphatase, and aminotransferase.

Adrenaline

- Promotes gluconeogenesis
- Increases glycogenolysis
- Favors release of glucose.

Growth Hormone

- Decreases glycolysis (inhibits PFK)
- Mobilizes FAs from adipose tissues
- Decreases uptake of glucose (releasing FA from adipose tissue).

Glucocorticoid

- The uptake of glucose by muscle
- Increases protein breakdown in muscle
- Increases gluconeogenesis.

Thyroxine

With the above-mentioned functions, thyroxine increases absorption of glucose.

INSULIN

Factors Stimulating Insulin Secretion

- Amino acids.
- Gastrointestinal hormones (GHs).
- Cortisol and estrogens.
- Glucose is the important stimulus for the insulin release.

Factors Inhibiting Insulin Secretion

Epinephrine suppresses insulin secretion and promotes energy metabolism by mobilizing energy-yielding compounds such as glucose from liver and FAs from adipose tissue.

Metabolic Effects of Insulin

Effects on Carbohydrate Metabolism

Normally half of the ingested glucose is utilized to meet the energy demands of the body (glycolysis), other 50% may be converted to fat or glycogen:

1. Insulin stimulates the uptake of glucose by muscle, adipose, tissue, leukocytes, and mammary glands. About 80% of glucose uptake is not dependent on insulin. Tissues into which glucose can freely enter include brain, kidney, erythrocytes, retina, nerve, blood vessels, and intestinal mucosa. The entry of glucose into hepatocytes does not depend on insulin. However, it stimulates the glucose utilization in liver and indirectly promotes its uptake.
2. Effect on glucose utilization: Increases glycolysis in muscle and liver. It stimulates:
   - Glucokinase
   - PFK
   - Pyruvate kinase
   - Glycogen synthase
   - HMP shunt through glucose-6-phosphate DH.

3. Effect on glucose production:
   - Decreases gluconeogenesis by inactivating pyruvate carboxykinase and glucose-6-phosphatase
   - Decreases glycogenolysis by inactivating glycogen phosphorylase.

Effects on Lipid Metabolism

1. Lipogenesis: Favors triglyceride (TG) synthesis (providing more glycerol-3-phosphate and NADPH). Increases activity of acetyl-CoA carboxylase, a key enzyme of FA synthesis
2. Lipolysis: Decreases the activity of hormone-sensitive lipase
3. Ketogenesis: Decreases ketogenesis. Increases the utilization of acetyl-CoA
4. Lipoprotein metabolism: Helps to utilize VLDL and LDL.

Effects on Protein Metabolism

- Increases protein synthesis
- Decreases protein breakdown.

MECHANISM OF ACTION OF INSULIN IN REGULATING THE BLOOD GLUCOSE

Mechanism of Action of Insulin

Insulin binds to specific plasma membrane receptors present on the target tissues (muscle and adipose tissue). This results in a series of reaction ultimately leading to the biological action. There are three mechanisms known:
1. Signal transduction
2. Insulin-mediated glucose transport
3. Insulin-mediated enzyme synthesis.

Insulin Receptor-mediated Signal Transduction

Insulin receptor: This is a tetramer consisting of four subunits of two types (α2, β2) of glycosylated form, held together by disulfide linkages. The β-subunit is extracellular and it contains insulin binding site. The β-subunit is a transmembrane protein, which is activated by insulin. The cytoplasmic domain of β-subunit has tyrosine kinase activity.

Signal transduction **(Fig. 7.33)**: Binding of insulin causes dimerization of the receptor. It is then internalized, so that the signal is transmitted. Then the tyrosine kinase phosphorylates tyrosine residues on the cytoplasmic side of insulin receptor. This in turn phosphorylates insulin receptor substrate (IRS).

Insulin-mediated Glucose Transport

The binding of insulin to insulin receptors signals the translocation of vesicles containing glucose transporters from intracellular pool to the plasma membrane. The vesicles fuse with the membrane recruiting the glucose transporters. The glucose transporters are responsible for the insulin-mediated glucose uptake by the cells. As the insulin level falls,

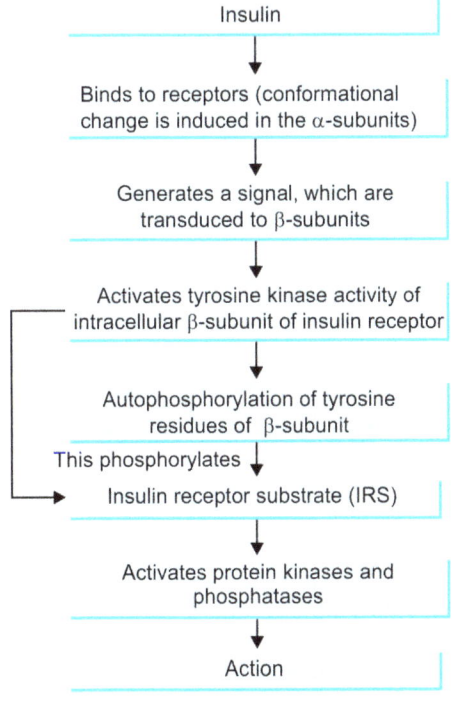

Fig. 7.33: Signal transduction.

the glucose transporters move away from the membrane to the intracellular pool for storage and recycle.

Insulin-mediated Enzyme Synthesis

Insulin promotes the synthesis of enzymes such as glucokinase, PFK, and pyruvate kinase. This is brought about by increased transcription (mRNA synthesis) followed by translocation.

HYPERGLYCEMIC HORMONES AND THEIR ROLE IN REGULATING THE BLOOD GLUCOSE

The following lists the features of glucagon:
- Anti-insulin in nature and it is secreted from the α-cells of pancreas.
- Liver is the primary target for the glycogenolytic effect of glucagon.
- Promotes the glycogenolysis and gluconeogenesis.
- Decreases glycogen synthesis.
- Inhibits glycolysis.
- Promotes FA oxidation, energy production, and ketone body synthesis.
- Increases amino acid uptake by liver and promotes gluconeogenesis through PEPCK, glucose-6-phosphatase, and fructose-1,6-bisphosphatase.

Mechanism of Action of Glucagon

Adrenaline or epinephrine increase liver glycogenolysis and increase lipolysis (**Fig. 7.34**).

DIABETES MELLITUS

Diabetes Mellitus and Its Major Types

Diabetes mellitus is a group of metabolic diseases in which a person has high blood sugar (>126 mg/dL), either because the body does not produce enough insulin (**Fig. 7.35**) or because cells do not respond to the insulin that is produced.

Types: It is broadly divided into two types:
1. Type I: Insulin-dependent diabetes mellitus (IDDM)
2. Type II: Non-IDDM (NIDDM).

Signs and Symptoms

- Frequent urination (polyuria)
- Excessive thirst (polydipsia)
- Extreme hunger or constant eating (polyphagia)
- Unexplained weight loss
- Presence of glucose in the urine
- Tiredness or fatigue
- Changes in vision
- Numbness or tingling in the extremities.
- Slow-healing wounds or sores.
- Abnormally high frequency of infection.
- Polyuria (large amount of glucose and water excretion).
- Polydipsia: Loss of fluid stimulates the thirst center; person drinks more and more water.
- Polyphagia: Lipid and protein breakdown with weight loss; person eats more frequently.
- Patient may show boils, abscesses, and cellulitis; complications of this type are retinopathy, neuropathy, and nephropathy.

Type I or Insulin-dependent Diabetes Mellitus

Usually onset in childhood and early teenage years (12–15 years of age). Genetic predisposition may also be a factor.

Cause: Total deficiency of insulin due to destruction of β-cells in pancreas.

Clinical complications: Complications of this type are retinopathy, neuropathy, and nephropathy.

Type II or Noninsulin-dependent Diabetes Mellitus

Type II comprises 90–95% of all diabetic population. The patients have minimum symptoms:

Metabolism of Carbohydrates

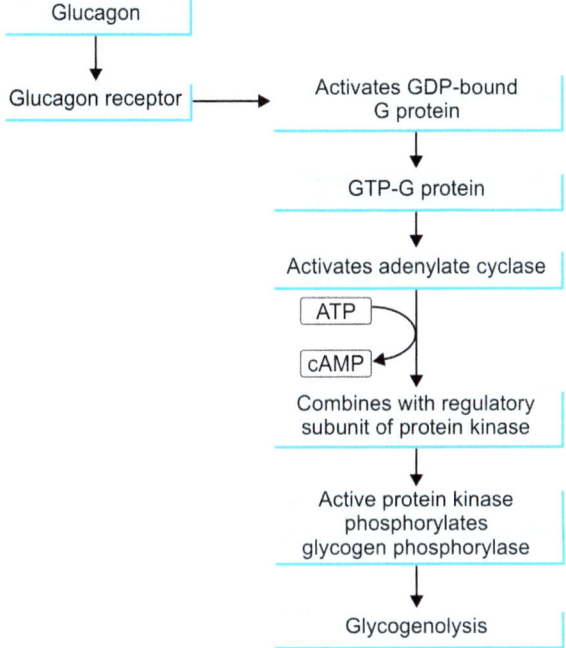

Fig. 7.34: Action of glucagon.

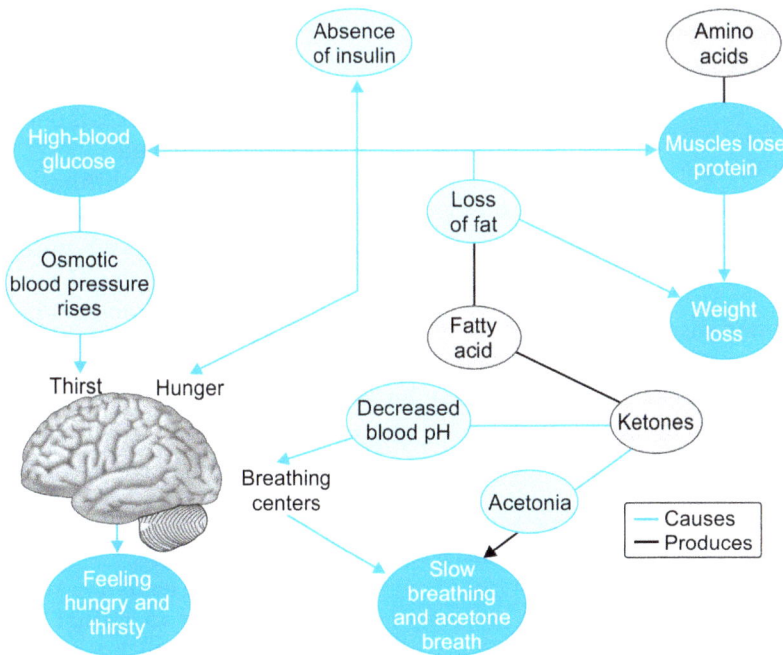

Fig. 7.35: Signs and symptoms of insulin deficiency.

- Not dependent on insulin.
- Obesity is common with NIDDM
- Usually occurs after the age of 40 years.
- Sometimes in young person also.

CRITERIA USED TO DIAGNOSE THE DIABETES MELLITUS

Diagnosis

Type I can be known by serious metabolic disturbances with increased blood glucose.

Criteria for the Diagnosis

- All adults older than 45 years of age should have a measurement of fasting blood glucose for every 3 months.
- Person with BMI of 27 kg/m^2
- Persons with family history of diabetes mellitus.
- Individual with history of gestational diabetes mellitus or delivery of large baby.
- With high-density lipoprotein (HDL) <35 mg/dL.
- Persons with impaired glucose tolerance.
- Elevated fasting glucose on more than one occasion.

Diabetes due to Secondary Causes

- Pancreatic disease
- Cushing's syndrome
- Acromegaly (-GH)
- Increased secretion of glucagon (tumor of pancreas)
- Hyperaldosteronism.

Metabolic Changes in Diabetes Mellitus

Carbohydrate Metabolism

- Hyperglycemia (decreased or impaired transport and uptake of glucose in muscles, and adipose tissue)
- Key glycolytic enzymes decrease
- Increased gluconeogenesis
- Glycogen synthesis decreases
- Glycosylated Hb increases in uncontrolled diabetes mellitus
- Sorbitol pathway: Hyperglycemia → Glucose → Sorbitol
- Increased breakdown of amino acids.

Protein Metabolism

Protein synthesis decreases.

Fat Metabolism

Fatty acid synthesis decreases and lipid breakdown increases.

Fatty acid → Acetyl-CoA → Cholesterol synthesis or ketone body formation.

Gestational Diabetes Mellitus and Its Complications

If the carbohydrate intolerance is noticed for the first time during pregnancy in nondiabetic women, it is referred to as gestational diabetes mellitus.

- Strong family history of diabetes mellitus, a history of stillbirth or neonatal death, a history of bearing an infant with congenital anomaly are the clues suggesting gestational diabetes mellitus.
- Delivery of large babies is one of the results of gestational diabetes.
- Symptoms of gestational diabetes are mild and it is not expressed in the mother. But it is associated with increased incidence of congenital malformations, increased risk of recurrence of diabetes after 10 years of parturition and prenatal mortality.

CLINICAL COMPLICATIONS OF DIABETES MELLITUS

Retinopathy

- Hyperglycemia leads to sorbitol formation.
- This may lead to retinal microvascular abnormalities, which leads to retinopathy and blindness.

Neuropathy

- A common complication
- Identified by symptoms such as pain, numbness, tingling, or burning sensation in extremities.

Angiopathy

1. Damage of basement membrane of blood vessels.
2. It increases risk of stroke and coronary artery disease.
3. It may cause atherosclerosis in medium-sized cerebral arteries (leading to paralysis), coronary arteries (leading to myocardial infarction), or peripheral vessels (leading to gangrene of limbs).
4. If small vesicles are affected, it is called microangiopathy, which leads to diabetic retinopathy and nephropathy.

Nephropathy

- Damage to the glomerulus of nephron of kidney and associated capillaries.
- This leads to decreased filtering capacity.
- Capillary damage is caused by angiopathy.
- Urinary protein detection is useful in the diagnosis of nephropathy.

Factors that Increase the Risk of Atherosclerosis

Hyperlipidemia and Atherosclerosis

- Serum triglyceride, cholesterol, and VLDL levels increases in type II.
- HDL decreases.
- All these factors increase the risk of atherosclerosis.

Diabetic Ketoacidosis

Deficiency of insulin increases the lipid breakdown, which increases acetyl-CoA further leading to increased cholesterol and ketone bodies. In this condition, acetone smell of breath, ketonuria, and ketonemia are seen. Whole condition is called ketosis. This leads to the decreased blood pH. Metabolic acidosis is seen due to diabetes, so it is called diabetic ketoacidosis.

Features of Hyperglycemic Hyperosmolar Nonketotic Coma

Hyperglycemic Hyperosmolar Nonketotic Coma

- Characterized by the glucose level above 600 mg%.
- Blood pH slightly decreases or normal.
- Serum osmolality more than 350 mOsm/kg; osmotic diuresis due to glucosuria causes severe H_2O and electrolyte depletion.
- Coma results from dehydration of cerebral cells.
- Hyperglycemic hyperosmolar nonketotic coma (HHNC) is primarily seen in type II.

GLUCOSE TOLERANCE TEST AND ITS CLINICAL SIGNIFICANCE

Glucose Tolerance Tests

The following list shows the significance of glucose tolerance test:
1. Normal person should be able to remove a glucose load from blood within a specified time. This is known as normal tolerance.
2. If the person have elevated blood glucose concentration for longer than the normal time, the condition is called reduced tolerance.
3. If the glucose concentration becomes very low or normal very early than the normal time, then the condition is called increased tolerance.
4. The tests that are used to measure these changes in blood glucose after a glucose load are called glucose tolerance tests (GTT).

Types of Glucose Tolerance Tests and the Reason for Performing Oral Glucose Tolerance

- Oral
- Intravenous.
  They are mainly used in the detection of diabetes. Oral GTT (OGTT) is the one commonly used in all the laboratories. It is convenient to give glucose through oral route.

Indications of Glucose Tolerance Tests

- To know the family history of diabetes mellitus
- Signs and symptoms comparable with diabetics without any complications
- Glucosuric patients with normal fasting blood sugar
- Border line of glucose in PPBS
- Reactive hypoglycemia for 3 hours or longer period after food intake
- Pregnancy with history of abortions, stillbirth and large baby.

Procedure for Performing Oral Glucose Tolerance Test

Preparation of the Patients

1. Patient should not be under fear or anxiety about the possibility of being a diabetic; if so, it leads to false-positive results. So it is the duty of the technician to prepare the patient psychologically or mentally and convince the patients.
2. Adequate carbohydrate intake. Before the test, the patient should have been on a diet containing at least 150 g of carbohydrate per day with low fat for at least 3 days. An adequate deposit of glycogen in the liver and other tissues is essential for the production of a normal response. If the subject is in a state of relatively low-carbohydrate diet for some time before the test, the rise in blood sugar levels following the ingestion of glucose will be more pronounced and its fall to the normal level is delayed.
3. It is desirable for the subject too fast for 10–12 hours before the test.
4. The test patient must not have taken a cup of tea or coffee on the day of test.
5. The patient should not have excess amount of exercise.
6. If the patient is not well, the test should be postponed.
7. The patient should not receive any drugs at least for 3 days before the test.

Factors Affecting Glucose Tolerance Tests

1. Factors associated with hyperglycemia: Aldosterone, catecholamines, diphenylhydantoin (DPH), nicotine, oral contraceptives, thiazides, glucagon, and growth hormone.
2. Factors associated with hypoglycemia: Ethanol, isoniazid (INH), and sulfonamide drugs.
3. The glucose tolerance tends to become lower in old age; hence, age factor is also important.

Method

1. The test is usually carried out in the early morning after an overnight fasting.
2. Fasting blood sample and urine is also collected. Then 75 g (or 100 g) of glucose dissolved in about 150–200 mL of water is given to drink.
3. Venous blood for the estimation of blood glucose is collected at half hourly intervals for 2–2.5 hours or hourly intervals for 3 hours after the ingestion of glucose. Urine specimens are also collected at the same time.
4. Blood glucose is estimated in each samples and the urine is tested for the presence of the sugar.

Comments

1. Some prefer administration of 1.75 g/kg body weight of glucose. However, amount of glucose makes very little difference in the response of the test.

2. It is preferable to give 100 mL of water after the ingestion of glucose, which takes away the sweet taste and decreases the risk of vomiting.
3. Plasma specimens are more satisfactory, than whole blood for glucose analysis, because plasma gives more reliable results and it is independent of hematocrit values.
4. Variation in hematocrit values can be accounted for differences in whole blood glucose values.

Normal and Abnormal Glucose Tolerance Tests

Normal Glucose Tolerance Curve

The normal curve has the following features:
- The fasting blood glucose in this category is usually within the range of 60–100 mg/dL (**Fig. 7.36 and Table 7.4**).
- The blood glucose does not rise above 160 mg/dL.
- The blood glucose at 2 hours after the load is 110 mg/dL.
- The urine remains free of glucose throughout the test.
- The timing of the peak value is not defined as a part of the normal pattern of response, but it is usually seen either in the 30 or 60 minutes blood sample.

Abnormal Glucose Tolerance

The main features are as follows:
- The fasting level is above 120 mg (**Fig. 7.37 and Table 7.5**).
- The glucose level crosses 200 mg/100 mL in 30–60 minutes.
- Blood glucose level is more than 110 mg/dL even after 2 hours.
- There may be glucose in at least two of the urine specimen.

Conditions Associated with Diminished Glucose Tolerance

1. Due to lack of insulin, there will be decreased tissue utilization of glucose, which is seen in diabetes mellitus.

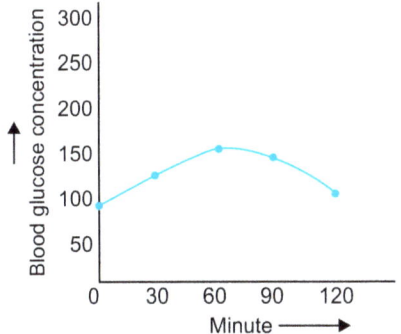

Fig. 7.36: Normal glucose tolerance test.

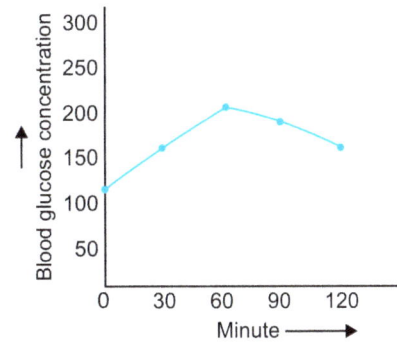

Fig. 7.37: Abnormal glucose tolerance test.

Table 7.4: Features of normal glucose tolerance test.

Samples	Glucose 100 mg/mL blood	Urine glucose
Fasting	90	Negative
30 minutes	120	Negative
60 minutes	150	Negative
90 minutes	140	Negative
120 minutes	90	Negative

Table 7.5: Features of abnormal glucose tolerance test.

Samples	Glucose 100 mg/mL blood	Urine glucose
Fasting	120	Negative
30 minutes	160	Positive
60 minutes	200	Positive
90 minutes	180	Positive
120 minutes	150	Negative

2. Increased glycogenolysis and gluconeogenesis. This is seen in glucocorticoid excess and hyperthyroidism.
3. Increased rate of absorption, which is seen in thyrotoxicosis.
4. Decreased glycogen storage, which is seen in severe hepatic diseases and glycogen storage diseases.

Increased Glucose Tolerance

Increased glucose tolerance curve is characterized by a flat response. Conditions associated with increased tolerance:
- Hypothyroidism.
- Hypoadrenalism.
- Hypopituitarism.
- Malabsorption from the gastrointestinal tract (GIT).
- Renal glycosuria.
- Hyperinsulinism: This is also characterized by:
  - Fasting hypoglycemia
  - Slight increase in blood glucose following glucose ingestion.

Intravenous Glucose Tolerance Test

Preparation of patient: Poor absorption of orally given glucose may result in a flat tolerance curve. Some patients are unable to tolerate a large amount of carbohydrate load. In these patients, an intravenous GTT may be performed to eliminate the factors related to the rate of the glucose absorption. This test is also used to monitor the first phase of insulin response in clinical studies. The preparation of patient is as that of OGTT. The dose of glucose is 0.5 g/kg body weight (25 g/dL solution). The dose is administered intravenously over 3 minutes through one hand and blood is collected at every 10 minutes from the opposite arm after the midinjection time for 1 hour and rate of glucose clearance is calculated.

> **What is lactic acidosis and mention the cause for it**
>
> *Lactic acidosis*
>
> *Cause:* Accumulation of lactic acid due to overproduction or underutilization. If diabetic patients are treated with hypoglycemic drugs (phenformin) lactic acidosis is seen.
>
> *Infection:* Susceptible to infection.
>
> *Pregnancy:* Fetal abnormalities, premature birth, big babies, and chances of absorption if they are not treated for diabetes.

SUMMARY

Carbohydrates are the essential component of our diet. The pancreatic and intestinal enzymes hydrolyze the polysaccharides of our diet into simple monosaccharides. The galactose and glucose are absorbed very rapidly by active transport mechanism, (energy and sodium dependent). Fructose and mannose are absorbed through sodium-independent facilitative diffusion transport mechanism. Glucose is the main source of energy to our body. Glucose undergoes glycolysis to generate the energy in the form of ATP. Pyruvate formed in aerobic glycolysis converted to acetyl-CoA, which enters TCA cycle to generate large number of ATPs. The anaerobic glycolysis generates lactate and this anaerobic glycolysis provides energy during strenuous exercise. The acetyl-CoA is also required to synthesize cholesterol, fatty acids, ketone bodies, and steroid hormones. Insulin stimulates the glycolytic enzymes after we consume food. Insulin stimulates the dephosphorylation of glycogen synthase to make it active and through which excess glucose absorbed will be converted to glycogen and stored in muscle and liver. Hyperglycemic hormones stimulate the glycogen breakdown (through the phosphorylation of glycogen phosphorylase) and gluconeogenesis (through the activation of gluconeogenic enzymes) whenever glucose level goes down. Glycogenesis and glycogenolysis are regulated by glycogen synthase and glycogen phosphorylase, respectively. Hexose monophosphate pathway generates a large number of NADPH, which is required to maintain the active reduced glutathione peroxidase and to synthesize fatty acids. Pathway also produces ribose sugars, which is the essential component for the synthesis of nucleic acids. The insulin deficiency results in diabetes mellitus, which are of two types: IDDM and NIDDM. The symptoms of diabetes are polyuria, polydipsia, and polyphagia. The major complications of diabetes are retinopathy, nephropathy, and neuropathy. The fasting blood glucose and HbA1c are used to detect and monitor diabetes. OGTT is preferred to detect the diabetes mellitus during pregnancy and other conditions.

SELF-ASSESSMENT QUESTIONS

Digestion and Absorption

1. Briefly describe the process of digestion and absorption of carbohydrates.
2. Explain the process of sodium-dependent glucose transport.
3. Mention the enzymes of gastrointestinal tract.
4. Add a brief note on absorption of glucose.
5. List the enzymes, which play a role in the digestion of carbohydrates.
6. Describe why cellulose is not digested. What is the importance of it in the diet?

Carbohydrate Metabolism

1. Outline the reactions of anaerobic glycolysis. Give its energetics.
2. Briefly discuss the aerobic glycolysis under the following headings:
   a. Reactions
   b. Energetics
   c. Regulation.
3. Explain the steps involved in TCA cycle. Give the energetics.
4. Mention the importance of TCA cycle.
5. Describe how glycogen is formed and utilized in human body.
6. Discuss the metabolism, which follows the strenuous exercise.
7. Explain the significance of HMP shunt.
8. Give the key reactions of gluconeogenesis.
9. How pyruvate is converted to acetyl-CoA?
10. How the glycogenolysis operates in muscles to meet the energy demand?
11. Add a note on the pentose pathway and write its importance.
12. Briefly discuss the synthesis of glycogen from glucose and mention the condition it is active.
13. What are the two types of diabetes mellitus? Discuss them briefly.
14. How the glycogenolysis operates in muscles to meet the energy demand?
15. How the hormones play a major role in the regulation of glucose?
16. Which pathway is referred to as amphibolic pathway?
17. Name the linkage present in glycogen at branching point.
18. Glucose-6-phosphatase deficiency leads to what?
19. Which enzyme converts glucose to glucose-6-phosphate during fed state?
20. What do we call, if conversion of muscle lactate into liver glucose occurs?
21. Which pathway helps in the detoxification of bilirubin?
22. Which enzyme deficiency leads to galactosemia?
23. Name the deficient enzyme of von Gierke's disease.
24. Which enzyme deficiency leads to McArdle's disease?
25. Name the enzyme, which is deficient in lactose intolerance.
26. Discuss the regulation of glycogenesis and glycogenolysis.

MULTIPLE-CHOICE QUESTIONS

Digestion and Absorption

1. **All the following enzymes help in the digestion of carbohydrates, *except*:**
   a. Amylase   b. Lipase
   c. Sucrase   d. Maltase
2. **Following statements are true with the absorption of glucose, *except*:**

a. Occurs against the concentration gradient
b. Requires a carrier protein
c. Does not require ATP
d. Sodium-dependent transport mechanism
3. The ouabain is the:
   a. Inhibitor of lipid absorption
   b. Carrier protein
   c. Inhibitor of carbohydrate absorption
   d. Enzyme

Answers

1. a   2. c   3. c

Carbohydrate Metabolism

1. All of the following are inhibitors of the TCA cycle, *except*:
   a. Aconitase   b. Malonate
   c. Fluoroacetate   d. Fluoride
2. Which of the following enzymes catalyzes substrate-level phosphorylation?
   a. Hexokinase
   b. Enolase
   c. Phosphoglycerate kinase
   d. Succinate dehydrogenase
3. The noncompetitive inhibitor that inhibits glyceraldehyde-3-phosphate dehydrogenase is:
   a. Fluoride
   b. Bromohydroxyacetone-phosphate
   c. Malonate
   d. Arsenite
4. The number of ATP molecules produced on complete oxidation of glucose under aerobic condition is:
   a. 38 ATP   b. 10 ATP
   c. 2 ATP   d. 8 ATP
5. All the following are the rate-limiting enzymes of gluconeogenesis, *except*:
   a. Pyruvate kinase
   b. Glucose-6-phosphatase
   c. Fructose-1,6-phosphatase
   d. Phosphoenolpyruvate carboxykinase
6. Which of following organ does not contain glucose-6-phosphatase?
   a. Kidney   b. Liver
   c. Muscle   d. Intestine
7. Which of the following is not a symptom of von Gierke's disease:
   a. Liver enlargement
   b. Fasting hypoglycemia
   c. Ketosis
   d. Hypouricemia
8. The hexose monophosphate shunt is located in the:
   a. Cytosol   b. Mitochondrion
   c. Lysosome   d. Golgi apparatus
9. Hexokinase:
   a. Presents in all the tissues
   b. Phosphorylates glucose only
   c. Is not inhibited by glucose-6-phos-phate
   d. Has low affinity for substrates
10. The end product of muscle glycolysis is:
    a. Pyruvate
    b. Fructose-6-phosphate
    c. Glyceraldehyde-3-phosphate
    d. Lactate
11. Regarding 2,3-BPG, the following statements are true, *except*:
    a. It binds to oxyhemoglobin and helps in unloading of oxygen
    b. It reduces the affinity of hemoglobin to oxygen
    c. It does not bind to hemoglobin
    d. Its concentration increases in hypoxic conditions
12. All of the following enzymes catalyze irreversible steps of glycolysis, *except*:
    a. Pyruvate kinase
    b. Hexokinase
    c. Enolase
    d. Phosphofructokinase
13. All of the following inhibits the enzyme glycogen phosphorylase, *except*:
    a. Glucose-6-phosphate
    b. ATP
    c. AMP
    d. Liver glucose
14. The pathway that predominantly produces NADPH is:
    a. TCA Cycle   b. Glycolysis
    c. HMP shunt   d. Gluconeogenesis
15. A classic example of exergonic reaction is the hydrolysis of:
    a. ADP   b. GMP
    c. ATP   d. GTP
16. The end product of anaerobic glycolysis is:
    a. Glycerol
    b. Fructose-6-phosphate
    c. Glyceraldehyde-3-phosphate
    d. Lactate

17. The glycolytic enzyme inhibited by fluoride is:
    a. Pyruvate kinase
    b. Enolase
    c. Glyceraldehyde-3-phosphate dehydrogenase
    d. Hexokinase
18. Which of the following hormone inhibits gluconeogenesis:
    a. Glucagon   b. Insulin
    c. Adrenaline   d. Cortisol
19. One of the following is not a clinical complication of Type II diabetes:
    a. Nephropathy   b. Retinopathy
    c. Neuropathy   d. Cardiomyopathy
20. The fate of pyruvate in aerobic condition is its conversion to:
    a. Lactate   b. Cholesterol
    c. Acetyl-CoA   d. Ribose
21. The common pathway for the oxidation of carbohydrates, fats, and proteins is:
    a. Gluconeogenesis
    b. TCA cycle
    c. Hexose monophosphate shunt
    d. Glycogenesis
22. One molecule of glucose on complete oxidation in anaerobic condition generates:
    a. 30 molecules of ATP
    b. 24 molecules of ATP
    c. 2 molecules of ATP
    d. 38 molecules of ATP
23. Cori cycle involves the conversion of:
    a. Pyruvate to lactate in muscle
    b. Muscle lactate to glucose in the liver
    c. Pyruvate to glucose in the liver
    d. Liver glucose to lactate
24. All of the following are essential for the pyruvate dehydrogenase to convert pyruvate to acetyl-CoA, *except*:
    a. TPP   b. NAD
    c. PLP   d. CoA-SH
25. A hormone that stimulates the activation of glycogen phosphorylase is:
    a. Glucagon   b. Insulin
    c. Progesterone   d. Estrogen
26. Which of the following enzyme deficiency results in McArdle's disease?
    a. Liver glycogen phosphorylase
    b. Liver glycogen synthase
    c. Lysosomal glucosidase
    d. Muscle glycogen phosphorylase
27. Glucose-6-phosphate dehydrogenase catalyzes the conversion of glucose to:
    a. Fructose-6-phosphate
    b. 6-phosphogluconolactone
    c. Xylulose-5-phosphate
    d. Ribulose-5-phosphate
28. HMP shunt helps in the generation of all the following, *except*:
    a. Pentose production
    b. NADH production
    c. NADPH production
    d. Ribose-5-phosphate production
29. All of the following inhibits the enzyme citrate synthase, *except*:
    a. ATP   b. NADH
    c. Acyl-CoA   d. ADP
30. Which of the following enzymes catalyzes substrate-level phosphorylation of the TCA cycle:
    a. Fumarase
    b. Malate dehydrogenase
    c. Succinate thiokinase
    d. α-Ketoglutarate dehydrogenase
31. All of the following stimulate the gluconeogenesis, *except*:
    a. Glucagon   b. ADH
    c. Acetyl-CoA   d. Adrenalin
32. The complete oxidation of one molecule of acetyl-CoA in the TCA cycle generates:
    a. 12 ATP   b. 10 ATP
    c. 38 ATP   d. 8 ATP
33. Malonate is a competitive inhibitor of:
    a. Aconitase
    b. α-Ketoglutarate dehydrogenase
    c. Succinate dehydrogenase
    d. Fumarase
34. All the following are the rate-limiting enzymes of gluconeogenesis, *except*:
    a. Pyruvate dehydrogenase
    b. Glucose-6-phosphatase
    c. Fructose-6-phosphatase
    d. Phosphoenolpyruvate carboxykinase
35. During glycogenesis the α-1,6 linkage is introduced by:
    a. Amylo-(1,4→1,6)-transglucosidase
    b. 1,4-glucan transferase
    c. Phosphorylase
    d. Glycogen synthase
36. Glucose-6-phosphatase is absent in:
    a. Kidney   b. Liver
    c. Muscle   d. Intestine

37. Which of the following enzyme deficiency results in von Gierke's disease?
    a. Liver phosphorylase
    b. Liver glucose-6-phosphatase
    c. Glycogen synthase
    d. Muscle phosphorylase
38. The TCA cycle is located in the:
    a. Cytosol   b. Mitochondrion
    c. Lysosome   d. Golgi apparatus
39. One of the following processes requires NADPH:
    a. Synthesis of fatty acids
    b. Reduction of protein
    c. Synthesis of glycogen
    d. Synthesis of glucagon
40. Which of the following conditions supports the formation of F-2,6-BP:
    a. High blood glucose
    b. Low blood glucose
    c. Normal blood glucose
    d. High blood cholesterol
41. Regarding glucokinase, all of the following statements are true, *except*:
    a. It is present in all the tissues
    b. It is present in liver
    c. It is not inhibited by glucose-6-phosphate
    d. It has high K_m value for glucose
42. The synthesis of glucose from non-carbohydrate sources is called:
    a. Gluconeogenesis
    b. Glycogenesis
    c. Glycolysis
    d. Glycogenolysis
43. Hers disease is due to the deficiency of:
    a. Liver phosphorylase
    b. Liver glucose-6-phosphatase
    c. Glycogen synthase
    d. Muscle phosphorylase
44. All of the following are the examples for noncompetitive inhibitors, *except*:
    a. Iodoacetate   b. Arsenite
    c. Malonate   d. Fluoride
45. Total number of ATP formed during aerobic glycolysis is:
    a. 10   b. 8
    c. 4   d. 2
46. Net ATP formed during anaerobic glycolysis:
    a. 8   b. 4
    c. 2   d. 10
47. Hormone, which stimulates the enzymes of glycolysis, is:
    a. Glucagon   b. Insulin
    c. Thyroxine   d. Cortisol
48. Glycolysis operates in:
    a. Cytosol   b. Mitochondria
    c. Ribosomes   d. Nucleus
49. Number of ATP formed in TCA cycle from acetyl-CoA (from a molecule of glucose) is:
    a. 30   b. 32
    c. 24   d. 40
50. All the following are the examples for hyperglycemic hormones, *except*:
    a. Glucagon   b. Insulin
    c. Epinephrine   d. Growth hormone
51. Glutathione (GSH):
    a. Protects RBCs from oxidative damage
    b. When oxidized decomposes H_2O_2
    c. Once oxidized is converted back to reduced form by glutathione transferase
    d. Is reduced by FADH and NADH
52. Which of the following is inhibited by arsenate poisoning?
    a. Aconitase
    b. Malonate dehydrogenase
    c. α-Ketoglutarate dehydrogenase
    d. Succinate dehydrogenase
53. Which of the following is not a gluconeogenic substrate?
    a. Glycerol   b. Tryptophan
    c. Lactate   d. Fructose
54. A healthy 20-year-old boy had a carbohydrate-rich meal. After 2 hours the activities of the following enzymes would increase, *except*:
    a. Hexokinase
    b. Phosphofructokinase
    c. Glycogen synthase
    d. Glycogen phosphorylase
55. One of the following enzymes becomes active during strenuous exercise:
    a. Glycogen synthase
    b. Glucose-6-phosphatase
    c. Glycogen phosphorylase
    d. Fructose-6-phosphatase
56. Concerning glycogen metabolism, all of the following statements are true, *except*:
    a. Glycogen synthesis takes place in liver and muscle
    b. Glycogen is stored in liver and muscle
    c. Glucose-6-phosphatase is present in muscle
    d. Muscle glycogen serves as a fuel reserve for the supply of ATP during muscle contraction

Metabolism of Carbohydrates

57. Insulin activates the key enzymes of:
    a. Gluconeogenesis   b. Glycolysis
    c. Glycogenolysis   d. None of the above
58. The enzyme, which is very active during hyperglycemia, is:
    a. Pyruvate carboxykinase
    b. Fructose-2,6-bisphosphatase
    c. Fructose-1,6-bisphosphatase
    d. Phosphofructokinase-2
59. The conversion of α-ketoglutarate to succinyl-CoA requires all of the following, *except*:
    a. TPP   b. NAD
    c. FAD   d. PLP
60. A 12-year-old child was playing football for the first time. He immediately got tired, he was given electrolytes dissolved in water to drink. But his tiredness did not reduce and he told the coach that he could not tolerate any more exercise. The possible defect in this child may be the absence of:
    a. Liver glycogen synthase
    b. Glucose-6-phosphatase
    c. Amylo-α-1,6-glucosidase
    d. Muscle glycogen phosphorylase
61. Which of the following determination helps to diagnose and to know the past history of diabetes is:
    a. Insulin
    b. C peptide
    c. Hemoglobin A1c (HbA1c)
    d. Cholesterol
62. All of the following are necessary for glucose absorption, *except*:
    a. Na^+ b. ATP
    c. Carrier protein   d. K^+
63. One of the following is not an enzyme of pancreatic origin:
    a. Amylase   b. Sucrase
    c. Lipase   d. Ribonuclease
64. All the following are the criteria for the diagnosis of diabetes, *except*:
    a. Persons family history of diabetes
    b. Persons with BMI of 27 kg/m²
    c. Persons with elevated creatinine
    d. Persons with impaired glucose tolerance
65. One of the following enzyme deficiency leads to galactosemia:
    a. Galactose-1-phosphate dehydrogenase
    b. Galactose-1-phosphate uridyl transferase
    c. Galactose-1-phosphate kinase
    d. Galactose-1-phosphate uridyl transpeptidase
66. One of the following enzymes is absent in humans:
    a. Pepsin
    b. Lipase
    c. Cellulose
    d. Carboxypeptidase
67. A 4-year-old child has massive liver enlargement and severe persistent hypoglycemia and ketosis. Which of the following disease classes should be suspected?
    a. Diabetes
    b. Glycogen storage disease
    c. Lysosomal storage disorder
    d. Mucopolysaccharidoses
68. For very high-force contractions lasting 1–2 seconds, the initial energy source is from:
    a. Glycolysis
    b. Glycogenolysis
    c. Phosphocreatine stores
    d. ATP stores
69. The most rapid method to resynthesize ATP during exercise is through:
    a. Glycolysis
    b. TCA cycle
    c. Glycogenolysis
    d. Phosphocreatine breakdown
70. Energy released from the breakdown of the high-energy phosphates, ATP and phosphocreatine, can sustain maximal exertion exercise for about:
    a. 2–4 seconds   b. 5–10 seconds
    c. 50–60 seconds   d. 100–220 seconds
71. The conversion of one molecule of glucose to two molecules of pyruvate results in the net formation of:
    a. 6 molecules of water
    b. 2 molecules of ATP
    c. 8 molecules of ATP
    d. 38 molecules of ATP
72. All of the following enzymes catalyze the irreversible steps of glycolysis, *except*:
    a. Hexokinase
    b. Pyruvate kinase
    c. Phosphofructokinase
    d. Phosphoglycerate kinase
73. Glycogen breakdown in exercising muscle is activated by:
    a. Insulin   b. Cortisol
    c. Epinephrine   d. Hexokinase

74. More hydrogen ions are formed when:
    a. Glycogen becomes reduced
    b. Phosphocreatine catabolism occurs
    c. Pyruvate is converted to lactate
    d. Glycolysis is being used as a major means of resynthesizing ATP
75. The net production of ATP via substrate-level phosphorylation in glycolysis is:
    a. 8   b. 2
    c. 3   d. 4
76. Muscle lactate production increases when:
    a. Glycolysis is activated at the onset of exercise
    b. Oxygen is readily available
    c. Pyruvate cannot be formed from glucose breakdown
    d. Muscle glycogen becomes depleted
77. Embedded in the inner membrane of the mitochondrion are:
    a. The enzymes of the TCA cycle (Krebs cycle)
    b. Triacylglycerol molecules
    c. GLUT-2 molecules
    d. The components of the ETC
78. Glucose enters muscle cells mostly by:
    a. Simple diffusion
    b. Facilitated diffusion using a specific glucose transporter
    c. Cotransport with sodium
    d. Cotransport with amino acids
79. Aerobic resynthesis of ATP occurs:
    a. In the mitochondria by a process called glycogenolysis
    b. In the cytosol
    c. In the mitochondria via oxidative phosphorylation
    d. In the sarcoplasmic reticulum
80. The synthesis of glucose from lactate and amino acids is called:
    a. Gluconeogenesis   b. Glycogenolysis
    c. Glycolysis   d. Glycogenesis
81. The energy for all forms of muscle contraction is provided by:
    a. ADP   b. Phosphocreatine
    c. GDP   d. ATP
82. Liver glycogen breakdown is stimulated by:
    a. Insulin   b. Glucagon
    c. Adrenaline   d. b and c
83. The major source of carbohydrate in a typical Western diet is:
    a. Starch   b. Cellulose
    c. Glycogen d. Lactose
84. Substrate-level phosphorylation differs from oxidative phosphorylation in that:
    a. Oxidative phosphorylation involves the transfer of electrons
    b. Substrate-level phosphorylation involves the transfer of electrons
    c. Substrate-level phosphorylation only occurs in the cytosol
    d. Oxidative phosphorylation only occurs in the cytosol
85. Which of the following promotes glucose and amino acid uptake by muscle?
    a. Adrenaline   b. Glucagon
    c. Insulin   d. Cortisol
86. During prolonged exercise, increased amounts of interleukin-6 are released from:
    a. Exercising muscle and influence carbohydrate and fat metabolism
    b. Macrophages and cause suppression of fibroblast functions
    c. Lymphocytes and inhibit macrophage function
    d. All muscles in the body and influence carbohydrate metabolism
87. A 14-year-old male patient who suspect has a deficiency of muscle glycogen phosphorylase, indicate a test based in exercising his forearm by squeezing a rubber ball. Compared with the normal person performing the same exercise, this patient would exhibit which of the following?
    a. Exercise for a longer time without fatigue
    b. Increased glucose levels in blood drawn from his forearm
    c. Decreased lactate levels in blood drawn from his forearm
    d. Hyperglycemia
88. A 3-year-old boy was transferred to hospital for further investigation of hepatomegaly. His parents were first cousins. It was learned that he was hospitalized for recurrent vomiting at 2 months of age, but no obvious cause was found and the symptoms then disappeared spontaneously. When he was 3 years old, his parents noticed his failure to thrive and hepatomegaly was noted on physical examination. Laboratory tests showed fructosemia and fructosuria. Other tests confirmed a hereditary fructose intolerance. Besides fructose, which of

the following carbohydrates should be obviously forbidden in this patient diet?
a. Glucose
b. Starch
c. Lactose
d. Sucrose

89. A 20-month-old baby boy presents with convulsions after a history of frequent morning fatigue before feeding. As RBS shows 25 mg%, so the hypoglycemia is treated accordingly. At the physical examination found a liver span of 14 cm and a grade III systolic murmur. The patient is hospitalized for further study. ECG shows a left ventricular hypertrophy. While hospitalized, blood test shows normal RBS, but elevated alanine aminotransferase (ALT), aspartate aminotransferase (AST), gamma-glutamyl transpeptidase (GGT), and creatine kinase. Given the history of the case a glycogen storage disease was suspected and specific test were indicated. The following results were obtained:
- During a fasting challenge, the time to hypoglycemia was 3 hours.
- Blood glucose increased after the administration of glucagon.
- Liver biopsy showed fibrosis with glycogen-filled hepatocytes.

With this information, which of the following enzymes activity do you expect to find decreased in this patient's hepatocytes?
a. Phosphoglucomutase
b. UDP-glucose uridyl transferase
c. Glycogen synthase
d. Debranching enzyme

90. A 69-year-old man with Alzheimer's disease and a 12-year history of type 2 diabetes is brought to a family practice clinic by his elder son. The patient is unable to give a clear account of how carefully he controls his blood glucose. Which of the following laboratory parameters could be used to assess glycemic control over the past 3–4 months?
a. Fasting blood glucose
b. Blood insulin levels
c. Glycosylated HbA1c
d. Urinary glucose

Answer is c: The amount of glycosylated HbA1c is directly related to the level of glucose in the blood. Since HbA1c is a stable product, its concentration reflects glucose levels over the past 3–6 months. HbA1c forms as a result of nonenzymatic glycosylation, a fundamental biochemical abnormality that accounts for most of the histopathologic alterations in diabetes mellitus. At first, glucose forms reversible glycosylation products with proteins by formation of Schiff bases. Rearrangement of Schiff bases leads to more stable, but still reversible, Amadori products and subsequently to irreversible advanced glycosylation end products (AGE) of which HbA1c is an example. Blood ketones, blood glucose, urinary glucose, and blood insulin do not reflect long-standing metabolic abnormalities of diabetes mellitus and cannot be used to assess long-term glycemic control.

91. Which one of the following statements is false?
a. The enzymes of the TCA are located in the mitochondria
b. TCA cycle is of no metabolic significance for the oxidation of fatty acids or amino acids
c. TCA cycle is an oxidative process
d. The cycle functions irreversibly

92. Gastric secretion is:
a. Inhibited by cholecystokinin
b. Stimulated by gastric inhibitory peptide
c. Stimulated by sympathetic stimulation
d. Stimulated by nicotinic agonists

93. Patient having McArdle's disease suffers from painful muscle cramping after brief exercise. The condition results from a deficiency of the following enzymes in glycogen breakdown:
a. Muscle glycogen phosphorylase
b. Muscle amylo-1,6-glucosidase
c. Liver glycogen phosphorylase
d. Liver amylo-1,6-glucosidase activity

Answers

1. d	2. c	3. b	4. a	5. a
6. c	7. d	8. a	9. b	10. d
11. c	12. c	13. c	14. c	15. c
16. d	17. b	18. b	19. d	20. c
21. b	22. c	23. b	24. c	25. a
26. d	27. b	28. b	29. d	30. c
31. b	32. a	33. c	34. a	35. a
36. c	37. b	38. b	39. a	40. a
41. a	42. a	43. a	44. c	45. b

46. c	47. b	48. a	49. c	50. b
51. a	52. c	53. d	54. d	55. c
56. c	57. b	58. d	59. d	60. d
61. c	62. d	63. b	64. c	65. b
66. c	67. b	68. d	69. d	70. b
71. d	72. d	73. c	74. d	75. b
76. a	77. d	78. b	79. c	80. a
81. d	82. d	83. a	84. a	85. c
86. a	87. b	88. d	89. c	90. c
91. b	92. a	93. a		

CASE STUDY

1. A 30-year-old man with a history of IDDM was treated for a urinary tract infection. 2 weeks later, he presented with persistent flank pain. The examination showed that he was a moderately ill-appearing person who was afebrile with a heart rate of 100, respiratory rate of 16, and BP of 180/95 mm Hg. He did not appear to be dehydrated. There was costovertebral angle tenderness on the left and left lower quadrant tenderness with guarding, but without rebound tenderness. Laboratory results:

Serum electrolytes

Sodium	127 mEq/L
Potassium	5
Chloride	92
Bicarbonate	17
Glucose	640 mg/dL
BUN	32
Creatinine	1.6

Urinalysis

Appearance	Pink/cloudy
Glucose	3+
Ketones	2+
Protein	3+
Sediment	RBCs found plenty
WBCs	Many

a. What is the probable cause of the patient thought about rebound tenderness?
b. How does the urinalysis support this diagnosis?
c. What do you think the decreased bicarbonate value means?
d. What do you think of the patient's BUN and creatinine values?

Acute Pyelonephritis

Diabetic patients are generally susceptible to infections and this patient has a potential source for a kidney infection in the previous UTI, which can ascend the ureters to reach the kidneys.

She has pain in her flank and appears ill, with an elevated white cell count and an increased number of immature white cell forms (bands). The physical examination reveals pain on palpation in the left lower back and abdomen. These signs point to a localized infection; back pain is suggestive of a retroperitoneal location. Patients with acute pyelonephritis will generally be febrile, but this patient has been treated for a UTI and may still be on oral antibiotics. This could be partially suppressing the infection.

The urinalysis is consistent with infection in the urinary tract. Pink urine is consistent with blood, the cloudiness is consistent with bacteria and/or tissue debris, more than 20 WBCs/HPF confirm infection. Protein is commonly elevated in urinary tract and kidney infections and may be derived from the inflammatory response and tissue destruction.

The elevated glucose and ketones suggest that the patient's diabetes may not be in good control. This result is confirmed by the plasma glucose of 700 mg/dL.

This urinalysis could occur in a bladder infection, but it also consistent with a kidney infection. It would more strongly support a kidney infection, if it contained casts, particularly white cell casts.

Metabolic Acidosis

Bicarbonate is reduced in metabolic acidosis or metabolic compensation of respiratory alkalosis. In this case, the serum glucose is markedly elevated and there are glucose and ketones in the urine. These findings in combination with the decreased bicarbonate suggest a mild diabetic ketoacidosis. Diabetic ketoacidosis is one of the forms of metabolic acidosis that produces an increased anion gap. If you calculate the anion gap for this patient, you will find that it is mildly elevated at 18, consistent with the hypothesis of a mild ketoacidosis.

The patient's creatinine is mildly elevated, suggesting some decrease in glomerular filtration rate (GFR). However, the BUN is disproportionately increased, leading to a BUN/creatinine ratio over 15. Part of this prerenal azotemia could be related to hypovolemia as a result of osmotic diuresis from elevated glucose (but the patient appears well hydrated) or to increased urea production related to tissue destruction in the infected area.

CHAPTER 8

Chemistry of Lipids

OBJECTIVES

At the end of this chapter, students should be able to:
- Classify the lipids with specific examples
- Explain the different phospholipids and glycolipids with their importance.

INTRODUCTION

Lipid or fat is characterized by their physical property with water, it says, "touch me not," but it goes well into solution with organic solvents. To the tongue it is tasteful; within limits, it is good for the life, but makes it danger when it is in excess.

Lipids are heterogeneous group of naturally occurring compounds, which are relatively insoluble in water, but freely soluble in nonpolar organic solvents such as benzene, chloroform, ether, and alcohol. Lipids are:
- Obtained from animals and plants living or fossilized
- Formed of long-chain hydrocarbon groups (carbon and hydrogen) but may also contain oxygen, phosphorus, nitrogen, and sulfur.

FUNCTIONS OF LIPIDS

Biomedical Importance of Lipids

1. Triglycerides are the major storage form of energy.
2. They provide essential fatty acids, phospholipids, hormones (prostaglandins), and they form important constituents of cell membrane.
3. Absorption of vitamins A, D, E, and K depends on the presence lipids in the diet.
4. The basic unit of lipids, i.e. acetyl coenzyme A (acetyl-CoA) (the active forms of acetic acid) is used for the synthesis of cholesterol and hence steroid hormones.
5. The lipids maintain the membrane structure and integrity.
6. Since lipids are hydrocarbon organic compounds, its insulating effect has been utilized in the body for protecting internal organs from shock.
7. They help in blood coagulation.
8. Dipalmitoyl lecithin, a phospholipid, acts as surfactant and is required for the normal functioning of the lung alveoli.

CLASSIFICATION OF LIPIDS WITH SPECIFIC EXAMPLES

Simple lipids	Compound lipids	Derived lipids
They are esters of fatty acid with glycerol or higher alcohols Examples: Fats and waxes	They are esters of fatty acid with one of the various alcohols, and in addition, it contains other groups (nonlipid component). Examples: Phospholipids: 1. *Glycerophospholipids*: Lecithin, cephalin, phosphatidylserine, phosphatidylinositol, cardiolipins, plasmalogens 2. *Sphingophospholipids* ➢ Glycolipids: Cerebrosides and gangliosides ➢ Lipoproteins: Chylomicron, very low density lipoprotein (VLDL), low density lipoprotein(LDL) and high density lipoprotein (HDL)	Derived from simple or compound lipids Examples: Fatty acid, glycerol, alcohol, and cholesterol

Chemistry of Lipids

SIMPLE LIPIDS

They are esters of fatty acid with glycerol or higher alcohols.

Example: fats and waxes.

Fats: Esters of fatty acids with glycerol. A fat in the liquid state is known as oil. Fat is also called triglyceride or triacylglycerol.

Composition and Importance of Triacylglycerol (Triglyceride)

- Nearly all the commercially important fats and oils of animal and plant origin consist almost exclusively of the simple lipid class triacylglycerols (often termed triglycerides).
- They consist of a glycerol moiety with each hydroxyl group esterified to a fatty acid. In nature, they are synthesized by enzyme systems, which determine that a center of asymmetry is created about carbon-2 of the glycerol backbone, so they exist in enantiomeric forms, i.e. with different fatty acids in each position.
- They are esters of fatty acid with the trihydric alcohol glycerol.
- Glycerol with one molecule of fatty acid is called monoacylglycerol.
- Glycerol with two molecules of fatty acid is called diacylglycerol.

$$\begin{array}{c} CH_2OH \\ R^n-COO-CH \\ CH_2OH \end{array}$$
2-monoacylglycerol

- Triglyceride is a glycerol attached with three fatty acids.

$$\begin{array}{l} \alpha_1 CH_2-OH \\ \beta CH-OH \\ \alpha_2 CH_2-OH \end{array} + 3\ Fatty\ acids \longrightarrow \begin{array}{l} \alpha_1 CH_2-O-CO-R_1 \\ \beta CH-O-CO-R_2 \\ \alpha_2 CH_2-O-CO-R_3 \end{array}$$
Glycerol   Triacylglycerol

- R_1, R_2, and R_3 indicate the fatty acids. The fatty acids may be same or may differ. Usually, R_2 is an unsaturated fatty acid.

Waxes

Waxes are esters of fatty acids with monohydric long-chain alcohols. In their most common form, wax esters consist of fatty acids esterified to long-chain alcohols with similar chain lengths. The latter tends to be saturated or have one double bond only. Such compounds are found in animals, plants, and microbial tissues, and they have a variety of functions, such as acting as energy stores, waterproofing, and lubrication.

$$\sim\sim\sim\sim\sim\sim\sim COO \sim\sim\sim\sim\sim\sim\sim$$

In some tissues, such as skin, avian preen glands, or plant leaf surfaces, the wax components can be much more complicated in their structures and compositions. They can contain aliphatic diols, free alcohols, hydrocarbons (e.g. squalene), aldehydes, and ketones.

COMPOUND LIPIDS

Compound lipids are esters of fatty acid with one of the various alcohols, and in addition, it contains other groups (nonlipid component). These are classified again on the basis of prosthetic group present in the lipid:
- Phospholipids
- Glycolipids
- Lipoproteins.

Types of Phospholipids and their Clinical Importance

Phospholipids are compound lipids containing alcohol, fatty acid, phosphoric acid, and a nitrogenous base or other alcoholic group. Phospholipids may be classified on the basis of the type of alcohol presented as:
1. Glycerophospholipids: The alcohol present in glycerophospholipids is glycerol. The different types of glycerophospholipids are:
   - Phosphatidylcholine (lecithin)
   - Phosphatidylethanolamine (cephalin)
   - Phosphatidylserine

- Phosphatidylinositol (PI)
- Cardiolipins
- Plasmalogens.
2. Sphingophospholipids: The alcohol present is sphingosine.

Glycerophospholipids

Phosphatidylcholine (lecithin): It contains alcohol, fatty acid, phosphoric acid, and choline. The fatty acid part of R_1 is a saturated fatty acid and R_2 at β position is an unsaturated fatty acid.

Lecithin is present in brain, nervous tissue, sperm, and egg yolk.

Lecithins are surface-active agent and help in emulsification of fats.

> *Dipalmitoyl lecithin* is a lung surfactant (lowers surface tension) that prevents the collapse of lung alveoli. Absence of dipalmitoyl lecithin in premature infants may produce **respiratory distress syndrome** or hyaline membrane disease.

$$\begin{array}{ll} CH_2-O-CO-R_1 & CH_2-O-CO-R_1 \\ CH-O-CO-R_2 & CH-O-CO-R_2 \\ CH_2-O-\text{Phosphoric} & CH_2-O-\text{Phosphoric} \\ \quad \text{acid} & \quad \text{acid-choline} \\ \text{Phosphatidic acid} & \text{Lecithin (phosphatidyl choline)} \end{array}$$

Phosphatidylethanolamine (cephalin): It contains alcohol, fatty acid, phosphoric acid, and ethanolamine as a nitrogenous base instead of choline present in lecithin. Cephalins are present in brain, erythrocytes, and many other tissues.

Phosphatidylserine: It contains alcohol, fatty acid, phosphoric acid, and serine as a nitrogenous base.

Phosphatidylinositol: It is a phospholipid-containing phosphatidic acid, bound to the alcohol inositol instead of a nitrogenous base. They are important components of cell membrane. The action of certain hormones (e.g. oxytocin and vasopressin) is mediated through PI. In response to hormonal action, PI is cleaved to diacylglycerol (DAG) and inositol triphosphate. Both these compounds act as second messenger for hormonal action.

$$\begin{array}{c} CH_2-OOCR' \\ R''COO-CH \quad O \\ CH_2-O-P-O \\ H^+ \; O^- \end{array} \quad \begin{array}{c} OH \\ OH \quad OH \\ OH \quad OH \end{array}$$

Phosphatidylinositol

Cardiolipin: It is diphosphatidylglycerol. It contains two molecules of phosphatidic acid held by glycerol. It is present in the inner mitochondrial membrane and has antigenic properties.

Phosphatidic acid —— G l y c e r o l —— Phosphatidic acid

Plasmalogen: These differ from lecithin or cephalin in α-1 position of glycerol where the fatty acid is replaced by a long-chain unsaturated aliphatic aldehyde such as palmitic or stearic aldehyde. Plasmalogens are present in large quantities in the skeletal muscle, cardiac muscle, and in semen.

Sphingophospholipids

Sphingomyelin: This is a sphingophospholipid. It does not contain glycerol but an unsaturated amino alcohol, i.e. sphingosine. They contain a molecule of choline, phosphoric acid, and a fatty acid. Sphingomyelin makes up a large part of the myelin sheath. These are also present in brain, lungs, nerve, and other tissues.

$$\begin{array}{c} \quad\quad\quad\quad\quad\quad\quad O \\ R''CHOHCHCH_2-O-P-O-CH_2CHN^+(CH_3)_3 \\ \quad | \quad\quad\quad\quad\quad\quad | \\ NHOCR' \quad\quad\quad O^- \end{array}$$

> Deposition of sphingomyelin in liver, lymph nodes, bone marrow, and central nervous system results in Niemann–Pick disease. It

may be due to the deficiency of sphingomyelinase enzyme in these tissues.

Ceramide: It is formed by the esterification of sphingosine (an amino alcohol) with a fatty acid of high molecular weight. It is principally found in white matter of brain in myelin sheath and medullated nerves. Ceramide is common for all glycolipids and sphingomyelin.

Glycolipids

Glycolipids contain fatty acid, sphingosine (alcohol), carbohydrate, or carbohydrate derivative.
1. Cerebrosides
2. Gangliosides.

Cerebrosides

These contain a molecule of fatty acid, an amino alcohol sphingosine, and a sugar (usually galactose). They are present in white matter of brain and myelin sheath of nerves. Their level is increased in Gaucher's disease in tissues such as reticuloendothelial cells of spleen, liver, lymph node, and bone.

Gangliosides

These are designated as GM1, GM2, etc. and are found in gray matter of the brain and contain *N*-acetylneuraminic acid (sialic acid), fatty acid, alcohol sphingosine, and three molecules of hexoses (such as glucose or galactose). The Tay–Sachs disease is characterized by elevated ganglioside level.

> *Case*
> The pediatrician noticed the infant admitted in his hospital with difficulty in breathing and the skin started turning blue. The pediatrician diagnosed it as respiratory distress syndrome which is due to the deficiency of lung surfactant. Which of the following is the phospholipid of primary importance in surfactant?
> a. Dipalmitoyl phosphatidylethanolamine
> b. Dipalmitoyl phosphatidylserine
> **c. Dipalmitoyl phosphatidylcholine**
> d. Dipalmitoyl phosphatidylinositol

Lipoproteins

Structure and function

Lipoproteins are conjugated proteins, composed of core and surface **(Fig. 8.1)**:
- Lipoprotein core has:
  - Triglycerides
  - Cholesterol esters.
- Lipoprotein surface has:
  - Phospholipids
  - Proteins
  - Cholesterol.
- Lipids are water insoluble.
- This is present in the blood in the form of lipoproteins, which are water soluble.
- They have an outer polar surface, which makes them water soluble.

Composition and Characteristics of Lipoproteins (Table 8.1)

Separation of lipoproteins by ultracentrifugation **(Fig. 8.2A)** and electrophoresis **(Fig. 8.2B)**.

Plasma Lipoprotein Classes and Functions

Chylomicron—transports dietary triglycerides from intestine to liver extrahepatic tissues.

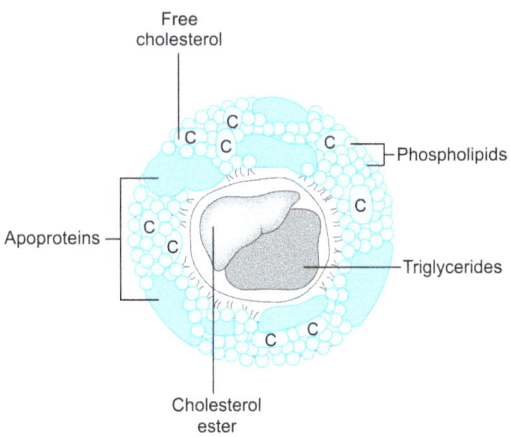

Fig. 8.1: Structure of lipoprotein.

Table 8.1: Composition and characteristics of lipoproteins.

Characteristics	Chylomicron	Very low density lipoprotein (VLDL)	Low-density lipoprotein (LDL)	High-density lipoprotein (HDL)
Density	<0.96	d=0.96–1.006	1.006–1.063	0.063–1.21
Electrophoretic mobility	Origin	Pre β	β	α
Protein (%)	2	10	22	40
Cholesterol (%)	8	22	46	30
Triacylglycerol (%)	83	50	10	8
Phospholipid (%)	7	18	22	22
Apoproteins	A, B, C and E	B, C and E	B	A and E

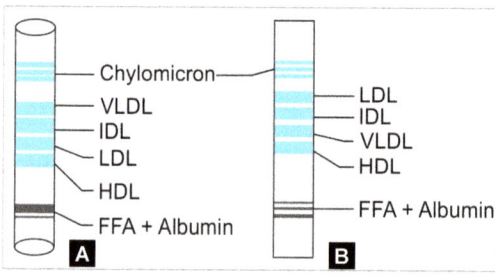

Figs. 8.2A and B: Separation of lipoproteins. (A) Ultracentrifugation. (B) Electrophoresis. (FFA, free fatty acid).

Very low density lipoprotein (VLDL)—transports endogenous triglycerides from liver to peripheral tissues.

Low-density lipoprotein (LDL)—transports cholesterol from liver to extrahepatic tissues.

High-density lipoprotein (HDL)—transports cholesterol from extrahepatic tissues to liver for further metabolism.

APOPROTEINS

The protein part of the lipoprotein is called apoprotein or apolipoprotein. The following types of apoproteins are seen in blood:
- Apo A-I
- Apo A-II
- Apo B-100
- Apo B-48
- Apo C-I
- Apo C-II
- Apo C-III
- Apo D
- Apo E
- Apo J.

Apo A-I
- Apo A-I is synthesized in the intestine and liver.
- It is a component of HDL-2.
- It is antiatherogenic, since it activates LCAT.
- Normal blood level is about 150 mg/dL.

Apo A-II
- Apo A-II is also synthesized in the intestine and liver.
- It is a component of HDL-3.
- It stimulates hepatic lipase and inhibits LCAT.
- Normal blood level is about 30 mg/dL.

Apo B-100
- Apo B-100 is synthesized in liver.
- It is a component of VLDL and LDL.
- It binds to LDL receptors.
- Normal level in blood is about 100 mg/dL.

Apo B-48
- Apo B-48 is synthesized in the intestine.
- It is a component of chylomicron.
- It has 48% size of Apo B-100.

Apo C-I
- Apo C-I is synthesized in liver.
- It is a component of chylomicron and VLDL.

- It activates lecithin-cholesterol acyltransferase (LCAT).
- Normal level in blood is about 10 mg/dL.

Apo C-II
- Apo C-II is synthesized in liver.
- It is a component of chylomicron and VLDL.
- It activates lipoprotein lipase in vessel wall of adipose tissues and skeletal muscles.
- Due to its action, triglycerides from chylomicrons and VLDL are broken down to give fatty acids and glycerol.
- Normal level in blood is about 5 mg/dL.

Apo C-III
- Apo C-III is synthesized in liver.
- It is a component of chylomicron and VLDL.
- It is antiatherogenic.
- It inhibits lipoprotein lipase (LPL).
- Normal level in blood is about 10 mg/dL.

Apo D
- Apo D is a component of HDL-3.
- It transfers cholesterol from tissues to HDL.

Apo E
- Apo E is synthesized in liver.
- It is a component of chylomicron, VLDL, and intermediate-density lipoprotein (IDL).
- It acts as ligand for hepatic uptake.
- Normal level in blood is about 2 mg/dL.

Apo J
- Apo J is synthesized in liver.
- It is a component of HDL-2.
- It is antiatherogenic.
- It inhibits macrophage-mediated cell damage.
- Normal level in blood is about 10 mg/dL.

Clinical Importance of Lipoprotein(a)

Lipoprotein(a)
1. Lipoprotein(a) [LP(a)] consists of LDL-like particle and the specific Apo A, which is covalently bound to the Apo B of the LDL-like particle.
2. Normal human being contains very small amount of LP(a).
3. They interfere with the action of plasminogen, impairing the process of clot resolution (fibrinolysis).
4. Its structure is similar to plasminogen and tissue plasminogen activator, and it competes with plasminogen for its binding site, leading to reduced fibrinolysis. Also because LP(a) stimulates secretion of plasminogen activator inhibitor-1, it leads to thrombogenesis.
5. In addition, because of LDL cholesterol content, LP(a) contributes to atherosclerosis.
6. High LP(a) in blood is a risk factor for coronary heart disease, cerebrovascular disease, atherosclerosis, thrombosis, and stroke.
7. LP(a) levels:
   - Desirable: <14 mg/dL
   - Borderline risk: 14–30 mg/dL
   - High risk: 31–50 mg/dL
   - Very high risk: >50 mg/dL.

DERIVED LIPIDS

Substances derived from the previous groups by hydrolysis, e.g. fatty acid, glycerol, alcohol, and cholesterol.

Fatty Acid

Fatty acids are aliphatic monocarboxylic organic acid with chain length usually ranging from C4 to C24 and it is a constituent of lipid. The fatty acids have the general formula R–CO–OH.

Nomenclature

Fatty acids are named after the name of the hydrocarbon with the same number of carbon atoms, with suffix "oic acid" for saturated fatty acid and the suffix "enoic acid" for the unsaturated fatty acid.

Numbering of a Fatty Acid

- The carbon atoms of fatty acids are numbered from carboxyl group (-COOH group).
- Carboxyl group carbon is C1 and then next carbon atom is C2. The carbon atom adjacent to the -COOH group is also called α-carbon atom; next carbon atom is β and so on. The last carbon atom or CH_3 group is designated as a carbon. For example, oleic acid is written as 18:1; 9 or Δ9, 18:1:

$$\overset{\omega}{C}H_3-(CH_2)_7-\underset{10}{C}H=\underset{9}{C}H-(CH_2)_5-\overset{\beta}{\underset{3}{C}H_2}-\overset{\alpha}{\underset{2}{C}H_2}-\underset{1}{C}OOH$$

- Oleic acid (18:1; 9) or Δ9; 18:1 indicates fatty acid having 18 carbons with one double bond at carbon atom 9. The position of the double can also be indicated by the symbol Δ followed by the position of the double bond in superscript.
- The fatty acids are numbered from the carbon.
- The linoleic acid is called omega (ω)-6 series because of the presence of first double bond from ω-6 carbon at the sixth carbon.

$$\underset{\omega}{\overset{18}{C}H_3}-\overset{17}{(CH_2)_4}-\underset{5}{\overset{13}{C}H}=\underset{6}{\overset{12}{C}H}-\overset{11}{C}H_2-\overset{10}{C}H=\overset{9}{C}H-\overset{8}{(CH_2)_7}$$
$$-\underset{1}{C}OOH$$

- Likewise linolenic acid is ω-3 series:

$$\underset{\omega}{\overset{18}{C}H_3}-\underset{2}{C}H_2-\underset{3}{C}H=CH-CH_2-CH=CH-CH_2-CH$$
$$=CH-(CH_2)_7-\underset{1}{C}OOH$$

- Arachidonic acid is ω-6 series:

$$\underset{\omega}{\overset{20}{C}H_3}-(CH_2)_4-\underset{5}{\overset{14}{C}H}=\underset{6}{C}H-CH_2-\overset{11}{C}H=CH-CH_2-\overset{8}{C}H$$
$$=CH-CH_2-\overset{5}{C}H=CH-(CH_2)_3-COOH$$

Classification of Fatty Acid

Saturated Fatty Acids

- No double bond present. For example:
  - Acetic acid (2 carbon atoms)
  - Butyric acid (4 carbon atoms)
  - Palmitic acid (16 carbon atoms)
  - Stearic acid (18 carbon atoms)
  - Lignoceric acid (24 carbon atoms).

Unsaturated Fatty Acids

The fatty acids, which have double bonds, are called unsaturated fatty acids. They are further classified into:

1. Monounsaturated fatty acid: Contains one double bond, e.g. palmitoleic acid (C16, Δ9) and oleic acid (C18, Δ9).
2. Polyunsaturated fatty acid (PUFA): Contains more than one double bond. For example:
   - Linoleic acid (C18, Δ9)
   - Linolenic acid (C18, Δ9, 12, 15)
   - Arachidonic acid (C20, Δ5, 8, 11, 14).

Essential Fatty Acids or Polyunsaturated Fatty Acids with Specific Examples

Fatty acids, which are not synthesized in the body and should be supplied through diet, are called essential fatty acids. They contain more than one double bond, for example, linoleic acid, linolenic acid, and arachidonic acid, i.e. PUFAs. These fatty acids are not synthesized in the human body because of the lack of the desaturase enzyme, which introduces double bonds beyond 9th and 10th carbon atoms.

1. Linoleic acid, represented as (18:2; 9,12) or [Δ⁹, 12; 18]. It means that this fatty acid contains 18 carbon atoms and two double bonds at positions C9 and C12.

$$-CH_3-(CH_2)_4-CH=CH-CH_2-CH=CH-(CH_2)_7$$
$$-COOH$$

2. Linolenic acid, represented as (18:3; 9, 12, 15) or [Δ⁹, 12, 15; 18].

$$-CH_3-CH_2-CH=CH-CH_2-CH=CH-CH_2-$$
$$CH=CH-(CH_2)_7-COOH$$

3. Arachidonic acid represented as (20:4; 5, 8, 11, 14) or [Δ⁵, 8, 11, 14; 20].

$$-CH_3-(CH_2)_4-CH=CH-CH_2-CH=CH-CH_2-$$
$$CH=CH-(CH_2)_3-COOH$$

Functions of Fatty Acids

1. Essential fatty acids are involved in the esterification of cholesterol and thus help in its transport and metabolism. So essential fatty acid lowers cholesterol level and hence decreases the risk of heart disease.
2. Essential fatty acids are constituent of the cell membrane and membranes of cell organelle (e.g. mitochondria).
3. They are essential for maintaining normal growth and health.
4. Fatty acids are components of simple and compound lipids, which are present in various tissues, e.g. **a**dipose tissue.
5. They are responsible for the hydrophobic nature of the compounds contained in them. They provide energy when they are oxidized in human body.
6. Prostaglandins and leukotrienes are formed from PUFA (arachidonic acid). They act as local hormones.
7. They protect the liver from accumulation of fat (prevent fatty liver).
8. Essential fatty acids help to prevent skin disease.

Cis versus Trans Fatty Acid

Cis: Both H atoms are on the same side of the C=C double bond, which causes a bend in their structure. Most naturally occurring unsaturated fatty acids in food are of cis type.

Trans: Both H atoms are on opposite sides of the C=C double bond:
- They do not bend and have physical properties similar to saturated fatty acids.
- They are not commonly found in nature.
- This form occurs in partially hydrogenated foods when hydrogen atoms shift around some double bonds and change the configuration from cis to trans.

- Major sources of trans fatty acids are as follows:
  - Margarine
  - Cakes and cookies
  - Snack chips
  - Meat and dairy products
  - Peanut butter
  - Fried foods.

Chaulmoogric Acid

Chaulmoogric acid is a special type of fatty acid. It contains a cyclic ring and used in the treatment of leprosy.

Glycerol

- Glycerol is a trihydric alcohol as it contains three hydroxyl groups.
- It is a gluconeogenic substance because on lipolysis of dietary lipid releases glycerol, which is converted into glucose in liver.

Steroids and Cholesterol

Steroids are often found in association of lipids. They are compounds having special ring called cyclopentanoperhydrophenanthrene nucleus, e.g. steroid hormone, bile acid, and vitamin D.

Cholesterol is one of the important steroids present in the body. It has 27 carbons, an –OH group, a double bond, two methyl groups at C10 and C13, and a side chain at C17 (**Fig. 8.3**). Other properties are:

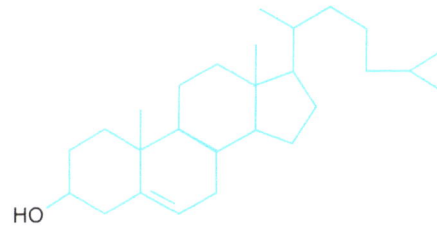

Fig. 8.3: Structure of cholesterol.

1. It is the precursor of various compounds such as vitamin D_3, bile acids, and adrenocortical and sex hormones.
2. Cholesterol is widely distributed in all cells of the body, but nervous tissue is rich in cholesterol.
3. Steroids containing one or more –OH groups are known as sterols.
4. Normal fasting serum cholesterol level is 150–200 mg/dL.
5. It is synthesized in our body using acetyl-CoA as precursor (1 g/day).
6. Cholesterol exists in free and ester form. It gets esterified through esterase enzymes.
7. Excess cholesterol is harmful to body in that it gets deposited in the intima of the arteries producing atherosclerosis. This can narrow the lumen of blood vessel impeding blood flow, which causes thrombosis.

Functions of Cholesterol

Cholesterol, if maintained in normal level, has number of good effects:
1. It is a precursor for the synthesis of bile acids in liver.
2. The steroid hormone in adrenal cortex and sex hormones in gonads are mainly synthesized from cholesterol.
3. Cholesterol form 7-dehydrocholesterol in skin, and it is converted to vitamin D_3 by ultraviolet rays.
4. Cholesterol is a poor conductor of heat and hence acts as an insulator.
5. Cholesterol is a poor conductor of electricity. It is abundant in brain and nervous tissue where it functions as an insulating covering for structure, which generates and transmits electrical impulse.

PROPERTIES OF LIPIDS

Physical Properties

Oils and fats (lipids) are similar in nature. Oils and lipids are different only in their physical property. Triglycerides, which contain a higher proportion of unsaturated fatty acid or short-chain fatty acid, are liquid at 20°C and are usually called oils, e.g. vegetable oils.

On the other hand, fats are solid at room temperature and contain saturated long-chain fatty acid, e.g. animal fat, dalda.

Amphipathic Nature of Lipids

The lipid that possess both hydrophobic (nonpolar) and hydrophilic (polar) groups is known as an amphipathic lipid. These include fatty acid, phospholipids (e.g. lecithin), sphingolipid, and bile salts.

Phospholipids have a hydrophilic head (phosphate group) attached to choline or ethanolamine, or inositol, etc. and a long hydrophobic tail. The general structure may be represented as polar head with a nonpolar tail.

$$\text{Triacylglycerol (tripalmitin)} \xrightarrow[\text{(Sodium salt)}]{\text{Acid/Alkali/\textit{Lipase}}} \text{Glycerol} + \text{3-palmitic acid}$$

When amphipathic lipids are mixed in water, the polar heads face toward aqueous phase, while nonpolar tails face in opposite direction. This nature leads to the formation of a micelle. Amphipathic lipids are important constituents of the lipid bilayer of biological membranes **(Fig. 8.4)**. Triglycerides (triacylglycerol) can be hydrolyzed by acids, alkali, or enzymes such as lipases.

Saponification

Saponification is nothing, but the hydrolysis of triglyceride by alkali, which forms soap.

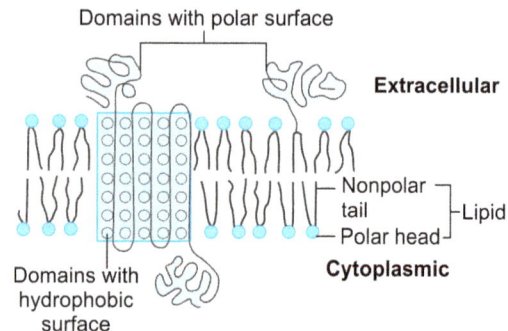

Fig. 8.4: Lipid bilayer of membrane.

Sodium and potassium soaps are soluble in water, whereas magnesium and calcium soaps form insoluble soaps. The number of milligram of potassium hydroxide required to completely saponify 1 g of the oil or fat is called saponification number. This is the measure of chain length of a fatty acid or average molecular size of the fatty acids present. The value is higher for fats-containing short-chain fatty acids.

$$\text{Triacylglycerol} + \text{Alkali [sodium hydroxide (NaOH)]} \longrightarrow \text{Glycerol} + \begin{matrix} R_1\text{—COONa} \\ R_2\text{—COONa} \\ R_3\text{—COONa} \end{matrix} \text{ Soap formaton}$$

Iodine Number

Iodine number is a measure of the degree of unsaturation of a fat. It is defined as the number of grams of iodine that combines with 100 g of a fat. High iodine numbers indicate higher degree of unsaturation. Iodine is incorporated into the double bonds present in the fatty acids. Determination of iodine number will help to know the degree of adulteration of given oil.

Rancidity

Naturally occurring fats particularly from animal sources, on storage in the presence of moist air give unpleasant smell and develop a characteristic taste and odor. It is due to the partial hydrolysis of fats, which are further oxidized into aldehyde and ketones. This process is called rancidity. Bacteria and lipolytic enzymes cause hydrolytic rancidity. Presence of oxygen or intermediates such as peroxides causes oxidative rancidity. Butter contains volatile (free) fatty acids and hence more prone to rancidity. Antioxidants such as vitamin E, vitamin C, butylated hydroxytoluene, and butylated hydroxyanisole can prevent oxidation of fats and thus help in the development of rancidity.

Peroxidation

Peroxidation (autooxidation) of lipids when exposed to oxygen is responsible not only for deterioration food but also for damage to tissues in vivo. Lipid peroxidation is a chain reaction generating continuously free radicals that initiate further peroxidation. To reduce this peroxidation, humans make use of antioxidants, which prevents the oxidative damage.

Reichert–Meissl Number

The number of milliliter of alkali required to neutralize the volatile fatty acids from 5 g of fat, for example, Reichert-Meissl value for butter is 26 and coconut oil is 7.

SUMMARY

Lipids are heterogeneous group of naturally occurring compounds insoluble in water and soluble in nonpolar organic solvents. Lipids are the major form of energy, provide essential fatty acids, maintain membrane structure and integrity, act as lung surfactant and essential for the absorption of fat soluble vitamins. Lipids are classified into simple, compound, and derived lipids. Fats and waxes are simple lipids. Phospholipids, glycolipids, and lipoproteins are the examples for compound lipids. Fatty acids and cholesterol are derived lipids. Compound lipids, i.e. lipoproteins are of different types such as chylomicron, VLDL, LDL, and HDL. The protein part of the lipoprotein is called apoprotein. HDL is good cholesterol and LDL is a bad one, because it transports cholesterol from extrahepatic tissues to liver and liver to extrahepatic tissues, respectively. Fatty acids are of saturated and unsaturated. The essential fatty acids are those which have to be supplied through diet, and they are linoleic acid, linolenic acid, and arachidonic acid. Most of the naturally occurring unsaturated fatty acids are of cis type. Triglyceride is a simple lipid, which is made of glycerol, one unsaturated and two saturated fatty acids. Lipids are amphipathic in nature. Cholesterol is formed from acetyl-CoA, which is required for steroid hormone synthesis.

SELF-ASSESSMENT QUESTIONS

Essay-type Questions

1. Classify the lipids with suitable example for each.
2. List the biomedical importance of lipids.
3. Describe the structure, classification, and functions of phospholipids.
4. Discuss the saturated and unsaturated fatty acids of biological importance.
5. Describe the structure of steroids and add a note on functions of cholesterol.
6. What are lipoproteins? On what basis are they classified? What is the clinical significance of their level detection in blood?
7. Briefly explain the following:
    a. Structure of triacylglycerol
    b. Glycolipids
    c. Essential fatty acids
    d. Rancidity
    e. Saponification number
    f. Iodine number
    g. Lecithin
    h. Atherosclerosis
    i. Sphingomyelin
    j. Prostaglandins
    k. Lipoproteins
    l. Lipotropic factors
    m. Amphipathic nature of the lipids.

Short Answer Questions

1. Which lipid serves as fuel reserve in animals?
2. Which cholesterol is good for health and why?
3. Name the phospholipid that produces second messenger in hormonal action.
4. Name the glycolipid containing N-acetylneuraminic acid.
5. What is the importance of forming chylomicron in our body?
6. Give an example for an antioxidant.
7. Explain the following:
    a. Vegetable oil is liquid at room temperature, whereas animal fat is solid.
    b. Lecithin is amphipathic molecule.
    c. Butter becomes rancid faster than ghee.
    d. Saponification number decreases with increase in molecular weight of fat.

MULTIPLE-CHOICE QUESTIONS

1. The nitrogenous base present in lecithin is:
   a. Ethanolamine   b. Inositol
   c. Serine   d. Choline
2. The number of double bonds present in arachidonic acid is:
   a. 1   b. 2
   c. 3   d. 4
3. Which of the following is an amphipathic lipid?
   a. Phospholipid   b. Fatty acid
   c. Bile salts   d. All the three
4. Name of the test employed to check the adulteration of butter:
   a. Iodine number
   b. Saponification number
   c. Zak's method
   d. Reichert–Meissl number
5. All the following alcohols are present in phospholipids, *except*:
   a. Sphingosine   b. Inositol
   c. Mannitol   d. Glycerol
6. Which of the following is not a phospholipid?
   a. Plasmalogen   b. Lecithin
   c. Sphingomyelin   d. Ganglioside
7. Which of the following is an essential fatty acid:
   a. Oleic acid   b. Arachidic acid
   c. Linoleic acid   d. Palmitic acid
8. Sphingomyelin contains which of the following component?
   a. Glycerol, phosphoric acid, two fatty acids, and choline
   b. Sphingosine, phosphoric acid, one fatty acid, and choline
   c. Sphingosine, phosphoric acid, and two fatty acids
   d. Glycerol, phosphoric acid, and two fatty acids

Chemistry of Lipids

9. The plasma lipoprotein, which is least dense:
   a. VLDL   b. LDL
   c. HDL   d. Chylomicron
10. The plasma lipoprotein, which moves fast toward the anode during electrophoresis is:
    a. VLDL   b. LDL
    c. HDL   d. Chylomicron
11. The PUFA is richly present in:
    a. Sunflower oil b. Butter
    c. Ghee   d. Coconut oil
12. Deficiency of which phospholipid causes respiratory distress syndrome:
    a. Cardiolipin
    b. Phosphatidic acid
    c. Dipalmitoyl lecithin
    d. Cephalin
13. Triglycerides have:
    a. One saturated and two unsaturated fatty acids
    b. Glycerol and three unsaturated fatty acids
    c. Three saturated fatty acids and glycerol as the backbone
    d. Two saturated and one unsaturated fatty acid
14. Phospholipids consist of:
    a. Glycerol and fatty acid esters
    b. Alcohol, cholesterol, and phosphoric acid
    c. Alcohol, phosphoric acid, fatty acids, and a nitrogenous base
    d. Alcohol, fatty acids, and a nitrogenous base
15. Concerning lecithin, all the following statements are true, *except*:
    a. It has both saturated and unsaturated fatty acids
    b. The dipalmitoyl lecithin is a lung surfactant
    c. Presence of dipalmitoyl lecithin in premature infants may produce respiratory distress syndrome
    d. Present in brain and nervous tissue
16. Phosphatidylinositol:
    a. Is absent in cell membrane
    b. Consists of glycerol and phosphatidic acid
    c. Has antigenic properties
    d. Acts as a second messenger for hormonal action
17. All the following are the examples of compound lipids, *except*:
    a. Glycolipids   b. Plasmalogen
    c. Cholesterol   d. Lipoprotein
18. The structure shown below is:
    $CH_3-CH_2-CH=CH-CH_2-CH=CH-CH_2-CH=CH-(CH_2)_7-COOH$
    a. Arachidonic acid   b. Linolenic acid
    c. Linoleic acid   d. Oleic acid
19. Concerning lipoproteins, one of the following statements is false:
    a. The LDL cholesterol transports cholesterol from extrahepatic tissues to liver
    b. It consists of triglyceride and cholesterol ester, proteins, phospholipid, and free cholesterol
    c. Chylomicron transports dietary triglyceride and cholesterol esters from intestine to peripheral tissues and liver
    d. It separates into four different types on the basis of their density
20. One of the following is the nonessential fatty acid:
    a. Arachidonic acid b. Linolenic acid
    c. Palmitic acid   d. Linoleic acid
21. The precursor essential for the cholesterol synthesis is:
    a. Pyruvate   b. Acetyl-CoA
    c. Glucose   d. Triacylglycerol
22. Phospholipase:
    a. Is involved in the synthesis of PG
    b. Is the key enzyme in the hormone action where Ca^{2+} is necessary
    c. Activation of protein kinase
    d. Is activated by adenylyl cyclase
23. The physical property that allows lipids to form membranes:
    a. Inherent flexibility
    b. They are amphipathic and have hydrophobic tails and hydrophilic heads
    c. Tight binding to proteins
    d. High degree of reactivity
24. All the following compounds are esterified with membrane phospholipids, *except*:
    a. Serine   b. Inositol
    c. Ethanolamine   d. Ribose
25. According to the chemical and biological classifications of fatty acids, we can classify palmitic acid as:
    a. Monounsaturated and essential
    b. Monounsaturated and nonessential
    c. Polyunsaturated and nonessential
    d. Saturated and essential

26. Different compounds included in this classificatory group of lipids, can act as pulmonary surfactant, component of membranes and precursors of second messengers. This is the group of:
    a. Steroids
    b. Sphingolipids
    c. Triacylglycerols
    d. Fatty acids
    e. Phosphoglycerides
27. A premature baby, shortly after birth, presents with rapid breathing, intercostal retractions and grunting sounds while breathing. A blood gas analysis reveals low oxygen and acidosis. A diagnosis of respiratory distress syndrome is quickly made. This syndrome is seen in newborns with immature lungs whose pneumocytes do not synthesize enough:
    a. Phosphatidylinositol
    b. Phosphatidylcholine
    c. Sphingosine
    d. Sphingomyelin
28. Polymers of polysaccharides, fats, and proteins are all synthesized from monomers by:
    a. Connecting the monosaccharides together
    b. Addition of water to each monomer
    c. The formation of disulfide bridges between monomers
    d. The condensation or dehydration reaction

Answers

1. d	2. d	3. a	4. a	5. c
6. d	7. a	8. b	9. a	10. c
11. a	12. c	13. d	14. c	15. c
16. d	17. c	18. b	19. a	20. c
21. b	22. b	23. d	24. d	25. c
26. b	27. b	28. d		

CHAPTER 9

Metabolism of Lipids

OBJECTIVES

At the end of this chapter, students should be able to:
- Explain the process of digestion and absorption of lipids
- Know about the β-oxidation of fatty acids (FAs) and its importance
- Explain the process of FA synthesis and its regulation in postabsorptive and fasting conditions
- Explain the process of ketone body formation and their utilization
- Know about the metabolism of various lipoproteins, including hyperlipoproteinemias.

DIGESTION AND ABSORPTION OF LIPIDS

Introduction

- Most of the fat in the human diet is in the form of **triacylglycerol (TAG)**, which consists of three FAs linked to glycerol. In the digestive tract, TAG is hydrolyzed by the enzyme **pancreatic lipase**, to release free FAs and monoglycerides.
- The process of lipid digestion is dependent on bile salts for emulsification. Before fat digestion to occur, it must be converted into fine droplets as an emulsion, which facilitates the digestion of lipids.
- The lipids delay the rate of emptying stomach, by way of the hormone enterogastrone, which inhibits gastric motility and retards the discharge of food from the stomach. Therefore fats have the satiety value.
- The heat of the stomach is important in liquefying dietary lipids.
- The enzymes of stomach, gastric lipase and lingual lipase, present in the chyme are active only at neutral pH.
- In adults no digestion of fat takes place in stomach due to acidic pH. These enzymes may be active in infants and act on short- and medium-chain FAs due to the pH of the stomach content, which is nearer to neutral pH.
- The hydrophilic short- and medium-chain FAs are absorbed via stomach wall and enter the portal vein.
- The long-chain FAs dissolve in the diet and pass on into the duodenum.

Process of Lipid Digestion and Absorption

- Entry of acidic chyme from the stomach into the duodenum stimulates the secretion of enteric hormones such as gastrin and cholecystokinin by the mucosal cells of duodenum.
- This cholecystokinin acts on the gallbladder, causing it to contract and release of bile salts into the small intestine.
- Cholecystokinin also acts on the exocrine cells of the pancreas, causing them to release digestive enzymes, including lipase.
- The same cholecystokinin also decreases gastric motility, which results in a slow

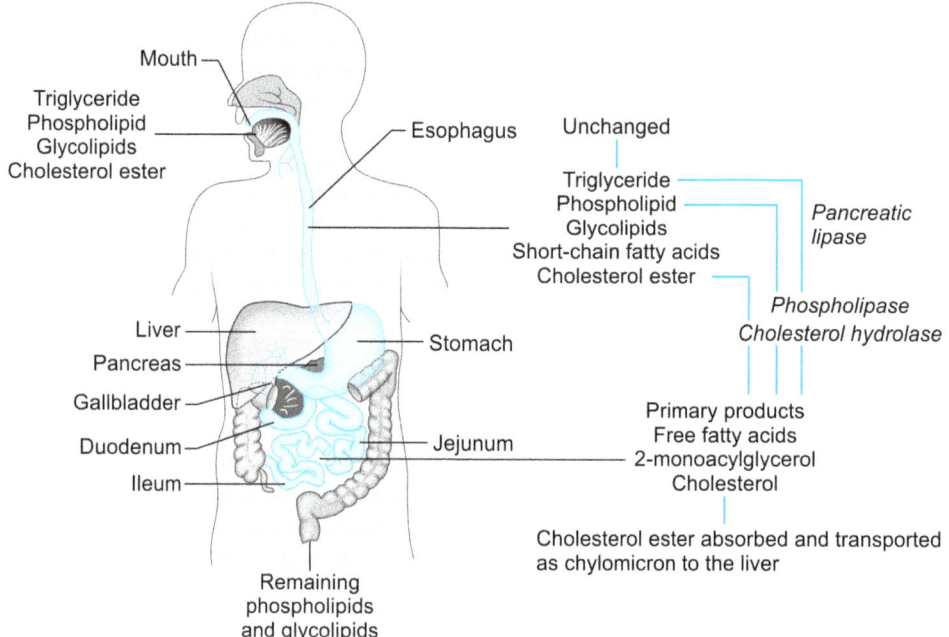

Fig. 9.1: Digestion of lipids.

release of the gastric contents into small intestine.
- The other hormone secretin causes the pancreas to release a bicarbonate-rich solution, which neutralizes the acidic chyme and changes the pH to the alkaline side. The formation of alkaline pH of the content is very important for the action of lipase and intestinal enzymes. The bile (with bile salts and phosphatidylcholine) enters the duodenum and provides the emulsifying action. After emulsification, the lipolytic enzymes such as lipase, phospholipase A2, and cholesterol esterase present in the pancreatic juice hydrolyze lipids (**Fig. 9.1**).
- Dietary glycerophospholipids are digested by pancreatic phospholipase A2. This enzyme catalyzing the hydrolysis of FA residues at the second position of the glycerophospholipid, leaving lysophospholipids. This lysophospholipid enters the mucosal cell or degraded further by lysophospholipase enzyme (secreted by intestinal cells) to remove final FA residue.
- Inside the mucosal cells, fats are resynthesized and converted to chylomicron, and transported to blood via lymphatic vessel.
- Fatty acids less than 10 carbon atoms along with glycerol are carried by portal blood to the liver.
- The long-chain free FAs, free cholesterol, 2-monoglyceride, 1-monoglyceride, and lysophospholipid together with bile salts form mixed micelles. The bile salts aggregate with their hydrophobic region placed internally and hydrophilic region facing the water medium and make the micelle water soluble. The glycerides and long-chain FAs in these micelles are transported into the intestinal mucosal cells leaving bile salts in the medium itself. The bile salts are reabsorbed in the intestine and returned to liver by portal vein for resecretion into bile. This process is called ***enterohepatic circulation*** of bile salts.

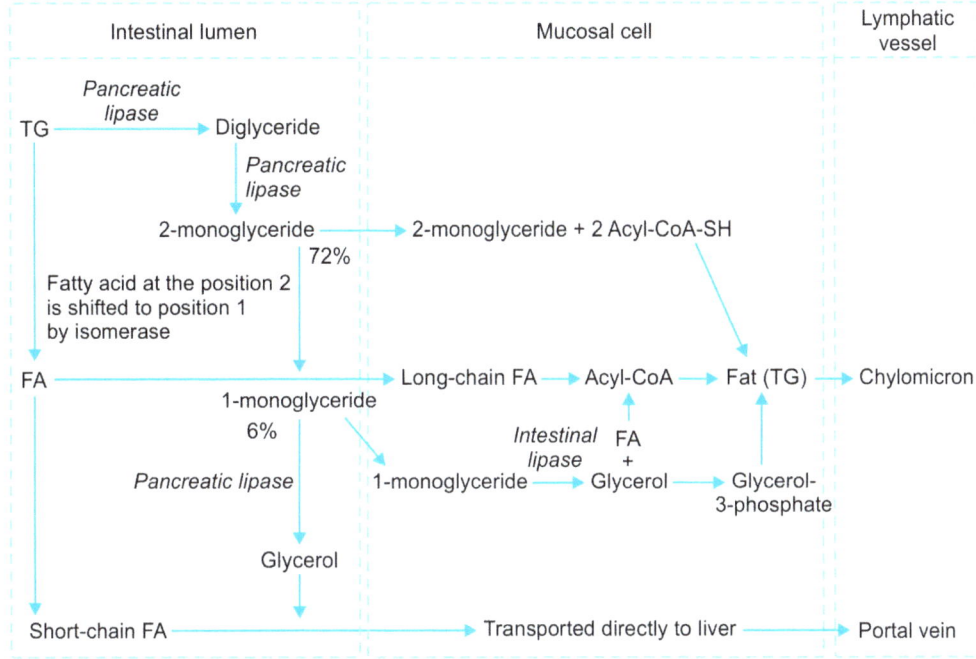

Fig. 9.2: Absorption of lipids.

- The short- and medium-chain FAs are absorbed directly into the intestinal epithelial cells and enter the portal blood to reach the liver.
- The 1-monoacylglycerol is further hydrolyzed in the intestinal mucosal cell by intestinal lipase.
- The 2-monoacylglycerol is reconverted to triglyceride (TG) as shown in **Figure 9.2**. The utilization of FAs inside the mucosal cell for the resynthesis of TAG needs the activation to acyl-CoA by thiokinase enzyme.
- The absorbed lysophospholipids and cholesterol are also recycled with acyl-CoA to regenerate phospholipids, and cholesterol esters.
- The phospholipid, cholesterol ester, TAG, synthesized in the intestinal mucosal cell, and the absorbed fat-soluble vitamins are transported from the mucosal cells into the lymph in the form of chylomicron.
- After absorption lipids are either oxidized mainly in the liver or stored in the depots (adipose tissue). For utilization by the body, TGs are first hydrolyzed by lipase to release glycerol and free FAs. Glycerol is converted into glucose by gluconeogenesis or enters glycolysis. Fatty acids are oxidized to carbon dioxide (CO_2) and water (H_2O) with the liberation of large amount of energy.
- The abnormalities of fat absorption occur during the diseases affecting intestinal mucosa, inhibition of pancreatic lipase by low pH and decreased synthesis of bile salts in liver cirrhosis.

Fate of Triacylglycerol in Adipose Tissue

1. In response to energy demands, the FAs of stored TAGs can be mobilized for use by peripheral tissues.
2. The release of metabolic energy, in the form of FAs, is controlled by a complex series of interrelated cascades that result in the activation of hormone-sensitive lipase.

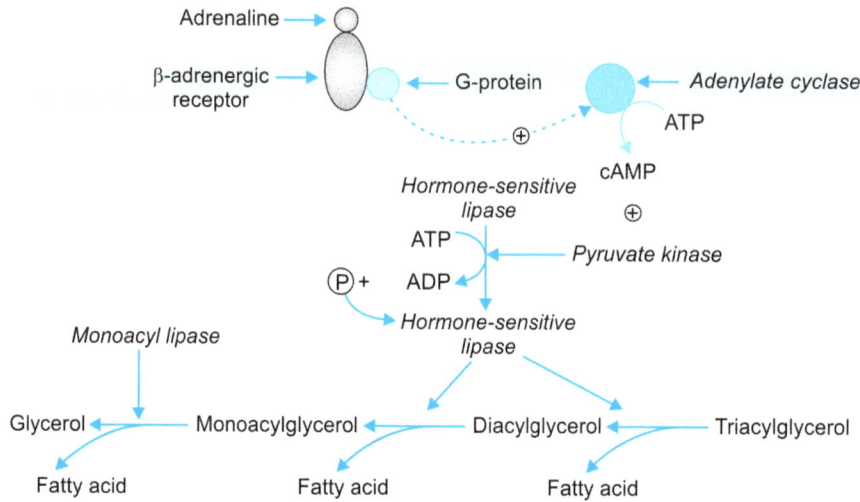

Fig. 9.3: Activation of hormone-sensitive lipase by epinephrine.

3. The stimulus to activate this cascade, in adipocytes, can be glucagon, epinephrine, or α-corticotropin (**Fig. 9.3**).
4. These hormones bind to the cell-surface receptors that are coupled to the activation of adenylate cyclase upon ligand binding. The resultant increase in cyclic adenosine monophosphate (cAMP) leads to activation of pyruvate kinase, which in turn phosphorylates and activates hormone-sensitive lipase. This enzyme hydrolyzes FAs from carbon atoms 1 or 3 of TAGs. The resulting diacylglycerols are substrates for either hormone-sensitive lipase or for the noninducible enzyme diacylglycerol lipase.
5. Finally, the monoacylglycerols are substrates for monoacylglycerol lipase. The net result of the action of these enzymes is three moles of free FA and one mole of glycerol. The free FAs diffuse from adipose cells, combine with albumin in the blood, and are thereby transported to other tissues, where they passively diffuse into cells.
6. The glycerol, released in adipose tissue, cannot be processed further by adipocytes, because they lack glycerol kinase. Therefore it is transported through the blood to the liver phosphorylation. The glycerol phosphate formed can be used to form TAG in the liver or to be converted to dihydroxyacetone phosphate.

Steatorrhea

Steatorrhea is the presence of excess fat in feces. Stools may be bulky and difficult to flush have a pale and oily appearance and can be especially foul smelling. An oily anal leakage or some level of fecal incontinence may occur.

Causes

Too much fat in the stool suggests that our digestive system is not digesting (breaking down) food sufficiently. Our body may not absorb the essential components of the food we eat, including dietary fat. One of the most common causes of malabsorption is cystic fibrosis.

Lack of enzymes due to **pancreatitis** results in poor digestion and absorption of food, especially fats. Thus weight loss is characteristic of chronic **pancreatitis**. Patients may notice bulky smelly bowel movements due to too much fat (**steatorrhea**).

Treatment:
- Intravenous fluids to restore electrolytes and stop dehydration
- Antidiarrheal medications
- Pancreatic enzyme replacement therapy
- Proton-pump inhibitors or PPIs.

METABOLISM OF LIPIDS

β-Oxidation of Lipids and Its Regulation during Fed and Fasting States

Oxidation of Fatty Acids

- Oxidation of FA takes place in mitochondria where the various enzymes for FA oxidation are present close to the enzymes of the electron transport chain.
- Most important theory of the oxidation of FA is the β-oxidation of FA.
  The primary sources of FAs for oxidation are dietary and mobilization from cellular stores. Fatty acids from the diet are delivered from the gut to cells via transport in the blood. Fatty acids are stored in the form of TAGs primarily within adipocytes of adipose tissue.
- Fatty acids are rich sources of energy.
- Energy is released when FA undergoes β-oxidation and it is a cyclic process.
- Oxidation of FA occurs at the β-carbon atom resulting in the elimination of two terminal carbon atoms as acetyl-CoA leaving fatty acyl-CoA, which has two carbon atoms less than the original FA.
- Active form of FA is called fatty acyl-CoA.
- If the starting FA is palmitic acid, which has 16 carbon atoms, at a time 2 carbon atoms are removed as acetyl-CoA, then seven cycles of β-oxidation occurs to convert palmitic acid (16C) into eight acetyl-CoA (2C) molecules.
  1. First step in FA is the activation to its fatty acyl-CoA form:

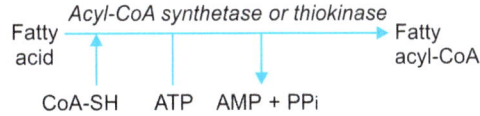

This reaction occurs outside the mitochondria.
2. Fatty acyl-CoA formed inside the mitochondria cannot cross the inner mitochondrial membrane. "Carnitine," a carrier substance, carries the acyl group into the mitochondrial membrane (**Fig. 9.4**).
3. Once the activated FA enter the mitochondria, flavoprotein-linked acyl-CoA dehydrogenase (DH) removes two hydrogen atoms from fatty acyl-CoA forming α,β-unsaturated fatty acyl-CoA. This contains a double bond at α and β positions (**Fig. 9.5**).
4. Enoyl-CoA hydratase enzyme adds a molecule of water at the double-bond position of α,β-unsaturated fatty acyl-CoA forming β-hydroxyacyl-CoA.
5. In the presence NAD+, β-hydroxyacyl-CoA DH enzyme oxidizes β-hydroxyacyl-CoA to form β-ketoacyl-CoA.

   Thiolase in the presence of CoA-SH cleaves β-ketoacyl-CoA to yield acetyl-CoA and fatty acyl-CoA having two carbon atoms less than the original FA. Newly formed acyl-CoA undergoes another six more cycles starting from step one and is finally degraded into acetyl-CoA molecules.

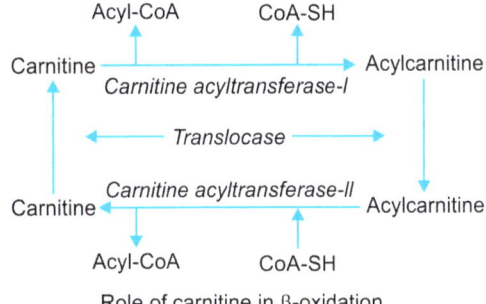

Fig. 9.4: Transport of acyl-CoA carnitine.

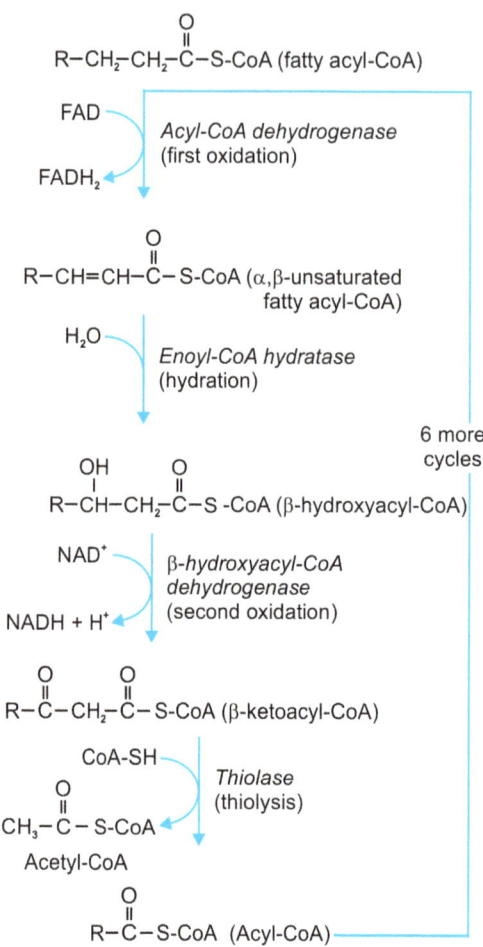

Fig. 9.5: Steps of β-oxidation of palmitic acid.

Energetics of β-oxidation of Palmitic Acid

Palmitic acid when undergoes β-oxidation, it releases eight molecules of acetyl-CoA in seven cycles of the oxidative process. In each round of β-oxidation, one molecule of flavin adenine dinucleotide ($FADH_2$) and one molecule of $NADH+H^+$ are produced, which generate 2-3 molecules of adenosine triphosphate (ATP), respectively, through oxidative phosphorylation in electron transport chain. The total number of ATPs produced in seven rounds of oxidation process is 35. In addition when each acetyl-CoA molecule oxidized in tricarboxylic acid (TCA) cycle, 12 ATPs are generated. Energetics of palmitic acid oxidation is given by: Per cycle of β-oxidation

Step I ($FADH2$)	= 1.5 ATP
Step II ($NADH + H^+$)	= 2.5 ATP
	= 4 ATP
7 cycles of β-oxidation	= 28 ATP
Number of ATPs produced in tricarboxylic acid (TCA) cycle/acetyl-CoA	= 10 ATP
Total number of acetyl-CoA formed from palmitic acid	= 8
Total number of adenosine triphosphate (ATP) produced by complete oxidation of palmitic acid	= (8 × 10) + 28 = 80 + 28 = 108 ATP
Number of ATPs utilized for activation of fatty acid	= – 2 ATP
Net ATPs produced by complete oxidation of palmitic acid	= 106 ATP
The standard free energy of palmitate	= 2,340 cal
106 × 7.3 cal = 773.8 cal	
The efficiency of energy conservation by fatty acid (FA) oxidation:	$\dfrac{773.8 \times 100}{2340}$ = 33%

Fatty acids are predominantly oxidized by the process of β-oxidation in mitochondria.

Oxidation of Odd-chain Fatty Acids

It is similar to β-oxidation with a difference in the final step, a three-carbon fragment, propionyl-CoA is left behind (in place of two-carbon unit for saturated FAs), which is converted to succinyl-CoA (**Fig. 9.6**).

Regulation of β-oxidation

The rate-limiting step in the β-oxidation is the formation of fatty acylcarnitine catalyzed by carnitine acyltransferase-1 (CAT-1). It is an

Metabolism of Lipids

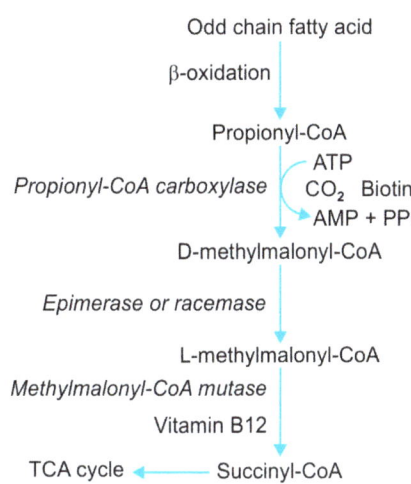

Fig. 9.6: Oxidation of odd-chain fatty acids.

allosteric enzyme and inhibited by malonyl-CoA (first intermediate in the biosynthesis of FA from acetyl-CoA catalyzed by acetyl-CoA carboxylase) **(Fig. 9.7)**.

Malonyl-CoA concentration increases in a well-fed state, which inhibits CAT-1 and leads to decrease in the FA oxidation.

In starvation, due to decrease in the insulin/glucagon ratio, acetyl-CoA carboxylase is inhibited and concentration of malonyl-CoA decreases, releasing the inhibition of CAT-1 and permitting more acetyl-CoA for oxidation.

Case
A 20-year-old female has been diagnosed with anorexia nervosa. In this female, the oxidation of FA is required to provide energy. Prior to oxidation, activation and the transport of activated fatty from cytosol to mitochondria takes place: which of the following is essential for the transport of activated FA to mitochondria?
a. Acetyl-CoA
b. Carnitine
c. Acetoacetate
d. Glucose

Answer is b.

Jamaican vomiting sickness
Jamaican vomiting sickness is characterized by:
- Severe hypoglycemia, vomiting, convulsions, coma, and death

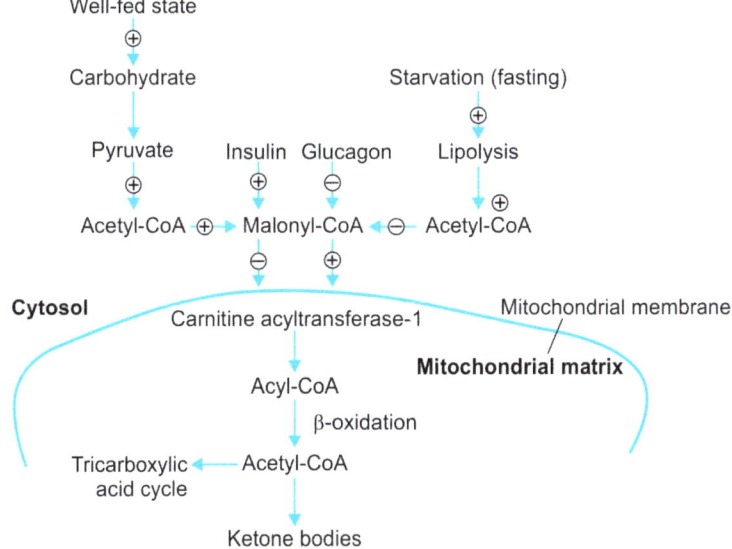

Fig. 9.7: Regulation of fatty acid metabolism.

- Cause: Eating unripe ackee fruit, which contains unusual toxic amino acid, hypoglycin-A
- This inhibits the enzyme acyl-CoA dehydrogenase and thus β-oxidation of fatty acid is blocked, leading to various complications.

Peroxisomal Fatty Acid Oxidation (Lipolysis)

1. Peroxisomes are subcellular organelles found in all nucleated cells.
2. Peroxisomes are able to conduct oxidation of long-chain FAs. Oxidation of very long-chain FAs (20–26 carbon atoms) begins in peroxisomes by a process similar to β-oxidation (completed in the mitochondria).
3. The action of acyl-CoA DH differs, it produces hydrogen peroxide (H_2O_2) rather than $FADH_2$.
4. Catalase located in peroxisomes converts this H_2O_2 to water and molecular oxygen. This process is not linked directly to phosphorylation and the generation of ATP. Once the long-chain FAs reduced to octanoyl-CoA (with eight carbons in its fatty acyl chain) leave the peroxisomes, it is transferred to carnitine through which it enters mitochondria, where they undergo β-oxidation:

```
        Fatty acyl-CoA
              │  ┌─ FAD      ┌─ H₂O₂
Acyl-CoA      │  │           │         Catalase
dehydrogenase │  └─ FADH₂    └─ O₂ ──► H₂O
              ▼
        Octanoyl-CoA
              │
              ▼
     β-oxidation in mitochondria
```

Clinical Importance

Clofibrate, a drug used to treat certain types of hyperlipoproteinemias, stimulates proliferation of peroxisomes, and causes induction of the peroxisomal FA **oxidation**.

Zellweger syndrome
- Rare inborn error of peroxisomal oxidation of FA oxidation
- Cause: Inherited absence of functional peroxisomes in all tissues
- The syndrome is caused by defect in the transport of enzymes into the peroxisomes; thus long-chain FAs (with 26–38 carbons) are not oxidized and accumulate in tissues such as brain, kidney, and muscle.

α-Oxidation

1. α-Oxidation of FA can also occur in human body mainly in liver and brain by removing one carbon from carboxyl end. There is no activation step.
2. Hydroxylation occurs at α-carbon atom done by monooxygenase system and then oxidized to ketoacid.
3. Ketoacid undergoes decarboxylation.
4. It liberates a molecule of CO_2 and a FA.
5. It does not require any CoA and it does not release energy.
6. Defect in enzyme system leads to Refsum disease.

Refsum disease
- Refsum disease, a rare but severe neurological disorder.
- Patients with this disease accumulate large quantities of an unusual fatty acid, phytanic acid derived from phytol, a constituent of chlorophyll.
- Also present in milk and animal fats.
- Phytanic acid cannot undergo β-oxidation due to the presence of a methyl group on carbon 3.
- This fatty acid undergoes initial α-oxidation to remove α-carbon, and this is followed by β-oxidation.
- Refsum disease is caused by a defect in the α-oxidation due to the deficiency of the enzyme phytanic acid oxidase.

- So phytanic acid cannot be converted to a compound that can be degraded by β-oxidation.
- In this condition, the patients should avoid diet containing chlorophyll.

Omega-Oxidation

- Omega-oxidation is a minor pathway of oxidation of long-chain FA in microsomes.
- It occurs from both the ends of FA chain.
- It needs hydroxylase enzymes with nicotinamide adenine dinucleotide phosphate (NADPH) and cytochrome P-450.
- Dicarboxylic acids are produced during this process.
- It is important when β-oxidation is defective. The dicarboxylic acids are excreted in urine causing dicarboxylic aciduria.
- Unsaturated FA can also be activated and transported across the inner mitochondrial membrane and undergo β-oxidation.

COMPOUNDS FORMED FROM ACETYL-COA

Metabolic Fates of Acetyl-CoA

Acetyl-CoA is produced by aerobic glycolysis of glucose, oxidation of FA via β-oxidation. Acetyl-CoA is mainly used in citric acid cycle (**Fig. 9.8**).

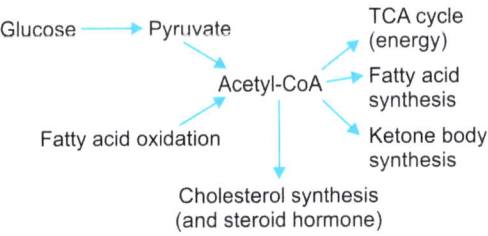

Fig. 9.8: Metabolic fates of acetyl-CoA.

Case

A 10-year-old boy was brought to the emergency department with a complaint of tiredness and severe abdominal pain in the semiconscious state. The blood glucose of this boy showed 40 mg/dL, and his sample showed negative for protein, glucose, and ketone bodies. Glucose was given intravenously and the condition improved within 5 minutes. The doctor sent blood sample for several investigations to know the exact cause for his condition. The laboratory investigation showed elevated acylcarnitine. The doctor diagnosed it as enzyme deficiency, which helps in the oxidation of fatty acids. So the doctor instructed the parents to feed the child more frequently. The deficient enzyme in this by might be:
a. Acyl-CoA synthetase
b. Translocase
c. Carnitine acyltransferase
d. Acyl-CoA dehydrogenase

Answer is d.
Acyl-CoA dehydrogenase is the first enzyme in the β-oxidation of fatty acids. So the deficiency of this enzyme results in the impairment of β-oxidation of fatty acids. The impaired β-oxidation results in impaired synthesis of ketone bodies. So the body has to meet the energy demands through glucose and the glucose requirement increased and there will be imbalance between the demands and the supply of glucose that leads to hypoglycemia in acyl-CoA dehydrogenase deficiency.

Biosynthesis or De Novo Synthesis of Fatty Acid

The majority of the FAs required by the body are supplied by our diet. Fatty acids are synthesized whenever there is a caloric excess in our diet. This excess amount of carbohydrate and protein obtained from the diet can be converted to FAs, which are stored as glycerol:

- Fatty acid synthesis involves the similar steps involved in β-oxidation of FA, but in a reverse way.
- Mammals can synthesize major portion of the saturated FA as well as monounsaturated FAs.
- The system for the fresh synthesis of FA is known as de novo synthesis of FA, occurs in liver, adipose tissue, kidney, and lactating mammary glands.
- The enzyme machinery is located in cytoplasm.
- It is referred to as extramitochondrial or cytoplasmic fatty acid synthase (FAS) system.
- Palmitic acid is the major FA synthesized.
- All the 16 carbon atoms are from acetyl-CoA.
- Acetyl-CoA and NADPH are the prerequisites for FA synthesis.
- Acetyl-CoA produced in the mitochondria cannot enter cytoplasm through inner mitochondrial membrane. So acetyl-CoA condenses with oxaloacetate in mitochondria to form citrate. Citrate is freely transported to cytosol where it is cleaved by citrate lyase to liberate acetyl-CoA and oxaloacetate (**Fig. 9.9**):

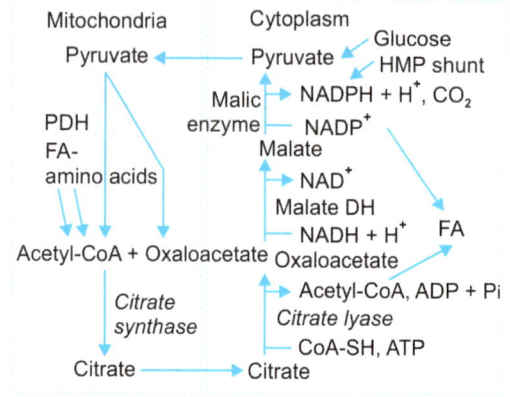

Fig. 9.9: Entry of acetyl-CoA into cytoplasm.

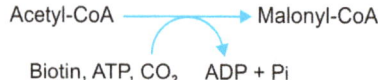

For the synthesis of FA, eight acetyl-CoAs are transported from the mitochondria to cytosol, which is linked with the synthesis of eight NADPHs. As such 14 NADPHs are needed to synthesize one molecule of palmitate. The remaining six NADPHs are supplied from hexose monophosphate shunt:

- Acetyl-CoA carboxylase, regulatory enzyme in FA synthesis.
- The remaining reactions of FA synthesis are catalyzed by multifunctional enzyme known as FAS complex (**Fig. 9.10**).

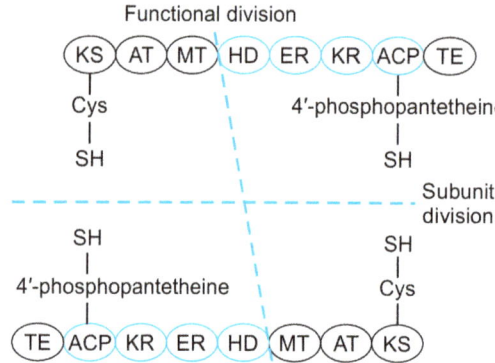

Fig. 9.10: Fatty acid synthase enzyme complex.

- It is a dimer with two identical subunits.
- Each monomer possesses the activities of seven different enzymes and an acyl carrier protein (ACP) bound to 4-phosphopantetheine-SH group.
- Two subunits lie in antiparallel (head-to-tail) orientation.
- The SH group of phosphopantetheine of one subunit is in close proximity with the SH of cysteine residue of the other subunit.
- Each monomer of FAS contains all the enzyme activities of FA synthesis.
- But only the dimer form is functionally active because the functional unit consists half of each subunit.

- Subunit interacts with the complimentary half of the other.

Components of FAS complex are:
- Acetyltransferase
- Malonyl transferase
- β-ketoacyl synthase
- β-ketoacyl reductase
- β-hydroxyacyl dehydratase
- Enoyl reductase
- Thioesterase (TE).

Acyl Carrier Protein

1. Fatty acid synthesis starts with the transfer of an acetyl-CoA to cysteinyl SH group of ACP (**Fig. 9.11**).
2. Malonyl-CoA-ACP transferase transfers malonate from malonyl-CoA to bind to ACP.
3. The acetyl unit attached to cysteine is transferred to malonyl group attached to ACP. Malonyl moiety loses CO_2, which was added by acetyl-CoA carboxylase and form b-ketoacyl enzyme.
4. β-Ketoacyl enzyme is reduced to β-hydroxybutyryl enzyme complex using $NADPH^+ H^+$.
5. Molecule of water (H_2O) is removed from β-OH butyryl enzyme to form α,β-unsaturated acyl enzyme.
6. The unsaturated bond in α,β-unsaturated acyl enzyme is again reduced using $NADPH^+ H^+$ to form butyryl or acyl enzyme. The carbon chain attached to ACP is transferred to cysteine residue and the reactions 2-6 are repeated six more times, and finally palmitic acid is synthesized.

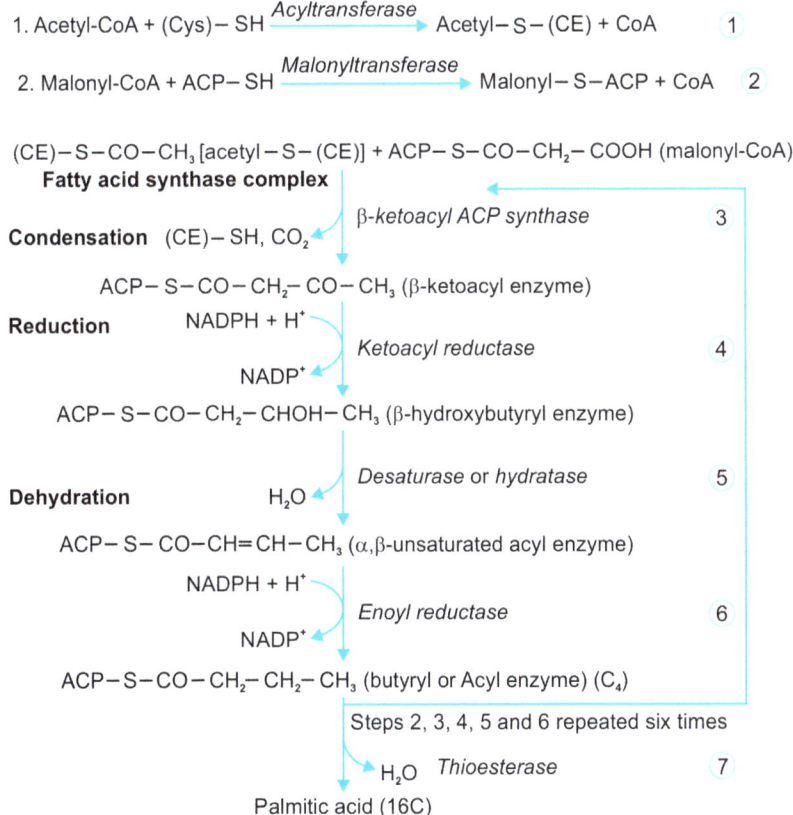

Fig. 9.11: Steps of fatty acid synthesis.

7. The completely synthesized FA is released from the enzyme system by the action of TE enzyme.
8. Chain elongation of FA occurs in the mitochondria and liver microsomes.
9. Of the 16 carbons present in palmitate, only 2 come from acetyl-CoA directly. The remaining 14 are from malonyl-CoA, which, in turn, is produced by acetyl-CoA.
10. During elongation in microsomes, palmitate is activated to palmitoyl-CoA. Malonyl-CoA serves as the donor of two carbons at a time in series of reactions.
11. The major elongation reaction occurs in the body involves the formation of stearoyl-CoA (C18) from palmitoyl-CoA (C16).
12. Elongation of this stearoyl-CoA in brain increases during myelination to provide C22 and C24 FAs present in the sphingolipids.
13. Mitochondrial elongation is less active and uses acetyl-CoA as the source of two-carbon units.
14. 8 Acetyl-CoA+7 ATP+14 NADPH+14 H$^+$ → palmitate+8 CoA+7 ADP+7 Pi+6 H$_2$O+14 NADP$^+$.

Regulation

1. Acetyl-CoA carboxylase enzyme controls a committed step in FA synthesis. This enzyme exists as an inactive protomer (monomer) or as an active polymer. Citrate promotes polymer formation, hence FA synthesis increases. Palmitoyl-CoA and malonyl-CoA causes depolymerization of the enzyme and inhibits FA synthesis.
2. Hormonal influence: Glucagon, epinephrine, and norepinephrine inactivate the enzyme by cAMP-dependent phosphorylation.
3. Insulin dephosphorylates and activates the enzyme.
4. Insulin promotes and glucagon inhibits FA synthesis.
5. Dietary regulation: High carbohydrate or fat-free diet increases the synthesis of acetyl-CoA carboxylase and FAS, which promotes FA synthesis.
6. Fasting or high-fat diet decreases FA production.
7. NADPH influences FA synthesis.

Cholesterol Metabolism

- Cholesterol is a sterol, present in cell membrane, brain, and lipoprotein:

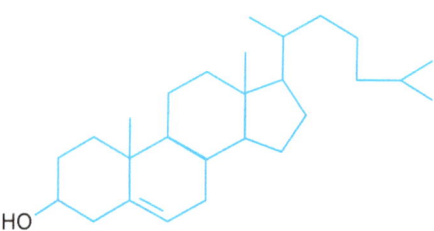

- It is a precursor for all steroids.
- It is amphipathic in nature (hydrophilic and hydrophobic).
- About 1 g of cholesterol is synthesized/per day in humans.
- About 80% of the liver cholesterol converted to bile acids.
- Vitamin D$_3$ is formed from 7-dehydrocholesterol.
- All the steroids have cyclopentanoperhydrophenanthrene ring made up of three cyclohexane rings, A, B, and C, and a cyclopentane ring D.
- Normal blood level is 200 mg/dL.
- Hypercholesterolemia is seen in nephrosis, diabetes mellitus, hypothyroidism, and obstructive jaundice.
- Increased cholesterol level leads to atherosclerosis.
- The OH group in the third position can get esterified with FAs to form cholesterol esters; this esterification occurs in the body by transfer of polyunsaturated fatty acid (PUFA) moiety by lecithin–cholesterol acyltransferase (LCAT), this step is important in the regulation of cholesterol level.
- It is a poor conductor of electricity.

Synthesis

Site: Extramitochondrial enzymes involved are found in cytosol and microsomal fractions of the cell (**Figs. 9.12A and B**):

- Synthesis takes place in liver, skin, and intestine, and also in adrenal cortex and testis.
- All the 27 carbon atoms are derived from acetyl-CoA.

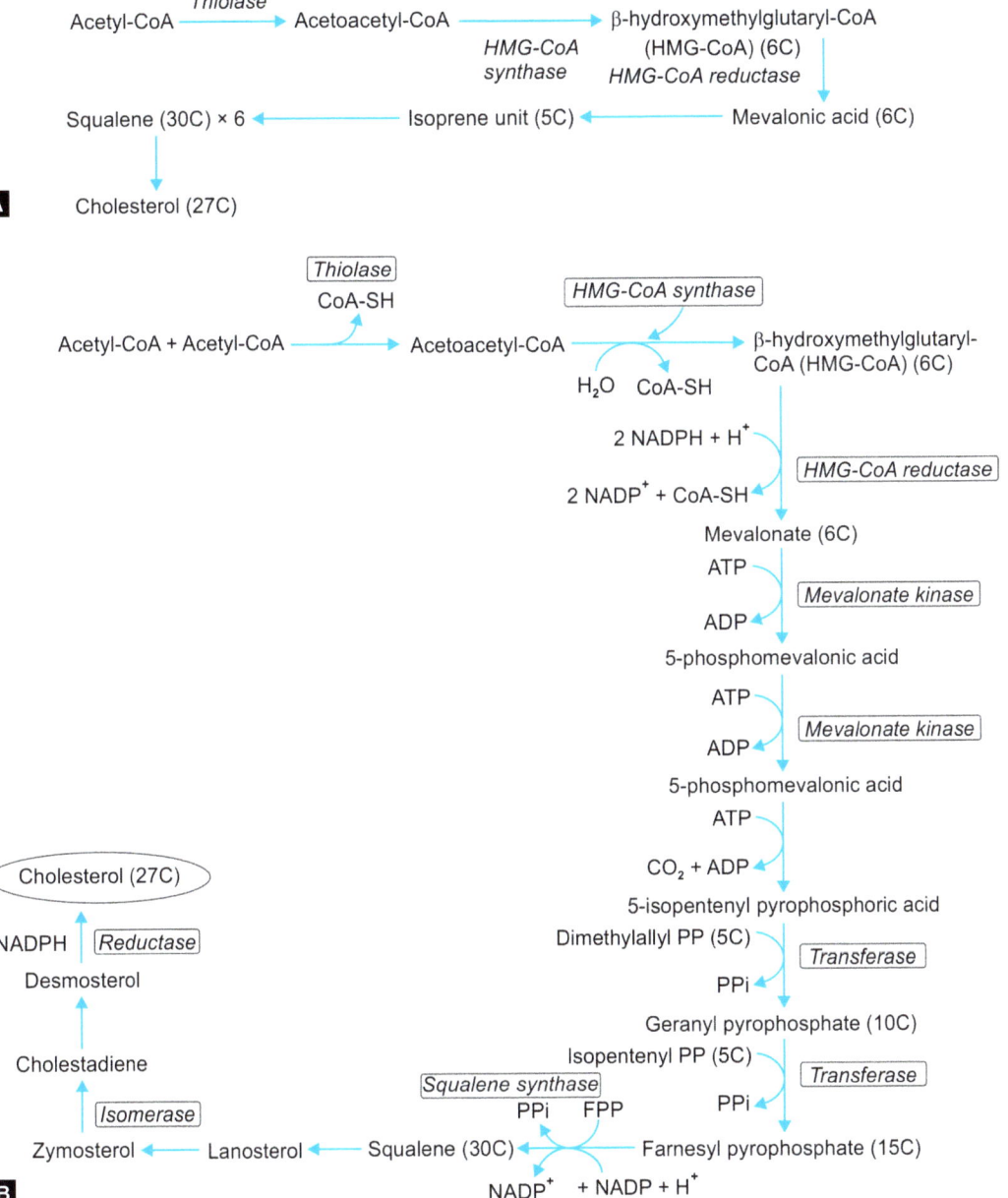

Figs. 9.12A and B: Cholesterol synthesis.

- About 18 acetyl-CoA are required.
- Acetyl-CoA formed by the glycolysis and oxidation of FA are the precursors for the cholesterol synthesis.

REGULATION OF CHOLESTEROL BIOSYNTHESIS AND SIGNIFICANCE OF BIOCHEMICAL BASIS OF USE OF HYPOLIPIDEMIC DRUGS

Regulation of Cholesterol Synthesis

Cholesterol biosynthesis is controlled by the rate-limiting enzyme HMG-CoA reductase (**Fig. 9.13**):

1. Feedback control: The end product of cholesterol controls its own synthesis of the enzyme by a feedback mechanism. Increase in the cellular concentration of cholesterol reduces the synthesis of the enzyme by decreasing the transcription of the gene responsible for the production of HMG-CoA reductase.
2. Hormonal regulation: The HMG-CoA reductase exists in two interconvertible forms. The dephosphorylated form of the enzyme is more active, whereas phosphorylated form is less active. Hormones exert their influence through cAMP.
3. Inhibition by drugs: The drugs compactin, lovastatin, mevastatin, and simvastatin, which inhibit HMG-CoA reductase, and which are used to decrease the cholesterol level.
4. The HMG-CoA reductase is inhibited by bile acids.
5. Low-density lipoprotein (LDL) transports cholesterol from the liver to peripheral tissues.
6. High-density lipoprotein (HDL) transports cholesterol from peripheral tissues to the liver.

> *Case*
> A 55-year-old obese woman presented with severe tiredness and join pain. The laboratory investigations revealed abnormal lipid profile values with a cholesterol level of 280 mg/dL. The doctor prescribed 10 mg statin tablet every day. This statin reduces cholesterol synthesis by inhibiting the enzyme:
> a. **HMG-CoA reductase**
> b. Thiolase
> c. Acyl-CoA dehydrogenase
> d. Thiophorase

Role of Lecithin–Cholesterol Acyltransferase

1. HDL and the enzyme LCAT are responsible for the transport and elimination of cholesterol from the body.
2. The LCAT is a plasma enzyme, synthesized by the liver.
3. The LCAT catalysis the transfer of FA from the second position of phosphatidylcholine (lecithin) to the OH group of cholesterol.

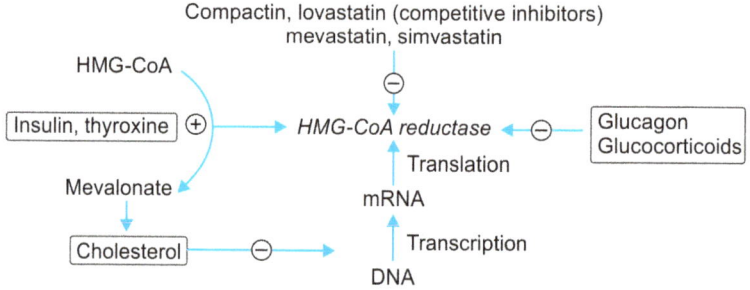

Fig. 9.13: Regulation of cholesterol synthesis.

4. The HDL cholesterol is the real substrate for LCAT and this reaction is freely reversible.
5. The LCAT activity is associated with apolipoprotein A1 of HDL:

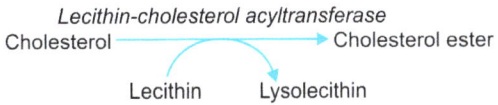

Metabolic Fate of Cholesterol

1. Cholesterol is mainly excreted in the form of bile salts in stool.
2. Increased plasma cholesterol results in the accumulation of cholesterol under the tunica intima of the arteries causing atherosclerosis. The progression of the disease process leads to narrowing of the blood vessels. Dietary intake of PUFA helps in transport and metabolism of cholesterol and prevents atherosclerosis.
3. Cholesterol is converted into following compounds as shown below:

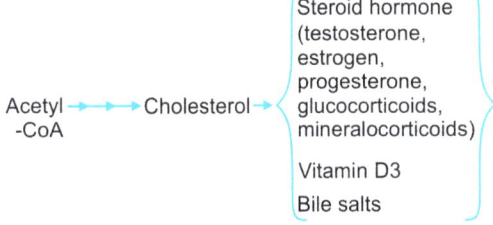

Bile Acid Synthesis and Utilization

1. The end products of cholesterol utilization are the bile acids, synthesized in the liver.
2. Synthesis of bile acids is one of the predominant mechanisms for the excretion of excess cholesterol. However, the excretion of cholesterol in the form of bile acids is insufficient to compensate for an excess dietary intake of cholesterol.
3. The most abundant bile acids in human bile are:
   a. Chenodeoxycholic acid (45%)
   b. Cholic acid (31%).

These two are referred to as the primary bile acids:
1. Before secretion they will be conjugated with either glycine or taurine, which increases their polarity and water solubility.
2. This mechanism of conjugation leads to the formation of four bile acids, within cholesterol:
   a. Glycocholic acid
   b. Taurocholic acid (TCA)
   c. Glycochenodeoxycholic acid
   d. Taurochenodeoxycholic acid.
3. Within the intestines the primary bile acids are acted upon by bacteria and converted to the secondary bile acids, identified as deoxycholate (from cholate) and lithocholate (from chenodeoxycholate).
4. Both primary and secondary bile acids are reabsorbed by the intestines and delivered back to the liver via the portal circulation.

Clinical Significance of Bile Acid Synthesis

Bile acids perform four physiologically significant functions:
1. Synthesis and subsequent excretion in the feces represent the significant mechanism for the elimination of excess cholesterol.
2. Bile acids and phospholipids solubilize cholesterol in the bile, thereby preventing the precipitation of cholesterol in the gallbladder as gallstones.
3. They facilitate the digestion of dietary TGs by acting as emulsifying agents that render fats accessible to pancreatic lipases.
4. They facilitate the intestinal absorption of fat-soluble vitamins.

KETONE BODY METABOLISM

Acetoacetate, β-hydroxybutyrate, and acetone are collectively called ketone bodies.

Synthesis of Ketone Bodies

Site: Liver mitochondria.

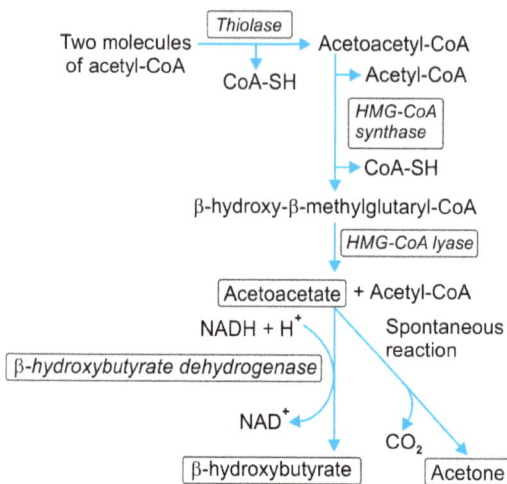

Fig. 9.14: Ketone body synthesis.

Both acetoacetate and β-hydroxybutyrate are weak acids, which slowly deplete alkali reserves (bicarbonate) of the body and cause metabolic acidosis. This condition is known as ketoacidosis.
- The process of formation of ketone bodies in the liver is called ketogenesis (**Fig. 9.14**).
- Ketone body level in the blood is usually less than 2 mg% in well-fed state.
- The ketone body excretion in the urine is approximately around 100 mg/day.
- Increased production of ketone bodies is known as ketosis.
- High level of ketone bodies in blood is referred to as ketonemia.
- If the level of ketone bodies is high in the urine, it is called ketonuria.
- Lungs mainly eliminate acetone.
- The acetyl-CoA formed in FA oxidation enters TCA cycle only if fat and carbohydrate degradation are appropriately balanced.

CONDITIONS IN WHICH KETONE BODY FORMATION OCCURS

Prolonged Starvation

During starvation, the carbohydrate level will be low. So the stored fat of the adipose tissue break down to free FAs. The free FAs formed enter the liver and undergo α-oxidation to release acetyl-CoA, which cannot be utilized by the liver through TCA cycle due to lack of oxaloacetate. In starvation, TCA cycle is impaired due to the deficiency of oxaloacetate, which is diverted to glucose synthesis (gluconeogenesis). Therefore acetyl-CoA is converted to ketone bodies to meet the energy needs.

Uncontrolled Diabetes Mellitus

- Because of the lack of insulin the carbohydrate metabolism is impaired.
- The adipose tissue fat becomes the main source of energy and its degradation is generally accelerated.
- This results in the excessive production of acetyl-CoA, leading to accumulation of acetyl-CoA and its conversion to ketone bodies.

Feeding High-Fat Diet

- Excess breakdown of FAs in the liver takes place.
- The abovementioned condition results in the formation of more acetyl-CoA.
- Once the acetyl-CoA formation exceeds more than the requirement of the liver tissues, it is converted to ketone bodies and exported to muscle, heart, and kidney to meet the energy requirement.
- So the peripheral tissues switch over to utilize ketone bodies.

Utilization of Ketone Bodies (Ketolysis)

Acetoacetate and β-hydroxybutyrate are weak acids, which slowly deplete alkali reserves (bicarbonate) of the body, and cause metabolic acidosis. This condition is known as ketoacidosis:
1. The liver cannot utilize ketone bodies because it lacks the enzyme thiophorase or CoA transferase, which is required for

Metabolism of Lipids

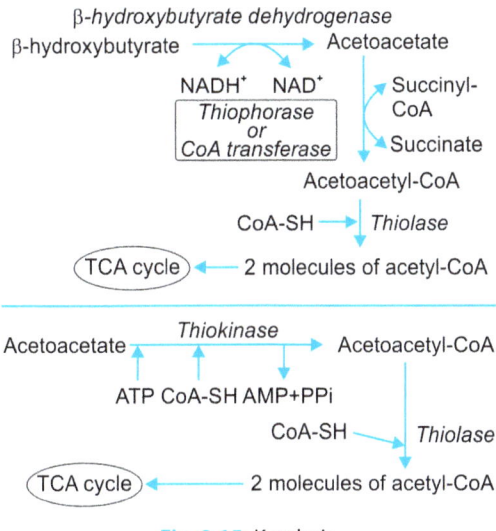

Fig. 9.15: Ketolysis.

the activation of ketone bodies (**Fig. 9.15**). Acetoacetate and β-hydroxybutyrate can be used as a source of energy in peripheral tissues (kidney, muscle).
2. The β-hydroxybutyrate is reconverted to acetoacetate and the acetoacetate is then reactivated to acetoacetyl-CoA.
3. Acetoacetyl-CoA formed is cleaved by thiolase to yield two molecules of acetyl-CoA, which can be oxidized in the TCA cycle to H_2O and CO_2.
4. During prolonged starvation brain utilizes ketone bodies.
5. Acetoacetate and β-hydroxybutyrate serve as an important source of energy for skeletal muscle, cardiac muscle, renal cortex, etc.
6. Ketone bodies are water soluble.
7. They are easily transported from the liver to various tissues.
8. During starvation ketone bodies can meet 50–70% energy needs of brain.

Regulation

- Glucagon stimulates ketogenesis.
- Insulin inhibits ketogenesis.
- The increased ratio of glucagon/insulin in diabetes mellitus promotes ketone body formation.

Ketogenic substances: Fatty acids, amino acids.

Antiketogenic substances: Glucose, glycerol, and glucogenic amino acids (glycine, alanine, serine, glutamate, etc.).

Case

Mr Raju a 58-year-old man with type II diabetes and hypertension is referred to the nephrologist for the evaluation of renal function. The nephrologist performed physical examination and requested for fasting blood glucose (FBS), HbA1c, and renal function tests. The laboratory results showed the following results:
- FBS—208 mg/dL
- HbA1c—8.0% of Hb
- Urea—20 mg/dL
- Creatinine—1.2 mg/dL
- Urine ketones positive
- Urine glucose positive

Which of the following enzymes most strongly associated with ketone body formation in Mr Raju?
a. Thioesterase
b. HMG-CoA synthase
c. Thiokinase
d. Hexokinase

Answer is b. There are three types of ketone bodies—acetoacetate, β-OH butyrate, and acetone. Two molecules of acetyl-CoA condense to form the acetoacetyl-CoA and this reaction is catalyzed by the enzyme thiolase. Acetoacetyl-CoA then combines with a molecule of acetyl-CoA to form hydroxymethylglutaryl-CoA, and this reaction is catalyzed by HMG-CoA synthase.

PHOSPHOLIPID METABOLISM

- Phospholipids are the compound lipids and found in membranes.
- There are two classes of phospholipids—glycerophospholipids (glycerol as the

backbone) and sphingophospholipids (contains amino alcohol, sphingosine).

Synthesis of Glycerophospholipids

The main structural components of biological membranes are the phospholipids. The biosynthesis of phospholipid depends on the synthesis of diacylglycerol. Diacylglycerol in liver comes from phosphatidic acid (1,2-diacyl-glycerol-3-phosphate).

Phosphatidic acid can be derived from glycerol by phosphorylating it at the expense of ATP to glycerol-3-phosphate. The enzyme catalyzing the reaction is glycerol kinase. Glycerol-3-phosphate can also be obtained from reduction of the glycolytic intermediate dihydroxyacetone phosphate (DHAP) by glycerol-3-phosphate DH. Glycerol-3-phosphate is then twice esterified using acyl-CoA precursors as FA donors to phosphatidic acid. The first acylation to 1-acyl-*sn*-glycerol-3-phosphate is catalyzed by glycerol-3-phosphate-*O*-acyltransferase and the second fatty acylation is catalyzed by 1-acylglycerol-3-phosphate-*O*-acyltransferase to 1,2-diacylglycerol-3-phosphate or phosphatidic acid (**Fig. 9.16**).

The first acylation of glycerol phosphate takes place at either the endoplasmic reticulum membrane or the mitochondrial membrane. The latter reaction is significant in liver, an organ with a large numbers of mitochondria. The product of this acylation is lysophosphatidic acid. Note that at this time all the following metabolites are membrane components, including all enzymes catalyzing the synthesis of membrane lipids.

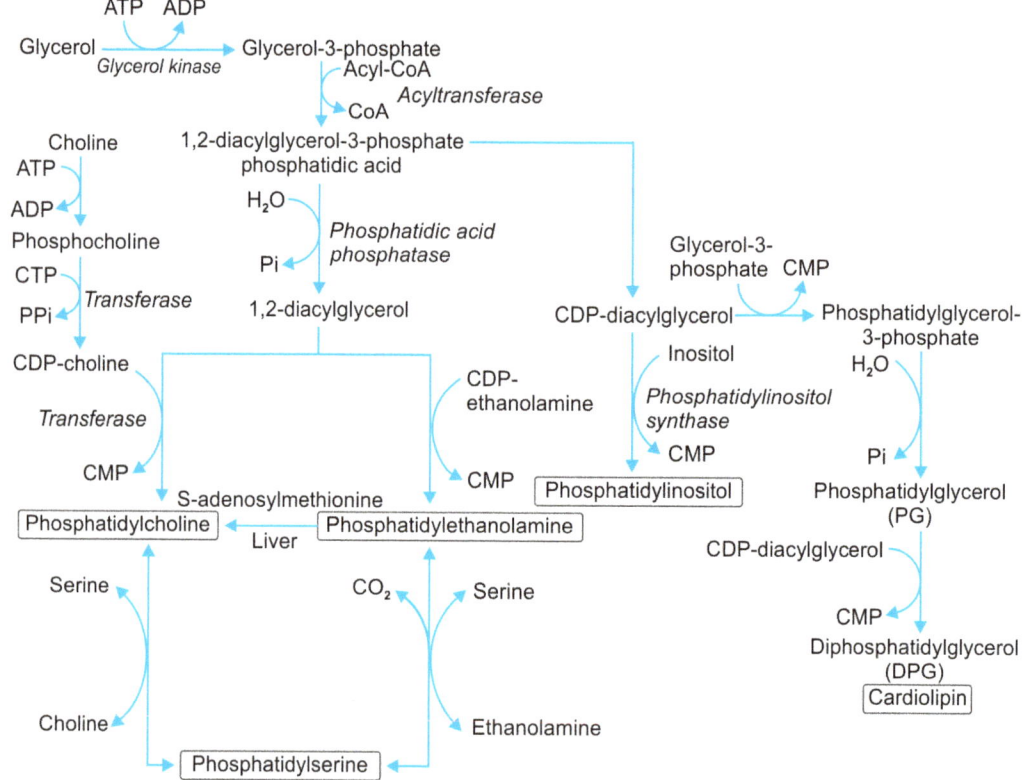

Fig. 9.16: Synthesis of glycerophospholipids.

Metabolism of Phosphatidylethanolamine and Phosphatidylcholine

1. Phosphatidylethanolamines (PEs) and phosphatidylcholine are the phospholipids found in biological membranes.
2. PEs are synthesized by the addition of cytidine diphosphate-ethanolamine to diglycerides, releasing cytidine monophosphate (CMP). S-adenosylmethionine can subsequently methylate the amine of PEs to yield phosphatidylcholines. It can mainly be found in the inner (cytoplasmic) leaflet of the lipid bilayer.
3. PEs play a role in membrane fusion and in disassembly of the contractile ring during cytokinesis in cell division. Additionally, it is thought that PE regulates membrane curvature.
4. The PE acts as an important precursor, substrate, or donor in several biological pathways.
5. As a polar head group, PE creates a more viscous lipid membrane compared to phosphatidylcholine.
6. As a lecithin, PE consists of a combination of glycerol esterified with two FAs and phosphoric acid. Whereas the phosphate group is combined with choline in phosphatidylcholine, it is combined with the ethanolamine in PE. The two FAs may be same, or different, and are usually in the positions 1 and 2.

LIPOPROTEIN METABOLISM

Lipoprotein Structure and Function

Chylomicrons

- Chylomicron is synthesized in small intestine (mucosal cells).
- It mobilizes and transports dietary lipids.
- It has 98% lipid, large sized, lowest density (**Fig. 9.17**).
- It has apolipoprotein B-48: Receptor binding.
- It has apolipoprotein C-II: Lipoprotein lipase (LPL) activator.

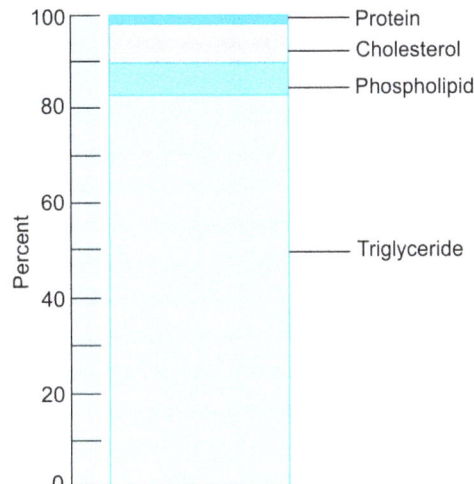

Fig. 9.17: Chylomicron composition.

- It has apolipoprotein E: Remnant receptor binding.
- Nascent chylomicron (Apo B-48, Apo A) before they enter circulation.
- Mature chylomicron (Apo C and Apo E in addition to Apo B-48, Apo A).
- LPL found on the surface of endothelial cells lining the capillaries in muscle and adipose tissues removes the FAs of TGs.
- Chylomicron remnant (CR):
  - Apolipoprotein C removed
  - Removed in liver.
- Substantial portion of the phospholipid and of Apo A and Apo C is transferred to HDLs during the process of FA removal.
- CR containing primarily cholesterol.
- Apo E and Apo B-48 are then delivered to taken up by the liver though the interaction with the CR receptor (**Fig. 9.18**).

Very Low Density Lipoprotein

- Synthesized in liver.
- Transport endogenous TGs (liver to peripheral tissues).
- 90% lipid, 10% protein (**Fig. 9.19**).
- Apo B-100: Receptor binding.
- Apo C-II: LPL activator liberates free FAs that are taken up by the adipose tissue and muscle.

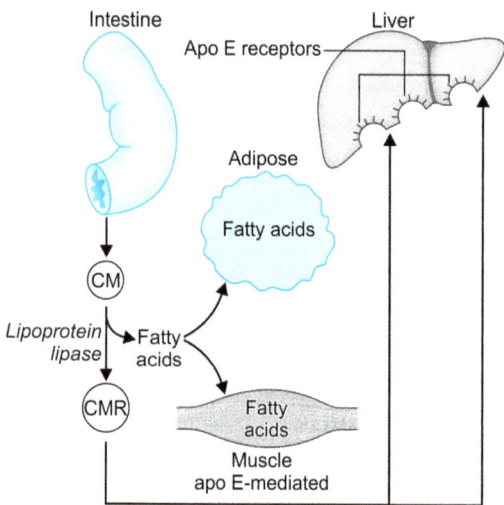

Fig. 9.18: Transport of chylomicron.
(Apo: apolipoprotein; CM: chylomicron;
CMR: chylomicron remnant.)

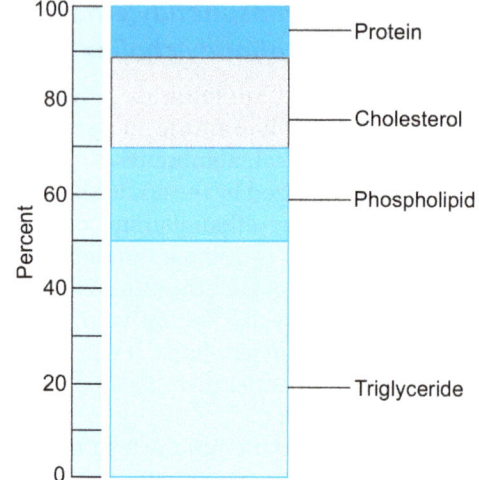

Fig. 9.19: Composition of very low density lipoprotein.

- Apo E: Remnant receptor binding.
- Nascent very low density lipoprotein (VLDL) (B-100)+HDL (Apo C and Apo E) = VLDL.
- LPL hydrolyzes TGs forming intermediate-density lipoprotein (IDL) and loses Apo C-II (reduces affinity for LPL).
- About 75% of IDL removed by liver: Apo E– and Apo B–mediated receptors.
- About 25% of IDL converted to LDL by hepatic lipase: Loses Apo E to HDL.
 The remnant is designated as IDL and contains less of TGs and more of cholesterol, thus IDL contains Apo B-100 and Apo E. A small part of IDL is taken up by the liver, by receptor-mediated endocytosis, helped by Apo B-100 and Apo E, and converted to LDL (**Fig. 9.20**).

Intermediate-density Lipoprotein

- Synthesized from VLDL during VLDL degradation
- TG transport and precursor to LDL
- Apo B-100: Receptor binding
- Apo C-II: LPL activator
- Apo E: Receptor binding.

Low-density Lipoprotein

- Synthesized from IDL.
- Half-life of LDL in blood is 2 days.

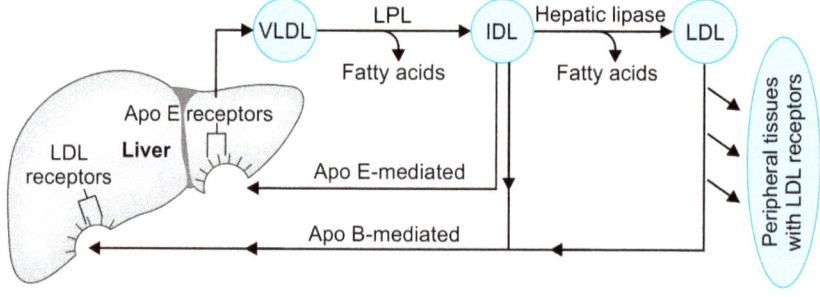

Fig. 9.20: Metabolism of VLDL.
(Apo: apolipoprotein; IDL: intermediate-density lipoprotein; LDL: low-density lipoprotein; VLDL: very low density lipoprotein)

Metabolism of Lipids

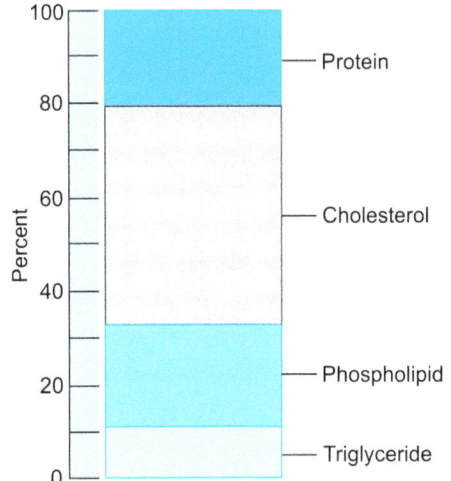

Fig. 9.21: Composition of low-density lipoprotein.

- Cholesterol transport liver to peripheral tissues.
- About 75% of the plasma cholesterol is incorporated into the LDL particles are derived from VLDL, a small part is directly released from liver.
- About 78% lipid, 58% cholesterol and cholesteryl ester (CE), Apo B-100 (**Fig. 9.21**) receptor binding interaction of LDL with LDL receptor.
- LDL receptor–mediated endocytosis:
- About 75% of LDLs are taken up by the liver, adrenal, and adipose tissue cells by LDL receptor-mediated endocytosis (**Fig. 9.22**).
- The LDL receptors on "coated pits" clathrin, a protein polymer that stabilizes pit.
- Endocytosis:
  - Loss of clathrin coating
  - Uncoupling of receptor, returns to surface.
- Fusing of endosome with lysosome: Free cholesterol and amino acids.

High-density Lipoprotein

- Synthesized in liver and intestine as protein-rich discoid particles
- Reservoir of apoproteins
- Reverse cholesterol transport

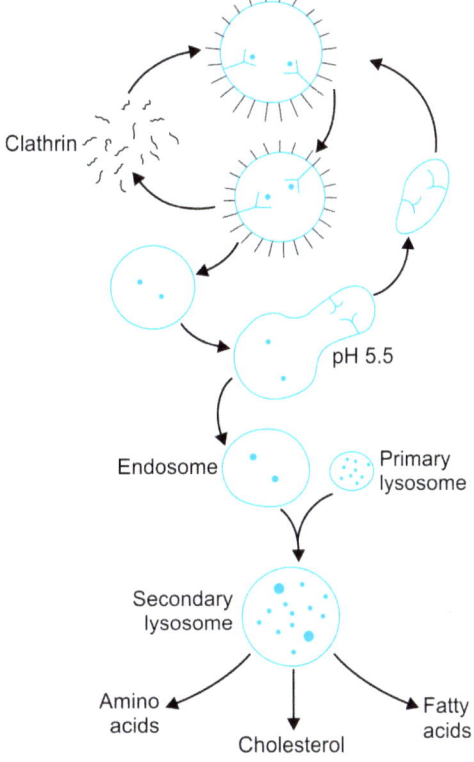

Fig. 9.22: Endocytosis.

- About 52% protein, 48% lipid, 35% cholesterol, and CE (**Fig. 9.23**)
- Apo A: Activates LCAT

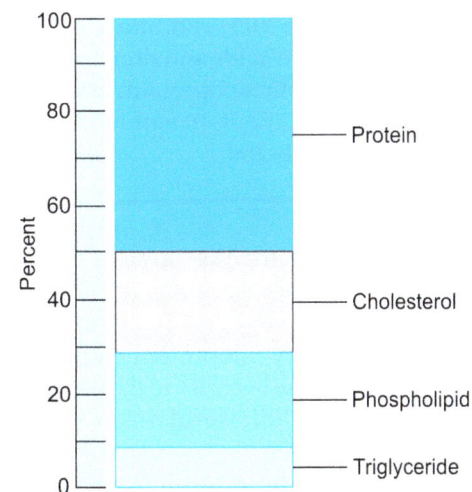

Fig. 9.23: Composition of high-density lipoprotein.

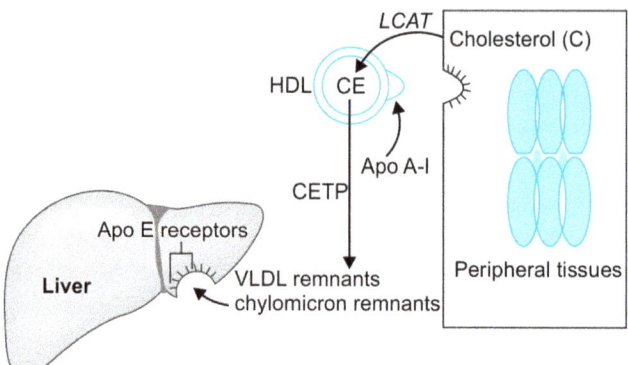

Fig. 9.24: Reverse cholesterol transport.
(Apo: apoprotein; CE: cholesteryl ester; CETP: cholesteryl ester transfer protein; HDL: high-density lipoprotein; LACT: lecithin–cholesterol acyltransferase; VLDL: very low density lipoprotein.)

- Apo C: Activates LPL.
- Apo E: Remnant receptor binding.
- Apoprotein exchange: This provides Apo C and Apo E to/from VLDL, and chylomicrons.
- Reverse cholesterol transport: Discoid HDLs are converted into spherical lipoprotein through the accumulation of CE.
- Uptake of cholesterol from peripheral tissues (binding by Apo A-I).
- Esterification of HDL-C by LCAT: LCAT activated by Apo A-I.
- Transfer of CE to lipoprotein remnants (IDL and CR) by CE transfer protein (CETP) (**Fig. 9.24**)
- Removal of CE-rich remnants by liver converted to bile acids and excreted.
The characteristic apoproteins present in chylomicron is Apo B-48 and in LDL, and VLDL, it is Apo B-100.

Functions of Lipoproteins

1. Chylomicrons are the largest, lightest lipoproteins. They carry dietary TGs to be hydrolyzed by peripheral tissues LPL.
2. Very low density lipoprotein carries TGs synthesized in the liver also to the periphery.
3. LDL carries cholesterol from liver to peripheral tissues.
4. HDL carries cholesterol from liver to peripheral tissues.

Case
An 8-year-old boy was brought to the hospital with a complaint of abdominal and epigastric pain. The surgeon noticed eruptive xanthomas and hepatosplenomegaly. The doctor asked the nurse to collect the blood sample for lipid profile and liver function tests. The sample was milky in appearance, and he contacted one of the clinical biochemists to discuss this. Which of the following is most likely lipoprotein elevated in this patient blood sample?
a. Chylomicron
b. HDL
c. Chylomicron remnant
d. LDL

Answer is c.

Hyperlipoproteinemias

Hyperlipoproteinemias occur due to the presence of excessive amounts of lipoproteins such as VLDL, LDL, or chylomicrons in the plasma following a 10–12 hours of fasting.

Fredrickson's Classification

Type I hyperlipoproteinemia: High TG and chylomicron

Cause: LPL absence

- *Type II a hyperlipoproteinemia:* High LDL with high cholesterol
- *Type II b hyperlipoproteinemia:* High LDL (cholesterol) and VLDL (TG)
- *Type III hyperlipoproteinemia:* High IDL + LDL
- *Type IV hyperlipoproteinemia:* High level of VLDL (high level of cholesterol and TG)
- *Type V hyperlipoproteinemia:* High chylomicrons and VLDL (high TG).

Causes

- Obesity
- Diabetes mellitus
- Alcoholism
- Nephrotic syndrome.

Familial Hypercholesterolemia

It is a genetic disorder characterized by high cholesterol levels, specifically very high levels of LDL, in the blood and early cardiovascular disease.

Many patients have mutations in the *LDLR* gene that encodes the LDL receptor protein (which normally removes LDL from the circulation), or apolipoprotein B (ApoB), which is the part of LDL that binds with the receptor.

Patients who have one abnormal copy (are heterozygous) of the *LDLR* gene may have premature cardiovascular disease at the age of 30–40. Having two abnormal copies (being *homozygous*) may cause severe cardiovascular disease in childhood.

Physical Signs

High cholesterol levels normally do not cause any symptoms. Cholesterol may be deposited in various places in the body that are visible from the outside, such as in yellowish patches around the eyelids, the outer margin of the iris, and in the form of lumps in the tendons of the hands, elbows, knees, and feet.

FATTY LIVER

1. Fatty liver, also known as fatty liver disease (FLD), is a reversible condition wherein large vacuoles of TG fat accumulate in liver cells via the process of steatosis.
2. Accumulation of fat (TAG) may also be accompanied by a progressive inflammation of the liver (hepatitis) called steatohepatitis. By considering the contribution by alcohol, fatty liver may be termed "alcoholic steatosis" or "nonalcoholic FLD" and the more severe forms as alcoholic steatohepatitis (part of alcoholic liver disease), and nonalcoholic steatohepatitis.
3. Fatty liver occurs when excess TAG accumulates inside liver cells. This means normal, healthy liver tissue becomes partly replaced with fatty tissue. The fat starts to invade the liver, gradually infiltrating the healthy liver areas, so that less healthy liver tissue remains. The fatty liver has a yellow greasy appearance and is often enlarged, and swollen with fat. This fatty infiltration slows down the metabolism of body fat stores, which means that the liver burns fat less efficiently, resulting in weight gain and inability to lose weight. However, some people can have a fatty liver without being overweight.
4. Fatty liver is slightly enlarged and yellow in color, and "shiny" or "greasy" in appearance because it is congested with fat (**Fig. 9.25**).

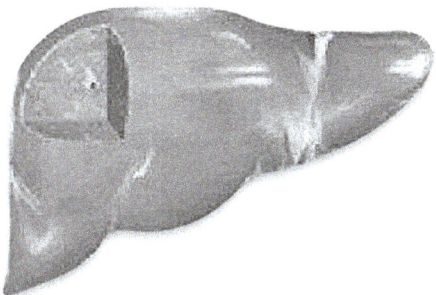

Fig. 9.25: Fatty liver.

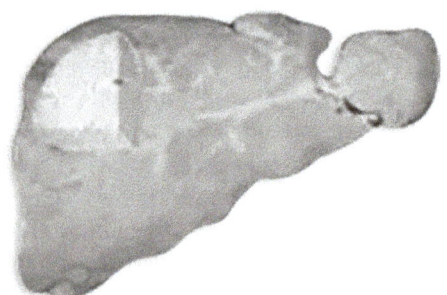

Fig. 9.26: Severe fatty liver.

5. Severe fatty liver (**Fig. 9.26**): The condition is more severe degree of fatty liver and is more often due to incorrect diet, alcohol excess, or obesity.

Causes of Fatty Liver

1. Increased synthesis of TAG: Mobilization of free FAs from adipose tissue and their entry into liver is higher than utilization. This leads to overproduction of TG and their accumulation in liver. The conditions in which increased mobilization of FAs takes place are diabetes mellitus, starvation, obesity, and alcoholism.
2. Impaired synthesis of lipoproteins: The synthesis of VLDL takes place in liver and its formation requires phospholipids and ApoB. Fatty liver due to impaired lipoproteins synthesis may be due to:
    a. A defect in phospholipids synthesis.
    b. A block in apoprotein formation.
    c. Failure in the formation/secretion of lipoprotein.
    d. Fatty liver due to impairment in phospholipids is associated with the dietary deficiency of lipotropic factors such as choline, betaine, and inositol. Deficiency of essential FAs leads to decreased formation of phospholipids.
    e. Some chemicals such as puromycin, ethionine, carbon tetrachloride (CCl_4), chloroform, and lead, which inhibit protein synthesis, cause fatty liver. This is due to blockage in the synthesis of ApoB required for VLDL production.
    f. Certain hormones such as adrenocorticotropic hormone, insulin, thyroid, and adrenocorticoids promote deposition of fat in liver.

How to Identify the Fatty Liver?

1. Many people with a fatty liver are unaware that they even have a liver problem, as the symptoms can be vague and nonspecific, especially in the early stages.
2. Most people with a fatty liver feel generally unwell and find they are becoming increasingly fatigued and overweight for no apparent reason.
3. They may have elevated liver enzymes on a blood test for liver function.
4. Fatty liver is diagnosed with a blood test and liver ultrasound scan.

Possible Symptoms of Fatty Liver (Nonalcoholic Steatohepatitis or Nonalcoholic Fatty Liver Disease)

- Weight excess in the abdominal area
- Inability to lose weight
- Elevated cholesterol and/or TG levels
- Fatigue
- Nausea and/or indigestion
- Overheating of the body
- Excessive sweating
- Red itchy eyes
- Discomfort over the liver area.

Fate of Triacylglycerol Formed in Liver and Adipose Tissue

1. In the liver very small amount of TAG is stored. The most is packaged with cholesterol, phospholipids, and proteins to form VLDL and released into the bloodstream.
2. This TAG of VLDL is hydrolyzed by LPL, which is located in the walls of blood capillaries. This enzyme clears the TAG and glycerol.
3. In adipose tissue, TAG is stored in the cells, and it serves as fat depot ready for mobilization when the body requires energy.

Biosynthesis of Triacylglycerol

Biosynthesis of Triacylglycerol is shown in **Figure 9.27**.

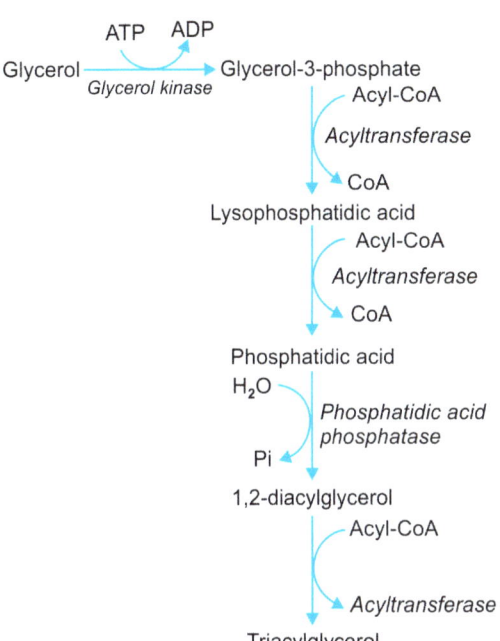

Fig. 9.27: Triacylglycerol synthesis.

Lipotropic Factors

1. Lipotropic factors are substances, which facilitate mobilization of fat from liver.
2. The various lipotropic factors (agents) are choline, betaine, methionine, and inositol.
3. They are required for the conversion of TG to phospholipid and thus help in normal transport and utilization of lipids especially in liver.
4. The deficiency of lipotropic factors leads to a condition known as fatty liver, i.e. increased accumulation of fat content in liver.

Synthesis of Plasmalogen

Synthesis of Plasmalogen is shown in **Figure 9.28**.

Role of Liver in Lipid Metabolism

1. Lipids are mainly stored in the adipose tissue.
2. Liver has a central role in the lipid metabolism (**Fig. 9.29**):
   a. Plasma lipoproteins such as VLDL, LDL, and HDL are synthesized in liver.
   b. Ketone bodies are synthesized in the liver.
   c. Fatty acid chain elongation (medium chain to long-chain FA).
   d. Synthesis of bile acid and bile salts.
   e. β-Oxidation of FA happens in the liver.

REGULATION OF LIPID METABOLISM

Action of Insulin

- Insulin stimulates HMP shunt and increases the supply of $NADPH^+ H^+$.
- It increases the peripheral utilization of glucose and depresses ketogenesis.
- TG synthesis is stimulated.

Glucocorticoids

These hormones increase the release of FA from adipose tissue, which in turn leads to ketogenesis and increase cholesterol synthesis.

ALCOHOL METABOLISM

Excess of alcohol produces cirrhosis in liver:
- It is readily absorbed from the gastrointestinal tract.
- It cannot be stored and the body must oxidize it to get rid of it.
- Alcohol can only be oxidized in the liver, where enzymes are found to initiate the process.
- Alcohol directly contributes to malnutrition.
- Ethanol does not have any minerals, vitamins, carbohydrates, fats, or proteins associated with it.
- It causes inflammation of the stomach, pancreas, and intestines, which impairs the digestion of food, and absorption into blood.
- The acetaldehyde (the oxidation product) can interfere with the activation of vitamins.

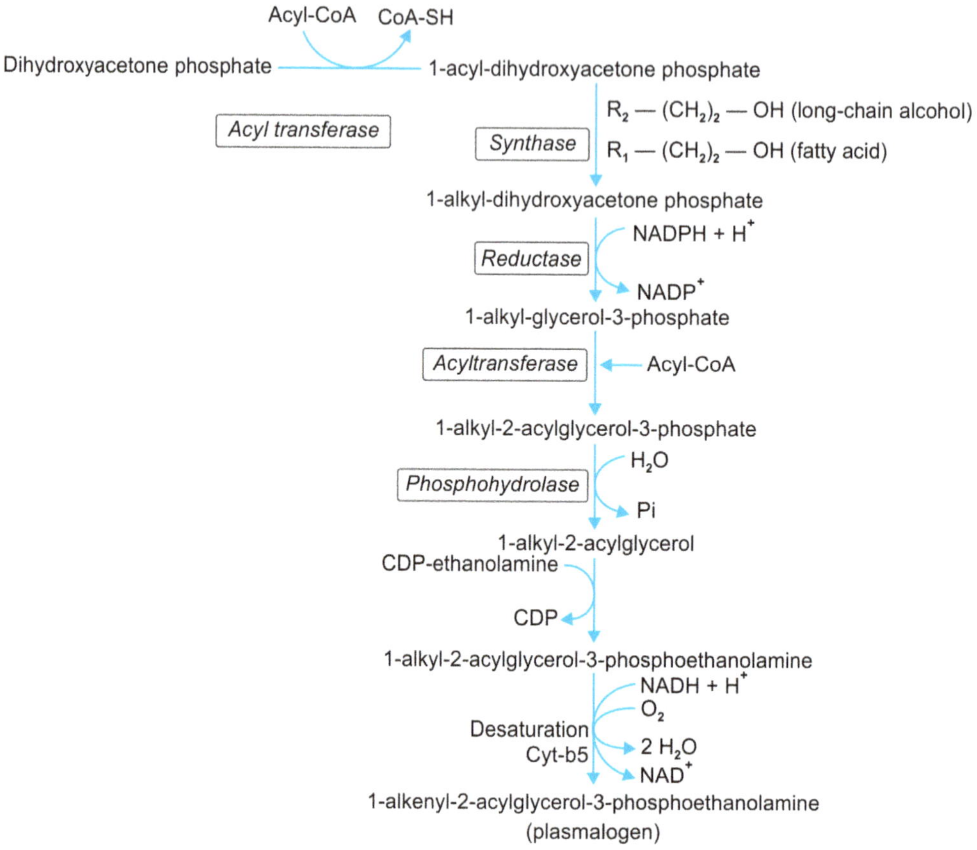

Acyl-CoA
CoA-SH
Dihydroxyacetone phosphate
1-acyl-dihydroxyacetone phosphate
Acyl transferase
Synthase
R_2 — $(CH_2)_2$ — OH (long-chain alcohol)
R_1 — $(CH_2)_2$ — OH (fatty acid)
1-alkyl-dihydroxyacetone phosphate
Reductase
NADPH + H^+
$NADP^+$
1-alkyl-glycerol-3-phosphate
Acyltransferase
Acyl-CoA
1-alkyl-2-acylglycerol-3-phosphate
Phosphohydrolase
H_2O
Pi
1-alkyl-2-acylglycerol
CDP-ethanolamine
CDP
1-alkyl-2-acylglycerol-3-phosphoethanolamine
NADH + H^+
O_2
Desaturation
Cyt-b5
2 H_2O
NAD^+
1-alkenyl-2-acylglycerol-3-phosphoethanolamine
(plasmalogen)

Fig. 9.28: Synthesis of plasmalogen.

1. Fatty acid synthesis (glucose → acetyl-CoA → fatty acid)
2. Cholesterol synthesis:
Glucose
Fatty acid breakdown
Ketogenic amino acid
Acetyl-CoA
Cholesterol

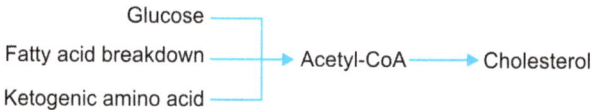

Fig. 9.29: Role of liver in lipid metabolism.

- The first step in the metabolism of alcohol is the oxidation of ethanol to acetaldehyde catalyzed by alcohol DH and the coenzyme NAD^+.
- The acetaldehyde is further oxidized to acetic acid and finally to CO_2, and water (citric acid cycle).
- Metabolic effects from alcohol are directly linked to the production of an excess of both NADH and acetaldehyde:

$$CH_3CH_2\,OH + NAD^+ \rightarrow CH_3\,CH{=}O + NADH + H^+.$$

Metabolic Fates of NADH

Pyruvic Acid to Lactic Acid

The conversion of pyruvic acid to lactic acid requires NADH:

$$\text{Pyruvic acid} + NADH + H^+ \rightarrow \text{Lactic acid} + NAD^+$$

This pyruvic acid normally made by transamination of amino acids is intended for conversion into glucose by gluconeogenesis. This pathway is inhibited by low concentrations of pyruvic acid, since it has been converted to lactic acid. The final result may be acidosis from lactic acid buildup and hypoglycemia from lack of glucose synthesis.

Synthesis of Lipids

Excess NADH may be used as a reducing agent in two pathways—one to synthesis glycerol and the other to synthesis FAs. As a result, heavy drinkers may initially be overweight.

Electron Transport Chain

The NADH may be used directly in the electron transport chain to synthesize ATP as a source of energy. This reaction has the direct effect of inhibiting the normal oxidation of fats in the FA and citric acid cycle. Fats or acetyl-CoA may accumulate resulting in the production of ketone bodies. Accumulation of fat in the liver can be alleviated by secreting lipids into the bloodstream. The higher lipid level in the blood is responsible for heart attacks.

Alcoholism Effects

A central role in the toxicity of alcohol may be played by acetaldehyde itself. Although the liver converts acetaldehyde into acetic acid, it reaches a saturation point where some of it escapes into the bloodstream. The accumulated acetaldehyde exerts its toxic effects by inhibiting the reactions and functions of mitochondria. When the metabolism of acetaldehyde to acetic acid decreases, more acetaldehyde accumulates and causes further liver damage—hepatitis and cirrhosis (**Fig. 9.30**).

SYNTHESIS OF PROSTAGLANDINS

Prostaglandins and Related Compounds

1. Prostaglandins (PGs) and their related compounds such as prostacyclins (PGI),

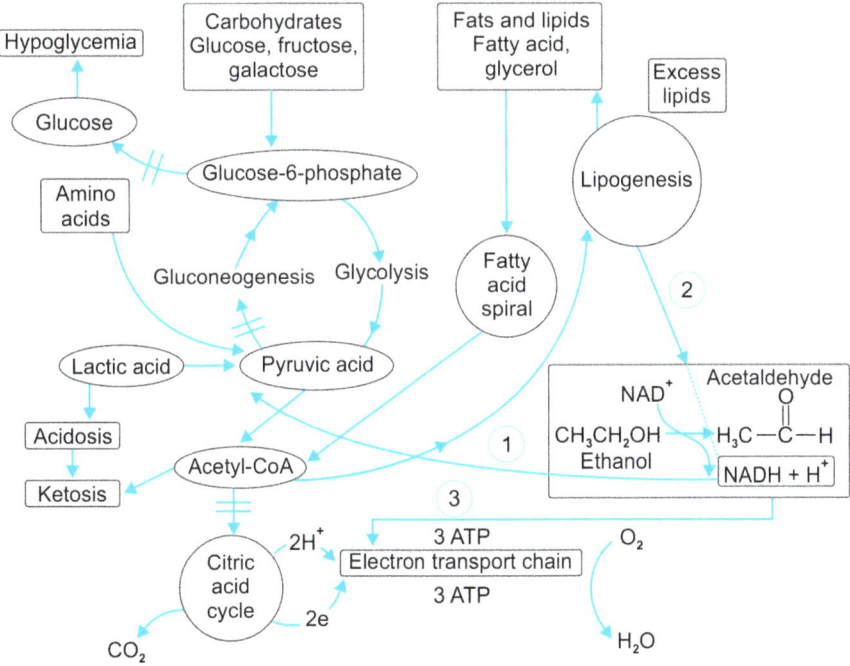

Fig. 9.30: Effects of alcohol.

thromboxanes (TXAs), and leukotrienes (LT) are collectively known as eicosanoids.
2. Eicosanoids are considered as locally acting hormones with a wide range of biochemical functions.
3. PGs are derivatives of a hypothetical 20-carbon FA, namely prostanoic acid.
4. The various prostanoids are:
   - PGs, e.g. PGE1, PGE2, and PGE3
   - PGI, e.g. PGI2 and PGI3
   - TXAs, e.g. TXA1 and TXA2.
5. PGs are named as PG plus a third letter (E, F, A, D), which corresponds to the type and arrangement of functional group in the molecule, and the subscript indicates the number of double bonds (PGE1).
6. PGs are synthesized from arachidonic acid, which is released from membrane-bound phospholipids.
7. Corticosteroid and aspirin inhibit the PG synthesis.
8. They act as local hormones and are involved in a wide range of biochemical function. In general, PGs are involved in the lowering of blood pressure (BP), induction of inflammation, medical termination of pregnancy, induction of labor, inhibition of gastric hydrochloric acid (HCl) secretion, decrease in immune response, and increase in glomerular filtration rate (GFR).

Synthesis

Arachidonic acid is the precursor for most of the PGs in humans:
1. Release of arachidonic acid from membrane-bound phospholipids by phospholipase A2, this is due to the stimuli by epinephrine or bradykinin.
2. Oxidation and cyclization of arachidonic acid to PGG2, which is then converted to PGH2 by a reduced glutathione-dependent peroxidase.
3. The PGH2 serves as the immediate precursor for the synthesis of a number of PGs, including PGI and TXAs (**Fig. 9.31**).

Inhibition of Prostaglandin Synthesis

- A number of structurally unrelated compounds can inhibit PG synthesis.
- Cortisol inhibits the enzyme phospholipase A2.
- Aspirin irreversibly inhibits the cyclooxygenase.

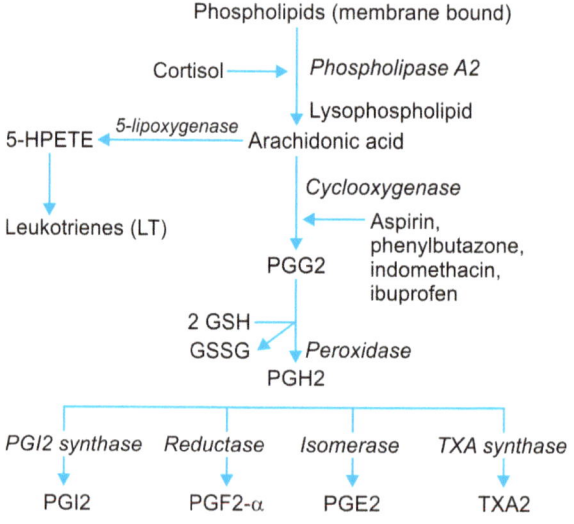

Fig. 9.31: Prostaglandin synthesis.
(GSSG: glutathione disulfide; GSH: glutathione; 5-HEPT: 5-hydroperoxyeicosatetraenoic acid; PG: prostaglandin; TXA: thromboxane.)

Degradation

- Almost all the eicosanoids are metabolized rapidly.
- Lung and liver are the major sites of PG degradation.
- 15-β-Hydroxy PG DH and 13-PG reductase convert hydroxyl group at C15 to keto group and then to C13, and C14 dihydro derivative.

BIOCHEMICAL ACTIONS OF PROSTAGLANDINS

- PGs act as local hormones.
- They differ from the true hormones in many ways.
- They are produced in almost all the tissues.
- They are not stored and they are degraded to inactive products at the site of their production.
- They are produced in small amounts with low half-lives.

Regulation of Blood Pressure

- PGs (PGE, PGA, and PGI2) are vasodilator in function, this results in increased blood flow and decreased peripheral resistance to lower the BP
- These serve as agents in the treatment of hypertension.

Inflammation

- The PGs (PGE1 and PGE2) induce the symptoms of inflammation (redness, swelling, edema, etc.) due to arteriolar vasodilation.
- Corticosteroids are usually used to treat inflammation, which inhibits PG synthesis.

Reproduction

The PGE2 and PGF2 are used for the medical termination of pregnancy, and induction of labor.

Pain and Fever

1. Pyrogens (fever-producing agents) may promote PG synthesis leading to the formation of PGE2 in the hypothalamus, the site of regulation of body temperature.
2. The PGE2 along with histamine and bradykinin causes pain. The cause for migraine is increased PGE2 level.
3. Aspirin and other nonsteroidal drugs inhibit PG synthesis and thus control fever and pain.

Prevention of Gastric Ulcer

- PGs are important in the pathophysiology of gastric ulcer.
- It is used in its prevention and treatment.

Effects on Respiratory Function

PGE is a bronchodilator, whereas PGF acts as constrictor of smooth muscles. PGE1 and PGE2 are used in the treatment of asthma.

Influence on Renal Function

- PGE increases GFR and promotes urine output.
- It increases the excretion of sodium and potassium.

Metabolism

The PGE:
- Decreases lipolysis
- Increases glycogenesis
- Promotes mobilization of calcium from the bone.

Platelet Aggregation and Thrombosis

- The PGs, namely PGI, i.e. PGI2, inhibit platelet aggregation.
- TXAs A2 and PGE2 promote platelet aggregation and blood clotting that might lead to thrombosis; thus they are antagonistic in their action.
- In the overall effect, PGI2 acts as a vasodilator, while TXA2 as a vasoconstrictor.

- TXA A2 and PGE1 promote platelet aggregation and PGI2 inhibits the platelet aggregation.
- Inhibitors of PG synthesis (aspirin, ibuprofen) are used in controlling fever, pain, migraine, and inflammation.
- PGs are found in seminal fluid, plasma, and other tissues; they have pharmacological and biochemical action and act on smooth muscle, blood vessel, and adipose tissue.

LEUKOTRIENES

1. LT are the mediators of allergic reactions and inflammation.
2. They also cause bronchoconstriction and increase vascular permeability and mucus secretion (e.g. LTA3 and LTA4).

Certain fish foods contain an unsaturated FA, namely eicosapentaenoic acid (20 carbon atoms and 5 double bonds), which inhibits the synthesis of TXAs, i.e. TXA2, thus decreases platelet aggregation and thrombosis, and therefore lowers the risk of myocardial complications as seen in the Eskimos.

LIPID STORAGE DISORDERS

Definition: Lipid storage diseases, or the lipidoses, are a group of inherited metabolic disorders in which harmful amounts of fatty materials called lipids accumulate in some of the body's cells and tissues. People with these disorders either do not produce enough of one of the enzymes needed to metabolize lipids or produce enzymes that do not work properly. Over time, this excessive storage of fats can cause permanent cellular and tissue damage, particularly in the brain, peripheral nervous system, liver, spleen, and bone marrow.

Many lipid storage disorders can be classified into the subgroup of sphingolipidoses, as they relate to sphingolipid metabolism. Members of this group include:
- Niemann–Pick disease
- Fabry disease
- Krabbe disease
- Gaucher disease
- Tay–Sachs disease
- Metachromatic leukodystrophy
- Multiple sulfatase deficiency
- Farber's disease.

They are generally inherited in an autosomal recessive fashion, but Fabry disease is X-linked. Lipid storage diseases are inherited from one or both parents who carry a defective gene that regulates a particular protein in a class of the body's cells. They can be inherited two ways:

1. Autosomal recessive inheritance occurs when both parents carry and pass on a copy of the faulty gene, but neither parent is affected by the disorder. Each child born to these parents has a 25% chance of inheriting both copies of the defective gene, a 50% chance of being a carrier, and a 25% chance of not inheriting either copy of the defective gene. Children of either gender can be affected by an autosomal recessive this pattern of inheritance.
2. X-linked (or sex-linked) recessive inheritance occurs when the mother carries the affected gene on the X chromosome that determines the child's gender and passes it to her son. Sons of carriers have a 50% chance of inheriting the disorder. Daughters have a 50% chance of inheriting the X-linked chromosome but usually are not severely affected by the disorder. Affected men do not pass the disorder to their sons, but their daughters will be carriers for the disorder.

Diagnosis is made through clinical examination, biopsy, genetic testing, and molecular analysis of cells or tissue to identify inherited metabolic disorders, and enzyme assays.

Gaucher Disease

Gaucher disease is a rare, inherited disorder. It occurs due to the deficiency of glucocerebrosidase. This causes too much of a fatty substance to build up in the spleen, liver, lungs, bones, and, sometimes, brain, which prevents these organs from working properly.

There are three types of Gaucher disease:
1. Type 1, the most common form, causes liver and spleen enlargement, bone pain and broken bones, and, sometimes, lung and kidney problems. It does not affect the brain. It can occur at any age.
2. Type 2, which causes severe brain damage, appears in infants. Most children who have it die by age 2.
3. In type 3, there may be liver and spleen enlargement. The brain is gradually affected. It usually starts in childhood or adolescence.

Niemann–Pick Disease

It is a group of autosomal recessive disorders caused by an accumulation of fat and cholesterol in cells of the liver, spleen, bone marrow, lungs, and, in some patients, brain. Neurological complications may include ataxia, eye paralysis, brain degeneration, learning problems, spasticity, feeding and swallowing difficulties, slurred speech, loss of muscle tone, hypersensitivity to touch, and some corneal clouding. A characteristic cherry-red halo develops around the center of the retina in 50% of patients.

Niemann–Pick disease is subdivided into four categories:
- **Type A**, the most severe form, begins in early infancy and occurs most often in Jewish families. Additional symptoms include weakness, an enlarged liver and spleen, swollen lymph nodes, and profound brain damage by six months of age. Children with this type rarely live beyond 18 months.
- **Type B** (also called juvenile onset) usually occurs in the preteen years, with symptoms that include ataxia and peripheral neuropathy. The brain is generally not affected. Other symptoms include enlarged liver and spleen, and pulmonary difficulties. In types **A** and **B**, insufficient activity of an enzyme called *sphingomyelinase* causes the buildup of toxic amounts of *sphingomyelin*, a fatty substance present in every cell of the body.

Types C and D may appear early in life or develop in the teen or even adult years. Niemann–Pick disease types C and D are not caused by a deficiency of sphingomyelinase but by a lack of the NPC1 or NPC2 proteins. As a result, various lipids and cholesterol accumulate inside nerve cells and cause them to malfunction. Patients with types C and D have only moderate enlargement of their spleens and livers. Brain involvement may be extensive, leading to inability to look up and down, difficulty in walking and swallowing, and progressive loss of vision and hearing.

Onset of type A, the most severe form, is in early infancy.

There is currently no cure for Niemann–Pick disease. Treatment is supportive. Children usually die from infection or progressive neurological loss.

Fabry Disease

Fabry disease, also known as α-galactosidase-A deficiency, causes the buildup of fatty material in the autonomic nervous system, eyes, kidneys, and cardiovascular system. Fabry disease is the only X-linked lipid storage disease. Males are primarily affected although a milder form is common in females, some of whom may have severe manifestations similar to those seen in affected males. Onset of symptoms is usually during childhood or adolescence.

Neurological symptoms include burning pain in the arms and legs, which worsens in hot weather or following exercise, and the buildup of excess material in the clear layers of the cornea (resulting in clouding but no change in vision). Fatty storage in blood vessel walls may impair circulation, putting the patient at risk for stroke or heart attack. Other symptoms include heart enlargement, progressive kidney impairment leading to renal failure, gastrointestinal difficulties, decreased sweating, and fever. Angiokeratomas (small, noncancerous, reddish-purple elevated spots on the skin) may develop on the lower part of the trunk of the body and become more numerous with age.

Patients with Fabry disease often die prematurely of complications from heart disease, renal failure, or stroke. Drugs such as phenytoin and carbamazepine are often prescribed to treat pain that accompanies Fabry disease. Metoclopramaide or Lipisorb (a nutritional supplement) can ease gastrointestinal distress that often occurs in Fabry patients, and some individuals may require kidney transplant or dialysis. Recent experiments indicate that enzyme replacement can reduce storage, ease pain, and improve organ function in patients with Fabry disease.

Farber's Disease

It is also known as Farber's lipogranulomatosis and describes a group of inherited metabolic disorders called lipid storage diseases, in which excess amounts of lipids (oils, FAs, and related compounds) build up to harmful levels in the joints, tissues, and central nervous system. The liver, heart, and kidneys may also be affected. Disease onset typically begins in early infancy but may occur later in life. Symptoms of the classic form may have moderately impaired mental ability and difficulty with swallowing. Other symptoms may include chronic shortening of muscles or tendons around joints, arthritis, swollen lymph nodes and joints, hoarseness, nodules under the skin (and sometimes in the lungs and other parts of the body), and vomiting. Some people may need a breathing tube. In severe cases, the liver and spleen are enlarged. Farber's disease is caused by a deficiency of the enzyme ceramidase. The disease occurs when both parents carry and pass on the defective gene that regulates the protein sphingomyelin. Children born to these parents have a 25% chance of inheriting the disorder and a 50% chance of carrying the faulty gene. The disorder affects both males and females.

Gangliosidoses

The gangliosidoses are a group of inherited metabolic diseases caused by a deficiency of the different proteins needed to break down fatty substances called lipids. Excess buildup of these fatty materials (oils, waxes, steroids, and other compounds) can cause permanent damage in the cells and tissues in the brain and nervous systems, particularly in nerve cells. There are two distinct groups of the gangliosidoses, which affect males and females equally.

The GM1 gangliosidoses are caused by a deficiency of the enzyme β-galactosidase and has three clinical subtypes:

1. Early infantile GM1 gangliosidosis is the most severe subtype, with onset shortly after birth which has symptoms of nerve function degeneration, seizures, liver and spleen enlargement, coarsening of facial features, skeletal irregularities, joint stiffness, distended abdomen, muscle weakness, exaggerated startle response, and problems with gait. About half of affected persons develop cherry-red spots in the eye. Children may be deaf and blind by age 1.
2. Onset of late infantile GM1 gangliosidosis typically between ages 1 and 3 years. Signs include an inability to control movement, seizures, dementia, and difficulties with speech.
3. Adult GM1 gangliosidosis strikes between ages 3 and 30, with symptoms that include the wasting away of muscles, cloudiness in the corneas, and dystonia (sustained muscle contractions that case twisting and repetitive movements or abnormal postures). Noncancerous skin blemishes may develop on the lower part of the trunk of the body. Adult GM1 is usually less

severe and progresses more slowly than other forms of the disorder.

The GM2 gangliosidoses include Tay–Sachs disease and its more severe form, called Sandhoff disease, both of which result from a deficiency of the enzyme β-hexosaminidase. Symptoms begin by age 6 months and include *progressive mental deterioration, cherry-red spots in the retina, marked startle reflex, and seizures*. Children with Tay–Sachs may also have *dementia, progressive loss of hearing, some paralysis, and difficulty in swallowing*. A rarer form of the disorder, which occurs in individuals in their twenties and early thirties, is characterized by an unsteady gait and progressive neurological deterioration. Additional signs of Sandhoff disease include weakness in nerve signaling that causes muscles to contract, early blindness, spasticity, muscle contractions, an abnormally enlarged head, and an enlarged liver and spleen.

There is no specific treatment for Sandhoff disease. As with Tay–Sachs disease, supportive treatment includes keeping the airway open and proper nutrition and hydration. Anticonvulsant medications may initially control seizures. Children generally die by age 3 from respiratory infections

Krabbe disease (also known as globoid cell leukodystrophy and galactosylceramide lipidosis): This is an autosomal recessive disorder caused by deficiency of the enzyme galactosylceramidase. The disease most often affects infants, with onset before age 6 months, but can occur in adolescence or adulthood. The buildup of undigested fats affects the growth of the nerve's protective myelin sheath and causes severe degeneration of mental and motor skills. Other symptoms include muscle weakness, hypertonia (reduced ability of a muscle to stretch), myoclonic seizures (sudden, shock-like contractions of the limbs), spasticity, irritability, unexplained fever, deafness, optic atrophy and blindness, paralysis, and difficulty when swallowing. Prolonged weight loss may also occur. The disease may be diagnosed by its characteristic grouping of certain cells, nerve demyelination and degeneration, and destruction of brain cells. In infants the disease is generally fatal before age 2. Patients with a later onset form of the disease have a milder course of the disease and live significantly longer. No specific treatment for Krabbe disease has been developed, although early bone marrow transplantation may help some patients.

RISK FACTORS FOR CARDIOVASCULAR DISEASE

Cardiovascular diseases are the leading cause of illness and death in the world. The majority of cases stem from atherosclerosis (a condition in which cholesterol, fat, and fibrous tissue build up in the walls of large- and medium-sized arteries). In coronary heart disease (CHD), the arteries to the heart muscle (myocardium) are narrowed, which leads to reduced blood supply to the heart and can result in chest pain (angina pectoris) or other symptoms, typically triggered by physical exertion. If a narrowed blood vessel is completely blocked by a blood clot, the area of the heart just beyond the blockage is denied oxygen and nourishment, resulting in a heart attack (myocardial infarction). The 10 risk factors help to predict the likelihood of CHD are:

- Heredity
- Gender
- Age
- Cigarette smoking
- High BP
- Diabetes
- Obesity
- Lack of physical activity
- Abnormal blood cholesterol
- Homocysteine levels.

The more risk factors a person has, the greater the likelihood of developing heart disease. Heredity, gender, and age cannot be modified, but the others can be influenced by the individual's behavior.

Risk of Cardiovascular Diseases

Major Risk Factors (Cannot be Modified)

Major risk factors are detailed below:
1. Age: About 83% of people who die of coronary heat disease (CHD) are 65 or older.
2. Gender: Men have a greater risk of heart attack than women do and they have attacks earlier in life.
3. Heredity (including race): Children of parents with heart disease are more likely to develop it themselves. African-Americans have more severe high BP than Caucasians and a higher risk of heart disease. Heart disease risk is also higher among Mexican-Americans, American-Indians, native Hawaiians, and some Asian-Americans. This is partly due to higher rates of obesity and diabetes. Most people with a strong family history of heart disease have one or more other risk factors.

Major Risk Factors (Can be Modified)

Major risk factors can be modified through treatment or control by changing lifestyle or taking medicine:
1. Tobacco smoke: Smokers' risk of developing CHD is two to four times more than that of nonsmokers. Cigarette smoking is a powerful independent risk factor for sudden cardiac death in patients with CHD; smokers have about twice the risk of nonsmokers. Cigarette smoking also acts with other risk factors to greatly increase the risk for CHD. People who smoke cigars or pipes seem to have a higher risk of death.
2. High blood cholesterol: As blood cholesterol rises, so does risk of CHD. When other risk factors (such as high BP and tobacco smoke) are present, this risk increases even more. A person's cholesterol level is also affected by age, sex, heredity, and diet. Total blood cholesterol is classified by levels:
   a. Desirable: **Under 200** mg/dL
   b. **Borderline: 200–239** mg/dL
   c. High risk: 240 mg/dL and above.
3. Low-density level cholesterol:
   a. Optimal (ideal): Less than 100 mg/dL
   b. Near optimal/above optimal: 100–129 mg/dL
   c. Borderline high: 130–159 mg/dL
   d. **High: 160–189** mg/dL (high risk)
   e. Very high: 190 mg/dL and above (very high risk).
4. High-density level cholesterol:
   a. Major heart disease risk factor: Less than 40 mg/dL.
   b. Protection against heart disease: 60 mg/dL and above.
5. High BP: It increases the heart's workload, causing the heart to thicken and become stiffer. It also increases stroke, heart attack, kidney failure, and congestive heart failure. When high BP exists with obesity, smoking, high blood cholesterol levels or diabetes, the risk of heart attack or stroke increases several times.
   Note: Healthy adult (at rest) should have a systolic pressure below 120 and a diastolic pressure below 80.
6. Physical inactivity: An inactive lifestyle is a risk factor for CHD. Regular, moderate-to-vigorous physical activity helps prevent heart and blood vessel disease. Physical activity can help control blood cholesterol, diabetes, and obesity, as well as lower BP in some people.
7. Obesity and overweight: People who have excess body fat especially at the waist are more likely to develop heart disease and stroke even if they have no other risk factors. Excess weight increases the heart's work. It also raises BP and blood cholesterol and TG levels and lowers HDL cholesterol levels. It can also make diabetes more likely to develop.

8. Diabetes mellitus: Diabetes seriously increases risk of developing cardiovascular disease. Even when glucose (blood sugar) levels are under control, diabetes increases the risk of heart disease and stroke, but the risks are even greater if blood sugar is not well controlled. About three quarters of people with diabetes die of some form of heart or blood vessel disease. If you have diabetes, it is extremely important to work with your health-care provider to manage it and control any other risk factors you can.

Other Factors Contribute to Heart Disease Risk

1. Stress may be a contributing factor. For example, people under stress may overeat, start smoking, or smoke more than they otherwise would.
2. Too much alcohol can raise BP, cause heart failure, and lead to stroke:
    a. It can contribute to high TG s. It contributes to obesity, alcoholism.
    b. Experts say that moderate intake is an average of one to two drinks per day for men and one drink per day for women.
    c. One drink is defined as 1.5 fluid ounces (fl oz) of 80 proof spirits (such as scotch, vodka, and gin), 1 fl oz of 100 proof spirits, 4 fl oz of wine, or 12 fl oz of beer. But drinking more than a moderate amount of alcohol can cause heart-related problems such as high BP, stroke, irregular heartbeats, and cardiomyopathy (disease of the heart muscle).

SUMMARY

The lipids are hydrolyzed to small- and long-chain fatty acids with the help of several enzymes. The hormone-sensitive lipase is the major enzyme, which digests triacylglycerol. The short- and medium-chain fatty acids are absorbed directly into the intestinal epithelial cells and enters the portal blood to reach the liver and the long-chain fatty acids form mixed micelle with bile salts and then absorbed. The absorbed fatty acids undergo β-oxidation to generate energy and acetyl-CoA. The β-oxidation starts with an activation step and then transfer of activated fatty acyl-CoA into the inner mitochondrial membrane through carnitine cycle. Carnitine acyltransferase I is the regulatory enzyme in the β-oxidation of fatty acids. The majority of the fatty acids required by the body are supplied through diet. Fatty acids are synthesized whenever there is a caloric excess in our diet. The fresh synthesis of fatty acid is the de novo synthesis. Acetyl-CoA and NADPH are required for the de novo synthesis of fatty acids, which takes place in cytoplasmic portion of the cell. Fatty acid synthase (FAS) complex enzyme catalyzes the synthesis of fatty acids. The dimer form of the FAS enzyme complex is active. Each monomer of FAS enzyme complex has seven different enzyme activities. Acetyl-CoA carboxylase enzyme catalyzed step is a committed step in fatty acid synthesis regulation. Cholesterol synthesis depends on acetyl-CoA. HMG-CoA reductase is the regulatory enzyme of cholesterol synthesis. Most of the statin drugs used, control the cholesterol synthesis by inhibiting the HMG-CoA reductase. Lecithin–cholesterol acyl transferase (LCAT) is responsible for the esterification, transportation, and elimination of cholesterol from the body. Cholesterol metabolized to bile acids and bile salts in the liver. Uncontrolled diabetes mellitus and starvation are the two conditions in which the ketone bodies are formed. Ketone bodies (acetoacetate, β-hydroxybutyrate, and acetone) are produced in the liver but utilized by the extrahepatic tissues. There are several factors contributing for fatty liver such as increased synthesis of TAG, VLDL, certain chemicals, and hormones promotes the fatty liver formation. There are several risk factors that are responsible for the development of cardiovascular disorders, such as obesity, hypertension, diabetes, high cholesterol, low HDL, high homocysteine levels, smoking, and alcohol consumption. Prostaglandins and their related compounds are prostacyclins (PGI), thromboxanes (TXAs), and leukotrienes (LT) are collectively known as eicosanoids.

Cardiovascular diseases are the leading cause of illness and death in the world. There are several risk factors that increase the risk of getting heart diseases. Heredity, gender, and age cannot be modified but cigarette smoking, high blood pressure (BP), diabetes, obesity, lack of physical activity, abnormal blood cholesterol, and homocysteine levels can be modified with change in the lifestyle.

SELF-ASSESSMENT QUESTIONS

Short Notes

1. Briefly discuss the digestion and absorption of lipids in the gastrointestinal tract.
2. Outline the steps of b-oxidation of fatty acids.
3. How many ATPs are produced when one mole of palmitic acid is completely metabolized to acetyl-CoA?
4. Explain the de novo synthesis of fatty acid.
5. Name the compounds formed from cholesterol.
6. What is atherosclerosis? Explain.
7. Name the ketone bodies and mention the conditions in which ketone bodies are formed.
8. Briefly discuss on the formation and utilization of ketone bodies.
9. Discuss the e following:
   a. Role of liver in lipid metabolism.
   b. Metabolic fate of acetyl-CoA.
   c. Carnitine cycle.
   d. Ketoacidosis.
10. What is ketonemia, ketonuria, and ketolysis.

Fill in the Blanks

1. Net ATP produced during complete oxidation palmitic acid is _____.
2. The _____ is required for the transport of activated fatty acid inside the mitochondria.
3. The _____ enzyme digest triglycerides.
4. Lipid absorption requires _____ for emulsification.

Match the Following

Enzyme	Action
1. Thiokinase	a. Splits HMG-CoA
2. Thiolase	b. β-Ketoacyl-CoA synthesis
3. HMG-CoA reductase	c. Interconverts β-OH-butyrate and acetoacetate
4. HMG-CoA reductase	d. Required for the activation of fatty acid
5. β-OH butyrate DH	e. Synthesis of mevalonic acid
6. β-OH acyl-CoA DH	f. β-Ketoacyl-CoA to acyl-CoA and acetyl-CoA

MULTIPLE-CHOICE QUESTIONS

1. **Concerning cholesterol, all the following statements are correct, *except*:**
   a. It is a low water-soluble lipid found in blood
   b. It exists in only one form in plasma
   c. It is a major structural component of cell surfaces
   d. It is esterified to some long-chain fatty acids, which enhances its hydrophobicity

2. **Regarding cholesterol determination on serum, the following statements are true, *except*:**
   a. It is determined by a modified method of Zak reaction
   b. The reddish brown color produced is due to the action of the $FeCl_3 H_2SO_2$

c. The color is directly proportional to the concentration of the substance present and quantitated spectrophotometrically at 550 nm
d. The color is inversely proportional to the concentration of the substance present and quantitated spectrophotometrically at 550 nm

3. If 20 mg standard cholesterol dissolved in 100 mL absolute ethanol then concentration of cholesterol in 1.0 mL solution is:
   a. 0.02 mg
   b. 0.8 mg
   c. 0.2 mg
   d. 2.0 mg

4. All the following are synthesized from cholesterol, *except*:
   a. Bile acids
   b. Vitamin C
   c. Vitamin D
   d. Steroid hormones

5. In all the following clinical conditions in which we find high blood cholesterol, *except*:
   a. Pernicious anemia
   b. Nephrosis
   c. Obstructive jaundice
   d. Diabetes mellitus

6. Concerning the structure of cholesterol, all of the following statements are true, *except*:
   a. It has a molecular formula of $C_{27}H_{46}O$
   b. It has five rings
   c. It has cyclopentanoperhydrophenanthrene ring
   d. It has three cyclohexane and one cyclopentane rings

7. Which one of the following statements best describes the cholesterol?
   a. Low-density lipoprotein is responsible for the transport and elimination of cholesterol from the body
   b. In healthy individuals the total plasma cholesterol is in the range of 90–150 mg%
   c. Cholesterol is not found in animals
   d. High-density lipoproteins and lecithin–cholesterol acyltransferase are responsible for the transport and elimination of cholesterol from the body

8. Which of the following is an accurate description of ketone bodies?

   a. Their synthesis is stimulated by insulin and inhibited by glucagon
   b. They are a water-soluble form of acetyl units that are synthesized in the liver and used by many other tissues in the body as a fuel source
   c. They are the major fuel source for the brain under basal metabolic conditions
   d. They are not produced during starvation

9. Which of the following accurately describes fatty acid synthesis in humans?
   a. Fatty acid synthase sequentially adds two-carbon units from malonyl-CoA until palmitate is made
   b. Complex of seven enzymes makes 16-carbon palmitate directly from eight molecules of acetyl-CoA
   c. Acetyl-CoA is transported out of the mitochondrial matrix as the three-carbon-activated molecule malonyl-CoA
   d. Fatty acid synthesis generates large quantities of NADPH, which can be used by the electron transport chain and ATP synthase to generate ATP.

10. Net amount of ATP formed when one molecule of palmitic acid undergoes β-oxidation is:
    a. 29
    b. 140
    c. 129
    d. 130

11. The regulatory enzyme of cholesterol synthesis is:
    a. Glucosyltransferase
    b. HMG-CoA reductase
    c. HMG-CoA synthase
    d. Mevalonate kinase

12. Which of the following is *not* a biochemical action of prostaglandin?
    a. Regulation of blood pressure
    b. Reproduction
    c. Development of bone
    d. Inflammation

13. Regarding fatty acid synthase complex, all the following statements are true, *except*:
    a. It is a dimer with identical subunits
    b. Monomer form is functionally active
    c. Monomer has seven different enzymes and an acyl carrier protein
    d. Two subunits lie in antiparallel orientation

14. All of the following involve acetyl-CoA, *except*:
    a. Ketone body synthesis
    b. Cholesterol synthesis
    c. Nucleotide synthesis
    d. Fatty acid synthesis
15. During prolonged starvation the brain mainly depends on one of the following for energy:
    a. Glucose residues
    b. Ketone bodies
    c. Amino acids
    d. Lactose molecules
16. For the synthesis of 16-carbon palmitic acid, number of acetyl-CoA transported from mitochondria to cytosol is:
    a. 10 b. 20
    c. 2 d. 8
17. Net amount of ATP formed one cycle of β-oxidation of fatty acid is:
    a. 29 b. 140
    c. 5 d. 130
18. Reduced glutathione is required for the formation of:
    a. PGH_2 from PGG_2
    b. PGI_2 from PGH_2
    c. PGG_2 from arachidonic acid
    d. PGE_2 from PGH_2
19. The substance, which carries acyl-CoA into the inner mitochondrial membrane for oxidation is:
    a. β-Carotene b. Carnitine
    c. Malate d. Creatinine
20. The main regulatory enzyme of fatty acid synthesis is:
    a. Acetyl-CoA carboxylase
    b. Hexokinase
    c. Phosphofructokinase
    d. Thioesterase
21. All the following are the biochemical actions of prostaglandins, *except*:
    a. Regulation of blood pressure
    b. Reproduction
    c. Inhibition of platelet aggregation
    d. Destruction of free radical
22. Regarding starvation, all the following statements are true, *except*:
    a. Increased gluconeogenesis
    b. Increased glycogen degradation
    c. Decreased fatty acid oxidation
    d. Increased fatty acid oxidation
23. All the following are the ketone bodies, *except*:
    a. Acetoacetate
    b. b-Hydroxybutyrate
    c. HMG-CoA
    d. Acetone
24. Ketosis occurs in all of the following conditions, *except*:
    a. Starvation
    b. In controlled diabetes mellitus
    c. In the well-fed state
    d. Feeding high-fat diet
25. In humans, most of the prostaglandins are predominantly formed from:
    a. Linoleic acid b. Arachidonic acid
    c. Palmitic acid d. Stearic acid
26. All the following are the components of fatty acid synthase complex, *except*:
    a. Acetyltransferase (AT)
    b. Malonyltransferase (MT)
    c. β-Ketoacyl synthase (KS)
    d. Succinate dehydrogenase (SD)
27. Function of apoprotein C is:
    a. Activation of amylase
    b. Binding lipoprotein to its receptors
    c. Activation of lipoprotein lipase
    d. Remnant receptor binding
28. Which of the following enzymes mainly digests triglycerides:
    a. Amylase b. Lipase
    c. Chymotrypsin d. Pepsin
29. Micelle formation with bile salts is essential for:
    a. Lipid absorption
    b. Carbohydrate absorption
    c. Lipid digestion
    d. Protein transport
30. The enzyme that splits HMG-CoA is:
    a. Thiokinase
    b. Thiolase
    c. HMG-CoA lyase
    d. HMG-CoA reductase
31. Which of the following excreted through lungs when their blood levels high?
    a. Acetone b. Acetoacetic acid
    c. β-OH butyric acid d. Pyruvic acid
32. The enzyme that esterifies cholesterol is:
    a. Acyltransferase
    b. Acyl-CoA dehydrogenase
    c. Lecithin–cholesterol acyl
    d. Cephalin acyltransferase

33. The absorbed dietary cholesterol transported as:
    a. VLDL
    b. HDL
    c. Chylomicron
    d. LDL
34. The enzyme that hydrolyzes phospholipids is:
    a. Phospholipase
    b. Cholesterol hydrolase
    c. Pancreatic lipase
    d. Amylase
35. Oxidation of odd-chain fatty acid ends up with:
    a. Acyl-CoA
    b. Propionyl-CoA
    c. Malonyl-CoA
    d. Succinyl-CoA
36. Hormone-sensitive lipase acts on stored:
    a. Liver fat
    b. Adipose tissue fat
    c. Kidney fat
    d. Skin triacylglycerol
37. Insulin:
    a. Reduces the release of free fatty acids from adipose tissue
    b. Increases the release of triacylglycerol from adipose tissue
    c. Increases the release of alanine from muscle
    d. Reduces triglyceride synthesis
38. After 3 weeks of starvation, the brain:
    a. Gets glucose through glycogenolysis
    b. Completely depends on gluconeogenesis to generate ketone bodies
    c. Depends on muscle proteins
    d. Depends on acetyl-CoA to generate ketone bodies
39. Concerning insulin action, all of the following statements are true *except*, It:
    a. Activates pyruvate kinase
    b. Stimulates glycerol phosphate acyltransferase
    c. Increases HMG-CoA reductase activity
    d. Activates hormone-sensitive lipase
40. Density of lipoprotein depends on its
    a. Protein content
    b. Lipid content
    c. Carbohydrate content
    d. Fluid content
41. The enzyme responsible for prostaglandin synthesis is:
    a. 15-hydroxy prostaglandin dehydrogenase
    b. Cyclooxygenase
    c. Oxidoreductase
    d. Adenylate cyclase
42. Before fats can be acted upon by the digestive enzymes, they must be:
    a. Neutralized
    b. Esterified
    c. Emulsified
    d. Hydrolyzed
43. In liver, the metabolism of acetyl-CoA can lead to all of the following, *except*:
    a. Cholesterol
    b. β-Hydroxybutyrate
    c. Palmitic acid
    d. Oleate
44. Bile salts:
    a. Are synthesized from lipoprotein
    b. Contain bilirubin
    c. Increase the surface tension in fat particles in the small intestine
    d. Form micelles with lipids in the small intestine
45. A 40-year-old man presents with familial hypercholesterolemia undergoes a detailed serum lipid and lipoprotein analysis. Studies demonstrate elevated cholesterol in the form of increased LDL without elevation of triglyceride other lipids. This patient's hyperlipidemia is best classified as which of the following types?
    a. Type I
    b. Type IIa
    c. Type IIb
    d. Type IV
46. The blood level of total cholesterol concentration recommended by the international diabetic association is:
    a. Less than 240 mg/dL
    b. Less than 250 mg/dL
    c. Less than 150 mg/dL
    d. Less than 200 mg/dL
47. Which of the following constituents is not usually found in bile?
    a. Cholic acid
    b. Glycocholic acid
    c. Deoxycholate
    d. Phosphodeoxycholate
48. If a patient has inadequate bile secretion, which of the following could contribute to the condition?
    a. Excessive steroid hormones
    b. Excessive release of cholecystokinin
    c. Excessive release of pepsin
    d. Excessive release of secretin
49. A deficiency of colipase would result in which of the following?
    a. Lipase may not be able to bind to the oil–water interface of the lipid
    b. An inability to digest phospholipids

c. An inability to digest cholesterol
d. An inability to digest lipids in the stomach

50. Which of the following lipoprotein has 98% lipid?
    a. Chylomicron
    b. HDL
    c. VLDL
    d. LDL

51. High blood level of LDLc is considered as level is a bad cholesterol because:
    a. It transports cholesterol from liver to kidney
    b. It transports triglyceride from extrahepatic tissues to liver
    c. It transports cholesterol from liver to extrahepatic tissues
    d. It transports dietary triglycerides to liver

52. Which of the following has high protein content?
    a. Chylomicron
    b. HDL
    c. VLDL
    d. LDL

53. Familial hypercholesterolemia is due to the mutations in:
    a. *LDLR* gene
    b. *HDLR* gene
    c. *LPR* gene
    d. *VLDR* gene

54. All of the following are the risk factors for cardiovascular diseases, *except*:
    a. Cholesterol level of 260 mg/dL
    b. Blood pressure of 160/95
    c. Homocysteine level of 40 micromoles/L
    d. HDL cholesterol level of 80 mg/dL

55. Secretin stimulates the secretion of:
    a. Bicarbonate-rich fluid from pancreas
    b. Enzymes from intestine
    c. Pancreatic fluid with enzymes
    d. HCl-rich fluid from stomach

56. All of the following enzymes are from Pancreas, *except*:
    a. Amylase
    b. Lipase
    c. Trypsin
    d. Pepsin

57. Concerning the oxidation of fatty acids, all the following statements are correct, *except*:
    a. Odd-chain fatty acids generate succinyl-CoA in addition to acetyl-CoA
    b. Zellweger syndrome is an inborn error of peroxisomal oxidation of fatty acids
    c. Acetyl-CoA carboxylase and ADP are essential for the activation of fatty acid
    d. Vitamin B_{12} is essential for the oxidation of odd-chain fatty acid

58. A 55-year-old man presented with severe chest pain that radiated into his shoulder. His angiogram showed the presence of atherosclerotic plaques in his arteries. The plaques were formed due to the high blood level of:
    a. HDLc
    b. LDLc
    c. Chylomicron
    d. IDLc

59. A young Jamaican boy complained of vomiting and weakness. His mother took him to a doctor and, while his history was being taken, his mother mentioned that he ate unripe ackee fruit from the yard. The doctor immediately remembered from his year-I medical biochemistry lecture that ackee contains a toxin that impairs β-oxidation of fatty acids by inhibiting this enzyme:
    a. β-Hydroxymethylglutaryl-Co A reductase
    b. Lecithin–cholesterol acyltransferase
    c. Acyl-CoA dehydrogenase
    d. Acetyl-CoA carboxylase

60. The first two carbon atoms for the de novo synthesis of fatty acids come from:
    a. Malonyl-CoA
    b. Propionyl-CoA
    c. Butyryl-CoA
    d. Acetyl-CoA

61. Concerning cholesterol:
    a. Its synthesis depends on 28 acetyl-CoA molecules
    b. It is a saturated fatty acid, present in kidney and liver
    c. Its synthesis is regulated by HMG-CoA reductase
    d. Its level is normal in hypothyroidism and nephrosis

62. Concerning ketone bodies:
    a. They are formed during diabetes insipidus
    b. They are utilized in the muscle and brain
    c. They are produced and utilized in liver
    d. The ratio of hydroxybutyrate to acetoacetate depends on $FADH_2/FAD$

63. Concerning the hormonal regulation of fatty acid synthesis:
    a. Palmitoyl-CoA causes polymerisation of acetyl-CoA carboxylase
    b. Glucagon and epinephrine activate the regulatory enzyme of fatty acid synthesis
    c. Insulin promotes fatty acid synthesis through the activation of acetyl-CoA carboxylase
    d. A high carbohydrate diet decreases the synthesis of acetyl-CoA carboxylase

64. Concerning fatty acid synthase complex (FAS) enzyme:

a. It is a regulatory enzyme of fatty acid synthesis
b. The monomer form of FAS contains seven enzymatic activities
c. Only the dimer form of FAS has acyl carrier protein
d. Catalyses the formation of acetyl-CoA

65. High-density lipoprotein molecules:
a. Contain 78% protein and 22% lipid
b. Increases the risk of cardiovascular diseases
c. Are rich in apolipoprotein B-100
d. Transport cholesterol from peripheral tissues to the liver

66. Concerning the oxidation of fatty acids, all of the following statements are true, *except*:
a. Odd-chain fatty acids generate succinyl-CoA in addition to acetyl-CoA
b. Zellweger syndrome is an inborn error of peroxisomal oxidation of fatty acids
c. α-Oxidation of fatty acids go through the activation steps.
d. β-Oxidation of palmitic acid generates seven molecules each of NADH and FADH

67. What is the correct order of function of the enzymes of ketone body formation shown below (1–4)?
1. β-Hydroxybutyrate dehydrogenase
2. Thiolase
3. HMG-CoA synthase
4. HMG-CoA lyase
a. 3, 1, 4, 2
b. 4, 3, 1, 2
c. 1, 4, 3, 2
d. 2, 3, 4, 1

68. The major function of Apoprotein C-II is to:
a. Mobilize lipids
b. Bind LDL to its receptor
c. Stimulate LCAT receptor binding
d. Activate lipoprotein lipase

69. Which of the following is a risk factor for heart disease?
a. LDL cholesterol of 70–120 mg/dL
b. Total cholesterol of 100–170 mg/dL
c. HDL cholesterol of 30 mg/dL
d. Triglyceride level of 150 mg/dL

70. The apoprotein present in LDL cholesterol is:
a. Apo B48
b. Apo B100
c. Apo CII
d. Apo A

Answers

1. b	2. d	3. c	4. b	5. a
6. b	7. d	8. b	9. a	10. c
11. b	12. c	13. b	14. c	15. b
16. d	17. c	18. a	19. b	20. a
21. d	22. c	23. c	24. c	25. b
26. d	27. c	28. b	29. a	30. c
31. a	32. c	33. c	34. a	35. b
36. b	37. a	38. d	39. d	40. a
41. b	42. a	43. d	44. d	45. d
46. d	47. d	48. a	49. a	50. a
51. c	52. b	53. a	54. d	55. c
56. d	57. c	58. b	59. c	60. d
61. c	62. b	63. c	64. b	65. d
66. c	67. d	68. d	69. c	70. b

CHAPTER 10

Integration of Metabolism

OBJECTIVES

At the end of this chapter, students should be able to:
- Understand how the metabolism integrated themselves during well fed and fasting conditions
- Explain the role of hormones in integrating the metabolism during well-fed and fasting conditions
- Explain the role of adiponectin and leptin in hunger and satiety
- Know about the various artificial sweeteners and their metabolic effects
- Explain the cause for atherosclerosis
- Discuss the laboratory tests available to diagnose myocardial infarction.

INTRODUCTION

All organisms possess their variable energy demands; hence, the supply is also equally variable. The consumed metabolic fuel may be oxidized to carbon dioxide (CO_2) and water (H_2O) or stored to meet the energy requirements per the body needs **(Fig. 10.1)**. Adenosine triphosphate (ATP) serves as the energy currency of the cell. Any deficiency or reduced action of insulin causes diabetes. Obesity is one of the major causes for developing diabetes. Obesity is the deposition excess fat and inversely proportional to adiponectin and leptin. Artificial sweeteners are used by diabetic and obese people mainly to control their weight. It is better to monitor cholesterol status of our body by performing lipid profile testing. High level of cholesterol as well as low-density lipoprotein (LDL) cholesterol results in atherosclerosis and later myocardial infarction (MI). MI can be diagnosed by analyzing blood levels of troponin T (TnT) and cardiac enzymes.

PATHWAYS OF METABOLISM

Glycolysis

Glycolysis is the process of degradation of glucose to pyruvate (lactate under anaerobic) generating ATP.

Fatty Acid Oxidation

Fatty acid (FA) oxidizes to acetyl coenzyme A (acetyl-CoA). Energy is trapped in the form of nicotinamide adenine dinucleotide and flavin adenine dinucleotide.

Amino Acid Degradation

When amino acids consumed more than the required, they are degraded to meet the fuel demands of the body. The glucogenic amino acids can serve as the precursor for the synthesis of glucose via pyruvate or intermediates of tricarboxylic acid (TCA) cycle.

The ketogenic amino acids form the precursor for acetyl-CoA.

Clinical Scenarios/Case Studies

1. Briefly explain the role of different organs and tissues in integrating the metabolism after 2–4 hours of food intake.

Integration of Metabolism

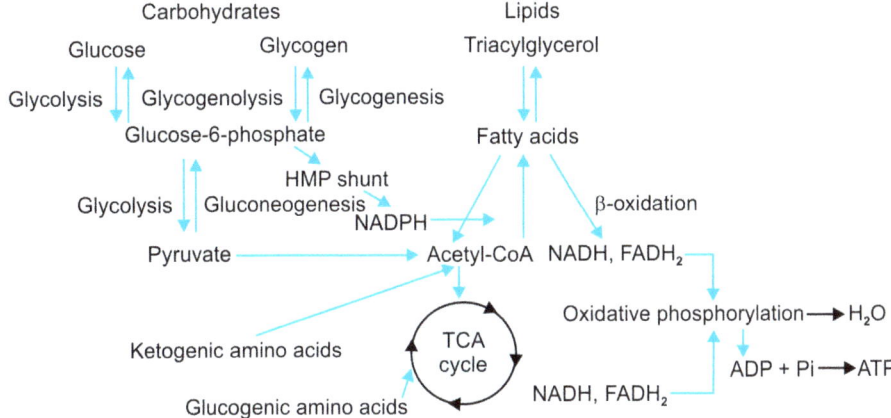

Fig. 10.1: Overview of metabolism.
(TCA: tricarboxylic acid)

Or
A 30-year-old man went to a marriage party and had nice lunch, which provided him enough carbohydrates, proteins, and fats. Explain how the various organs of his body work in a well-coordinated manner to meet his metabolic demands?

The various organs of the body work in a well-coordinated manner to meet its metabolic demands (usually 2–4 hours after food consumption) **(Fig. 10.2)**.

Liver
Liver is specialized to serve as the body's central metabolic clearing house. After a

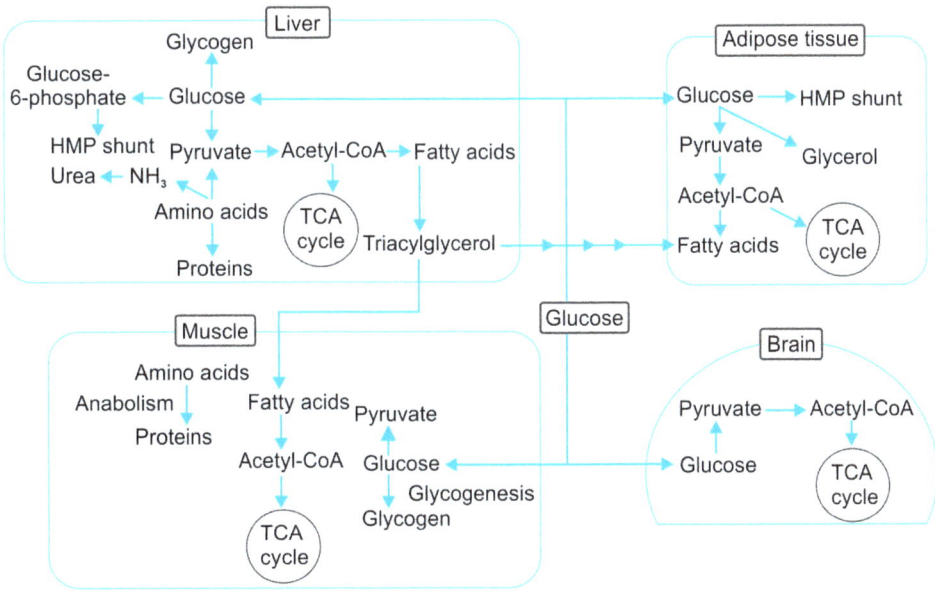

Fig. 10.2: Integration of metabolism during fed state.
(TCA: tricarboxylic acid)

meal, the liver takes up the carbohydrates, lipids, and amino acids; processes them; and routes to other tissues. The major metabolic functions of liver in absorptive state are:
- Carbohydrate metabolism: Increased glycolysis, glycogenesis, and hexose monophosphate pathway (HMP) shunt and decreased gluconeogenesis
- Lipid metabolism: Increased FA and triacylglycerol (TG) synthesis
- Protein metabolism: Increased degradation of amino acids and protein synthesis.

Adipose tissue

Adipose tissue is regarded as the energy storage tissue:
- Carbohydrate metabolism: Increases uptake of glucose, glycolysis, and HMP shunt
- Lipid metabolism: FA and TG synthesis increases
- Breakdown of TG inhibited.

Skeletal muscle

The major metabolic functions of skeletal muscle in absorptive state are:
- Carbohydrate metabolism: Uptake of glucose is higher and glycogenesis increased.
- Lipid metabolism: FA taken up from the circulation.
- Protein metabolism: Incorporation of amino acids into proteins is higher.

Brain
- Carbohydrate metabolism: Glucose is the only source of fuel in an absorptive state; about 120 g of glucose is utilized per day.
- Lipid metabolism: Free FAs cannot cross the blood–brain barrier; hence, their contribution for the supply of energy to the brain is insignificant.

2. **Briefly discuss the integration of metabolism during starvation.**
   Or
   Factory workers went on hunger strike on demanding the hike in their salary. **The management did not respond to their demand and the workers decided to continue their hunger strike. Discuss the different organs and tissues take part in integrating the metabolism during this condition to meet their energy requirement.**

This part explains how all the metabolism is integrated in different organs and tissues of our body followed by starvation (**Fig. 10.3**):
1. Starvation may be due to food scarcity or the desire to rapidly lose weight or during surgery and burns.
2. It is metabolic stress, which imposes certain metabolic compulsions on the organism.
3. The metabolism is reorganized to meet the new demands of starvation.
4. Glucose is the fuel of choice for brain and muscle. Unfortunately, the carbohydrate is not sufficient to meet the requirements.
5. The TG of adipose tissue is the predominant energy reserve of the body. Protein can also meet the fuel demands of the body.
6. Starvation is associated with decreased insulin and increased glucagon.

Liver in starvation
1. Carbohydrate metabolism: Increased gluconeogenesis and glycogen degradation.
2. Lipid metabolism: FA oxidation increased. The TCA cycle cannot cope with the excess production of acetyl-CoA, so it is diverted for ketone body formation. The fuel demands of the brain are met by ketone bodies.

Adipose tissue in starvation
1. Carbohydrate metabolism: Glucose uptake and its metabolism are lowered.
2. Lipid metabolism: Degradation of TG increased leading to increased release of FA from the adipose tissue, which serves as a fuel for various tissues (brain is an exception). Glycerol liberated during

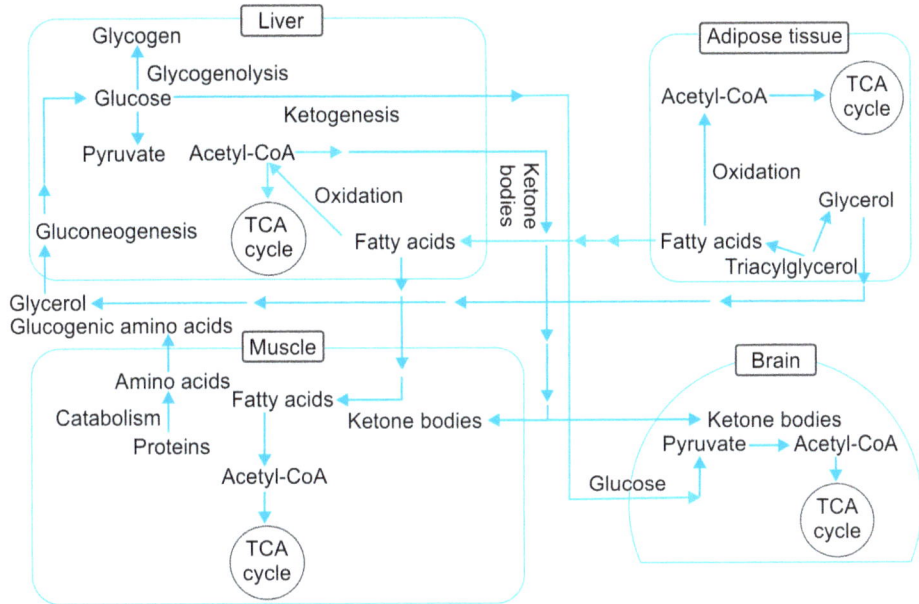

Fig. 10.3: Integration of metabolism during fasting condition.
(TCA: tricarboxylic acid)

lipolysis is used for glucose synthesis by the liver. The synthesis of FA and TG is completely stopped here.

Skeletal muscle in starvation
1. Carbohydrate metabolism: Glucose uptake and its metabolism are lowered.
2. Lipid metabolism: FA and ketone bodies are utilized as fuel by the muscle. Prolonged starvation adopted to utilize FA.
3. Protein metabolism: Muscle proteins are degraded and the amino acids are utilized for glucose synthesis by liver. Protein breakdown is reduced, if the starvation is prolonged.

Brain in starvation
In the early 2 weeks of starvation, the brain depends on glucose, supplied by liver gluconeogenesis. This, in turn, depends on the amino acids released from the muscle protein breakdown. Starvation beyond 3 weeks results in increased plasma ketone bodies and the brain adopts itself to depend on ketone bodies for the energy.

Hormonal Regulation of Metabolism during Well-fed State (Fig. 10.4)

Hormonal Regulation of Carbohydrate Metabolism

1. In the regulation of blood glucose, the liver, extrahepatic tissues, and hormones play a major role.
2. Increased level of circulating glucose releases insulin, which reduces the blood glucose level in many ways.
3. Insulin stimulates glucose transporter type 4 (GLUT-4) to increase the active transport of glucose across membranes of muscle and adipose tissue. Glucose is rapidly taken up into liver via GLUT-2 transporter.
4. In the liver, insulin increases the use of glycolysis by inducing the glycolytic enzymes such as glucokinase, phosphofructokinase, and pyruvate kinase.
5. Glucokinase is important in regulating blood glucose after meal.
6. In the liver and muscle, insulin stimulates glycogenesis by stimulating glycogen

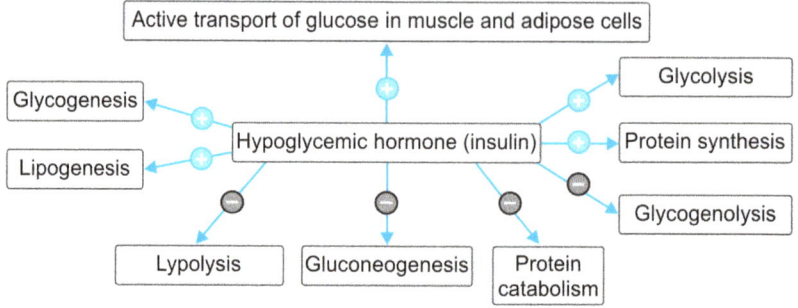

Fig. 10.4: Hormonal regulation of metabolism during well-fed state.

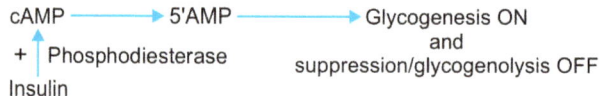

Fig. 10.5: Control of glycogen metabolism by insulin.

synthase by reducing the elevated cyclic adenosine monophosphate (cAMP) levels and thereby leading to suppression of glycogenolysis (Fig. 10.5).
7. Insulin inhibits gluconeogenesis by suppressing the action of key enzymes of gluconeogenesis, i.e. pyruvate carboxylase, phosphoenolpyruvate carboxykinase, fructose-1,6-bisphosphatase, and glucose-6-phosphatase.
8. In adipose tissue, glucose is converted to the glycerol-3-phosphate, which is required for the formation of TG and inhibits the lipolysis by inhibiting hormone-sensitive lipase.
9. Insulin increases protein synthesis and decreases protein catabolism, thereby decreasing the release of amino acids for gluconeogenesis.

Hormonal Regulation of Fat Metabolism

1. Insulin inhibits the activity of hormone-sensitive lipase and reduces the release of free FAs, and glycerol from the adipose tissue, resulting in fall in the circulating plasma-free FAs.
2. Insulin enhances TG synthesis.
3. Insulin enhances lipogenesis both in liver and adipose tissue by stimulating pyruvate dehydrogenase, acetyl-CoA carboxylase, and glycerol phosphate acyltransferase.

Hormonal Regulation of Metabolism during Fasting/Starvation

Regulation of Carbohydrate Metabolism in Fasting State

Glucagon
1. In the liver, it stimulates glycogenolysis by activating glycogen phosphorylase and inhibits glycogen synthase. It exerts its action on metabolic processes through the generation of cAMP.
2. It enhances gluconeogenesis from amino acids and lactate.
3. Alanine is the predominant amino acid released from muscle to liver by glucose alanine cycle.

Epinephrine
Epinephrine favors glycogenolysis in liver and muscle through cAMP-dependent activation of adenylyl cyclase, which converts ATP to cAMP (stimulates phosphorylase) (Fig. 10.6).

Glucocorticoids
It increases:
- Gluconeogenesis

Integration of Metabolism

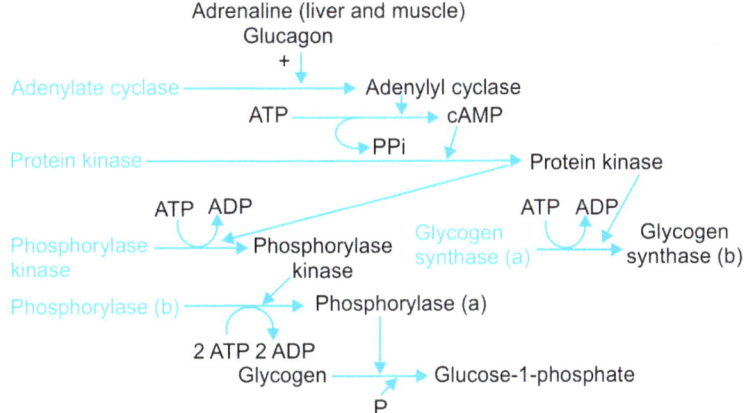

Fig. 10.6: Regulation of glycogen metabolism during fasting condition.

- Protein catabolism to provide amino acids for gluconeogenesis
- Activity of aminotransferase (to convert pyruvate to alanine).

Anterior pituitary hormones
- Growth hormone (GH) and adrenocorticotropic hormone (ACTH) antagonize the action of insulin by elevating the blood glucose level.
- GH decreases glucose uptake in the muscle and ACTH decreases glucose utilization by the tissue.

Thyroxine
It accelerates liver glycogenolysis and increases the rate of absorption of hexoses from the intestine.

Hormonal Regulation of Fat Metabolism

Starvation is associated with decreased insulin and increased glucagon; therefore the hyperglycemic hormones antagonize the action of insulin.

Norepinephrine, glucagon, ACTH, GH, and vasopressin accelerate the release of free FAs from adipose tissue and raise the plasma-free FA concentration by increasing the lipolysis of the TG (**Figs. 10.7 and 10.8**).

cAMP, by stimulating cAMP-dependent protein kinase, activates hormone-sensitive lipase, glucagon, epinephrine, and norepinephrine and inactivates the enzyme by cAMP-dependent phosphorylation and inhibits the FA synthesis.

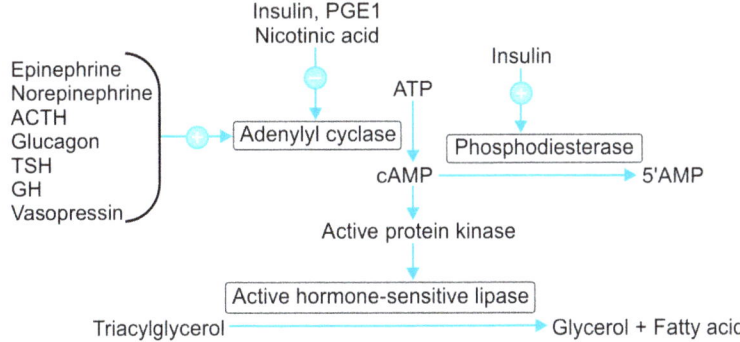

Fig. 10.7: Hormonal regulation of fat metabolism during fasting condition.

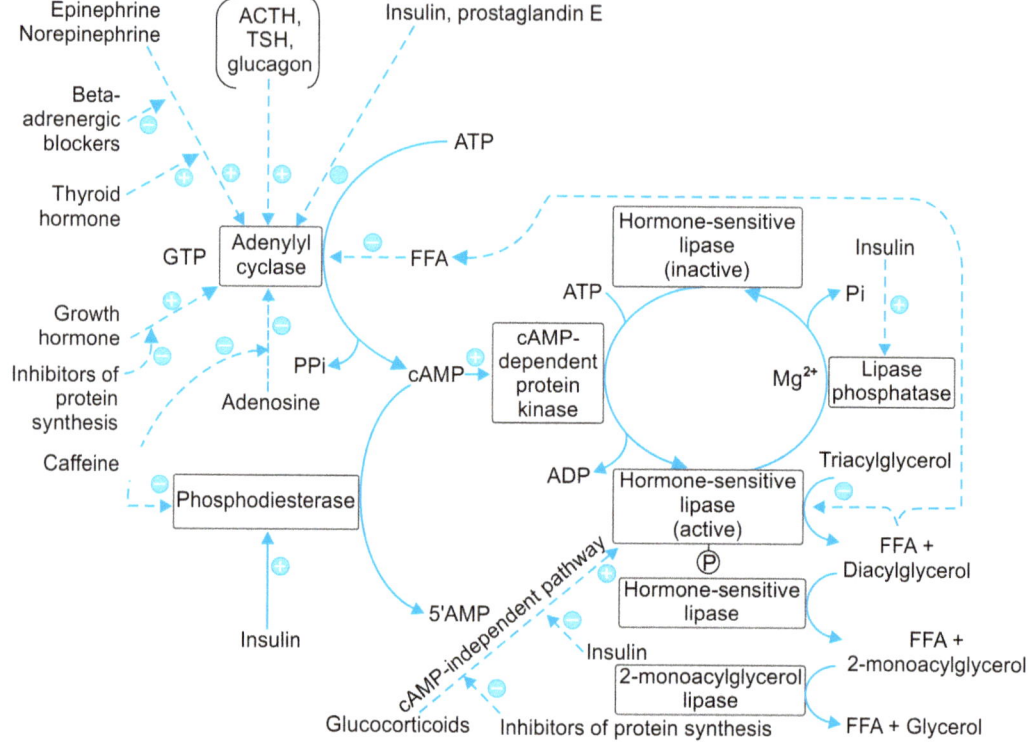

Fig. 10.8: Hormonal regulation of metabolism during fasting state.

Hormonal Regulation of Cholesterol Metabolism

The β-hydroxy-β-methylglutaryl-CoA (HMG-CoA) reductase is the regulatory enzyme of cholesterol synthesis. Insulin and thyroid hormones increase HMG-CoA reductase activity through dephosphorylation of the enzyme (active).

Glucagon and glucocorticoids decrease HMG-CoA reductase activity through cAMP-dependent phosphorylation (inactive) **(Fig. 10.9)**.

ADIPOSE TISSUE HORMONES

Adiponectin

Adiponectin is a 244-amino acid protein hormone and synthesized exclusively in adipose tissue. It is a major adipokine secreted by fat cells.

Functions

- Glucose flux: Decreases gluconeogenesis, increases glucose uptake
- Lipid catabolism: Increases β-oxidation
- Protection from endothelial dysfunction
- Improves insulin secretion
- Biomarker for insulin sensitivity
- Weight loss
- Antiinflammatory in action.

Leptin

Leptin is a hormone predominantly made by adipose cells and enterocytes in the small intestine that helps to regulate energy balance by inhibiting hunger, which in turn

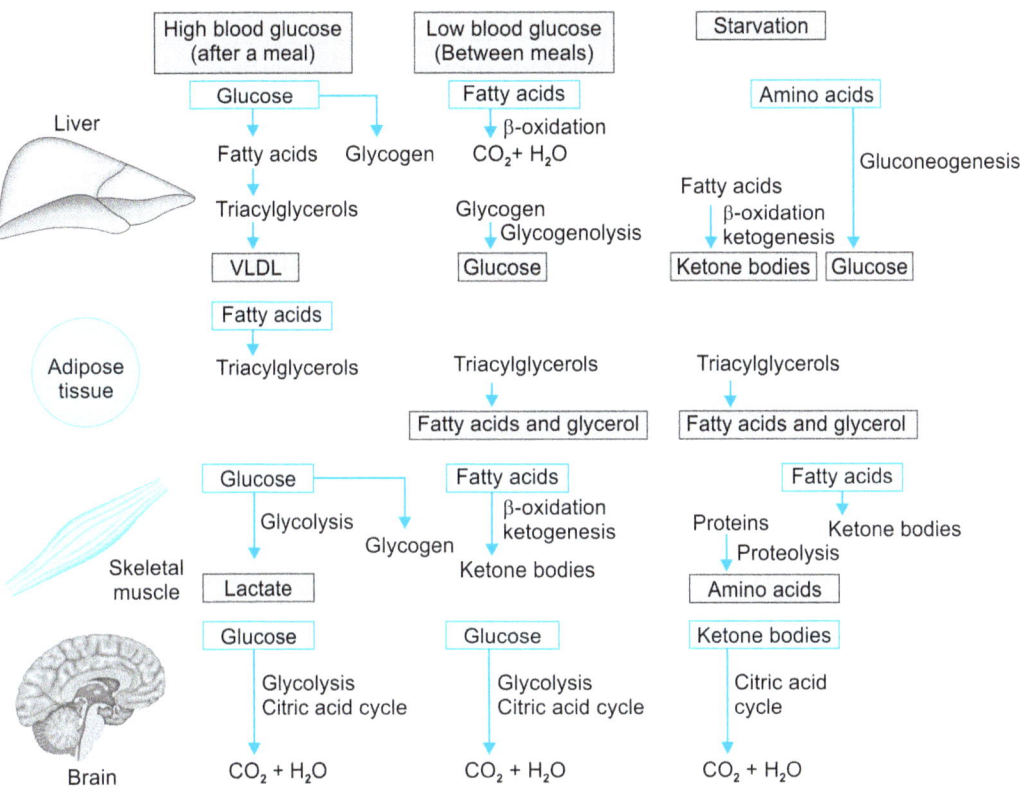

Fig. 10.9: Integration of metabolism after meal, between meals, and starvation.

diminishes fat storage in adipocytes. Leptin acts on cell receptors in the arcuate nucleus of the hypothalamus.

Leptin is a **hormone** that is produced by our body's fat cells. It is often referred to as the "**satiety hormone**" or the "**starvation hormone**."

Functions

- Helps to regulate the synthesis of thyroid hormones
- Decreases glucose stimulated insulin secretion
- Increases heart rate
- Regulates bone mass
- Regulates the menstrual cycle
- Regulates appetite, controls metabolism, and energy expenditure
- Helps in the activation of immune cells
- Increases blood pressure.

Studies have shown that an absence of **leptin** in the **body** or **leptin** resistance can lead to uncontrolled feeding and weight gain.

Role of Adiponectin and Leptin in Hunger and Satiety

Obesity: Obesity can be defined as a chronic condition with excess amount of body fat, or more specifically, a body mass index (BMI) of 30 and above. It is also shown to be inversely related to *adiponectin and leptin*.

Adipose tissue plays an important role in the effect that different environmental temperatures have on appetite. Adipokines are secreted by adipose tissue and are involved in homeostatic and appetite-regulating signaling in the body. Leptin and adiponectin are adipokines that play a major role in energy homeostasis and appetite regulation. Leptin signals the hypothalamus that energy requirements are being met and that no more food intake is required. Adiponectin also acts at the hypothalamus but works to stimulate food intake.

DIABETES MELLITUS: TYPES, METABOLIC CHANGES, AND COMPLICATIONS

Guidelines for Diagnosis of Diabetes Mellitus

Refer to Chapter 7.

Artificial Sweeteners

Artificial sweeteners or intense sweeteners are sugar substitutes that are used as an alternative to table sugar. They are many times sweeter than natural sugar and as they contain no calories, they may be used to control weight and obesity. Extensive scientific research has demonstrated the safety of the six low-calorie sweeteners currently approved for use in foods in the United States and Europe, which are as follows:

1. Stevia
2. Acesulfame K
3. Aspartame
4. Neotame
5. Saccharin
6. Sucralose.

Table sugar has been an essential component of human diet. Its excess can lead to unhealthy effect on the body, most notably diabetes mellitus. Therefore sugar substitutes were introduced as safer alternatives.

Uses

- Used in diabetes
- In controlling or reducing weight
- In dental caries
- In reactive hypoglycemia
- Flavor enhancement.

Potential risks: Malignancy (used at very high dose), hypertriglyceridemia (fructose), weight gain, and gastrointestinal symptoms.

Various natural sweeteners, which are safer, can be used instead of artificial sweeteners. Many of these include added benefits of being rich in minerals and vitamins. These include honey, coconut nectar, fruits, coconut sugar, maple syrup, molasses, sugar alcohols, stevia, dates, agave nectar, and apple sauce.

They are safe for people with diabetes, and they can be used to reduce both your calorie and carbohydrate intake. Sugar substitutes also can help curb those cravings you have for something sweet.

Lipid Profile

Lipids are a group of fats and fat-like substances that are important constituents of cells and sources of energy. A lipid panel measures the level of specific lipids in the blood.

To assess your risk of developing cardiovascular disease and to monitor the treatment of unhealthy lipid levels, the following tests of lipid profile should be done:
- Total cholesterol
- Triglyceride
- LDL cholesterol
- High-density lipoprotein (HDL) cholesterol
- Very-low-density lipoprotein (VLDL)
- Total cholesterol/HDL cholesterol ratio
- Lipoprotein electrophoresis.

Maintaining healthy levels of these lipids is important in staying healthy. While the body produces the cholesterol needed to function properly, the source for some cholesterol is the diet. Eating too much of foods that are high in saturated fats and trans unsaturated fats (trans fats) or having an inherited predisposition can result in a high level of cholesterol in the blood. The extra cholesterol may be deposited in plaques on the walls of blood vessels. Plaques can narrow or eventually block the opening of blood vessels, leading to hardening of the arteries (atherosclerosis) and increasing the

Integration of Metabolism

risk of numerous health problems, including heart disease and stroke.
Specimen: Blood collected in red top tube, fasting sample

Estimation of LDL Cholesterol and VLDL Cholesterol by Calculation

Commonly total cholesterol, HDL cholesterol, and triglycerides are estimated.

The remaining two (VLDL and LDL) are calculated from the above values as follows:

$$\text{VLDL cholesterol} = \frac{\text{Serum triglycerides}}{5}$$

LDL cholesterol=Total cholesterol-(HDL cholesterol+VLDL cholesterol).

Normal serum values
Total cholesterol=150–200 mg/dL
Triglyceride=40–160 mg/dL
HDL cholesterol
Males=28–61 mg/dL
Females=38–75 mg/dL
LDL cholesterol=60–130 mg/dL

Clinical Significance of Cholesterol Estimation

Increased levels of cholesterol in serum are called **hypercholesterolemia** that is seen in:
- Nephrosis
- Nephrotic syndrome
- Obstructive jaundice
- Myxedema
- Xanthochromatosis
- Coronary artery thrombosis and angina pectoris.

Decreased level is called **hypocholesterolemia** that is seen in:
- Hyperthyroidism
- Pernicious and other anemia
- Malabsorption syndrome
- Hemolytic jaundice.

Lipoprotein(a) and Its Importance in Cardiovascular Diseases

- A lipoprotein(a) [Lp(a)] is a heterogeneous macromolecule associated with early MI, coronary artery disease (CAD), and stroke.
- It composes 27% protein, 65% lipid, and 8% carbohydrates.
- Its composition is similar to that of LDL, but is usually present in much lower concentration.
- The structure of Lp(a) consists of an apolipoprotein(a) molecule linked to apolipoprotein B-100 on a lipid-rich LDL core.
- Its electrophoretic mobility is in the prebeta region.
- Although similar to LDL, Lp(a) is not affected by dietary factors.
- The Lp(a) determination is being recognized as a significant independent marker for assessment of the risk of coronary heart disease (CHD).
- The levels of Lp(a) is genetically controlled.
- It has a strong structural homology to plasminogen.

ATHEROSCLEROSIS

Atherosclerosis is the condition where LDL cholesterol deposited in the subintimal regions of arteries causes obstruction to the flow of blood **(Fig. 10.10)**. This may lead to extra burden on the heart, which may be one of the reasons for hypertension. If this condition is neglected for long time, it may lead to cardiac diseases and ischemia.

- Atherosclerosis leads to CHDs or CADs or ischemic heart diseases (IHDs). The deposited organic matter mainly composed of cholesterol and cholesterol ester. Hypercholesterolemia may be due to defects in transport, utilization, and excretion.

Risk Factors for Atherosclerosis

Serum Cholesterol

- Values **above 250 mg/dL increase the risk** and the person needs active treatment.
- Values **around 220 mg/dL** indicate **moderate risk**.
- Values **below 200 mg/dL are safer**.

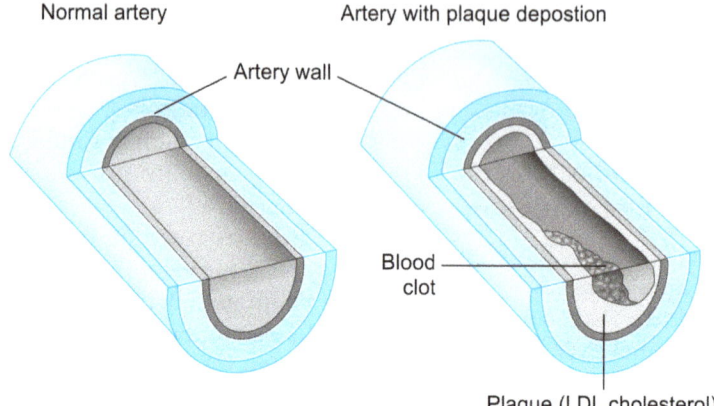

Fig. 10.10: Plaque formation.

LDL Cholesterol

- LDL cholesterol level is directly related to risk of atherosclerosis. So LDL is named as **bad cholesterol**.
- Values **above 190 mg/dL** indicate high-risk.
- Values **between 130 and 159 mg/dL** are in borderline risk.
- Values **below 130 mg/dL** are safer.

HDL cholesterol

- HDL cholesterol is inversely related to the risk of atherosclerosis. So it is named as **good cholesterol**.
- HDL cholesterol values **above 60 mg/dL** indicate very low risk for atherosclerosis.
- HDL **below 35 mg/dL** increases the risk of atherosclerosis. Below 35 mg/dL, with every 1 mg/dL decrease in HDL increase the risk of atherosclerosis by 3%.
- It is very important to note the ratio of total cholesterol to HDL cholesterol and to maintain the normal **ratio of below 4.5**. Increase in ratio increases the risk of atherosclerosis.
- It is also important to note the ratio of LDL cholesterol to HDL cholesterol and to maintain the normal ratio of less than 3.

- Women have higher HDL (due to the presence of estrogen), so they are less prone to heart diseases compared to men.

LABORATORY TESTS IN MYOCARDIAL INFARCTION

A diagnosis of MI is created by integrating the history of the presented illness and physical examination with electrocardiogram findings and cardiac markers.

Cardiac markers or cardiac enzymes are proteins that leak out of injured myocardial cells through their damaged cell membranes into the bloodstream.

The markers most widely used in detection of MI are creatine kinase-MB (CK-MB) subtype of the enzyme creatine kinase (CK) and cardiac TnT and troponin I (TnI) as they are more specific for myocardial injury. The cardiac TnT and TnI, which are released within 4–6 hours of an attack of MI and remain elevated for up to 2 weeks, have nearly complete tissue specificity and are now the preferred markers for assessing myocardial damage **(Fig. 10.11)**.

- Cardiac enzymes such as **CK, CKMB, lactate dehydrogenase (LDH), LDH1, and aspartate aminotransferase (AST)** are included in the cardiac enzyme panel.

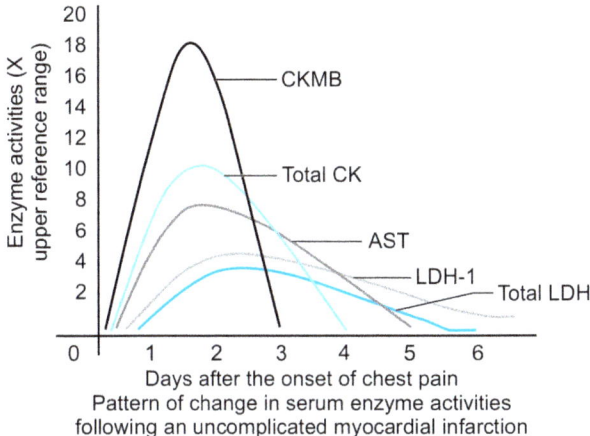

Days after the onset of chest pain
Pattern of change in serum enzyme activities
following an uncomplicated myocardial infarction

Fig. 10.11: Serum enzyme levels after myocardial infarction.

- Following MI, the first set of enzymes to increase is CK and CKMB. Immediately after the heart attack, CKMB starts increasing and reaches a maximum level by the end of the first day. After reaching the peak level, CK and CKMB decrease and reach normal level by the third day. In MI, CKMB may go up to 10–30% of total CK.
- AST levels in plasma increase after 6–8 hours of chest pain and reach the peak value by the second day and come to normal by the fourth or fifth day.
- Total LDH and LDH1 begin to increase 8–12 hours after the chest pain. They go on increasing and reach the maximum value by the third day and slowly come to normal by about the seventh day.
- The level of these enzymes in serum is related to the severe damage to heart muscle.
- CKMB and LD1 are the most sensitive and specific markers for the diagnosis of MI.

Troponins I and T

Troponin is a protein complex consisting of three subunits with different structure and function:

1. TnT: Tropomyosin-binding element. It is the myofibrillar protein of the striated muscle, which is the building block of the contractile apparatus.
2. TnI: Actinomyosin ATPase inhibitory element.
3. Troponin C: Calcium binding.
   - Troponins have been investigated as markers of acute cardiac ischemia.
   - *TnT* is normally measured because a small pool of it is not compartmentalized in the contractile apparatus and may be a precursor for synthesis of the troponin complex.
   - It is released into the blood within about 4 hours after the onset of symptoms, peaks at 12–16 hours, and remains elevated for 5–9 days post infarction.
   - Therefore cardiac troponin is very useful as a marker at any time interval after the heart attack, which is its great advantage.
   - A level >1.2 µg/L is indicative of myocardial damage.
   - TnT is the specific and sensitive test for the diagnosis of MI as compared to creatine phosphokinase (CPK) and LDH enzymes.

Its estimation indicates
- Acute MI
- Subacute MI
- Micro-infarction

- Size of infarction
- Monitoring the outcome of thrombolysis therapy.

SUMMARY

The human beings have variable demands of energy and therefore the supply is also equally variable. The absorbed metabolic fuel may be oxidized to CO_2 and H_2O or stored to meet the energy requirement as and when the body needs. In a well-fed state, the metabolism and organs integrate themselves to meet the energy demands and to metabolize or to store the consumed dietary components. The insulin becomes active to burn the carbohydrates as well as to store the excess. Well-fed state makes hormone-sensitive lipase inhibition through insulin to reduce the release of free FAs. During starvation, the metabolism gets reorganized to meet the energy demands. Starvation is a metabolic stress, which imposes certain metabolic compulsions on the organism. The glucagon activity increases to make an effort to build up the blood glucose level. The TG of adipose tissue is the predominant energy reserve of the body. The hormone-sensitive lipase becomes active to hydrolyze the TG. The prolonged starvation results in the production of ketone bodies to provide the energy to brain. Any deficiency or reduced action of insulin causes diabetes. Obesity is one of the major causes for developing type 2 diabetes. Obesity is the deposition of excess fat and a BMI of 30 and above is considered as obese. The obesity is inversely proportional to adipose tissue hormones such as adiponectin and leptin. There are several artificial sweeteners available and used by diabetic and obese people mainly to control their weight. It is better to monitor cholesterol status of our body by performing lipid profile testing. High level of cholesterol as well as LDL cholesterol results in atherosclerosis and later MI. MI can be diagnosed by analyzing blood levels of TnT and cardiac enzymes.

SELF-ASSESSMENT QUESTIONS

1. Describe the pathway for the storage of glucose in the liver in the fed state. How is this pathway regulated?
2. What pathway provides for the production of pyruvate to be used for FA synthesis in the fed state? How is this pathway regulated?
3. During the conversion of glucose to FA, how is pyruvate, produced from glycolysis, converted to citrate in the cytosol? In which compartment does each reaction take place?
4. What are the sources of the reducing agent used for the reductive biosynthesis of FAs?
5. Which enzyme controls the pathway for the synthesis of FAs from acetyl-CoA in the cytosol? How is this pathway regulated?
6. What keeps newly formed free FA from entering the mitochondria in the fed state?
7. What happens to the product of the FA synthase complex before it is found in the blood?
8. Compare the K_m for lipoprotein lipase in heart and adipose tissue. What implications does this have for the usage of blood TG in the fed and fasting state?
9. How does insulin affect the delivery of free FA into adipose cells in the fed state?
10. What are the pathways for the synthesis of TG in adipose from glucose and free FAs? How is the production of glycerol phosphate regulated?
11. What happens to the glycerol released in the lipoprotein lipase reaction in the fed state?
12. What pathways provide blood glucose during fasting? Why are these pathways active?
13. Why glycogen is not made in the liver during fasting?

14. Glycolysis does not function when gluconeogenesis is functioning. What factors turn on gluconeogenesis and turn off glycolysis?
15. What is the control enzyme for the release of free FAs during a fast and how is this enzyme regulated?
16. Why are ketone bodies produced during a fast?
17. Besides providing ATP, how does increased β-oxidation enable gluconeogenesis?
18. Explain how increased FA oxidation and decreased insulin spare blood glucose by muscle in the fasting, and resting state?
19. What is the effect of exercise upon the use of blood glucose by muscle in the fasting state? What is the mechanism?

MULTIPLE-CHOICE QUESTIONS

1. An 8-year-old male patient with type 1 diabetes mellitus feels nauseated, drowsy, and has been vomiting for a few hours. Clinical examination shows mild signs of dehydration and low blood pressure. You request laboratory tests and the results show the following results:
   - Blood glucose: 380 mg/dL (above the reference range)
   - Hemoglobin A: 11.8 g/dL (reference range: 13.5–17.0 g/dL)
   - Hemoglobin A1c: 12% of total hemoglobulin (reference range: <6%)
   - Urine ketones: Positive
   - Urine glucose: Positive
   - Blood pH: 7.29
   - Partial pressure of carbon dioxide in arterial blood (PaCO$_2$): Below reference range
   - Serum bicarbonate: Below reference range

   Which of the following best indicates that this patient has had hyperglycemia over a period of weeks?
   a. Ketonemia   b. Hemoglobin A1c
   c. Glucosuria   d. Blood pH

2. Insulin facilitates energy storage in liver. Which enzymes of carbohydrate metabolism are coordinately regulated in liver in response to insulin signaling?
   a. Glycogen synthase
   b. Phosphofructokinase-2
   c. Pyruvate kinase
   d. All the above

3. Which one of the following enzymes of carbohydrate metabolism is not dephosphorylated in liver in response to insulin signaling?
   a. Glycogen synthase
   b. Glycogen phosphorylase
   c. Phosphofructokinase-1
   d. Pyruvate kinase

4. Enzymes such as glycogen synthase, glycogen phosphorylase, the phosphofructokinase-2 (PFK-2)/fructose biphosphatase-2 (FBPase-2), and pyruvate kinase are phosphorylated by glucagon and/or epinephrine action. Which kinase is responsible for these phosphorylation events?
   a. Protein kinase A
   b. Calmodulin-dependent protein kinase
   c. Protein kinase C
   d. Receptor tyrosine kinase

5. The receptor to which epinephrine binds in order to stimulate phosphorylation of glycogen synthase and glycogen phosphorylase is:
   a. α-1   b. α-2
   c. β   d. γ

6. Insulin regulates all of the following enzymes in liver. Which of these enzymes are also regulated by insulin in muscle?
   a. Glycogen synthase
   b. Glucokinase
   c. Glycogen phosphorylase
   d. (a) and (c)

7. The hormone that increases the rate of absorption of hexoses from intestine is:
   a. Glucocorticoids
   b. Thyroxine
   c. Anterior pituitary hormones
   d. Epinephrine

8. In a fasting state, glucocorticoids:
   a. Decrease protein catabolism
   b. Decrease hepatic uptake of amino acids
   c. Stimulate the utilization of glucose in extrahepatic tissues
   d. Increase the activity of aminotransferase

9. Concerning insulin action, one of the following statements is incorrect, it:

a. Activates pyruvate kinase
b. Stimulates glycerol phosphate acyltransferase
c. Increases HMG-CoA reductase activity
d. Activates hormone-sensitive lipase

10. **Starvation associated with:**
    a. Increased insulin and decreased glucagon
    b. Decreased epinephrine and increased insulin
    c. Decreased insulin and increased glucagon
    d. Decreased insulin and decreased glucocorticoids

11. **Lipase phosphatase is stimulated by:**
    a. Insulin   b. Epinephrine
    c. Prostaglandin   d. ACTH

12. **During starvation:**
    a. Acetyl-CoA carboxylase remains active
    b. Hormone-sensitive lipase becomes active
    c. Fructose-1,6-bisphosphatase becomes inactive
    d. Glycogen phosphorylase becomes inactive through cAMP-dependent phosphorylation

13. **Prolonged starvation is associated with:**
    a. The formation of fructose from carbohydrates
    b. Reduced breakdown of muscle glycogen
    c. Formation of fatty acids using acetyl-CoA
    d. Increased breakdown of triacylglycerol

Answers

1. b	2. d	3. c	4. a	5. c
6. d	7. b	8. d	9. d	10. c
11. a	12. b	13. d		

CHAPTER 11

Hemoglobin

OBJECTIVES

At the end of this chapter, students should be able to:
- Understand the structure of hemoglobin (Hb) and its major function
- Know the difference between Hb and myoglobin
- Explain the basis for different types of abnormal Hb
- Explain the synthesis of Hb
- Know about different types of porphyrias, including their causes and symptoms.

INTRODUCTION

Hb is a conjugated protein. It is the red pigment present in red blood cell (RBC) and transports oxygen (O_2) from lungs to tissues. It transports carbon dioxide (CO_2) and H^+ from tissues to lungs and kidney. It acts as an intracellular buffer and then involves in acid–base balance. It is a globular, oligomeric protein made up of two parts, i.e. heme, a pigment, and a protein part called globin.

Hb synthesis takes place in the bone marrow. Its blood level is 12-16 g/dL. The synthesis of Hb depends on three important factors such as iron, folic acid, and vitamin B_{12} along with amino acids. Deficiency of any of these factors decreases the ability of the bone marrow to synthesize RBC, thus causing anemia.

STRUCTURE OF HEMOGLOBIN

- Heme consists of a porphyrin ring with one iron [ferrous (Fe^{2+})] at the center (**Figs. 11.1A and B**).
- Hb is a conjugated metalloprotein of molecular weight 68,000.
- It consists of four heme molecules linked to the protein portion called "globin," and this globin part has four polypeptide chains.

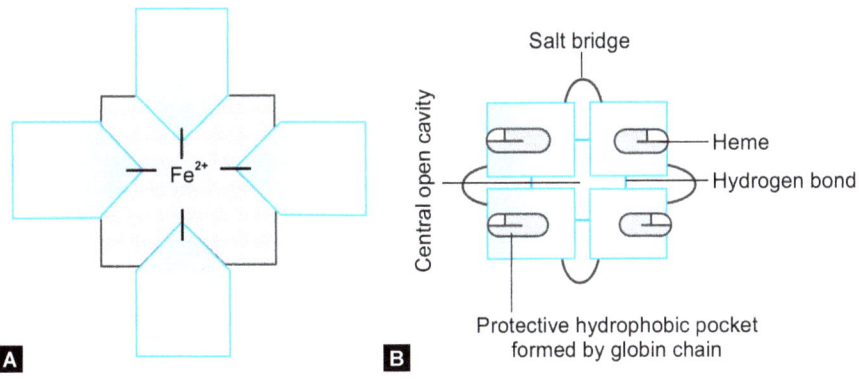

Figs. 11.1A and B: Structure of hemoglobin.

- Each heme molecule is located in a pocket formed by the folding of polypeptide chain.
- The quaternary structure of Hb is stabilized by hydrogen bonds, salt bridges, and van der Waals forces.
- The iron (Fe^{2+}) is held in the center of the protoporphyrin molecule by coordination bonds with the four nitrogen of the protoporphyrin ring.
- The iron has six coordination bonds:
  - Four bonds are formed between the iron and nitrogen atoms of the porphyrin ring system.
  - Fifth bond is formed between nitrogen atoms of histidine residue of the globin polypeptide chain, and it is the proximal histidine.
- The form of Hb is stabilized by hydrogen bond between O_2 and side chain of another histidine residue of the globin chain, and it is distal histidine. This distal histidine is not directly involved with the heme group but helps to stabilize the binding of O_2 to the heme molecule.
- Normal adult blood consists of two types of Hb, and they are Hb A1 (HbA1) and Hb A2 (HbA2).
- The HbA1 comprises 97% of the total Hb and HbA2 is about 3% of the total Hb.
- The newborn baby contains another type of Hb called fetal Hb (HbF). The amount of HbF is up to 90% in the neonatal stage and falls gradually by about 4–5 months.
- In normal adults, HbF concentration is about 1%.
- The polypeptide chain composition of various Hb is:
  - HbA1: $\alpha_2\beta_2$ chains
  - HbA2: $\alpha_2\delta_2$ chains
  - HbF: $\alpha_2\gamma_2$ chains.
- The number of amino acids in the polypeptide chains is as follows:
  - α-chain: 141
  - β-chain: 146
  - δ-chain: 146
  - γ-chain: 146.

Binding Sites for Oxygen, Hydrogen, and Carbon Dioxide

Oxygen bounds to the Fe^{2+} atoms of the heme to form oxyhemoglobin (HbO_2). Carbon dioxide bounds to α-amino group of N-terminal end of the polypeptide chains of Hb to form carbaminohemoglobin ($HbCO_2$) (**Fig. 11.2**).

COMPARISON OF MYOGLOBIN WITH HEMOGLOBIN

The following list shows the differences of myoglobin with hemoglobin:
- The heme proteins, myoglobin and Hb, maintain a supply of O_2, which is essential for oxidative metabolism.

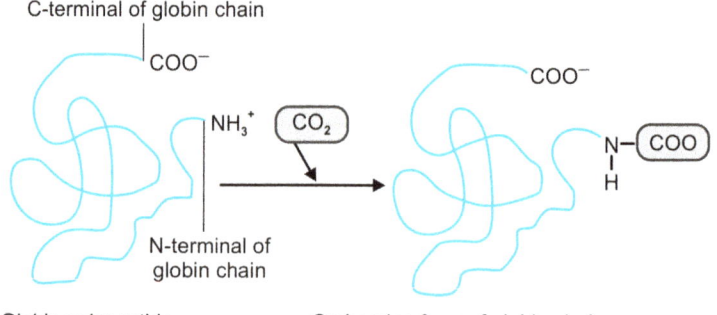

Fig. 11.2: Binding of carbon dioxide to hemoglobin.

- Myoglobin is a monomeric protein of red muscle and stores O_2 as a reserve against O_2 deprivation. It releases O_2 during severe exercise for use in muscle mitochondria for aerobic synthesis of adenosine triphosphate (ATP).
- The tertiary structure of myoglobin is that of a typical water-soluble globular protein. Its secondary structure is unusual in that it contains a very high proportion (75%) of α-helical secondary structure.
- Each myoglobin molecule contains one heme prosthetic group inserted into a hydrophobic cleft in the protein.
- Each heme residue contains one central coordinately bound iron atom that is normally in the Fe^{2+} oxidation state.
- The heme of myoglobin lies in a crevice between helices E and F oriented with its polar propionate groups facing the surface of the globin.
- The histidine, F8-linked iron, and E7 on the sides of the heme ring play important roles in O_2 binding.
- Hb, tetrameric protein of erythrocytes, transports O_2 to the tissues and returns CO_2 and protons to the lungs.
- The secondary structure of the polypeptide subunits of Hb resembles myoglobin.
- The heme and Fe^{2+} iron are responsible for storage and transport of O_2.

Oxygen Dissociation Curves for Myoglobin and Hemoglobin

- The oxygen binding curve for myoglobin is hyperbolic.
- Myoglobin therefore loads O_2 readily at the partial pressure of oxygen (PO_2) of the lung capillary bed (100 mm Hg).
  However, strenuous exercise lowers the PO_2 of muscle tissue to about 5 mm Hg, myoglobin releases O_2 for mitochondrial synthesis of ATP, to keep continuing the muscular activity.
- The myoglobin and α-subunit of HbA have almost identical secondary and tertiary

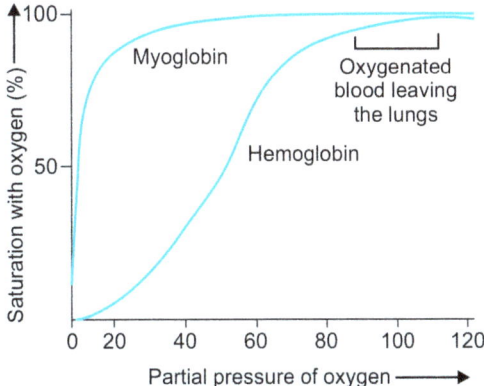

Fig. 11.3: Oxygen dissociation curve of hemoglobin and myoglobin.

structures except the number of amino acids.
- The cooperative binding nature of Hb (tetrameric) permits Hb to maximize both the quantity of O_2 loaded at the PO_2 of the lungs and the quantity of O_2 released at the PO_2 of the peripheral tissues (**Fig. 11.3**).

Formation of Oxyhemoglobin

- The binding of the first O_2 molecule to deoxyhemoglobin shifts the heme iron toward the plane of the heme ring from a position about 0.6 nm beyond it.
- This is transmitted to the proximal histidine and other residues lying next.
- The salt bridges between the carboxyl-terminal residues of all four subunits break.
- The pair of α- and β-subunits rotates 15° with respect to the other, compacting the tetramer. The changes in secondary, tertiary, and quaternary structure accompany the high-affinity O_2-induced transfer of Hb from the low-affinity, stressed or tense (T) or taut state to the high-affinity, relaxed (R) state (**Fig. 11.4**). These changes increase the affinity of the remaining unoxygenated hemes for O_2.

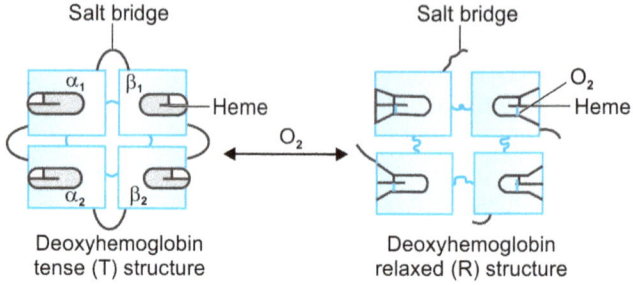

Fig. 11.4: Tense and relaxed structure of hemoglobin.

COOPERATIVE BINDING OF OXYGEN BY HEMOGLOBIN

The cooperative binding of oxygen by hemoglobin is shown below:
- The cooperative interaction between different binding sites makes Hb an unusually good O_2 transport protein because it enables the molecule to pick up as much O_2 as possible once the partial pressure of this gas reaches a particular threshold level and then gives off as much O_2 as possible when the partial pressure of O_2 drops significantly below this threshold level. The hemes are much too far apart to interact directly. But, changes that occur in the structure of the globin that surrounds a heme when it picks up an O_2 molecule are mechanically transmitted to the other globins in this protein (**Fig. 11.5**). These changes carry the signal that facilitates the gain or loss of an O_2 molecule by the other hemes.
- The cooperative binding of O_2 by Hb enhances O_2 transport. The shape of O_2 binding curve of Hb is sigmoidal (S-shaped) because O_2 binding is cooperative (refer to **Fig. 11.3**). This shape indicates that the affinity of Hb for binding the first molecule of O_2 is relatively very low, but subsequent O_2 molecules are bound with a very much higher affinity accounting for the steeply rising portion of the S-shaped curve.

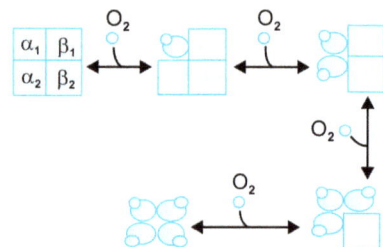

Fig. 11.5: Cooperative binding of oxygen to hemoglobin.

- The Hb also transports CO_2 (by-product of respiration) and protons from peripheral tissues to the lungs. Hb carries CO_2 as carbamates (15%) formed with the amino-terminal nitrogen of the polypeptide chains. $CO_2 + Hb - NH_2 \leftrightarrow H^+ + Hb - NH - COO^-$.
- This favors the salt bond formation between α- and β-chains of Hb. The remaining CO_2 is carried as bicarbonate (HCO_3), which is formed in erythrocyte by the hydration of CO_2 to carbonic acid (H_2CO_3), catalyzed by carbonic anhydrase. The venous blood pH dissociates H_2CO_3 into HCO_3 and a proton.
- Deoxyhemoglobin binds one proton for every two O_2 molecules released, contributing significantly to the buffering capacity of blood. In the lungs, the process reverses. As O_2 binds to deoxyhemoglobin, protons are released (due to rupture of salt bridges) and combine with HCO_3 to form H_2CO_3. Dehydration of H_2CO_3 catalyzed by

Hemoglobin

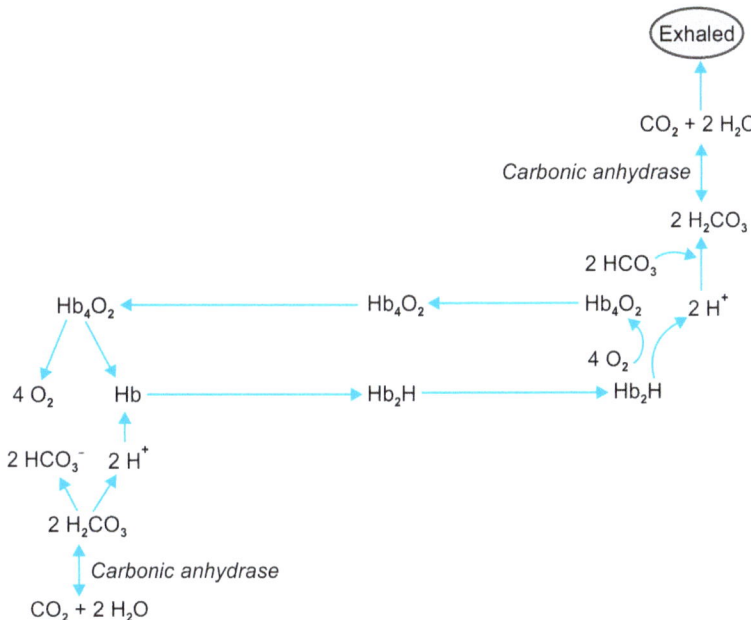

Fig. 11.6: Bohr effect.

carbonic anhydrase forms CO_2, which is exhaled. This reciprocal coupling of protons and O_2 binding is termed "Bohr effect." This effect mainly depends on cooperative interactions between the hemes of the Hb tetramer. Therefore myoglobin (monomer) does not exhibit Bohr effect (**Fig. 11.6**).

- Bohr effect increases in hydrogen ion concentration and decreases the amount of O_2 bound by Hb at any O_2 concentration (partial pressure). Coupled to the diffusion of HCO_3 out of RBCs in the tissues, there must be ion movement into the RBCs to maintain electrical neutrality. This is the role of chloride ion (Cl^-) and is referred to as the chloride shift. In this way, Cl^- plays an important role in HCO_3 production and diffusion and thus also negatively influences O_2 binding to Hb (**Fig. 11.7**).

Factors Affecting Oxygen Binding

The binding of O_2 to Hb can be dramatically altered by a small group of substances called allosteric effectors. Hydrogen ions (protons), CO_2, and 2,3-bisphosphoglycerate (2,3-BPG) are effectors that can promote the release of O_2 by favoring the deoxygenated form of Hb.

Role of 2,3-Bisphosphoglycerate

Low PO_2 in peripheral tissues promotes the synthesis of 2,3-BPG in erythrocytes from 1,3-BPG. This 2,3-BPG binds to deoxygenated Hb and stabilizes it. The BPG binds more weakly to HbF than to HbA. Therefore the HbF has higher affinity for O_2 than HbA.

Hemoglobin Synthesis

Heme Synthesis

The following list shows the heme synthesis:
- Heme is synthesized in a complex series of steps involving enzymes in the mitochondrion and in the cytosol of the cell (**Fig. 11.8**).
- The first step in heme synthesis takes place in the mitochondrion, with the condensation

Hemoglobin

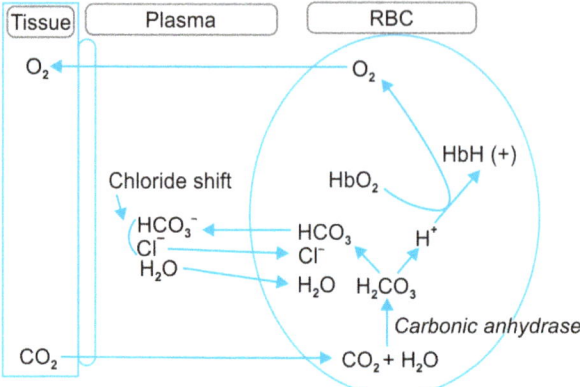

Fig. 11.7: Chloride shift.
(RBC: red blood cell)

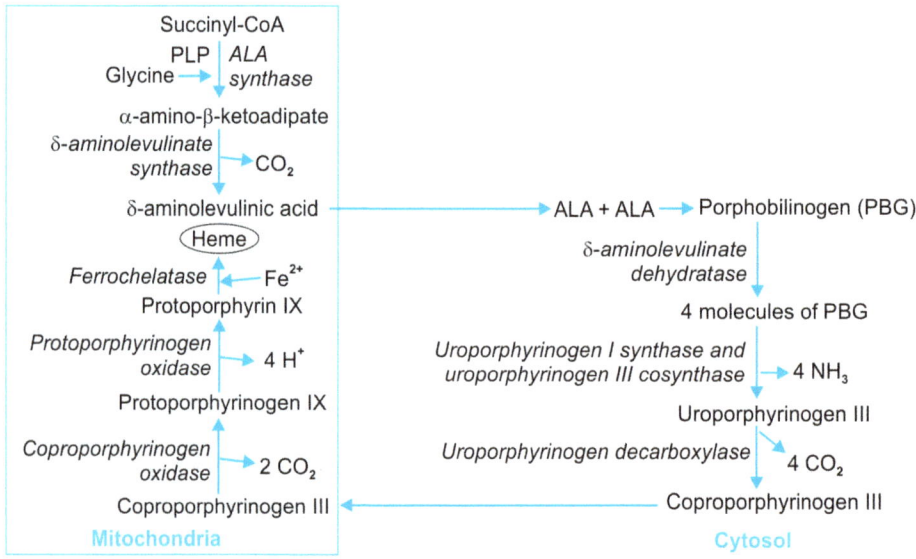

Fig. 11.8: Schematic diagram showing hemoglobin synthesis.
(ALA: delta or 5-aminolevulinic acid; PLP: pyridoxal 5′-phosphate)

of succinyl coenzyme A and glycine by 5-aminolevulinic acid (ALA) synthase to form ALA. This molecule is transported to the cytosol where a series of reactions produce a ring structure called coproporphyrinogen III. This molecule returns to the mitochondrion where an addition reaction produces protoporphyrin IX.

- The enzyme, ferrochelatase, inserts iron into the ring structure of protoporphyrin IX to produce heme.
- Deranged production of heme produces a variety of anemias.
- Iron deficiency, the world's most common cause of anemia, impairs heme synthesis, thereby producing anemia. A number of

drugs and toxins directly inhibit heme production by interfering with enzymes involved in heme biosynthesis. Lad commonly produces substantial anemia by inhibiting heme synthesis, particularly in children.

Globin Synthesis

Two distinct globin chains (each with its individual heme molecule) combine to form Hb. One of the chains is designated α. The second chain is called "non-α". With the exception of the very first week of embryogenesis, one of the globin chains is always α. A number of variables influence the nature of the non-α-chain in the Hb molecule. The fetus has a distinct non-α-chain called γ. After birth, a different non-α-globin chain, called β, pairs with the α-chain. The combination of two α-chains and two non-α-chains produces a complete Hb molecule (a total of four chains per molecule).

Regulation of Heme Biosynthesis

Although heme is synthesized in virtually all tissues, the principal sites of synthesis are erythroid cells (~85%) and hepatocytes. The differences between these two tissues and their needs for heme result in quite different mechanisms for the regulation of heme biosynthesis. In hepatocytes, heme is required for incorporation into the cytochromes, in particular, the P450 class of cytochromes that are important for detoxification. In addition, numerous cytochromes of the oxidative-phosphorylation pathway contain heme.

The rate-limiting step in hepatic heme biosynthesis occurs at the **ALA synthase** catalyzed step, which is the committed step in heme synthesis. The Fe^{3+} oxidation product of heme is termed "hemin." Hemin acts as a feedback inhibitor on ALA synthase. Hemin also inhibits transport of ALA synthase from the cytosol (its site of synthesis) into the mitochondria (its site of action) as well as represses synthesis of the enzyme.

In erythroid cells, all of the heme is synthesized for incorporation into Hb and occurs only upon differentiation when synthesis of Hb proceeds. When red cells mature, the synthesis of both heme and Hb ceases. The heme and Hb must, therefore, survive for the life of the erythrocyte (normally this is 120 days). In reticulocytes (immature erythrocytes), heme stimulates protein synthesis. Additionally, control of heme biosynthesis in erythrocytes occurs at numerous sites other than at the level of ALA synthase. Control has been shown to be exerted on ferrochelatase, the enzyme responsible for iron insertion into protoporphyrin IX and on porphobilinogen deaminase.

CLINICAL ASPECTS OF HEME METABOLISM

Porphyria and its Causes and Symptoms

Clinical problems associated with heme metabolism are of two types (**Table 11.1**). The inherited disorder of bilirubin metabolism results in hyperbilirubinemia. Disorders that arise from defects in the enzymes of heme biosynthesis are termed "porphyrias" and cause elevations in the serum and urine content of intermediates in heme synthesis. Bilirubin is potentially toxic waste product of heme catabolism. The body eliminates bilirubin by transporting it to the liver bound to albumin in the serum. In the liver, it is conjugated with glucuronate, which renders it water-soluble. The glucuronide conjugate is then excreted in the bile. Persons with extreme elevation in unconjugated bilirubin are susceptible to bilirubin encephalopathy, also referred to as kernicterus. Accumulation of bilirubin in the plasma and tissues results in jaundice. Gilbert's syndrome and Crigler–Najjar syndrome result from predominantly unconjugated hyperbilirubinemia. Dubin–Johnson syndrome and Rotor's syndrome result from conjugated hyperbilirubinemia. The porphyrias are both inherited and acquired disorders in heme synthesis. These disorders are classified

Table 11.1: Causes and features of porphyrias.

Porphyrias	Enzyme defect	Primary symptoms
Erythropoietic class		
Congenital erythropoietic porphyria	Uroporphyrinogen III cosynthase	Photosensitivity (itching and burning of skin when exposed to light), excrete more uroporphyrinogen and coproporphyrinogen I, which then oxidized to uroporphyrin and coproporphyrin (red pigments)
EPP	Ferrochelatase	Photosensitivity, protoporphyrin IX excreted into urine and feces
Hepatic class		
ALA dehydratase deficiency porphyria (ADP)	ALA dehydratase	Neurovisceral
AIP	PBG deaminase or uroporphyrinogen I synthase	Neurovisceral increased excretion of PBG and ALA, and urine gets darkened
HCP	Coproporphyrinogen oxidase	Neurovisceral, some photosensitivity, coproporphyrinogen, ALA and PBG are excreted in urine and feces
VP	Protoporphyrinogen oxidase	Neurovisceral, some photosensitivity; all the intermediates of heme synthesis accumulate and excreted in urine and feces
PCT	Uroporphyrinogen decarboxylase	Photosensitivity, increased excretion of uroporphyrins
HEP	Uroporphyrinogen decarboxylase	Photosensitivity, some neurovisceral

(AIP: acute intermittent porphyria; ALA: 5-aminolevulinic acid; EPP: erythropoietic protoporphyria; HCP: hereditary coproporphyria; HEP: hepatoerythropoietic porphyria; PBG: porphobilinogen; PCT: porphyria cutanea tarda; VP: variegate porphyria)

as either erythroid or hepatic, depending upon the principal site of expression of the enzyme defect. Eight different porphyrias have been classified (refer to **Table 11.1**).

Heme Catabolism

Breakdown of RBC releases heme and globin. The globin goes to globin pool and heme is converted to hemin. The hemin loses its iron and is converted to biliverdin. The biliverdin reductase reduces biliverdin to bilirubin, a yellow pigment (**Fig. 11.9**).

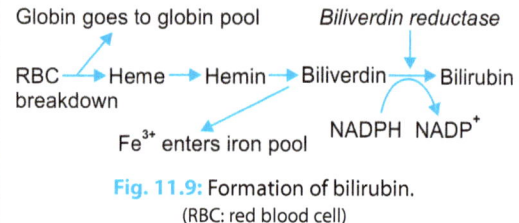

Fig. 11.9: Formation of bilirubin.
(RBC: red blood cell)

Bilirubin Transport, Conjugation, and Excretion

Transport, conjugation, and excretion of bilirubin is shown below:

- Once the bilirubin is formed, it binds to albumin and is transported to the liver.
- In the liver, it is separated from the albumin and the bilirubin is taken up by the liver parenchymal cells.
- In the liver, the uridine diphosphate (UDP)-glucuronyltransferase enzyme conjugates the bilirubin with two molecules of UDP glucuronic acid to form a conjugated bilirubin called bilirubin diglucuronide.
- The conjugated bilirubin is secreted into the bile through bile duct and reaches the intestine.
- The intestinal bacterial enzyme, β-glucuronidase, hydrolyzes the conjugated bilirubin and deconjugates it.
- The portion of this free bilirubin then gets reduced by fecal flora to a colorless tetrapyrrole urobilinogen.
- Then a small percent of this urobilinogen is reabsorbed from the intestine and returned to the liver by portal blood, and reexcreted through the liver known as enterohepatic urobilinogen cycle.
- More than 90% of the recirculated urobilinogen is taken up by the liver and reexcreted into the bile, the remainder is filtered by the kidneys and excreted in the urine.
- The urobilinogen is also excreted through blood, but it is negligible.
- The urobilinogen is further reduced to stercobilinogen and excreted through feces (around 200–300 mg/day).
- The urobilinogen and stercobilinogen are colorless compounds; but when they are exposed to atmospheric oxidation, they are converted to a colored urobilin and stercobilin, respectively.
- The conjugated water-soluble bilirubin when treated with diazo reagent [sodium nitrate ($NaNO_3$)+sulfanilic acid] gives a red color immediately. This is called direct van den Bergh's test. The conjugated bilirubin reacts directly without adding methanol, so it is also called direct bilirubin (direct positive).
- The water-insoluble unconjugated bilirubin gives a positive van den Bergh's test only if methanol is added to the serum. This is indirect van den Bergh's test. This also called indirect bilirubin (indirect positive).
- The water-soluble free conjugated bilirubin can be filtered through the glomerular membrane and excreted in the urine when there is increase in the blood levels of conjugated bilirubin.
- The water-insoluble unconjugated bilirubin is not filtered by the glomerular membrane as it is bound to albumin; hence, it does not appear in the urine, whenever a blood level of unconjugated bilirubin is increased.

DISORDERS OF HEMOGLOBIN CATABOLISM

The following list shows the disorders of hemoglobin catabolism:

Normal concentration of serum bilirubin is:
- Total bilirubin: 0.1–1.0 mg/dL
- Conjugated bilirubin: 0.1–0.2 mg/dL
- Unconjugated bilirubin: 0.2–0.8 mg.

The bilirubin metabolism is altered when there is:
- Increased load of bilirubin to the liver.
- Reduced hepatic uptake.
- Reduced intracellular transport.
- Reduced conjugation and excretion of bilirubin.
- Obstruction to the flow of bile.
- One or more of the above problems leads to elevated bilirubin and causing jaundice.

Jaundice

The following list shows the information about jaundice:

- Normal serum bilirubin concentration is around 1.2 mg/100 mL (**Table 11.2**).
- When the bilirubin level exceeds more than 1.2 mg/dL, it diffuses into the tissues. The skin and sclera of the eye turns yellow. The condition is called jaundice (icterus).
- The yellowish coloration is caused by an excess amount of bilirubin in the skin.
- Bilirubin is a yellowish-red pigment.
- Normally, small amounts of bilirubin are found in everyone's blood.
- When too much bilirubin is made, the excess is dumped into the bloodstream and is deposited in tissues for temporary storage.
- Jaundice in the infant appears first in the face and upper body and progresses downward toward the toes. Hyperbilirubinemia may be acquired or inherited.

Acquired Hyperbilirubinemia

- Prehepatic or hemolytic jaundice
- Hepatic jaundice
- Obstructive jaundice
- Neonatal or physiologic jaundice.

Prehepatic or hemolytic jaundice

Prehepatic or hemolytic jaundice mainly arises due to excessive breakdown of RBC. This excess hemolysis may be due to:
- Sickle cell Hb
- Deficiency of glucose-6-phosphate dehydrogenase
- Incompatible blood transfusions.

Table 11.2: Causes and laboratory findings of different types of jaundice.

Specimen	Prehepatic or hemolytic	Hepatic	Posthepatic or obstructive
Causes	Abnormal red cells; antibodies; abnormal hemoglobin	Viral hepatitis; toxic hepatitis; drugs and toxins	Extrahepatic cholestasis; gallstones; tumor of bile duct; carcinoma of pancreas
Blood			
Unconjugated bilirubin	Present (++)	Present (++)	Normal
Conjugated bilirubin	Normal	Increases in early phase and later decreases	Present (++)
Urine			
Bile salt (Hay's test)	Absent	Absent	Present
Conjugated bilirubin			
Fouchet's test	Absent	Present	Present
Urobilinogen			
Ehrlich's test	Present (+++)	Increases in early phase and later decreases	Absent
Feces			
Urobilins	Present (++)	In intrahepatic cholestasis decreases	Clay colored
Serum enzymes			
ALP	Normal	Moderately increased	Increased markedly
ALT	Normal	Increased markedly	Moderately increased
AST	Normal	Increased markedly	Moderately increased
GGT	Normal	Moderately increased	Increased

(ALP: alkaline phosphatase; ALT: alanine transaminase; AST: aspartate aminotransferase; GGT: gamma-glutamyltransferase)

Hepatic Jaundice

Hepatic jaundice mainly arises due to the damage of the parenchymal liver cells.

Obstructive or Posthepatic Jaundice

Obstruction to the flow of bile causes the conjugated bilirubin to return to the blood. Therefore the serum contains increased amount of direct bilirubin.

Neonatal or Physiologic Jaundice

Neonatal or physiologic jaundice mainly arises due to excessive breakdown of RBC. This type of jaundice is common in newborn babies, where there is increase bilirubin formed and released into the bloodstream when RBCs are broken down. Infants have too many RBCs. It is natural process for the baby's body to break down these excess RBCs, forming a large amount of bilirubin. It is this bilirubin that causes the skin to take on a yellowish color. A newborn's liver is immature and deficient in **UDP-glucuronyltransferase**, a conjugating enzyme, and cannot process bilirubin as quickly as it will be able to when it gets older. This slow processing of bilirubin has nothing to do with liver disease. It merely means that the baby's liver is not as fully developed as it will be and thus there is some delay in eliminating the bilirubin.

Occasionally, there are other factors that cause jaundice in an infant. Two of the conditions known are ABO incompatibility and rhesus incompatibility. Both of these conditions result in a very fast breakdown of RBCs. Also, jaundice may appear in infants with physical defects in the organs that work to eliminate the bilirubin from the body and decreased conjugating enzyme.

Congenital Hyperbilirubinemias

Inherited unconjugated hyperbilirubinemia

Crigler–Najjar syndrome

Crigler–Najjar syndrome is a rare autosomal recessive disorder due to deficiency of hepatic glucuronyltransferase enzyme. There are two types of this condition:
- Type I: It is characterized by the complete absence of the conjugating enzyme glucuronyltransferase. Therefore no conjugated bilirubin is formed in this condition. It leads to severe jaundice with kernicterus.
- Type II: It is a less severe form due to partial deficiency of the conjugating enzyme. The patient survives without any neurologic impairment.

Gilbert's syndrome

Gilbert's syndrome is an inherited disease characterized by mild benign unconjugated hyperbilirubinemia due to:
- Impaired hepatic uptake from the circulation
- Partial conjugation defect due to reduced activity of the conjugating enzyme.

Inherited conjugated hyperbilirubinemia

Dubin–Johnson syndrome

Dubin–Johnson syndrome is a benign autosomal recessive disorder, which causes an increase of conjugated bilirubin without elevation of liver enzymes. This condition is associated with a defect in the ability of hepatocytes to secrete conjugated bilirubin into the bile. It is usually diagnosed in early infancy. It is also characterized by abnormal black pigment in the hepatocytes, giving a dark brown-to-black color to the liver.

Rotor's syndrome

Rotor's syndrome has many things in common with Dubin–Johnson syndrome except that in Rotor's syndrome, the liver cells are not pigmented. The main symptom is a nonitching jaundice. There is a rise in bilirubin in the patient's serum, mainly of the conjugated type.

ROLE OF HEMOGLOBIN IN DISEASE

The role of hemoglobin is as follows:
- Decreased levels of Hb, with or without an absolute decrease of RBCs, leads to symptoms of anemia.

- Anemia has many different causes.
- The absence of iron decreases heme synthesis, RBCs in iron deficiency anemia are hypochromic (lacking the red Hb pigment) and microcytic (smaller than normal). Other anemias are rarer.
- In hemolysis (accelerated breakdown of RBCs), associated jaundice is caused by the Hb metabolite bilirubin and the circulating Hb can cause renal failure.
- Mutations in the globin chain are associated with the hemoglobinopathies, such as sickle cell disease and thalassemia.

Case study

Stan, a marathon runner, had been touring different places for many years. Recently he complained of feeling weak, tired, and unwell. He observed that he had occasional fever, no appetite, and his urine was dark. His brother Mathew also told him that his eyes looked yellow. Mathew took Stan to the outpatient clinic at the local hospital. On examination, Stan showed scleral icterus and an enlarged liver was palpable. The physician requested for liver function test from the laboratory. The lab results showed the elevated levels of alanine amino transaminase, aspartate amino transaminase, total bilirubin, direct and indirect bilirubin. Which of the following problems Mr Stan is suffering from?

a. Intrahepatic jaundice
b. Multiple myeloma
c. Prehepatic jaundice
d. Abstractive jaundice

Answer is a.

ABNORMAL HEMOGLOBIN

The abnormal Hb of sickle cell anemia was first demonstrated by Linus Pauling in 1949. Structurally each globin chain has its own genetic locus. The individual chain of Hb is under genetic control. Based on the genetics of the globin chain production, structural abnormalities can be divided into four groups:

1. Amino acid substitutions: HbS, HbC, HbD, and HbE
2. Amino acid deletion (deletion of three nucleotides in deoxyribonucleic acid): Hb Gun Hill
3. Elongated globin chains (resulted from chain termination, shift mutation, or other mutations)
4. Fused or hybrid chains (resulted from nonhomologous crossing over): Hb Lepore.

Most of the Hb variants arise by a single amino acid substitution, which is called "point mutations." Deletion of one or two nucleotide bases can shift the reading frame of all code words that follow. Such an event observed in microorganisms was called "frame-shift mutation."

Abnormal Hbs are inherited as autosomal codominants. Thus subjects who inherit one normal and one abnormal gene are heterozygous, and those who have two identical abnormal genes are homozygous.

HEMOGLOBINOPATHY

When biological functions of Hb are altered due to a mutation in Hb, the condition is known as hemoglobinopathy, which may be grouped into two types:

1. Quantitative hemoglobinopathies, characterized by decreased synthesis of either α- or β-globin chain, leading to altered combination of normal α, β, γ, or δ chains, e.g. thalassemia.
2. Qualitative hemoglobinopathies, characterized by an altered sequence of amino acids, usually in one of the constituent chains, e.g. sickle cell disease, HbC disease, HbD disease, and HbM disease.

In normal adults, amount of HbF is about 1%. Presence of the HbF more than 1% in adults and children above the age of 1 year is abnormal, and the condition is known as hemoglobinopathy.

THALASSEMIA AND ITS IMPORTANT TYPES

Thalassemia

The name derived from the Greek word, "thalassa," which means "sea." Greeks inherited this disease present around Mediterranean Sea. The absence or diminished synthesis of one of the polypeptide chains of human Hb is characterized as "thalassemia." The reduction in the α-chain synthesis is called α-thalassemia and decreased synthesis of β-chain synthesis is called β-thalassemia. The β-thalassemia is more common.

α-thalassemia: The α-globin chain is structurally normal, but the production of a globin chain is impaired, resulting in the production of excess β-globin and γ-globin chains, which results in the:
- Formation of β-globin tetramer, called HbH, and tetramer of γ-globin Hb Bart. These two forms cannot deliver O_2 to the tissues, leading to fetal death.
- Decreased production of Hbs, but contains α-chains, i.e. HbA1, HbA2, and HbF.

β-thalassemia: In this type, β-globin chain is structurally normal, but the production of β-globin chain is decreased. This decreased production of β-globin chain leads to a large excess of α-chain and form α-globin tetramer that precipitates immediately within the RBC as Heinz bodies and responsible for damage of the cell membrane, and premature breakdown of RBCs.

There are two types of β-thalassemia:
1. *β-thalassemia major*: Homozygous state for the β-thalassemia gene and a severe disease. Splenomegaly and skin pigmentation are the clinical pictures. Blood picture shows anemia and erythrocyte shows marked anisocytosis. The mean corpuscular volume and mean corpuscular hemoglobin decrease, whereas mean corpuscular hemoglobin concentration increases. Both HbA and HbF are present [HbF 10 (98%)].
2. *β-thalassemia minor*: Heterozygous state for the β-thalassemia gene. In this condition, both HbA and HbF are present with less symptoms.

SICKLE CELL HEMOGLOBIN AND ITS CAUSES AND SYMPTOMS

Sickle Cell Hemoglobin

Sickle cell hemoglobin shows the following causes and symptoms:
- The sickle cell hemoglobinopathies are hereditary disorders in which the red cells contain HbS.
- They include heterozygous (sickle cell trait, HbA and HbS present) and homozygous (sickle cell anemia, only HbS is present with the complete absence of HbA) for HbS.
- The HbS causes a condition called sickle cell anemia.
- The HbS differs from HbA in the substitution of **valine** for **glutamic acid** in the **sixth** position from the N-terminal end of the β **chain**:
- HbA—Val-His-Leu-Thr-Pro-**Glu**-Glu-Lys.
- HbS—Val-His-Leu-Thr-Pro-**Val**-Glu-Lys.
- The side chain of valine is distinctly nonpolar, whereas that of glutamate is highly polar. This generates hydrophobic contact point called sticky patch, at position six of the β-chain.
- This sticky patch is present on the outer surface of the oxygenated and deoxygenated HbS. This is not found in normal HbA.
- A complementary sticky patch is also present on the surface of the deoxygenated HbS. It is masked in oxygenated HbS.
- This alteration in polarity reduces the solubility of deoxygenated HbS.
- When this HbS is deoxygenated, the sticky patch can bind to the complementary patch on another deoxygenated HbS molecule. This binding causes polymerization of deoxyhemoglobin S-forming insoluble long tubular fibrous precipitates (**Fig. 11.10**).

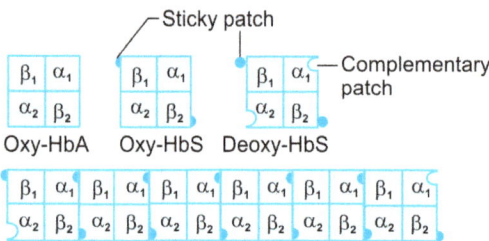

Fig. 11.10: Polymerization of deoxyhemoglobin.

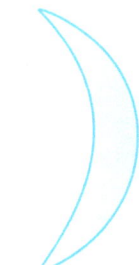

Fig. 11.11: Sickle red blood cells.

- The insoluble fibers of deoxygenated HbS distort the red cells into sickle-shaped (crescent-shaped) cells (**Fig. 11.11**). Hence, this condition is known as sickle cell anemia. The change in the shape of the cell causes hemolysis leading to anemia.

Clinical Symptoms

- Chronic hemolytic anemia.
- Hypoxia (breathlessness) due to less blood supply to the tissues and decreased O_2.
- Pain and swelling in the joints.
- Persons with sickle cell trait show an increased resistance to malaria specifically for *Plasmodium falciparum*. This parasite spends an obligatory part of its life cycle in the RBC.

TEST FOR THE DETECTION OF ABNORMAL HEMOGLOBIN

Electrophoresis of Hemoglobins

Different types of Hbs can be separated from each other by electrophoresis. The Hb variants

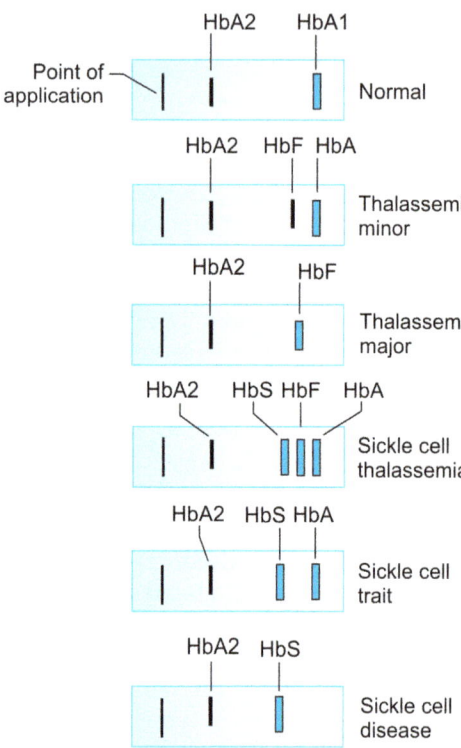

Fig. 11.12: Normal and abnormal hemoglobin patterns on cellulose acetate electrophoresis.

move with different speed in an electrical field and appear as separate bands (**Fig. 11.12**).

These differences in the migration are the result of different electrical charges of each Hb variant brought about by various amino acids in the polypeptide chains of Hb molecules.

Support medium used for Hb electrophoresis is cellulose acetate strip.

Detection of HbS

Sickling Test

Sickling test can be performed when red cells containing HbS is mixed with a freshly prepared solution of sodium metabisulfite (reducing agent). This can be detected under microscope. This test is simple and will detect both homozygous and heterozygous sickle gene. False results may be obtained if the

Table 11.3: Alkali denaturation test.

Parameter	Reference range (HbF%)
Normal	0.5–2
Thalassemia major	10–100
Thalassemia minor	0.5–8
Sickle cell β-thalassemia	5–20
Sickle cell anemia	5–30
Normal newborn	60–90

Table 11.4: Solubility test.

Parameter	Reference range (solubility %)
Normal	90–95
Hemoglobin A and hemoglobin S (Hb AS)	25–35
Sickle cell anemia (Hb SS)	3–10

patient has had a recent transfusion of normal red cells or if the blood sample is infected **Table 11.3**).

Solubility Test

The HbS is less soluble in concentrated buffer solution at a pH of 6.5, whereas normal Hb is soluble. This principle is used in differentiating HbS from normal Hb. When Hb is added to a solution of sodium hydrosulfite, a reducing agent in phosphate buffer, the solubility decreases and the solution becomes turbid if HbS is present (**Table 11.4**).

DERIVED HEMOGLOBIN COMPOUNDS

Carboxyhemoglobin, Sulphemoglobin, and Methemoglobin

Hemoglobin derivatives are formed by joining of different groups with the heme part or change in the oxidation state of iron.

Oxyhemoglobin

Oxyhemoglobin is the form of Hb present in the RBC, in the body. O_2 is combined to Hb through Fe^{2+}. It is dark red in color and the λ_{max} is 577 nm.

Reduced Hemoglobin or Deoxyhemoglobin

Deoxyhemoglobin is without O_2. This is purple red in color.

Carboxyhemoglobin

Carboxyhemoglobin (HbCO) is formed by binding CO with Hb. CO binds with the iron atom in the same way as O_2 binds. CO has more affinity toward Hb than O_2; hence, even a small quantity of CO present that will bind to the Hb λ_{max} of HbCO is 572 mm.

Exposure to CO occurs in the following conditions:
- In the mines (also deep wells).
- Heavy cigarette smoking.
- Incomplete burning of petrol.

Methemoglobin

A substitution of tyrosine for the histidine at either the proximal or distal histidine residues of either the α- or β-chains locks the heme iron into a trivalent state ferric (Fe^{3+}) or the action of oxidizing agents on Fe^{2+} form of Hb converts Fe^{2+} into Fe^{3+} state. Fe^{3+} cannot bind O_2; hence, O_2 transport is not possible. Increased methemoglobin (MetHb) in the blood is known as methemoglobinemia.

Causes of Methemoglobinemia

- Congenital MetHb reductase deficiency.
- Ingestion of nitrites, nitrates, sulfa drugs, or certain dyes (aniline dyes).
- Household substances such as shoe polishes (nitrobenzene) and furniture.

When MetHb in the blood increases up to 15% of the total pigment, cyanosis occurs (bluish color of the skin). Normally small amount of MetHb is produced in the blood. The enzyme MetHb reductase present in the RBC converts the Fe^{3+} to Fe^{2+}

form, thus converting the MetHb to normal Hb. Thus under through Fe. It is dark red in color and the RBC converts the Fe^{3+} to Fe^{2+} form, thus converting the MetHb to normal Hb. Thus under normal conditions MetHb concentration is less than 1% of the total Hb:

λ_{max} of MetHb = 630 nm.

Types

There are again two types of methemoglobinemia:
1. Hereditary methemoglobinemia associated with nicotinamide adenine dinucleotide-MetHb reductase deficiency. This is an autosomal recessive trait and affected subjects are persistently cyanotic.
2. Hereditary methemoglobinemia associated with HbM. This is associated with cyanosis. This disorder is transmitted as an autosomal dominant trait.

Sulfhemoglobin

Sulfhemoglobin is an abnormal sulfur containing Hb (attached to the porphyrin ring). It does not act as an O_2 carrier and it is not present in the normal RBCs. It is formed by the toxic action of drugs and chemical agents that contains sulfur. It results in cyanosis.

Cyanmethemoglobin

Hemoglobin is converted to cyanmethemoglobin by Drabkin's reagent (potassium ferricyanide+potassium cyanide). It is a complex formed by MetHb with cyanide and it is a stable compound having λ_{max} at 540 nm. This provides an accurate method for the estimation of Hb in the blood.

Carbaminohemoglobin

Carbaminohemoglobin is the form of Hb transporting CO_2 from tissues to the lungs.

SUMMARY

Hemoglobin is a conjugated iron-containing metalloprotein with four heme molecules linked to the protein portion called "globin." Globin part consists of four polypeptide chains. Normal Hb consists of two α and two β chains. Oxygen binds to the Fe^{2+} atoms of the heme to form HbO_2. Myoglobin is a monomeric protein of red muscle and stores O_2 as a reserve against O_2 deprivation. It releases O_2 during severe exercise for use in muscle mitochondria for aerobic synthesis of ATP. The oxygen binding curve for Hb is sigmoidal in shape, but myoglobin is hyperbolic. Defect in the synthesis or mutation of hemoglobin chain results in the formation of abnormal Hb (sickle cell hemoglobin). The reduction in the globin chain synthesis results in thalassemia. Hb can be differentiated by electrophoresis. Heme synthesis takes place in mitochondrion and cytosol, which depends on succinyl-CoA, glycine, ALA synthase, and iron. Disorders that arise from defects in the enzymes of heme biosynthesis are termed "porphyrias" and cause elevations in the serum and urine content of intermediates in heme synthesis. The porphyrias are both inherited and acquired disorders in heme synthesis. Catabolism of heme results in bilirubin. The body eliminates bilirubin by transporting it to the liver bound to albumin in the serum. In the liver, it is conjugated with glucuronate, which renders it water-soluble. The glucuronide conjugate is then excreted in the bile. Persons with extreme elevation in unconjugated bilirubin are susceptible to bilirubin encephalopathy, also referred to as kernicterus. Accumulation of bilirubin in the plasma and tissues results in jaundice. There are three types of it and they are hemoloytic, prehepatic, and posthepatic jaundice.

SELF-ASSESSMENT QUESTIONS

1. Briefly explain the structure of normal Hb.
2. What is sickle cell hemoglobin?
3. What is thalassemia? What are its types?
4. Name the tests used to detect abnormal Hb.
5. Write the significance of alkali denaturation test.
6. What are the different types of Hb derivatives?
7. Write short note on MetHb.

MULTIPLE-CHOICE QUESTIONS

1. The polypeptide chains of HbA1 are:
   a. $\alpha_2\beta_2$
   b. $\alpha_1\beta_2$
   c. $\alpha_2\beta_1$
   d. $\alpha_1\beta_1$
2. The rate-limiting step of Hb synthesis is catalyzed by:
   a. Ferrochelatase
   b. Porphobilinogen deaminase
   c. ALA synthase
   d. Protoporphyrinogen oxidase
3. Concerning fetal Hb, all are true, *except*:
   a. Compared to adult Hb, it is less sensitive to 2,3-BPG
   b. Its binding curve is to the right of myoglobin
   c. It consists of two α and two γ chains
   d. Compared to adult Hb, the critical substitution involves replacement of histidine with tryptophan
4. Concerning heme catabolism, all of the following statements are correct, *except*:
   a. Heme converted to hemin once it loses globin
   b. Hemin loses iron and converted to biliverdin
   c. Biliverdin reductase converts biliverdin to bilirubin
   d. Biliverdin gains H⁺ and changes to yellow pigment
5. Unconjugated hyperbilirubinemia results in:
   a. Dubin–Johnson syndrome
   b. Crigler–Najjar syndrome
   c. Rotor syndrome
   d. Metabolic syndrome
6. The porphyria, which does not show photosensitivity, is:
   a. Acute intermittent porphyria
   b. Variegate porphyria
   c. Porphyria cutanea tarda
   d. Erythropoietic protoporphyria
7. The erythropoietic protoporphyria results from the deficiency of:
   a. Coproporphyrinogen oxidase
   b. Protoporphyrinogen oxidase
   c. Ferrochelatase
   d. ALA dehydratase
8. Concerning sickle cell hemoglobin, one of the following statements is incorrect:
   a. It results from the substitution of valine for glycine
   b. It is determined by solubility test
   c. It moves just behind HbA1 during electrophoresis
   d. The substitution takes place at the sixth position of β-chain
9. All the following are the causes for metemoglobinemia, *except*:
   a. Congenital MetHb reductase deficiency
   b. Ingestion of nitrites
   c. Continuous exposure to nitrobenzene
   d. Exposure to lead
10. λ_{max} of MetHb is:
    a. 630 nm
    b. 540 nm
    c. 380 nm
    d. 700 nm
11. Which of the following trace elements may produce anemia in children by inhibiting Hb synthesis?
    a. Selenium
    b. Lead
    c. Iodine
    d. Fluorine
12. Hepatic glucuronyl transferase deficiency results in:
    a. Gilbert's syndrome
    b. Dubin–Johnson syndrome
    c. Lesch–Nyhan syndrome
    d. Crigler–Najjar syndrome

Answers

1. a	2. c	3. d	4. d	5. b
6. a	7. c	8. a	9. d	10. a
11. b	12. d			

CASE STUDY

1. A neonate developed unconjugated hyperbilirubinemia. No hemolysis can be demonstrated and other liver function tests are normal. There is no bilirubin found in the urine. This infant's condition continues to deteriorate and he or she dies at 2 weeks of age. To which of the following conditions did the infant most likely succumb?
   a. Crigler-Najjar syndrome type I
   b. Crigler-Najjar syndrome type II
   c. Dubin-Johnson syndrome
   d. Gilbert's syndrome

   Answer is a: The diseases listed in the answers are all inherited disorders of bilirubin metabolism that are usually discussed together. Crigler-Najjar syndrome and Gilbert's syndrome are both unconjugated hyperbilirubinemias, while Dubin-Johnson syndrome and Rotor syndrome are conjugated hyperbilirubinemias. Crigler-Najjar syndrome is rare and extremely serious, while Gilbert's syndrome is completely benign. The type II variant of Crigler-Najjar is intermediate in severity between Gilbert's syndrome and the type I. Dubin-Johnson and Rotor syndrome are also relatively benign. Dubin-Johnson syndrome is distinguished from Rotor's syndrome by the presence of a black pigment of unknown composition in the liver.

CHAPTER 12

Hormones

OBJECTIVES

At the end of this chapter, students should be able to:
- Classify the hormones and understand the mechanism of hormonal action
- Discuss the functions of pituitary hormones, including the pathophysiology
- Explain the actions and pathophysiology of various hormones such as thyroid, parathyroid, adrenal, pancreatic, ovarian, and testicular hormones.

INTRODUCTION

Hormones are the substances secreted by highly specialized cells and carried by the extracellular fluid (ECF) (mainly blood) and act through the receptor on the target organ to alter the activity of the cells quantitatively to influence:
- Metabolism
- Growth
- Reproduction
- Adaptation to the environment.

Hormones carry messages from glands to cells, to maintain chemical levels in the bloodstream that achieve homeostasis. Glands manufacture hormones that circulate freely in the bloodstream, waiting to be recognized by a target cell, their intended destination.

The target cell has a receptor that can only be activated by a specific type of hormone. Once activated, the cell knows to start a certain function within its walls. There are two types of hormones known, e.g. steroids and peptides. In general, steroids are sex hormones related to sexual maturation and fertility. Steroids are made from cholesterol. Cortisol is an example of a steroid hormone. Peptides regulate other functions such as sleep and sugar level. They are made from long strings of amino acids, so sometimes they are referred to as "protein" hormones.

Growth hormone (GH) helps us to burn fat and build up muscles. Insulin starts the process to convert sugar into cellular energy. As special categories, autocrine hormones act on the cells of the secreting gland, while paracrine hormones act on nearby, but unrelated, cells.

Chemical classes of hormones

Vertebrate hormones fall into three chemical classes:
1. *Amine-derived hormones*: Derivatives of the amino acids—tyrosine and tryptophan. Examples are catecholamines and thyroxine.
2. *Peptide hormones*: Consists of chains of amino acids. Examples of small peptide hormones are thyrotropin-releasing hormone (TRH) and vasopressin.
   - Peptides composed of hundreds of amino acids are referred to as proteins. Examples of protein hormones include insulin and GH.
   - More complex protein hormones bear carbohydrate side chains and are called glycoprotein hormones. Luteinizing hormone, follicle-stimulating hormone (FSH), and thyroid-stimulating hormone (TSH) are glycoprotein hormones.

3. *Lipid- and phospholipid-derived hormones*: Derived from lipids such as linoleic acid, arachidonic acid, and phospholipids. The main classes are the steroid hormones that derive from cholesterol and the eicosanoids. Examples of steroid hormones are testosterone and cortisol. The adrenal cortex and the gonads are primary sources of steroid hormones. Examples of eicosanoids are the widely studied prostaglandins.

MECHANISM OF HORMONAL ACTION

The mechanism behind the hormonal action is as follows:
- The hormone binds to a site on the extracellular portion of the receptor (**Fig. 12.1**).
- The receptors are transmembrane proteins that pass through the plasma membrane seven times, with their N-terminal exposed at the exterior of the cell and their C-terminal projecting into the cytoplasm.
- Binding of the hormone to the receptor activates a G protein.
- This initiates the production of a second messenger, i.e. cyclic adenosine monophosphate (cAMP), which is produced by adenylyl cyclase from adenosine triphosphate, inositol 1,4,5-trisphosphate (IP3).
- The second messenger, in turn, initiates a series of intracellular events such as phosphorylation and activation of enzymes; release of calcium ions (Ca^{2+}) into the cytosol from stores within the endoplasmic reticulum.
- In the case of cAMP, these enzymatic changes activate the transcription factor CREB (CREB stands for cAMP response element binding protein).
- Bound to its response element in the promoters of genes that are able to respond to the hormone, activated CREB turns on gene transcription, then to translation to produce the desired protein.
- The biochemical response is achieved finally.
- The cell begins to produce the appropriate gene products in response to the hormonal signal it has received at its surface.

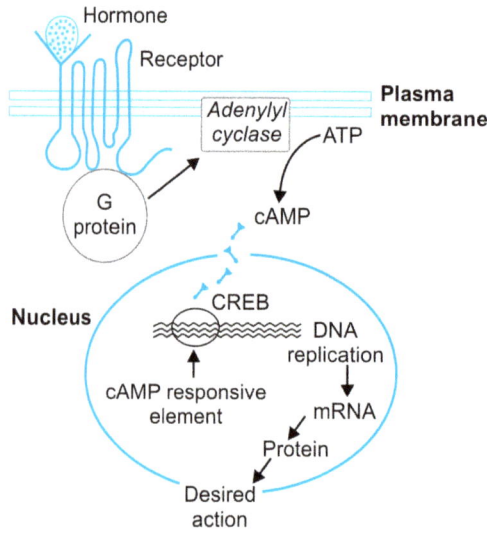

Fig. 12.1: Mechanism of hormonal action.
(ATP: adenosine triphosphate; cAMP: cyclic adenosine monophosphate; CREB: cAMP response element binding protein; DNA: deoxyribonucleic acid; mRNA: messenger ribonucleic acid)

Classification

In classical endocrinology, the hormones are classified as follows (**Fig. 12.2**):
- Pituitary hormones
- Thyroid hormones
- Parathyroid hormones (PTHs)
- Pancreatic hormones
- Suprarenal cortical hormones
- Suprarenal medullary hormones
- Ovarian hormones
- Posterior pituitary
- Intermediate lobe
- Testicular hormones
- Hypophyseal hormones.

PITUITARY HORMONES

The endocrine is a gland, which secretes hormone also called ductless glands, as the

Hormones

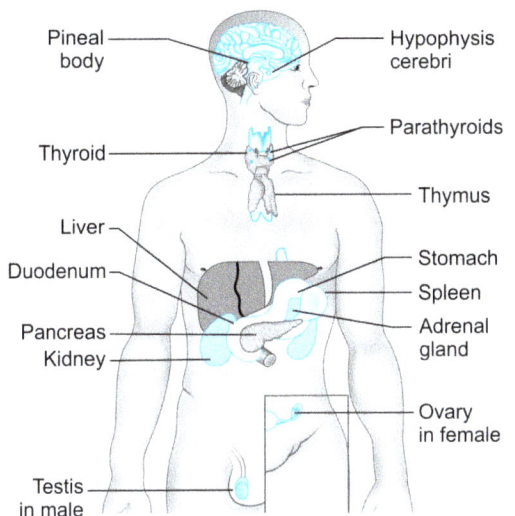

Fig. 12.2: Endocrine glands location in humans.

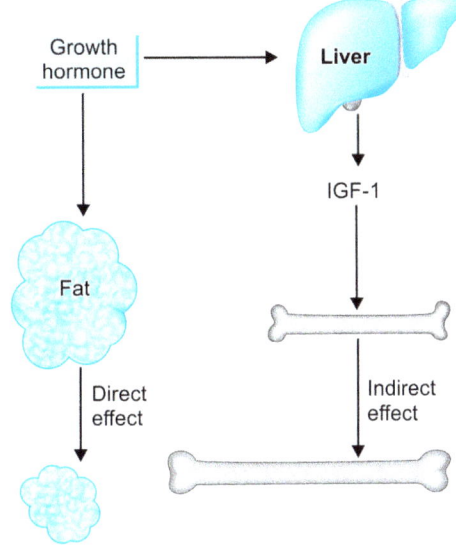

Fig. 12.3: Direct and indirect effects of growth hormones.
(IGF-1: insulin-like growth factor 1)

hormone is carried not by the duct, but by blood. Pituitary gland comprises:
- Anterior pituitary
- Posterior pituitary
- Intermediate lobe.

Anterior Pituitary Hormones

Following are the anterior pituitary hormones:
- GH
- TSH
- FSH
- Luteinizing hormone (LH)
- Adrenocorticotropic hormone (ACTH)
- Prolactin (PRL)
- Alpha-melanocyte-stimulating hormone.

Growth Hormone

Human GH (also called somatotropin) is a protein of 191 amino acids. The GH-secreting cells are stimulated to synthesize and release GH by the intermittent arrival of GH-releasing hormone (GHRH) from the hypothalamus.

Direct effects are the result of GH binding its receptor on target cells. Fat cells (adipocytes), for example, have GH receptors and GH stimulates them to break down triglyceride and suppresses their ability to take up and accumulate circulating lipids.

Indirect effects are mediated primarily by an insulin-like growth factor 1 (IGF-1), a hormone that is secreted from the liver and other tissues in response to GH. A majority of the growth-promoting effects of GH are actually due to IGF-1 acting on its target cells (e.g. on long bones) (**Fig. 12.3**).

Pathophysiology
- In childhood, hyposecretion of GH produces the stunted growth of a dwarf.
- Dwarfism can also result from an inability to respond to GH.
- This can result from inheriting two mutant genes encoding the receptors for:
  - GH-releasing hormone
  - GH.

Growth hormone deficiency symptoms
Symptoms of GH deficiency in children include the following:
- Short stature
- Low growth velocity (speed) for age and pubertal stage

- Increased amount of fat around the waist
- The child may look younger than other children of his age
- Delayed tooth development
- Delayed onset of puberty.

Symptoms of GH deficiency in adults include the following:
- Low energy
- Decreased strength and exercise tolerance
- Decreased muscle mass
- Weight gain, especially around the waist
- Feelings of anxiety, depression or sadness causing a change in social behavior.

Hypersecretion of GH

The effect of excessive secretion of GH is also very dependent on the age of onset and is seen as two distinctive disorders:

1. Hypersecretion leads to gigantism. It is the result of excessive GH secretion that begins in young children or adolescents. It is a very rare disorder, usually resulting from a tumor of somatotrophs.
2. In adults, a hypersecretion of GH leads to acromegaly. This results from excessive secretion of GH in adults, usually the result of benign pituitary tumors. The onset of this disorder is typically insidious, occurring over several years. Clinical signs of acromegaly include overgrowth of extremities, soft tissue swelling, abnormalities in jaw structure, and cardiac disease.
3. The excessive GH and IGF-1 also lead to a number of metabolic derangements, including hyperglycemia.

Thyroid-stimulating Hormone

Thyroid-stimulating hormone (also known as thyrotropin) is a glycoprotein, which consists of:
- β-chain with 112 amino acids.
- α-chain with 89 amino acids. The α-chain is identical to that found in two other pituitary hormones, FSH, and LH. Thus

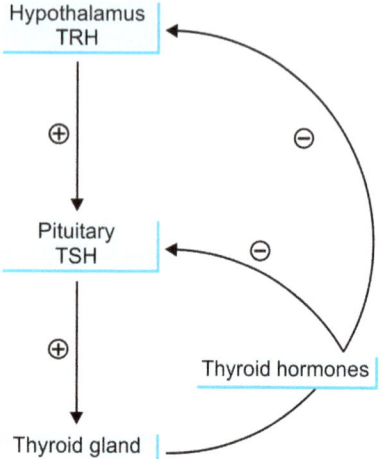

Fig. 12.4: Stimulation of TSH by TRH.
(TRH: thyroid-releasing hormone; TSH: thyroid-stimulating hormone)

it is its β-chain that gives TSH its unique properties.
- The secretion of TSH is:
  - Stimulated by the arrival of TRH from the hypothalamus
  - Inhibited by the arrival of somatostatin from the hypothalamus (**Fig. 12.4**).

As its name suggests, TSH stimulates the thyroid gland to secrete its hormone thyroxine (T4).

Follicle-stimulating Hormone

The role of FSH in females and males is given below:
- *In females*: FSH acts on the ovary to stimulate the development of ovarian follicle.
- *In males*: It acts on the testes for the maturation of sperm.

Luteinizing Hormone

The role of LH in females and males is given below:
- *In females*: LH stimulates the ovarian follicle to mature and also to secrete the estrogen.
- *In males*: It stimulates the secretion of testosterone.

Adrenocorticotropic Hormone

The role of ACTH is given below:
- The ACTH is a peptide of 39 amino acids.
- It is cut from a larger precursor proopiomelanocortin.
- It acts on the cells of the adrenal cortex stimulating them to produce their hormone.

Pathophysiology
- If ACTH secretion is increased by the pituitary or by ectopic production from a tumor, it results in Cushing's syndrome.
- The decreased ACTH production leads to Addison's disease.

Prolactin (Somatomammotropin)

The role of PRL is given below:
- PRL is a protein of 198 amino acids.
- During pregnancy, it helps in the preparation of the breasts for future milk production.
- After birth, PRL promotes the synthesis of milk.
- PRL secretion is stimulated by TRH and repressed by estrogens and dopamine.
Normal range: Females—5.4–22.5 ng/mL (midcycle), 4.5–15 ng/mL (menopausal women).
Men: 4.2–15 ng/mL.

Pathophysiology
- Hyperprolactinemia is a cause of infertility in females.
- Secretion of PRL is stimulated by TRH and inhibited by prolactin-inhibiting factor.

Posterior Pituitary Hormones

Vasopressin

Following list shows the information about vasopressin:
- Vasopressin was originally named because of its ability to control blood pressure when administered in pharmacological amounts.
- But more appropriately, it is called antidiuretic hormone (ADH), because of its important function to promote reabsorption of water from the distal convoluted tubules.

- Defect in the ADH secretion or the decreased action, it may lead to diabetes insipidus.
- Diabetes insipidus is characterized by excretion of large volumes of diluted urine.
  - *Primary diabetes insipidus*: An insufficient secretion of hormone, which is due to the destruction of the hypothalamo-hypophyseal tract.
  - Arises due to basal skull fractures.
  - Tumor or infection.
  - It may be hereditary also.

Biochemical findings
- Decreased specific gravity
- Decreased ADH
- Diluted urine
- Polyuria.

Oxytocin

Production and function of oxytocin are given below:
- Oxytocin is produced in hypothalamus and transported to posterior pituitary gland.
- Appropriate stimulation releases the hormones into the blood.
- The neural impulses that result from stimulation of the nipples are the primary stimuli for oxytocin release.
- Vaginal and uterine distention is the secondary stimuli.
- Estrogen also stimulates the production of oxytocin.
- Oxytocin causes contraction of uterine smooth muscles and thus is used in pharmacological amount to induce labor in humans.
- The most likely physiologic function of oxytocin is stimulation for the contraction of cells surrounding mammary alveoli.

- This promotes the movement of milk into the system and allows milk ejection.

THYROID HORMONES

The role of thyroid hormone is as follows:
- The thyroid gland synthesizes and secretes T4 and triiodothyronine (T3).
- Thyroxine is a derivative of the amino acid tyrosine with four atoms of iodine.
- In the liver, one atom of iodine is removed from T4 converting it into T3.
- The T3 is the active hormone.
- It has many effects on the body, among the most prominent of these are:
  - An increase in metabolic rate (seen by a rise in the uptake of oxygen)
  - An increase in the rate and strength of the heartbeat.
- The thyroid cells responsible for the synthesis of T4 take up circulating iodine from the blood.

Normal levels: As follows:
- T3 = 0.8 – 2.0 mg/mL
- T4 = 4.5 – 12.0 mg/dL.

Pathophysiology

Hypothyroid diseases

Hypothyroid diseases are caused by inadequate production of T3. This includes:
- *Cretinism*: Hypothyroidism in infancy and childhood leads to stunted growth and intelligence. It can be corrected by giving T4, if started early enough.
- *Myxedema*: Hypothyroidism in adults leads to lowered metabolic rate and vigor. It can be reversed by giving T4.
- *Goiter*: Enlargement of the thyroid gland can be caused by:
  - Inadequate iodine in the diet with resulting low levels of T4 and T3.
  - An autoimmune attack against components of the thyroid gland (called Hashimoto's thyroiditis).
  - The region for hypothyroid disease produces an enlarged gland.

- The activity of the thyroid is under negative feedback control.
- The synthesis and release of TRH and TSH is normally inhibited as the levels of T4 and T3 rise in the blood.
- When the iodine supply is inadequate, T4 and T3 levels fall:
  - Stimulates the hypothalamus and pituitary to increase TRH and TSH activity, respectively
  - Stimulates the thyroid gland to enlarge (fruitlessly).

Symptoms
- Decrease basal metabolic rate
- Slow heart rate
- Diastolic hypertension
- Sluggish behavior
- Sleepiness
- Constipation
- Sensitivity to cold
- Dry skin and hair.

Biochemical findings
- Decreased T3, T4 and increased TSH especially in primary hypothyroidism
- Decreased T3, T4 and decreased TSH in secondary hypothyroidism.

Hyperthyroid diseases

Hyperthyroid diseases are caused by excessive secretion of thyroid hormones.
- Graves' disease.
- *Osteoporosis*: High levels of thyroid hormones suppress the production of TSH through the negative feedback mechanism mentioned above. The resulting low level of TSH causes an increase in the numbers of bone-reabsorbing osteoclasts resulting in osteoporosis.

Symptoms
- Rapid heart rate
- Nervousness
- Inability to sleep
- Weight loss in spite of hyperthyroidism
- Weakness

- Excessive sweating
- Sensitivity to heat.

Biochemical findings: Increased T3 and T4 and decreased TSH.

PARATHYROID HORMONES

Functions

The function of PTHs is as follows:
- Calcium homeostasis (regulation): PTH restores normal calcium concentration by acting directly on bone and kidney and acting indirectly on intestinal mucosa (**Fig. 12.5**):
  - *Bone*: It increases the resorption in both organic and inorganic phases, which lose Ca^{2+} into ECF.
  - *Kidney*: It reduces renal clearance or excretion of calcium and hence increases ECF concentration of calcium.
  - *Gastrointestinal tract:* It increases efficiency of calcium absorption from the intestine by promoting the synthesis of calcitriol. It acts upon the intestine to increase Ca^{2+} absorption and plays a permissive role of PTH on bone, and kidney.
- The PTH also increases renal phosphate clearance. Thus the net effect of PTH on bone and kidney is to increase ECF Ca^{2+} concentration and decrease ECF phosphate (PO_4) concentration.

Hyperparathyroidism

Excessive secretion of PTH is seen in two forms:
1. Primary hyperparathyroidism is the result of parathyroid gland disease, most commonly due to a parathyroid tumor (adenoma), which secretes the hormone without proper regulation.
   Common manifestations of this disorder are chronic elevations of blood calcium concentration (hypercalcemia), kidney stones, and decalcification of bone.
2. Secondary hyperparathyroidism is the situation where disease outside of the parathyroid gland leads to excessive secretion of PTH. A common cause of this disorder is kidney disease. If the kidneys are unable to reabsorb calcium, blood calcium levels will fall, stimulating continual secretion of PTH to maintain normal calcium levels in blood. Secondary hyperparathyroidism can also result from inadequate nutrition, e.g. diets that are deficient in calcium or vitamin D or which contain excessive phosphorus. A prominent effect of secondary hyperparathyroidism is decalcification of bone.

Hypoparathyroidism

Inadequate production of PTH, i.e. hypoparathyroidism results in decreased concentrations of calcium and increased concentrations of phosphorus in blood. Common causes of this disorder include surgical removal of the parathyroid glands and disease processes that lead to destruction of parathyroid glands. The resulting hypocalcemia often leads to tetany and convulsions and can be acutely life threatening.

ADRENAL GLAND HORMONES

The adrenal gland comprises cortex and medulla. Cortex has three zones:

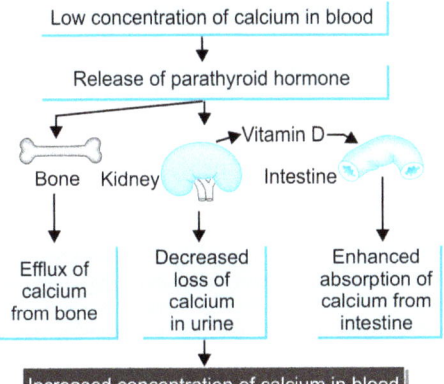

Fig. 12.5: Calcium regulation.

- *Zona glomerulosa*: It produces mineralocorticoids.
- *Zona fasciculata*: It produces glucocorticoids.
- *Zona reticularis*: It secretes sex steroids such as androgens and estrogens.

Glucocorticoids

Glucocorticoids are a class of steroid hormones. It is mainly derived from cholesterol. The functions of glucocorticoid in the human body are:
- The glucocorticoids get their name from their effect of raising the level of blood sugar. They do this by stimulating gluconeogenesis in the liver.
- The conversion of fat and protein into intermediate metabolites that are ultimately converted into glucose.
- The most abundant glucocorticoid is cortisol (also called hydrocortisone).
- Cortisol and the other glucocorticoid also have a potent anti-inflammatory effect on the body.
- They depress the immune response, especially cell-mediated immune response.
- They are widely used in therapy.
  - To reduce the inflammatory destruction of rheumatoid arthritis and other auto-immune diseases
  - To prevent the rejection of transplanted organs
  - To control asthma.

Control of Cortisol Secretion

- Cortisol and other glucocorticoids are secreted in response to a single stimulator, i.e. ACTH from the anterior pituitary. ACTH is itself secreted under control of the hypothalamic peptide corticotropin-releasing hormone (CRH). The central nervous system is thus the commander and chief of glucocorticoid responses, providing an excellent example of close integration between the nervous and endocrine systems.
- Virtually any type of physical or mental stress results in elevation of cortisol concentrations in blood due to enhanced secretion of CRH in the hypothalamus.
- Cortisol secretion is suppressed by classical negative feedback loops. When blood concentrations rise above a certain threshold, cortisol inhibits CRH secretion from the hypothalamus, which turns off ACTH secretion that leads to a turning off of cortisol secretion from the adrenal (**Fig. 12.6**). The combination of positive and negative control on CRH secretion results in pulsatile secretion of cortisol. Typically, pulse amplitude and frequency are highest in the morning, and lowest at night.
- The ACTH binds to receptors in the plasma membrane of cells in the zona fasciculata and reticularis of the adrenal. Hormone-receptor engagement activates adenylyl cyclase, leading to elevated intracellular

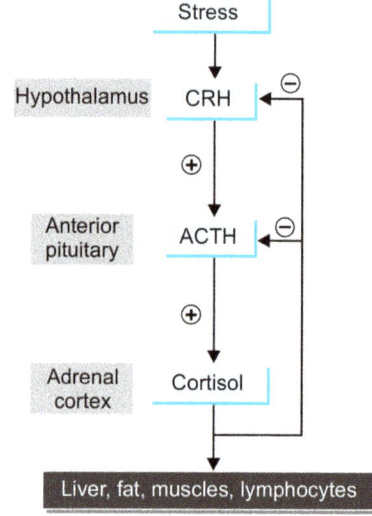

Fig. 12.6: Release of cortisol and its negative feedback control.
(ACTH: adrenocorticotropic hormone; CRH: corticotropin-releasing hormone)

levels of cAMP, which leads ultimately to activation of the enzyme systems involved in biosynthesis of cortisol from cholesterol.

Mode of Action

Glucocorticoids bind to the cytosolic glucocorticoid receptor. This type of receptor is activated by ligand binding. After a hormone binds to the corresponding receptor, the newly formed receptor–ligand complex translocates itself into the cell nucleus, where it binds to many glucocorticoid response elements in the promoter region of the target genes.

Pathophysiology

Addison's disease (adrenal insufficiency)
- Addison's disease is a rare endocrine or hormonal disorder that occurs in all age-groups.
- There is an insufficient amount of steroid hormones (glucocorticoids and often mineralocorticoids).
- The disease is also called adrenal insufficiency or hypocortisolism.

Causes

Failure to produce adequate levels of cortisol can occur for different reasons.
- The problem may be due to a disorder of the adrenal glands themselves (primary adrenal insufficiency).
  - Destruction of the adrenal glands by infection
  - Their destruction by an autoimmune attack.
- Inadequate secretion of ACTH by the pituitary gland (secondary adrenal insufficiency).
- An inherited mutation in the ACTH receptor on adrenal cells.
This form of adrenal insufficiency is much more common than primary adrenal insufficiency and can be traced to a lack of ACTH. Without ACTH to stimulate the adrenals, the production of cortisol of the adrenal glands drops, but not aldosterone.

A temporary form of secondary adrenal insufficiency may occur when a person who has been receiving a glucocorticoid hormone such as prednisone for a long time abruptly stops or interrupts taking the medication. Glucocorticoid hormones, which are often used to treat inflammatory illnesses such as rheumatoid arthritis, asthma, or ulcerative colitis, block the release of both CRH and ACTH. Normally, CRH instructs the pituitary gland to release ACTH. If CRH levels drop, the pituitary is not stimulated to release ACTH and the adrenals then fail to secrete sufficient levels of cortisol.

Another cause of secondary adrenal insufficiency is the surgical removal of benign or noncancerous ACTH-producing tumors of the pituitary gland (Cushing's disease).

Other causes

Less common causes of primary adrenal insufficiency are:
- Cancer cells spreading from other parts of the body to the adrenal glands
- Amyloidosis
- Surgical removal of the adrenal glands.

Symptoms
- Hypoglycemia
- Extreme sensitivity of insulin
- Intolerance to stress
- Weight loss
- Nausea
- Severe weakness
- Patients have low blood pressure.
  Replacement therapy with glucocorticoid and mineralocorticoids can permit a normal life.

Diagnosis

A diagnosis of Addison's disease is made by laboratory tests. The aim of these tests is to determine whether levels of cortisol are insufficient and then to establish the cause.

- *The ACTH stimulation test*: This is the most specific test for diagnosing Addison's disease. In this test, blood cortisol, urine cortisol, or both are measured before and after a synthetic form of ACTH is given by injection in the so-called short or rapid, ACTH test. Measurement of cortisol in blood is repeated 30–60 minutes after an intravenous.

  ACTH injection. The normal response after an injection of ACTH is a rise in blood and urine cortisol levels. Patients with either form of adrenal insufficiency respond poorly or do not respond at all.
- Routine investigation may show:
  - Hypoglycemia
  - Hyponatremia
  - Hypokalemia
  - Eosinophilia and lymphocytosis.

Cushing's syndrome

Cushing's syndrome is a hormonal disorder caused by prolonged exposure of the body's tissues to high levels of the hormone cortisol. In Cushing's syndrome, the level of adrenal hormones, especially of the glucocorticoids (cortisol), is too high (**Fig. 12.7**).

Causes
- Excessive production of ACTH by the anterior lobe of the pituitary.
- Excessive production of adrenal hormones themselves (e.g. because of a tumor).
  - *Ectopic ACTH syndrome*: Some benign or malignant (cancerous) tumors that arise outside the pituitary can produce ACTH. This condition is known as ectopic ACTH syndrome. Lung tumors cause over 50% of these cases.
  - As a result of glucocorticoid therapy for some other disorder such as rheumatoid arthritis or decreased glucocorticoid hormone synthesis.

Symptoms
- Hyperglycemia.
- High blood pressure.
- Severe protein catabolism results in thinning of skin, muscle-wasting disease, osteoporosis, and negative nitrogen balance.
- There is a peculiar redistribution of fat in trunks.
- Moon face.
- Central obesity and typical buffalo hump.
- Resistant to infection and inflammatory response is impaired.
- Facial hair growth.

Diagnosis

Diagnosis is based on a review of the patient's medical history, physical examination, and laboratory tests:
- *24-hour urinary free cortisol level*: This is the most specific diagnostic test. The patient's urine is collected over a 24-hour period and tested for the amount of cortisol. If the cortisol level is higher than 50–100 μg a day for an adult, it suggests Cushing's syndrome. The normal range may vary from laboratory to laboratory depending on the techniques they use.
- *Dexamethasone suppression test*: This test is used to distinguish patients with excess production of ACTH due to pituitary adenomas from those with ectopic ACTH-producing tumors. Patients

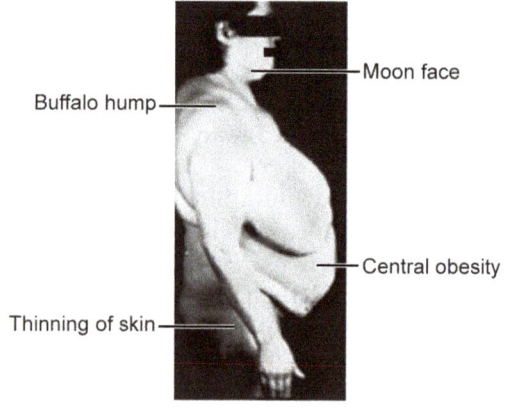

Fig. 12.7: Features of Cushing's syndrome.

are given dexamethasone, a synthetic glucocorticoid, by mouth every 6 hours for 4 days. For the first 2 days, low doses of dexamethasone are given and for the last 2 days, higher doses are given. 24-hour urine sample collections are made before dexamethasone is administered and on each day of the test. Since cortisol and other glucocorticoids signal the pituitary to lower secretion of ACTH, the normal response after taking dexamethasone is a drop in blood and urine cortisol levels. Different responses of cortisol to dexamethasone are obtained depending on whether the cause of Cushing's syndrome is a pituitary adenoma or an ectopic ACTH-producing tumor.

The dexamethasone suppression test can produce false-positive results in patients with depression, alcohol abuse, high estrogen levels, acute illness, and stress. Conversely, drugs such as phenytoin and phenobarbital may cause false-negative results in response to dexamethasone suppression. For this reason, patients are usually advised by their physicians to stop taking these drugs at least 1 week before the test.

- *The CRH stimulation test*: This test helps to distinguish between patients with pituitary adenomas and those with ectopic ACTH syndrome or cortisol-secreting adrenal tumors. Patients are given an injection of CRH, which causes the pituitary to secrete ACTH. Patients with pituitary adenomas usually experience a rise in blood levels of ACTH and cortisol. This response is rarely seen in patients with ectopic ACTH syndrome and practically never in patients with cortisol-secreting adrenal tumors.

Mineralocorticoids

- Mineralocorticoids are steroid hormones and mainly derived from the cholesterol.
- They get their name from their effect on mineral metabolism.
- The most important of them is the steroid aldosterone.

Functions

The function of aldosterone is as follows:
- Aldosterone acts on the kidney promoting the reabsorption of sodium ions (Na^+) into the blood.
- Water follows the salt and this helps maintain normal blood pressure.
- Aldosterone also acts on sweat glands to reduce the loss of Na^+ in perspiration.
- It acts on taste cells to increase the sensitivity of the taste buds to sources of Na.
- The secretion of aldosterone is stimulated by:
  - A drop in the level of Na in the blood
  - A rise in the level of potassium ions (K^+) in the blood.
  - Angiotensin II
  - ACTH.

Pathophysiology
Primary aldosteronism or Crohn's syndrome
- Results from an aldosterone-secreting tumor, which leads to elevated levels of plasma aldosterone
- The plasma pH in this condition increases because of hypokalemic alkalosis and the plasma osmolality also increases.

Hormones Secreted by Adrenal Medulla

Adrenal medulla secretes:
- Dopamine
- Adrenaline (epinephrine)
- Noradrenaline (norepinephrine).

Functions

- The adrenal medulla consists of masses of neurons that are part of the sympathetic branch of the autonomic nervous system.
- Instead of releasing their neurotransmitters at a synapse, these neurons release them into the blood. Thus, although part

of the nervous system, the adrenal medulla functions as an endocrine gland.
- The adrenal medulla releases:
  - Adrenaline (also called epinephrine)
  - Noradrenaline (also called norepinephrine); both are derived from the amino acid tyrosine.
- Release of adrenaline and noradrenaline is triggered by nervous stimulation in response to physical or mental stress. Some of the effects are:
  - Increase in the rate and strength of the heartbeat resulting in increased blood pressure
  - Blood shunted from the skin and viscera to the skeletal muscles, coronary arteries, liver, and brain
  - Rise in blood sugar
  - Increased metabolic rate
  - Bronchi dilate
  - Pupils dilate
  - Hair stands on end
  - Reduced clotting time
  - Increased ACTH secretion from the anterior lobe of the pituitary.

Pathophysiology
The tumor of the adrenal medulla results in oversecretion of its hormones and leads to a condition called pheochromocytoma.

PANCREATIC HORMONES

The α-cells of pancreas secrete glucagon and β-cells of islets of Langerhans of pancreas secrete insulin.

Insulin

- Insulin is a polypeptide hormone synthesized from the β-cells of islets of Langerhans of pancreas.
- It is synthesized as a larger precursor called preproinsulin. Preproinsulin has 109 amino acids. It is immediately converted into proinsulin in the endoplasmic reticulum by the removal of 23 amino acids. So, the proinsulin formed contains 86 amino acids. The proinsulin is transported to Golgi apparatus and is cleaved to form insulin, and C-peptide.
3. The C-peptide contains 33 amino acids. Insulin formed from proinsulin contains 53 amino acids from which 2 amino acids are cleaved to form insulin with 51 amino acids.

Functions

Insulin mainly controls blood glucose by the following mechanisms:
- Increases the uptake of glucose by the peripheral cells
- Increases the utilization of glucose by stimulating the glycolysis
- Stimulates glycogenesis and inhibits glycogenolysis
- Inhibits lipolysis
- Inhibits gluconeogenesis.

Glucagon

Glucagon is a polypeptide secreted by α-cells of islets of Langerhans of pancreas. It is called anti-insulin hormone since its actions are entirely opposite to that of insulin.

Functions

Glucagon stimulates the production of glucose in liver by promoting glycogenolysis and gluconeogenesis (refer to blood sugar regulation).

FEMALE SEX HORMONES

It is very important to know how hormones can affect the female body, mind, and emotions. Then we will be able to minimize their negative effects and enhance their positive ones.

Female Sex Hormones at Different Stages

The most important hormones made by the ovaries are known as female sex hormones, such as estrogen and progesterone. The ovaries also produce some of the male hormone, i.e. testosterone.

Infancy

Newborn babies (boys and girls) may have slightly enlarged breasts, sometimes accompanied by a little milk production, due to the female hormone, estrogen, in the mother's body passing through the placenta during pregnancy and stimulating breast development in the baby, and finally, disappearing during childhood.

Puberty

- At puberty, hormones will begin to make major, lasting changes to a girl's body.
- Breasts will get bigger and take on the shape of an adult woman's breasts.
- She will develop underarm and pubic hair and will get noticeably taller as a significant growth spurt occurs.
- Her periods will start, usually as the growth spurt is beginning to slow down.
- From beginning to end, the process of puberty usually takes at least 4 years.
- The hypothalamus starts to release hormone, which stimulates the pituitary gland to produce LH and FSH, which in turn cause a girl's ovaries to start producing other hormones.

During puberty, estrogen stimulates breast development and causes the vagina, uterus, and Fallopian tubes to mature. It also plays a role in the growth spurt and alters the distribution of fat on a girl's body, typically resulting in more being deposited around the hips, buttocks, and thighs. Testosterone helps to promote muscle and bone growth.

From puberty onward, LH, FSH, estrogen, and progesterone all play a vital role in regulating a woman's menstrual cycle, which results in her periods. Each individual hormone follows its own pattern, rising and falling at different points in the cycle, but together they produce a predictable chain of events. One egg (out of several hundred thousand in each ovary) becomes mature and is released from the ovary to and run toward Fallopian tube, and into the womb. If that egg is not fertilized, the levels of estrogen and progesterone produced by the ovary begin to fall. Without the supporting action of these hormones, the lining of the womb, which is full of blood, is shed, resulting in a period.

Pregnancy

If the egg released from the ovary is fertilized and a pregnancy results, a woman's hormones change dramatically. The usual fall in estrogen and progesterone at the end of the menstrual cycle does not occur, so no period is seen. A new hormone, human chorionic gonadotropin, produced by the developing placenta, stimulates the ovaries to produce the higher levels of estrogen and progesterone that are needed to sustain a pregnancy. By the fourth month of pregnancy, the placenta takes over from the ovaries as the main producer of estrogen and progesterone. These hormones cause the lining of the womb to thicken, increase the volume of blood circulating, and relax the muscles of the womb sufficiently to make room for the growing baby. Around the time of childbirth, other hormones such as oxytocin come into play that help the womb to contract during and after labor, as well as stimulate the production and release of breast milk.

After Childbirth

The levels of estrogen, progesterone, and other hormones fall sharply, causing a number of physical changes. The womb shrinks back to its nonpregnant size, pelvic floor muscle tone improves, and the volume of blood circulating round the body returns to normal.

Menopause

The next significant hormonal change for most women occurs around the time of the last period, i.e. the menopause. Over 3–5 years leading up to a woman's last period, the normal functioning of her ovaries begins to deteriorate. This can cause her menstrual cycle to become shorter or longer and sometimes it becomes quite erratic. Eventually, the ovaries produce so little estrogen and finally periods stop altogether.

Ovary

The ovarian follicles secrete the following hormones:
- Estrogen is secreted from the follicular tissue.
- Progesterone is secreted from the corpus luteum.
- Androgens.

Estrogen

Estrogens are primarily responsible for the conversion of girls into sexually mature women. It is also responsible for:
- Development of breasts
- Further development of the uterus and vagina
- Broadening of the pelvis
- Growth of pubic and axillary hair
- Increase in adipose (fat) tissue
- Participating in the monthly preparation of the body for a possible pregnancy
- Participating in pregnancy, if it occurs.

Progesterone

Progesterone plays the following roles:
- Progesterone is a steroid hormone synthesized from parent compound cholesterol.
- It causes the development of endometrium and prepares it for the implantation of fertilized ovum for conception.
- It stimulates the mammary glands.
- Normal range:
  - *Follicular and mid-cycle*: 0.175–0.7 ng/mL
  - *Luteal cycle*: 4.7–20 ng/mL.

Testes

Testes play the following roles:
- Secretes testosterone.
- Promotes the growth and function of epididymis, vas deferens, and prostate and seminal vesicles.

SUMMARY

Hormones are the substances secreted by highly specialized cells and carried by the ECF and act through the receptor on the target organ to alter the activity of cells quantitatively to influence metabolism, growth, reproduction, and adaptation to the environment. There are steroids and peptides hormones. Steroids are sex hormones related to sexual maturation and fertility. Peptides regulate sleep and sugar level. The pituitary hormones are of two types, i.e. anterior and posterior. GH, TSH, ACTH, FSH, LH, and PRL are the anterior pituitary hormones. Oxytocin and ADH are the posterior pituitary hormones. TSH stimulates the thyroid gland for the secretion of thyroid hormones T3 and T4. Low level of thyroid hormones seen in goiter, cretinism, and myxedema. High level of thyroid hormones seen Grave's disease. Parathyroid secretes PTH which helps in the regulation of calcium in the body. Mineralocorticoids, glucocorticoids, and sex steroids are secreted from the adrenal gland. Mineralocorticoids help in the regulation blood sodium and glucocorticoids work as hyperglycemic hormones, which become active during starvation or during fasting. Insulin and glucagon are secreted from pancreas. Excess secretion of glucocorticoids results in Cushing's syndrome, which is characterized by moon face, central obesity, and buffalo hump. Reduced level of glucocorticoids results in Addison's disease. Insulin is hypoglycemic hormone and an important hormone that regulates the blood sugar during well-fed state. Glucagon is a hyperglycemic in action and becomes active during fasting condition through its action on metabolism. Testes secrete testosterone, and progesterone and estrogen are secreted from ovary.

- Enhances and maintains the mobility and fertilizing power of the sperms.
- Promotes protein synthesis in the body.

SELF-ASSESSMENT QUESTIONS

1. What are hormones?
2. List the hormones secreted from anterior and posterior pituitary gland.
3. Describe the mechanism of hormonal action.
4. Explain the pathophysiology of GH.
5. List the hormones secreted from thyroid gland and which hormones stimulate the thyroid hormone release?
6. Briefly discuss the cretinism, goiter, and myxedema.
7. How do the PTHs work in maintaining calcium homeostasis?
8. State the hormones secreted from three zones of adrenal cortex.
9. List the functions of glucocorticoid and mineralocorticoid hormones.
10. Write the cause, signs and symptoms of:
    a. Addison's disease
    b. Cushing's syndrome.
11. List the adrenal medullary hormones and their functions.
12. Mention few functions of female sex hormones and mention on what influence they enter the circulation to act finally?
13. What are the hormones secreted from pancreas?

MULTIPLE-CHOICE QUESTIONS

1. Binding of hormones to receptor activates:
   a. Glycoprotein
   b. G protein
   c. M protein
   d. Lipoproteins
2. The hormonal action on the target organs depends on all the following factors, *except*:
   a. Cyclic AMP
   b. Adenylyl cyclase
   c. Receptor
   d. ADP
3. Which of the following is not an anterior pituitary hormone?
   a. Prolactin
   b. Follicular-stimulating hormone
   c. Antidiuretic hormone
   d. α-melanocyte-stimulating hormone
4. Human growth hormone is also called:
   a. Cortisol
   b. Somatomammotropin
   c. α-melanocyte-stimulating hormone
   d. Somatotropin
5. Concerning prolactin, all of the following statements are true, *except*:
   a. Hypoprolactinemia is a cause of infertility in females
   b. It is a protein of 198 amino acids
   c. Its secretion is stimulated by TRH
   d. Its secretion is repressed by dopamine
6. Vasopressin:
   a. Is secreted from anterior pituitary gland
   b. Its deficiency results in diabetes mellitus
   c. Its deficiency occurs due to basal skull fractures
   d. Its deficiency leads to oliguria
7. Which one of the following is not a hypothyroid disease?
   a. Cretinism
   b. Myxedema
   c. Graves' disease
   d. Goiter
8. Concerning the hypothyroidism, one of the following is incorrect:
   a. Sensitivity to heat
   b. Rapid heart rate
   c. Increased BMR
   d. Reduced TSH
9. Concerning calcium homeostasis by PTH, all of the following statements are true, *except*:
   a. It increases the resorption of bone
   b. It reduces renal clearance or excretion of calcium during hypocalcemia
   c. It acts upon the intestine to increase Ca^{2+} absorption
   d. It increases the renal phosphate clearance
10. Concerning the glucocorticoids all of the following statements are true, *except*:
    a. It stimulates glycolysis
    b. It has anti-inflammatory effect
    c. It prevents the rejection of transplanted organs
    d. It is used to control asthma
11. Cushing's syndrome:
    a. Results from deficiency of glucocorticoids
    b. Presents with low blood glucose

c. Is sensitive to infection
d. Patients have obesity
12. **Cohn's syndrome results from the deficiency of:**
   a. Elevated aldosterone
   b. Elevated cortisol
   c. Reduced mineralocorticoids
   d. Reduced dopamine
13. **Concerning the adrenal gland hormones, one of the following statements is incorrect:**
   a. They are derived from tyrosine
   b. They rise the blood pressure
   c. Elevated BMR
   d. Reduced ACTH secretion from the anterior pituitary
14. **Insulin:**
   a. Stimulates gluconeogenesis
   b. Is synthesized directly
   c. Inhibits lipolysis
   d. Increases the uptake of glucose from the peripheral cells
15. **Concerning the estrogen, all of the following are true, *except*:**
   a. Stimulates the mammary gland
   b. Increases the adipose tissue fat
   c. Participates in pregnancy if it occurs
   d. Broadens the pelvis
16. **All of the following are the adrenal gland hormones, *except*:**
   a. Epinephrine
   b. ADH
   c. Mineralocorticoids
   d. Glucocorticoids
17. **Which one of the following does not secret steroid hormones?**
   a. Ovary
   b. Testes
   c. Adrenal medulla
   d. Placenta
18. **Receptors within cell cytoplasm are specific to:**
   a. Peptide hormones
   b. Protein hormones
   c. Catecholamine
   d. Cortisol
19. **The maximum number of hormone-secreting cells of anterior pituitary is:**
   a. Thyrotrophs
   b. Corticotrophs
   c. Lactotrophs
   d. Somatotrophs
20. **Which of the following is rapid acting?**
   a. T4
   b. Thyroxine-binding globin
   c. T3
   d. Thyroglobulin
21. **In myxedema, serum findings are all, *except*:**
   a. Low T3, T4
   b. High TSH
   c. Low cholesterol
   d. Normal creatinine
22. **Conversion of vitamin D_3 to 1,25-dihydroxy-cholecalciferol occurs in:**
   a. Kidney
   b. Adrenal cortex
   c. Bone
   d. Intestine
23. **Thyroid hormone:**
   a. Decreases the absorption of carbohydrate from the intestine
   b. Exerts a positive feedback action on TSH production
   c. Indirectly increases the nitrogen excretion
   d. Has a does not have any action on the cardiac muscle
24. **Concerning aldosterone one of the following statements is incorrect:**
   a. Its deficiency results in hypotension
   b. Increases sodium reabsorption from urine
   c. Its release is stimulated by an increase in angiotensin II
   d. Is secreted by the zona fasciculata
25. **Concerning insulin all the following are true, *except*:**
   a. Stimulates glycolysis in liver
   b. Stimulates lipogenesis in liver and fat tissues
   c. Is synthesized in the endoplasmic reticulum of the β-cells
   d. Receptors are increased in the presence of uremia
26. **Calcitonin:**
   a. Is produced by the parafollicular cells outside the thyroid glands
   b. Is a steroid hormone
   c. Is decreased in the presence of hypercalcemia
   d. Increases incorporation of calcium into bone matrix
27. **Parathyroid hormone:**
   a. Is not a peptide hormone
   b. Is released in the response to hypocalcemia

c. Increases phosphate reabsorption in the kidneys
   d. Increases calcium excretion in the kidneys
28. Amyloidosis:
   a. The protein stained with eosin
   b. The deposition is intracellular
   c. Has a polymorphous structure
   d. Amyloid light-chain (AL) type is seen in 15% of patients with multiple myeloma

Answers

1. b	2. d	3. c	4. d	5. a
6. c	7. c	8. b	9. d	10. a
11. d	12. a	13. d	14. c	15. a
16. b	17. c	18. d	19. d	20. c
21. c	22. a	23. c	24. d	25. d
26. d	27. b	28. d		

CASE STUDIES

1. A patient presents with a blood pressure of 175/90 mm Hg, and complaints of tiredness and muscle weakness. The laboratory result reveals that plasma sodium is slightly increased and plasma potassium is significantly decreased compared to normal. Hematocrit is also low. Plasma renin activity is markedly decreased and serum aldosterone is increased. Which of the following is the most likely diagnosis?
   a. Addison's disease
   b. Conn's syndrome
   c. Cushing's syndrome
   d. Pheochromocytoma

   Answer is b: Conn's syndrome or primary hyperaldosteronism results from an adrenal tumor that secretes excessive aldosterone. The increased mineralocorticoid effects of aldosterone lead to renal sodium, water retention, and increased renal potassium excretion (hypokalemia). The volume expansion also explains the decrease in hematocrit. The increased blood volume, increased blood pressure, and hypernatremia will all tend to suppress renin secretion in an attempt to compensate for the increased aldosterone.

2. A 65-year-old woman presents to her physician prior to beginning chemotherapy for newly diagnosed small cell lung carcinoma. Her examination is notable for obesity, blood pressure of 170/100, facial hair, abdominal striae, and an acneiform rash on her chest and back. Laboratory values are normal except for serum glucose of 300 mg/dL. Her chest X-ray shows a right perihilar mass and severe diffuse osteoporosis. Which of the following accounts for her physical examination, laboratory and X-ray findings?
   a. Adrenal gland destruction by metastases
   b. Anterior pituitary gland disruption by metastases
   c. Ectopic production of PTH
   d. Ectopic production of ACTH

   Answer is d: This woman has all the classic findings of Cushing's syndrome such as obesity, hypertension, hirsutism, acne, striae, glucose intolerance, and osteoporosis. Cushing's syndrome may be caused by an excess production of cortisol by bilateral adrenal hyperplasia or an adrenal neoplasm; by excess production of ACTH by a pituitary adenoma; or by ectopic production of ACTH by a tumor, most commonly a small cell lung.

3. A 35-year-old woman with disseminated histoplasmosis complains of profound weakness, easy fatigability, anorexia, weight loss, and diarrhea. Laboratory investigation reveals serum sodium of 131 mEq/L, serum potassium of 5.8 mEq/L, and pH of 7.58. Skin hyperpigmentation is seen on physical examination. Which of the following is the most likely diagnosis?
   a. Primary adrenocortical insufficiency
   b. Conn's syndrome
   c. Cushing's syndrome
   d. Secondary adrenocortical insufficiency

   Answer is c: The evidences shown indicate that this patient has adrenal insufficiency due to diminished aldosterone production. The primary form of adrenocortical insufficiency results from any condition that destroys the adrenal cortex. Clinical manifestations of hypoaldosteronism appear when 90% of the adrenal cortex is destroyed. The most frequent form is due to an autoimmune process. The remaining cases are secondary to infections (such as tuberculosis or fungal infections) or metastatic disease involving both adrenals. Secondary adrenocortical insufficiency differs from the primary form:
   - It is caused by disorders affecting the pituitary gland or hypothalamus and leading to reduced ACTH production.

- It is not associated with skin hyperpigmentation. Skin hyperpigmentation results from increased production of ACTH precursor (which stimulates melanocytes), present in Addison's disease, but obviously lacking in secondary adrenocortical insufficiency.

4. A 50-year-old man is evaluated for congestive heart failure. In addition to a dilated cardiomyopathy, he displays multiple signs and symptoms, including intellectual function, fatigue, lethargy, cold intolerance, listlessness, thickened facial features, periorbital edema, dry and coarse skin, and peripheral edema. Serum studies demonstrate a T4 of 1.4 µg/dL and a TSH of 22 µU/mL. Which of the following diagnoses is supported by these data?
   a. Cretinism
   b. Graves' disease
   c. Hashimoto's thyroiditis
   d. Myxedema

Answer is d: The diagnosis of myxedema, due to long-standing hypothyroidism in adults, is warranted. The clinical manifestations are those listed in above with the question. Myxedema can result from the many causes of hypothyroidism such as Hashimoto's thyroiditis, idiopathic primary hypothyroidism, iodine deficiency, and drugs for pituitary lesions, hypothalamic lesions, and damage to the thyroid by surgery or radiation.

5. A 5-year-old female develops swelling in her neck and diarrhea. X-ray shows dense calcification in her thyroid. Physician asked her to have a nuclear scan and it showed a cold nodule that does not concentrate radioiodine. Her doctor does serum assays for several hormones. After the hormone is assayed, doctor tells her general practitioner that the patient probably has medullary carcinoma of the thyroid since one of the hormones is markedly raised. What hormone did the physician order?
   a. Calcitonin
   b. Thyroid-stimulating hormone
   c. Thyroid hormone
   d. Parathyroid hormone

Answer is a: Medullary thyroid cancer is a malignancy of the thyroid parafollicular cells. Thyroid parafollicular cells normally produce the hormone calcitonin. A malignancy of these cells, therefore, can also produce calcitonin. Assay of calcitonin is a very good diagnostic test for medullary carcinoma of the thyroid. TSH is an anterior pituitary hormone and is not produced by the thyroid gland at all.

6. A patient with small cell carcinoma of the lung complains of muscle weakness, fatigue, confusion, and weight gain. Serum sodium is found to be 115 mEq/L. Which of the following abnormal laboratory results would also be expected in this patient?
   a. Decreased plasma atrial natriuretic peptide concentration
   b. Decreased serum osmolarity
   c. Decreased urinary sodium concentration
   d. Increased plasma aldosterone concentration

Answer is b: Bronchogenic carcinomas can secrete ectopic vasopressin, i.e. ADH, leading to the syndrome of inappropriate ADH (SIADH). As long as water intake is not decreased, the increased plasma vasopressin causes excessive water reabsorption by the renal distal tubule and collecting duct. The increased total body water can explain the weight gain. Edema is usually absent because the extra free water is distributed to both intracellular and extracellular volumes. The extra plasma water produces a dilutional hyponatremia, which can explain the weakness, fatigue, and confusion. There will also be a dilutional decrease in serum osmolarity. With SIADH, the urine sodium is usually increased compared to normal. This leads to inappropriately concentrated urine. The volume expansion results from the excessive water retention, which may be responsible for the increased urinary sodium. Volume expansion would increase plasma atrial natriuretic peptide (ANP) and renal sodium excretion. The volume expansion would also inhibit renin secretion from the kidney with subsequent decrease in plasma aldosterone. Decreased plasma aldosterone would then allow for increased renal excretion of sodium.

7. A 48-year-old women presents with complaints of moderate weight loss over the past 4 months, heat intolerance, palpitations, and fine tremors in the hands. Physical examination reveals the presence of a diffuse goiter and exophthalmos. Which

of the following laboratory findings would be expected in this individual?
a. Decreased serum T4
b. Decreased resin T3 uptake
c. Increased plasma concentration of TSH
d. Increased plasma concentration of thyroglobulin

Answer is d: The abovementioned case is of an individual with Graves' disease. Hypersecretion of thyroid hormone because of stimulation of the TSH receptor by thyroid-stimulating immunoglobulins results in excessive movement of thyroglobulin from the colloid to the plasma. The presence of exophthalmos is thought to be part of the autoimmune disorder in Graves' disease. It is postulated that the thyroid and orbital muscles may share a common antigen.
Lymphocytic infiltration and inflammation of orbital muscle then produce the ophthalmopathy.

8. A 45-year-old man presents with the complaints of recurrent headaches. He also admits to impotence and loss of libido that has gradually worsened during the past year. Visual field examination reveals a bitemporal hemianopsia. Laboratory examination reveals an increase in serum prolactin, while serum LH and testosterone are decreased. Which of the following is the most likely diagnosis?
a. Idiopathic panhypopituitarism
b. Pituitary infarction
c. Prolactinoma
d. LH deficiency

Answer is d: Hyperprolactinemia is the most common hypothalamic-pituitary disorder. A tumor in the pituitary (prolactinoma) that secretes excessive prolactin is the most common functional pituitary tumor. The increase in serum prolactin suppresses the normal gonadotropin-releasing hormone (GnRH), gonadotropin-gonadal steroid axis. Hypogonadism, manifested as amenorrhea in females or loss of libido and/or impotence in males, is a prominent symptom. Blood levels of sex steroids are usually decreased. Although not present in this patient, galactorrhea may occur due to the action of prolactin on the mammary gland. Since the anterior pituitary is located just below the optic chiasm, space-filling tumors that compress this structure may produce visual field defects.

9. At 26 weeks of pregnancy, an unidentified infection greatly compromises the viability of a developing fetus. The level of which of the following hormones in the mother's blood is most likely to be affected?
a. Human chorionic gonadotropin
b. Human chorionic somatomammotropin
c. Progesterone
d. Estriol

Answer is d: Plasma levels of maternal estrogens during pregnancy are dependent on a functioning fetus. The fetal adrenal cortex and liver produce the weak androgens, dehydroepiandrosterone sulfate (DHEAS), and 16-hydroxydehydroepiandrosterone sulfate (16-OH DHEAS), which are carried to the placenta by the fetal circulation. The placenta then desulfates the androgens and aromatizes them to estrogens (16-OH DHEAS, estriol) prior to delivery to the maternal circulation. Both estradiol and estrone increase approximately 50-fold during pregnancy, whereas estriol increases about 1,000 fold. When estriol is assayed daily, a significant drop may be a sensitive early indicator of fetal jeopardy.

10. A patient with signs and symptoms consistent with hypothyroidism exhibits a decrease in both serum TSH and serum T4. Injection of TRH fails to produce the expected increase in TSH. Which of the following is the most likely cause of the patient's hypothyroidism?
a. Secondary hypothyroidism
b. Hashimoto's thyroiditis
c. Iodine deficiency
d. Tertiary hypothyroidism

Answer is a: A decrease in both serum T4 and TSH could result from either a pituitary defect or a hypothalamic defect. In the case of the hypothalamic defect, decreased secretion of TRH leads to decreased TSH secretion and, hence, decreased T4 secretion. In secondary hypothyroidism, a decrease in TSH secretion due to a pituitary defect is responsible for the decreased T4. The TRH stimulation test can be used to distinguish between these two possibilities. Failure of TSH to increase after injection of TRH indicates a pituitary defect.

CHAPTER 13

Acid-base Balance

OBJECTIVES

At the end of this chapter, students should be able to:
- List various buffer systems of our body playing their role in maintaining the acid-base status
- Understand the role of bicarbonate buffer system in maintaining the acid-base homeostasis
- Explain the renal and respiratory mechanism in regulating acid-base balance
- Understand the acid-base status in metabolic acidosis, metabolic alkalosis, respiratory acidosis, and respiratory alkalosis.

INTRODUCTION

- The human body can be described as a complex system, which consists of several levels and subsystems.
- At the chemical level, acids and bases are one of the essential compounds upon which all biochemical processes depend.
- The biochemical reactions taking place in our body are sensitive to even small changes in the acidity or alkalinity of the environment.
- The acid-base homeostasis should be maintained for cellular viability, enzymatic reactions, protein conformation, central nervous system (CNS) functions, etc.
- These functions are modified when there is change in the cellular and extracellular acid-base status. For these reactions, the acids and bases that are formed constantly should be kept in balance.

To understand acid-base homeostasis, a definition of some of the terms needed and are explained below.

Acids: Brønsted defined an acid as a chemical entity that donates protons in solution:

$$HCl \longleftrightarrow H^+ + Cl^-$$
$$H_2CO_3 \longleftrightarrow H^+ + HCO_3^-$$
$$NH_4 \longleftrightarrow H^+ + NH_3$$
$$H_2PO_4 \longleftrightarrow H^+ + HPO_4^-$$

Bases: Bases are those that accept protons.

pH: Sørenson expressed pH as the negative logarithm of hydrogen ion (H^+) concentration ($-\log [H^+]$).

Buffer: It is a solution that resists change in pH when acid or base is added. The effectiveness depends on its logarithm of K (pK) or (pKa). pK is the pH at which the buffer is 50% ionized, meaning that the acid concentration is exactly equal to that of the base conjugate. The buffer is very efficient at a pH of ±1 around its pK. For example, pK of phosphate buffer is 6.8. This buffer will have maximum buffer capacity between pH 5.8 and 7.8. A buffer solution is a mixture of a weak acid and its sodium (Na) or potassium (K) salt (base).

Henderson–Hasselbalch Equation

$$pH = pK_a + \log_{10}\left(\frac{[Base]}{[Acid]}\right)$$

The abovementioned equation indicates the relationship between the pH, pK of the buffer, and the ratio of conjugate base to the undissociated acid. It enables to relate

Acid-base Balance

quantitatively the changes in pH, [acid], and [base].

Hydrogen Ion Balance

- In a healthy individual, the normal pH of arterial blood is 7.4 ± 0.05 and that of venous blood is 7.4 ± 0.02.
- When the arterial pH increases above 7.45, then the individual is considered to have alkalosis, or if the pH is below 7.35, they considered to have acidosis.
- In a healthy subject, the pH of blood is always between 7.35 and 7.45. The change in pH leads to serious effects; therefore the control of pH is necessary.

Metabolic Acids

There are two types of metabolic acids such as fixed and volatile acids:
- Carbon dioxide (CO_2) is the volatile acid.
- Lactic acid, acetoacetic acid, β-hydroxybutyric acid, sulfuric acid (H_2SO_4), and phosphoric acid (H_3PO_4) are nonvolatile or fixed acids.
- Carbon dioxide is the major end product in the oxidation of carbohydrates, fats, and amino acids. It has the ability to react with water (H_2O) to form carbonic acid (H_2CO_3) and again they dissociate to H^+, and bicarbonate ion (HCO_3^-). The CO_2 can be regarded as an acid by virtue of its ability to react with H_2O to form H_2CO_3, which in turn can dissociate to form H^+ and HCO_3^-. In vivo, it is the carbonic anhydrase in tissues of liver and kidney, which catalyzes the following reaction either way depending on the blood pH:

$$CO_2 + H_2O \xleftrightarrow{\text{Carbonic anhydrase}} H_2CO_3$$

$$H_2CO_3 \xleftrightarrow{\text{Carbonic anhydrase}} H^+ + HCO_3^-$$

- The fixed acids H_2SO_4 and H_3PO_4 are the end product of sulfur-containing amino acids, phospholipids nucleic acids, phosphoproteins, and phosphoglycerides.
- Organic acids such as lactic acid and β-hydroxy butyric acids are formed during the metabolism of carbohydrates, and lipids.
- Accumulation of lactic acid is called lactic acidosis. Normally, lactic acid produced by the anaerobic glycolysis is taken up by the liver and converted to glucose through a Cori cycle.
- Pyruvate and lactate accumulate in conditions such as arsenic or mercury poisoning, and also in thiamine deficiency. Inherited enzyme pyruvate dehydrogenase deficiency also leads to lactic acidosis.

REGULATION OF ACID-BASE BALANCE

The pH of the plasma is 7.4 and is normally maintained within a narrow range from 7.35 to 7.45. Blood buffer system regulates small changes in acids or bases.

Next one is the respiratory system by increasing the expulsion of the CO_2 (hyperventilation) or by conservation of CO_2 (hypoventilation) regulates the blood pH. These two compensatory mechanisms cannot go longer, it is only temporary balance.

The renal system maintains acid-base balance of blood by adjusting the rate of reabsorption and excretion of H^+ or HCO_3^- or HPO_3^- in addition to formation, and excretion of ammonia (NH_3) and ammonium (NH_4^+).

BLOOD BUFFER SYSTEM

Describe the Regulation of pH of Blood by Buffers

The extracellular fluid (ECF) buffers are as follows:
- Bicarbonate buffer [carbonate bicarbonate—H_2CO_3/HCO_3^- (20:1)]
- Phosphate buffer [hydrogen phosphate (HPO_4)/dihydrogen phosphate ion ($H_2PO_4^-$) (4:1)]
- Basic/acidic proteins
- Organic base/organic acid.

Bicarbonate Buffer System

- The most important buffer system in the plasma is the bicarbonate and carbonate system.
- It accounts for 60% of buffering action in plasma and 40% in the whole body.
- The HCO_3^- level is regulated by the kidney; the acidic part of H_2CO_3 is under respiratory control.
- The buffer is most active when the ratio of salt and acid are equal according to the Henderson–Hasselbalch equation.
- The normal plasma bicarbonate level = 24 mmol/L, partial pressure of CO_2 (pCO_2) of arterial blood = 40 mm Hg, H_2CO_3 = 1.2 mmol/L, and the pKa of the H_2CO_3 is 6.1.
- Substituting these values in Henderson–Hasselbalch equation, one gets:

$$pH = pK_a + \log_{10}\left(\frac{[Base]}{[Acid]}\right)$$

$$pH \text{ of blood} = 6.1 + \log_{10}\left(\frac{[HCO_3^-]}{[H_2CO_3]}\right)$$

$$7.4 = 6.1 + \log [24]/[1.2]$$
$$= 6.1 + \log 20 \text{ (antilog of 20 is 1.3)}$$
$$= 6.1 + 1.3$$

So, the ratio between HCO_3^- and H_2CO_2 is 20:1, i.e. $HCO_3^-:H_2CO_2$ is 20:1.

Therefore the ratio of HCO_3^- to H_2CO_3 at pH 7.4 is 20 in normal conditions. The bicarbonate represents the alkali reserve and it is sufficient to meet the acid load. During the compensation if HCO_3^- is 24, then H_2CO_3 is adjusted to 1.2. This is how compensatory mechanism operates to bring the ratio back to 20:1.

Whenever metabolic acid is added to the blood, it reacts with the basic component of the buffer system producing salt, water and helps to prevent the fall in blood pH. Reversal of this mechanism takes place in the event of addition of base by metabolic processes.

Mechanism

- When a strong acid, e.g. HCl is added to the bicarbonate buffer solution, the increased hydrogen ions are buffered by HCO_3^-. This results in more H_2CO_3 formation and this in turn leads to more production of CO_2, and H_2O:

$$HCl \rightarrow H^+ + Cl^-$$
$$HCO_3^- + H^+ \rightarrow H_2CO_3$$
$$H_2CO_3 \rightarrow CO_2 + H_2O$$

- The net result is stimulation of respiration by CO_2 and this respiration tries to eliminate this CO_2 from the ECF.
- The opposite reaction takes place when a strong base such as sodium hydroxide (NaOH) is added to the bicarbonate buffer system. In this case, the hydroxyl ions (OH–) released combines with H_2CO_3 to form additional HCO_3^-. The sodium bicarbonate ($NaHCO_3$) replaces the strong base NaOH. At the same time, concentration of H_2CO_3 decreases because it reacts with NaOH causing more CO_2 to combine with H_2O to replace H_2CO_3:

$$NaOH \longrightarrow Na^+ + OH^- + H_2CO_3$$

$$\xrightarrow{\text{Carbonic anhydrase}} NaHCO_3 + H_2O$$

$$CO_2 + H_2O \xleftrightarrow{\text{Carbonic anhydrase}} H_2CO_3$$

- The decreased CO_2 concentration in the blood inhibits respiration and decreases the rate of CO_2 removal through respiration. The rise in blood HCO_3^- is compensated by increased renal excretion of HCO_3^-. The bicarbonate is considered as the alkali reserve because any stronger acid than H_2CO_3 is buffered by bicarbonate as long as any bicarbonate is present in the blood.

Phosphate Buffer System

Phosphate is the main intracellular buffer. The pKa value, 6.8 is nearer to the physiological pH 7.4. When equation is applied:

$$pH = pK_a + \log_{10}\left(\frac{[Base]}{[Acid]}\right)$$

$$7.4 = 6.8 + \log_{10}\left(\frac{[Base]}{[Acid]}\right)$$

$$\log\frac{[4]}{[1]}$$

$7.4 = 6.8 + \log_4$ (antilog of 4 is 0.6)

$7.4 = 6.8 + 0.6$

Therefore the ratio is 4:1.

The phosphate buffer system is effective at wide range of pH because of the more ionizable groups. It has different pK_a values:

$H_3PO_4 \xrightarrow{pK_a = 1.96} H^+ + H_2PO_4^-$

$H_2PO_4^- \xrightarrow{pK_a = 6.8} H^+ + HPO_4^-$

$HPO_4^- \xrightarrow{pK_a = 12.4} H^+ + PO_4^{2-}$

The disodium phosphate (Na_2HPO_4)/monosodium phosphate ($NaH_2PO_4^-$) is an effective buffer system in the human body because of its pK_a value nearer to the physiological pH.

Protein Buffer System

The buffering action of proteins mainly depends on the pK_a value of its ionizable side chains. The effective group is histidine with a pK_a value of 6.1. Therefore the albumin and hemoglobin (Hb) with more histidine residues play an important role in buffering action in the body.

Action of Hemoglobin Buffer in the Regulation of Blood pH

- Hb releases H^+ in the lungs when it gets oxygenated because the oxygenated from Hb is a stronger acid than deoxygenated Hb. This decreases the bicarbonate level and increases the H_2CO_3, and its anhydride CO_2, thus increasing pCO_2 of the blood.
- The lungs eliminate this increased pCO_2 through the elimination of CO_2 from the blood and bring back the ratio of HCO_3^- : H_2CO_3 to 20.
- Deoxy Hb neutralizes H_2CO_3 to raise the pH and causes an increase in the bicarbonate level, and a decrease in pCO_2. Some of the H^+ ions are bound by the deoxygenated Hb and the rest are bound by the proteins, and phosphate buffer in the plasma. Because all the H^+ ions formed are buffered, there is no change in the pH. This type of H^+ ion buffering action is called isohydric shift.
- The HCO_3^- formed in erythrocyte as a result of H^+ ion uptake diffuses out of the cells into the plasma in exchange for Cl^-, which diffuses into the red blood cell (RBC) from the plasma. This increase in Cl^- is termed "chloride shift." This chloride will come out of the RBC when CO_2 comes out of lungs **(Fig. 13.1)**.

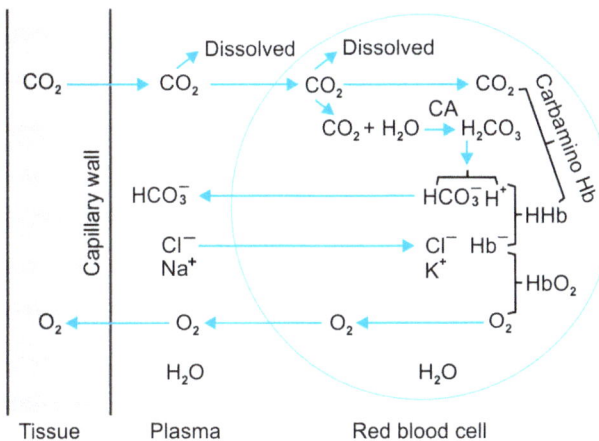

Fig. 13.1: Hemoglobin buffer system.
(CA: carbonic anhydrase)

ROLE OF RESPIRATORY AND RENAL MECHANISM IN REGULATING THE BLOOD PH

Respiratory Regulation of Acid-base Balance

- The second line of defense against acid-base disturbance is the control of CO_2 by the lungs by increasing or decreasing.
- The rate of respiration is known to be controlled by the receptors in the respiratory center, which are sensitive to changes in pH and pCO_2 of blood. When there is a fall in pH of plasma, the respiratory center is stimulated resulting in hyperventilation, which eliminates more CO_2 thus lowering H_2CO_3 concentration in blood. If the blood pH increases, the respiratory center is inhibited so that elimination of CO_2 is decreased by hypoventilation till the blood pH comes to normal.
- The Hb transports CO_2 formed in the tissues and also it serves to generate bicarbonate or alkali reserve by the activity of carbonic anhydrase system.

Renal Regulation of pH

An important function of kidney is to regulate the function by excreting either acidic or basic urine. The pH of urine ranges from 4.5 to 9.5 because the renal system plays a significant role in long-term pH maintenance of the blood at 7.4 ± 0.05. This is possible by its capacity of reabsorption, secretion, and excretion of the nonvolatile acids, e.g. lactic acid; lungs cannot excrete pyruvic acid, and inorganic acid, hydrochloric acid (HCl), H_3PO_4, and H_2SO_4, which are produced in the body. The first mechanism for removal of acids from the body is by renal excretion. The major mechanism by which the kidney regulates the level of HCO^- in plasma is reabsorption of filtered HCO_3^-, generation of new HCO_3^-, and by secreting HCO_3^- under condition of chronic alkalosis.

The filtered HCO_3^- combined with H^+ forming H_2CO_3, carbonic anhydrase presents in the brush border of the cell wall dissociate H_2CO_3 into H_2O and CO_2. The CO_2 diffuses into the cell; in the cell carbonic anhydrase again ionizes H_2CO_3 into HCO_3^- and H^+. It is secreted into the lumen in exchange for Na^+ and HCO_3^- and is reabsorbed into plasma along with Na^+. There is no net excretion of H^+ or generation of new HCO_3^-, so this mechanism helps to maintain a steady state of acid-base balance **(Fig. 13.2)**.

Another function of the kidney is to buffer acids and thus to conserve fixed base is through the production of NH_3 from amino acids with the help of an enzyme glutaminase. Whenever there is excess acid production, the NH_3 production is also increased, which combines with H^+ to form NH^+, which is excreted as ammonium chloride (NH_4Cl). This occurs in the event of acidosis. When alkali is in excess, H^+ is reabsorbed into the cell in exchange to Na^+/K^+.

Compensation

The body acid-base balance is tightly regulated. Several buffering agents exist, which reversibly bind H^+ ion and slow down any change in pH. Extracellular buffers include HCO_3 and NH_3, while proteins and phosphate act as intracellular buffers. The bicarbonate buffering system is especially key, as CO_2 can be shifted through H_2CO_3 and HCO_3^- as given below:

$$HCO_3^- + H^+ \longleftrightarrow H_2CO_3 \longleftrightarrow CO_2 + H_2O$$

Acid-base imbalances that overcome the buffer system can be compensated in the short term by changing the rate of ventilation. This alters the concentration of CO_2 in the blood. For instance, if the blood pH drops too low (acidemia), the body will compensate by increasing breathing, expelling CO_2.

The kidneys are slower to compensate, but renal physiology has several powerful mechanisms to control pH by the excretion of

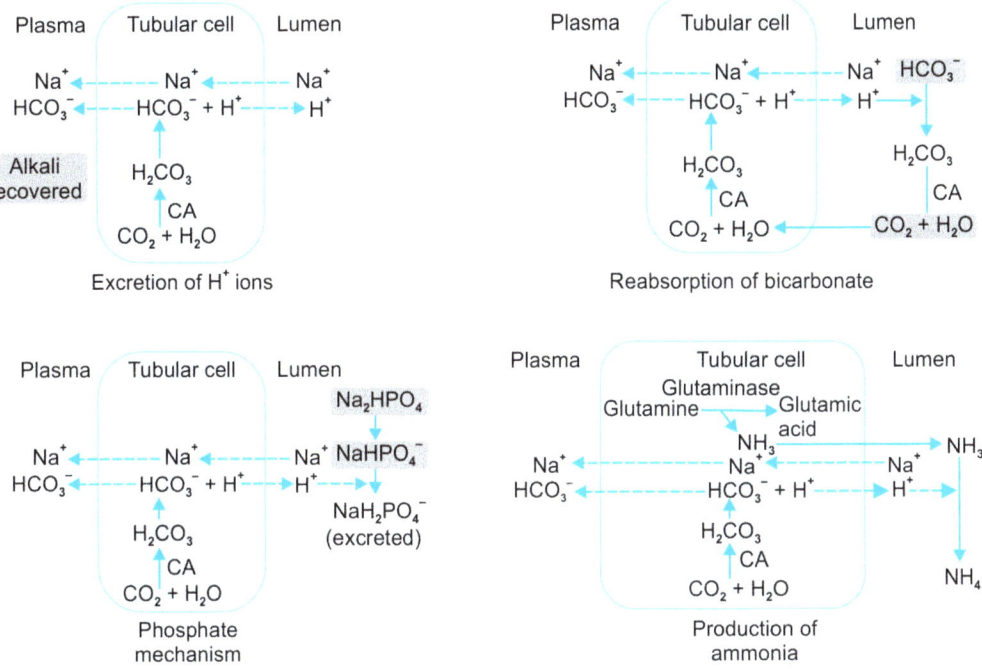

Fig. 13.2: Role of kidney in the regulation of acid-base balance.
(CA: carbonic anhydrase)

excess acid or base. In responses to acidosis, tubular cells reabsorb more HCO_3 from the tubular fluid, collecting duct cells secrete more hydrogen and generating more HCO_3, and ammoniagenesis leads to increased formation of the NH_3 buffer. In responses to alkalosis, the kidney may excrete more HCO_3 by decreasing H^+ ion secretion from the tubular epithelial cells and lowering rates of glutamine metabolism, and NH_3 excretion.

ACID-BASE DISORDERS

- Acid-base disorders result from a variety of pathological conditions. If the pH is more than the normal range, it is termed "alkalemia" and pH lesser than the normal range, it is called acidemia, and the conditions are called alkalosis and acidosis, respectively.

- There are two reasons for the pH abnormalities in blood, which are metabolic or respiratory causes. Metabolic causes are responsible for metabolic acidosis and alkalosis. The respiratory causes are responsible for respiratory acidosis and respiratory alkalosis.
- Laboratory findings in acid-base disturbances are detailed in **Table 13.1**.

Metabolic Acid-base Disorders

Metabolic Acidosis (HCO_3 Deficit or Fall in pH)

- Metabolic acidosis is the most common acid-base disturbance **(Fig. 13.3)**.
- In this condition, the HCO^- concentration is reduced. This is due to the increased production of acids. These acids dissociate

Table 13.1: Laboratory findings in acid-base disturbances.

Acid-base conditions	pH	pCO_2	HCO_3^-	HCO_3^-/H_2CO_3
Normal	7.4 ± 0.05	40 mm Hg	20 mm Hg	20
Metabolic acidosis	Decreased	Normal	Decreased	Decreased
Metabolic alkalosis	Increased	Normal	Increased	Increased
Respiratory acidosis	Decreased	Increased	Normal	Decreased
Respiratory alkalosis	Increased	Decreased	Increased	Increased

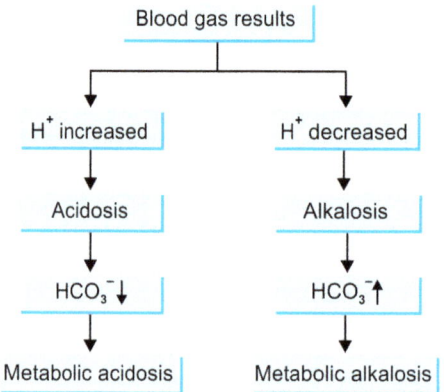

Fig. 13.3: Metabolic acidosis and alkalosis.

to give H⁺ ions, which are buffered by HCO_3^-.
- Metabolic acidosis is also due to ingestion of acids, e.g. NH_4Cl. The ammonia part after detoxified leaves behind the H⁺.
- It also occurs in diarrhea, which leads to loss of HCO_3^- from the intestinal fluid.
- The primary compensatory mechanism in metabolic acidosis is through hyperventilation that removes CO_2 and the deep, rapid, and gasping respiratory pattern is known as Kussmaul breathing.
- There is also elimination of acids in the urine and the urinary ammonia is also increased. For example:
  $[HCO_3^-]$ = 15 mEq/L, pCO_2 = 1.2 mEq/L
  $pH = pK_a + \log[HCO_3^-]/[pCO_2]$
     = 6.1 + log[15]/[1.2]
     = 6.1 + log 12.5
     = 6.1 + 1.2 = 7.3 (antilog of 12.5 is 1.2).

Causes

- Uncontrolled diabetes mellitus.
- *Lactic acidosis:* This results from a number of causes, particularly tissue anoxia. In acute hypoxia condition such as respiratory failure or cardiac arrest, lactic acidosis develops immediately. Lactic acidosis may also be caused by liver disease. The presence of lactic acidosis can be determined by plasma lactate.
- *Diabetic ketoacidosis*: It is a metabolic state associated with high concentrations of ketone bodies formed by the breakdown of fatty acids and the deamination of amino acids due to lack of insulin. The two common ketones produced in humans are acetoacetic acid and β-hydroxybutyrate. Ketoacidosis is most common in untreated type 1 diabetes mellitus, when the liver breaks down fat and proteins in response to a perceived need for respiratory substrate.
- Chronic renal failure (accumulation of sulfates, phosphates, and urea).
- *Intoxication*: It is as follows:
  - Organic acids [salicylates, ethanol, methanol, formaldehyde, ethylene glycol, paraldehyde, and isoniazid (INH)]
  - Sulfates and metformin (Glucophage).

Metabolic Alkalosis (HCO_3^- Excess or Rise in pH)

- This condition occurs due to the gain of more HCO_3^- **(Fig. 13.3)**.

- This occurs in:
  - Vomiting (loss of gastric HCl)
  - Ingestion of bicarbonate in the treatment of peptic ulcer
  - *Potassium depletion*: Hypokalemic alkalosis is caused by the kidneys response to an extreme lack or loss of potassium, which can occur when people take certain diuretic medications.
- The compensatory mechanism is through hypoventilation to prevent CO_2 loss. CO_2 is then consumed toward the formation of the H_2CO_3 intermediate, thus decreasing pH.
- The secondary compensatory mechanism by increasing the excretion of HCO_3^- by kidneys. For example:
  $[HCO_3^-] = 36$ mEq/L, $pCO_2 = 1.2$ mEq/L
  $pH = pK_a + \log [HCO_3^-]/[pCO_2]$
  $= 6.1 + \log [36]/[1.2]$
  $= 6.1 + \log 30$
  $= 6.1 + 1.45 = 7.55.$

Respiratory Acid-base Disorders

Respiratory Acidosis (Excess CO_2)

- The retention of CO_2 leads to change in HCO_3^- (**Fig. 13.4**).
- The ratio of $[HCO_3^-]:[CO_2]$ decreases.
- This is caused by hypoventilation, which occurs due to an obstruction of respiration, i.e. in pneumonia, emphysema, asthma, and depression of the respiratory centers in morphine bicarbonate poisoning, and alcohol ingestion.
- The primary compensatory mechanism is reabsorption of HCO_3^- from the kidney. For example:
  $[HCO_3^-] = 27$ mEq/L, $pCO_2 = 1.8$ mEq/L
  $pH = pKa + \log [HCO_3^-]/[pCO_2]$
  $= 6.1 + \log [27]/[1.8]$
  $= 6.1 + \log 15$
  $= 6.1 + 1.17 = 7.27.$

Respiratory Alkalosis (CO_2 Deficit)

- Respiratory alkalosis is caused by hyperventilation that leads to reduced concentration of CO_2 (**Fig. 13.4**).

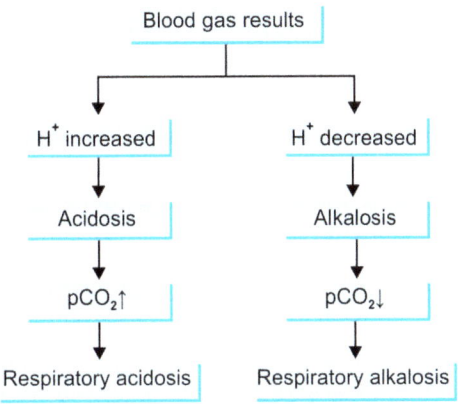

Fig. 13.4: Respiratory acidosis and alkalosis.

- The HCO_3^- level also slightly varies.
- This occurs when respiration is stimulated as in fever, hot bath, lack of oxygen at high altitude, and increased environmental temperature.
- Compensatory mechanism is by increasing the excretion of HCO_3^- by kidney. For example:
  $[HCO_3^-] = 27$ mEq/L, $pCO_2 = 0.68$ mEq/L
  $pH = pK_a + \log [HCO_3^-]/[pCO_2]$
  $= 6.1 + \log [27]/[0.68]$
  $= 6.1 + \log 39.7$
  $= 6.1 + 1.6 = 7.7.$

Mixed Acid-base Disorders

Mixed acid-base disorders occur when there is more than one primary acid-base disturbance present simultaneously. They are frequently seen in hospitalized patients, particularly in the critically ill. Mixed acid-base disorder occurs when:

- The expected compensatory response does not occur.
- Compensatory response occurs, but level of compensation is inadequate or too extreme.
- Whenever the pCO_2 and $[HCO_3^-]$ becomes abnormal in the opposite direction (i.e. one is elevated, while the other is reduced). In simple acid-base disorders, the direction of the compensatory response is always

the same as the direction of the initial abnormal change.
- pH is normal, but pCO_2 or HCO_3^- is abnormal.
- In anion gap metabolic acidosis, if the change in bicarbonate level is not proportional to the change of the anion gap. More specifically, if the delta ratio is greater than 2 or less than 1.
- In simple acid-base disorders, the compensatory response should never return the pH to normal. If that happens, suspect a mixed disorder.

Mixed acid-base disorders usually produce arterial blood gas results that could potentially be explained by other mixed disorders. Oftentimes, the clinical picture will help to distinguish. It is important to distinguish mixed acid-base disorders because management will depend on accurate diagnosis.

Types

- Chronic respiratory acidosis with super-imposed acute respiratory acidosis:
  - Acute exacerbation of chronic obstructive pulmonary disease (COPD) secondary to acute pneumonia
  - The COPD patient with worsening hypoventilation secondary to oxygen therapy or sedative administration.
- Chronic respiratory acidosis and anion gap metabolic acidosis:
  - The COPD patient, who develops shock and lactic acidosis.
- Chronic respiratory acidosis and metabolic alkalosis:
  - Pulmonary insufficiency and diuretic therapy.
  - The COPD patient treated with steroids or ventilation (important to recognize as alkalemia will reduce acidemic stimulus to breathe).
- Respiratory alkalosis and metabolic acidosis:
  - Salicylate intoxication
  - Gram-negative sepsis
  - Acute cardiopulmonary arrest
  - Severe pulmonary edema.

Anion Gap and the Clinical Significance of Measuring it

Anion Gap

- The sum of cations and anions in ECF is always equal so as to maintain the electrical neutrality.
- The 95% of the cations were maintained by Na^+ and K^+.
- Chloride and HCO_3^- account for 86% of anions.
- These are the commonly measured electrolytes and hence there is a difference between cations and anions.
- The difference between cations and anions or the unmeasured anions constitutes the anion gap, which is due to the presence of phosphorus, SO_4^{2-}, phosphate (PO_4^{3-}), and organic acid salts.
- The difference between Na^+ and K^+, and Cl^- and HCO_3^- is normally about 12 ± 5 mEq/L (mmol/L).
- Measurement of anion gap is extremely useful in the clinical assessment with acid-base disorders.

ASSESSMENT OF ACID-BASE ANALYSIS

The blood gas analyzers, which measure pH, pCO_2 and partial pressure of oxygen (pO_2) by means of electrodes is usually used to measure acid-base parameters of arterial blood (**Fig. 13.5**). Heparinized blood is collected and directly introduced into the analyzer. The blood should be analyzed within 20 minutes of collection. There should not be any contact of collected blood with the external air either during collection or analysis.

Procedure

- Usually, blood is taken from an artery. The blood may be collected from the radial

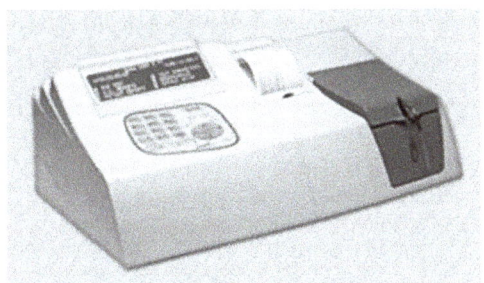

Fig. 13.5: Blood gas analyzer.

artery in the wrist, the femoral artery in the groin or the brachial artery in the arm.
- The health-care provider will insert a small needle through the skin into the artery. You can choose to have numbing medicine (anesthesia) applied to the site before the test begins.
- After the blood is taken, pressure is applied to the site for a few minutes to stop the bleeding. The health-care provider will watch the site for signs of bleeding or circulation problems.
- The sample must be quickly sent to a laboratory for analysis to ensure accurate results.
- There is no special preparation. If you are on oxygen therapy, the oxygen concentration must remain constant for 20 minutes before the test.
- The test is used to evaluate respiratory diseases and conditions that affect the lungs. It helps to determine the effectiveness of oxygen therapy. The test also provides information about the body acid-base balance, which can reveal important clues about lung and kidney function, and the body general metabolic state.
- In the absence of blood gas analyzer, venous blood may be collected under paraffin. Bicarbonate is estimated by titration to pH 7.4. If acid-base disturbance is suspected, the electrolytes should also be estimated. From the values of electrolytes and bicarbonate, the anion gap is calculated.

SUMMARY

The human body is a complex system, which consists of several levels and subsystems. At the chemical level, acids and bases are one of the essential compounds upon, which all biochemical processes depend. The acid-base homeostasis should be maintained for cellular viability, enzymatic reactions, protein conformation, CNS functions, etc. These functions are modified when there is change in the cellular and extracellular acid-base status. Carbonate-bicarbonate buffer, phosphate buffer and protein buffer (Hb) are the major buffer systems of our body, which helps to maintain the acid-base balance. The respiratory system also participates in the regulation of acid-base balance whenever there is a change in the acid-base concentration, either by eliminating or retaining CO_2. Kidney plays an important role in the regulation of acid-base concentration by excreting, either acidic or basic urine. Metabolic acidosis and alkalosis are the two acid-base disorders whenever there is a disturbance in the metabolism. Hypo- or hyperventilation causes respiratory acidosis and alkalosis.

SELF-ASSESSMENT QUESTIONS

1. Name the blood buffer systems.
2. Briefly discuss the bicarbonate buffer system to show how it helps to regulate the blood pH.
3. Explain the regulation of blood pH through renal mechanism.
4. Discuss the various acid-base disorders. Mention the causes and findings of each disorder.
5. Mention the laboratory findings of metabolic acidosis and respiratory alkalosis.
6. What is metabolic alkalosis and respiratory acidosis?

MULTIPLE-CHOICE QUESTIONS

1. **Concerning acid-base balance one of the following statements is incorrect:**
   a. Blood buffer system helps in maintaining the acid-base balance
   b. Respiratory system regulates the blood pH through expulsion of CO_2
   c. Renal mechanism regulates the pH through the absorption or excretion of H^+
   d. Carbon dioxide and bicarbonate buffer system is first mechanism, which regulates blood pH

2. **The buffering action of protein mainly depends on the:**
   a. pKa value of its ionizable side chains of histidine
   b. pKa value of tyrosine
   c. Basic amino acid content
   d. Neutral amino acid content

3. **Concerning renal regulation of acid-base balance, one of the following statements is incorrect:**
   a. Reabsorption of filtered HCO_3^-
   b. Generation of new HCO_3^-
   c. Generation of H^+
   d. Excretion of H^+

4. **Metabolic acidosis occurs in all the following conditions, *except*:**
   a. Vomiting
   b. Uncontrolled diabetes mellitus
   c. Starvation
   d. Severe exercises

5. **Deficit of HCO_3^- results in:**
   a. Metabolic alkalosis
   b. Metabolic acidosis
   c. Respiratory acidosis
   d. Respiratory alkalosis

6. **Respiratory acidosis results from:**
   a. Excess CO_2
   b. Excess HCO_3
   c. Excess H^+
   d. Excess H_2CO_3

7. **All of the following are the laboratory findings of metabolic alkalosis, *except*:**
   a. pH increased
   b. pCO_2 decreased
   c. HCO_3^- increased
   d. HCO_3/H_2CO_3 decreased

8. **In uncompensated metabolic alkalosis:**
   a. The plasma pH, the plasma HCO_3 concentration, and the arterial pCO_2 are all low
   b. The plasma pH is high and the plasma HCO_3^- concentration and arterial pCO_2 are low
   c. The plasma pH and the plasma HCO_3^- concentration are low, and the arterial pCO_2 is normal
   d. The plasma pH and the plasma HCO_3^- concentration are high, and the arterial pCO_2 is normal

9. **Concerning angiotensin II, one of the following statements is false:**
   a. It is produced from angiotensin I in the lungs
   b. It is a vasoconstrictor
   c. It stimulates aldosterone secretion
   d. It is a decapeptide

10. **One of the following is a recognized cause of metabolic acidosis with increased anion gap:**
    a. Diabetic ketoacidosis
    b. High fat diet
    c. Hyperparathyroidism
    d. Diarrhea

11. **Concerning metabolic acidosis, all of the following statement are true, *except*:**
    a. Caused by severe diarrhea is associated with a normal anion gap
    b. Caused by renal tubular acidosis is associated with a normal anion gap
    c. Caused by lactic acidosis is associated with an increase in the anion gap
    d. Caused by diabetic ketoacidosis is associated with a decrease in the anion gap

12. **The metabolism of the following amino acids results in the production of acids:**
    a. Histidine   b. Aspartate
    c. Glutamate   d. Alanine

13. **Respiratory alkalosis:**
    a. Occurs in hyperventilation
    b. Occurs in normal pregnancy
    c. Does not occur in type I respiratory failure
    d. May occur in type II respiratory failure

14. **A 19-year-old man has the following arterial blood results:**
    pH = 7.50
    pH = 7.50
    pCO_2 = 48 mm Hg
    $[HCO_3^-]$ = 37 mM
    Oxygen saturation = 98% on air
    His plasma potassium concentration is 2.5 mM:

a. There is a respiratory alkalosis
b. There is a metabolic alkalosis
c. His urine is likely to be alkaline
d. Pulmonary embolism is a likely diagnosis

15. Concerning renal regulation of acid-base balance, one of the following statements is false:
a. Ammonium ions are mainly produced in the loop of Henle
b. Glutamine metabolism by the kidneys results in bicarbonate production
c. Ammonia production by the kidneys is increased in acidosis
d. Secreted hydrogen ions are buffered by the phosphate buffer system in tubular fluid

16. Arterial blood gas analysis from a 20-year-old woman shows:
pH = 7.36
pCO_2 = 32 mm Hg [HCO^-] = 17 mM
Oxygen saturation = 99% on air:
a. Pulmonary embolism is a likely diagnosis
b. She is acidotic
c. Aspirin overdose is a possible diagnosis
d. The anion gap is likely to be decreased

17. Which of the following statement is false with respect to the bicarbonate buffer system?
a. Within extracellular fluid is made up of H_2CO_3 and sodium bicarbonate
b. Within intracellular fluid is made up of H_2CO_3 and potassium bicarbonate
c. The majority of H_2CO_3 exists as dissolved carbon dioxide
d. The pH is proportional to the logarithm of the bicarbonate ion concentration

18. With respect to acid-base status, the:
a. pH is calculated from (logarithm of hydrogen ion concentration)
b. pH of arterial blood is 7.35
c. pH of venous blood is 7.4
d. pH of interstitial fluid is 7.35

19. Respiratory acidosis:
a. Occurs in type I respiratory failure
b. If chronic, is associated with a fall in plasma bicarbonate concentration
c. Occurs in chronic bronchitis
d. Is associated with a high arterial pO_2

20. The following are recognized causes of metabolic acidosis with a normal anion gap:
a. Salicylate poisoning
b. Starvation
c. Diarrhea
d. Pancreatic secretion

21. A 36-year-old woman has the following arterial blood gas results:
pH = 7.33
[HCO^-] = 16 mM
pCO_2 = 30 mm Hg:
a. Pulmonary embolism is a likely diagnosis
b. She has a respiratory acidosis
c. She has a metabolic acidosis
d. There is a respiratory compensation to a metabolic acidosis

22. Concerning acid-base balance:
a. The plasma proteins represent the major extracellular buffer
b. The normal range for the plasma pH
c. The normal range for the plasma bicarbonate is 30–34 mmol/L
d. Most of the hydrogen that is excreted in the urine is in the form of free H^+ ions

Answers

1. d	2. a	3. c	4. a	5. b
6. a	7. d	8. d	9. d	10. a
11. d	12. a	13. a	14. b	15. a
16. c	17. d	18. d	19. c	20. c
21. c	22. b			

CASE STUDIES

1. A 30-year-old drug addict is found unconscious in a valley with an empty syringe beside. When victim blood gases are checked, which of the following would be expected?
a. Metabolic acidosis
b. Metabolic alkalosis
c. Respiratory acidosis
d. Respiratory alkalosis

Answer is c: Respiratory acidosis
Opioids, such as heroin, depress respiration centrally by reducing the responsiveness of brainstem respiratory centers to CO_2. The resulting hypoventilation leads to CO_2 retention because of the inability of the patient to "blow off" the CO_2. This increases the production of H_2CO_3 by carbonic anhydrase present in RBCs (which converts CO_2 to H_2CO_3). Dissociation of H_2CO_3 to bicarbonate and protons produces a respiratory acidosis.

2. Arterial blood gases (ABG) were obtained twice on the day of birth and 2 days later with the following results:
Day of birth: Serum bicarbonate 24 mEq/L.

	Day 1 (63% O_2 by hood)	Day 2	Day 3 (25% O_2)
pO_2	107	63	57
pCO_2	48	45	36
pH	7.35	7.37	7.44

a. What is the infant's initial acid-base status?
b. What does a comparison of the second day-1 measurement with the day-3 measurement suggest?
c. What clinical conditions could produce this pattern?

Initially it is respiratory acidosis
The pH is acidotic and the pCO_2 is greater than 40 mm Hg, indicating that the lung has retained acid in the body, and is at least a partial cause for the acidosis. The serum bicarbonate is 24, indicating that the kidney has not had time to compensate for the respiratory problem.

Pulmonary shunt may be present
The important thing to notice here is that the oxygen level in inspired air was dropped by more than half between the second specimen on day 1 and day 3, with essentially no change in the blood pO_2. If the pO_2 of 63 were due to a selective block in oxygen transfer [ventilation perfusion (VQ) mismatch or pulmonary fibrosis], decreasing the oxygen content of the inspired air should have dramatically affected pO_2.
Remember that shunts normally do not affect pCO_2 unless they are very large, because the lung has a lot of excess capacity to remove CO_2. Thus in this case where CO_2 retention is occurring, we would be postulating a very big shunt. Shunts might be produced in this setting by:
- Large cardiac defects
- Pulmonary vascular defects
- Lung tissue that is perused but not ventilated.

3. A 40-year-old woman was admitted to the hospital for evaluation. Her evaluation at admission including ABG obtained before, during, and after an exercise stress test, showed the following results:
   a. Serum bicarbonate: 27 mEq/L
   b. Arterial blood gases:

	At rest	During exercise	Rest/oxygen
pO_2	91	67	541
pCO_2	32	37	29
pH	7.46	7.41	7.49

Respiratory alkalosis
The pH is alkalotic and the pCO_2 is below 40 mm Hg indicating that the lung is producing the alkalosis by removing acid (CO_2) from the body. Interestingly, the bicarbonate concentration of 27 mEq/L is slightly higher than the normal of 24 mEq/L. This indicates that there is no renal response to the respiratory alkalosis. Perhaps the current alkalosis is partly triggered by stress or nervousness in the patient and his/her usual resting pH is nearer normal. Also note that the patient's pO_2 is adequate, indicating that the lungs can keep up with the body's oxygen demand, but it is probably lower than it should be for the patient's level of respiration.
Exercise uncovers patient basic defect in oxygen transfer by increasing the body's demand for oxygen. Under these conditions, the lungs cannot keep up with the oxygen demand and the pO_2 drops to 67 mm Hg. These results suggest VQ mismatch or pulmonary fibrosis. Other causes for hypoxemia do not really fit patient pattern. The patient's hypoxia corrects with oxygen, which would not occur if a shunt was present. Note that the patient's pCO_2 is still quite low (29 mm Hg), indicating that he/she is still breathing rapidly. Patient probably had not been on oxygen long when this sample was drawn.

CHAPTER 14

Biological Oxidation

OBJECTIVES

At the end of this chapter, students should be able to:
- Understand transport of reducing equivalents across mitochondria
- Know about the electron transport chain (ETC) organization and its components
- Explain the oxidative phosphorylation and chemiosmotic theory
- List the inhibitors of ETC and oxidative phosphorylation
- Know about the uncouplers and their significance.

INTRODUCTION

Oxidation-reduction Reactions

- Oxidation-reduction (redox) reactions are coupled chemical reactions in which one atom or molecule loses one or more electrons (oxidation), while another atom or molecule gains those electrons (reduction).
- The compound that loses electrons becomes oxidized.
- The compound that gains those electrons becomes reduced.
- In covalent compounds, however, it is usually easier to lose a whole hydrogen (H) atom; a proton and an electron rather than just an electron.
- An oxidation reaction during which both a proton and an electron are lost is called dehydrogenation.
- A reduction reaction during which both a proton and an electron are gained is called hydrogenation.

- The large quantity of reduced form of nicotinamide adenine dinucleotide (NADH) resulting from tricarboxylic acid (TCA) cycle activity can be used for reductive biosynthesis.
- The reducing potential of mitochondrial NADH is most often used to supply the energy for adenosine triphosphate (ATP) synthesis via oxidative phosphorylation.
- The oxidation of NADH with phosphorylation of adenosine diphosphate (ADP) to form ATP is a process supported by the mitochondrial electron transport assembly and ATP synthase, which are integral protein complexes of the inner mitochondrial membrane.
- The electron transport assembly comprised a series of protein complexes that catalyze sequential oxidation reduction reactions; some of these reactions are thermodynamically competent to support ATP production via ATP synthase provided a coupling mechanism, such as a common intermediate, is available. Proton translocation and the development of a transmembrane proton gradient provide the required coupling mechanism.

Principles of Redox Reactions

- Redox reactions involve the transfer of electrons from one chemical species to another.
- An example of a coupled redox reaction is the oxidation of NADH by the ETC.

$NADH + ½O + H^+ \rightarrow NAD^+ + HO$

- The description of ATP synthesis through oxidation of reduced electron carriers indicated three moles of ATP could be generated for every mole of NADH and two moles for every mole of reduced form of flavin adenine dinucleotide ($FADH_2$). However, direct chemical analysis has shown that for every two electrons transferred from NADH to oxygen, 2.5 equivalents of ATP are synthesized and 1.5 for $FADH_2$.

ELECTRON TRANSPORT CHAIN, ITS ORGANIZATION AND COMPONENTS

Respiratory Electron Transport Chain

Structure of the Mitochondria

- The mitochondrion consists of outer membrane, the inner membrane, the intermediate space, the cristae, and the matrix.
- The components of the ETC are located in the inner mitochondrial membrane. The inner mitochondrial membrane is a specialized structure that is impermeable to ions [hydrogen ion (H^+), sodium ion (Na^+) and potassium ion (K^+)], and small molecules such as ATP, ADP, pyruvate, and other metabolites. Therefore the specialized carriers or transport systems are required to move ions or molecules across membrane. The inner membrane is rich in protein and is highly folded to form cristae, and serve to increase greatly the surface area of the membrane.
- The inner membrane particles attached to the inner surface of the inner mitochondrial membrane are called ATP synthetase complexes.
- The gel-like solution in the interior of the mitochondria is mitochondrial matrix. This is rich in enzymes responsible for oxidation of fatty acid, pyruvate, amino acids, and TCA cycle.

Organization of the Electron Transport Chain

The inner mitochondrial membrane can be disrupted into five separate enzyme complexes called complex I, II, III, IV, and V. Complex I–IV are carriers of electrons, whereas complex V catalyzes ATP synthesis. There are certain mobile electron carriers in the respiratory chain. Each carriers of the ETC can receive electrons from an electron donor and donate subsequently to next carrier. The greater portion of the oxygen supplied to the body is utilized by the mitochondria for the operation of ETC (**Fig. 14.1**).

Reactions of the Electron Transport Chain

Formation of NADH

The NADH is more actively involved in the ETC. Oxidized form of nicotinamide adenine dinucleotide (NAD^+) is reduced to NADH and H^+ by removal of two hydrogen atoms from the substrate glyceraldehyde 3-phosphate, pyruvate, malate, etc. The reduced form of nicotinamide adenine dinucleotide phosphate is not a substrate for ETC (**Fig. 14.2**).

Flavoproteins

The NADH dehydrogenase [NADH-coenzyme ubiquinone (CoQ) reductase] is a flavoprotein with flavin mononucleotide (FMN), accepts two electrons and a proton to form $FMNH_2$. NADH dehydrogenase is a complex enzyme, which contains several iron atoms paired with sulfur.

Succinate dehydrogenase (succinate-coenzyme Q reductase) is an enzyme found in the inner mitochondrial membrane. It is a flavoprotein with flavin adenine dinucleotide

Biological Oxidation

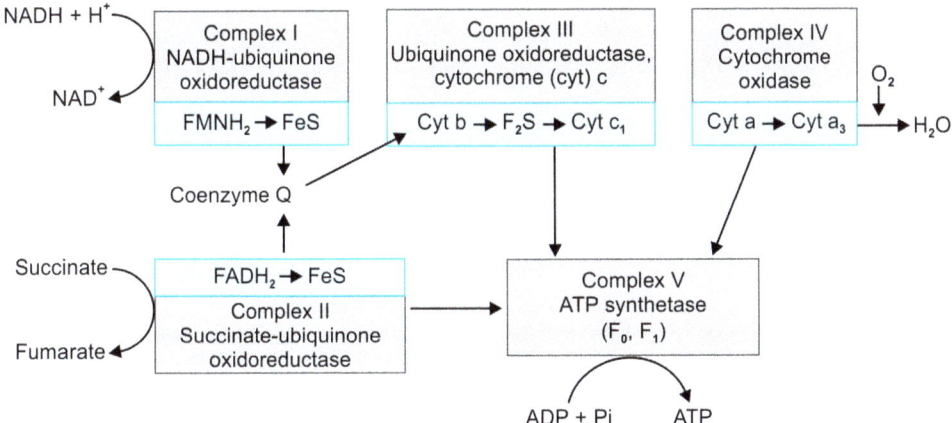

Fig. 14.1: Complexes in electron transport chain.
(NADH: nicotinamide adenine dinucleotide; ATP: adenosine triphosphate; ADP: adenosine diphosphate; FADH2: flavin adenine dinucleotide; Cyt: cytochrome; FMNH2: flavin adenine mononucleotide)

(FAD) as the coenzyme, which accepts two hydrogen atoms from succinate.

Iron–Sulfur Protein

It exists in the oxidized [ferric (Fe^{3+})] or reduced [ferrous (Fe^{2+})] state. One iron–sulfur (FeS) is involved in the transfer of electron.

Coenzyme Q

Coenzyme Q is a quinine derivative with a long isoprenoid tail. It is also called ubiquinone because it's ubiquitous in biological systems. It can accept hydrogen atoms both from $FMNH_2$ produced by NADH dehydrogenase and from $FADH_2$, which is produced by succinate dehydrogenase.

Cytochromes

Cytochromes are conjugated proteins containing heme group made of a porphyrin ring containing an atom of iron. Unlike the heme groups of hemoglobin and myoglobin, the cytochrome iron atom is reversibly converted from its Fe^{3+} to Fe^{2+}, which is essential for the transport of electrons in the ETC. Electrons are transported from coenzyme Q (ubiquinone) to cytochromes b, c_1, c, a, and a_3.

Cytochrome a and a_3: The term "cytochrome oxidase" is used to represent cytochrome a and a_3, which is the terminal component of ETC. This cytochrome is the only electron carrier, the heme iron of which can directly react with molecular oxygen. This also contains copper atoms that are required for this complex reaction to occur. Electrons from FMN CoQ and the other associated with cytochrome b, and c_1 transport to a and a_3.

Inhibitors of Electron Transport Chain

Inhibitors of electron transport chain are shown in **Figure 14.2**.

Oxidative Phosphorylation

The transfer of electrons through the ETC is linked with the release of free energy. The process of synthesizing ATP from ADP and Pi coupled with the ETC is called oxidative phosphorylation. The complex V is the site of oxidative phosphorylation (**Fig. 14.3**).

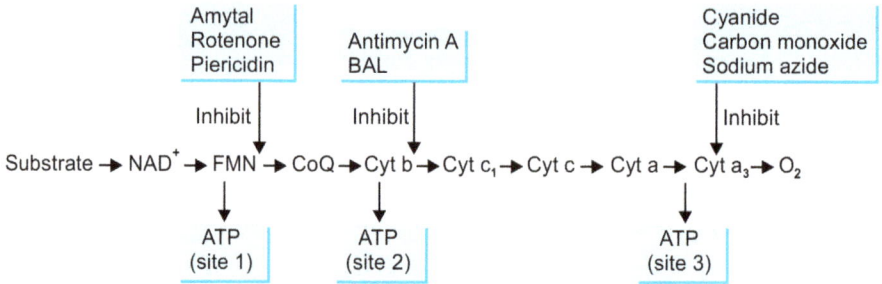

Fig. 14.2: Electron transport chain with inhibitors.
(BAL: 2,3-dimercaptopropanol; CoQ: coenzyme ubiquinone; Cyt: cytochrome; ATP: adenosine triphosphate; FMN: flavin mononucleotide; NAD+: nicotinamide adenine dinucleotide)

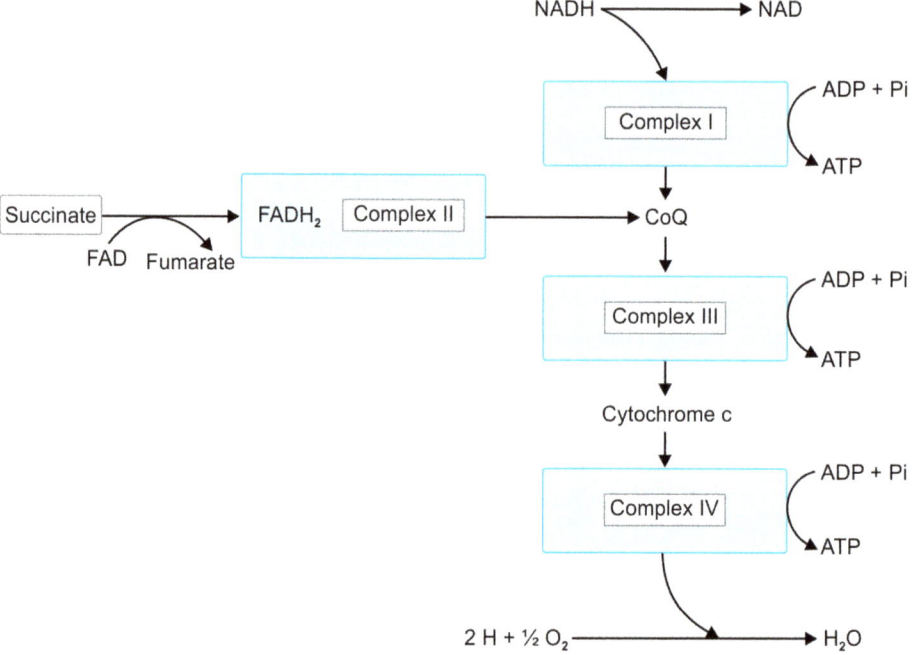

Fig. 14.3: Electron transport chain with adenosine triphosphate synthesis.
(CoQ: coenzyme ubiquinone ; NADH: nicotinamide adenine dinucleotide; ATP: adenosine triphosphate; ADP: adenosine diphosphate; FADH2: flavin adenine dinucleotide; NAD: nicotinamide adenine dinucleotide)

Phosphate/Oxygen Ratio

It refers to the number of inorganic phosphate utilized for ATP generation for every atom of oxygen consumed. It represents the number of molecules of ATP generated per pair of electrons carried through ETC.

- Phosphate/oxygen (P:O) ratio of three can be given to mitochondrial oxidation of NADH:

  $NADH + H + ½ O_2 + 3 ADP + 3 Pi^- \rightarrow NAD^+ + 3 ATP + 4 H_2O$

- The P:O ratio of two can be assigned to the oxidation of $FADH_2$.

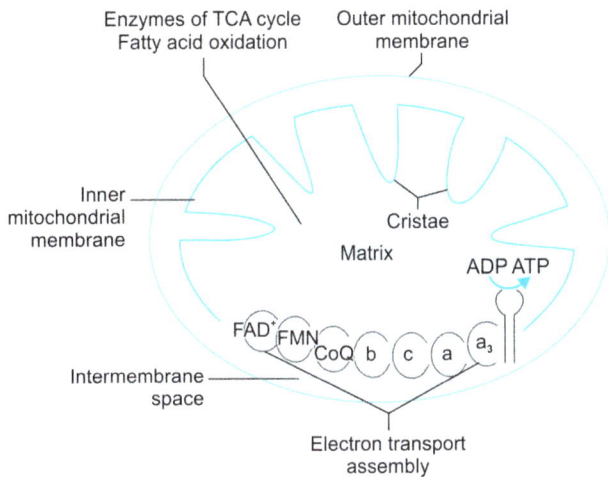

Fig. 14.4: Mitochondrion showing chemiosmotic hypothesis.
(CoQ: coenzyme ubiquinone; TCA: tricarboxylic acid; ATP: adenosine triphosphate; FMN: flavin mononucleotide)

- There are three sites of oxidative phosphorylation in ETC result in the synthesis of three ATP molecules.
  - Oxidation of $FMNH_2$ by CoQ
  - Oxidation of cytochrome by cytochrome c_1
  - Cytochrome oxidase reaction.

Each one of the previous reactions represents a coupling site for ATP production. The first reaction is bypassed for the oxidation of $FADH_2$ (two ATP molecules synthesized).

Mechanism

Important hypotheses to explain the process of oxidative phosphorylation are:
- Chemical coupling hypothesis
- Conformational coupling hypothesis
- Chemiosmotic hypothesis.

Chemical Coupling

According to chemical coupling, hypothesis during the course of electron transfer in respiratory chain a series of phosphorylated high-energy intermediates are first produced are utilized for the synthesis of ATP. However, this hypothesis does not have the experimental evidence.

Conformational Coupling

According to this hypothesis, induced conformational change in the membrane protein may be responsible for the synthesis of ATP.

Chemiosmotic Hypothesis

Chemiosmosis is the movement of ions across a selectively permeable membrane, down their electrochemical gradient. More specifically, it relates to the generation of ATP by the movement of H^+ ion across a membrane during cellular respiration. This hypothesis explains how the free energy generated by the transport of electrons by the ETC is used to produce ATP **(Figs. 14.4 and 14.5)**.

Proton Gradient

Electron transport is coupled to transport protons (H^+) across the inner mitochondrial membrane from the matrix to the intermembrane space. This process creates across the inner mitochondrial membrane an electrical

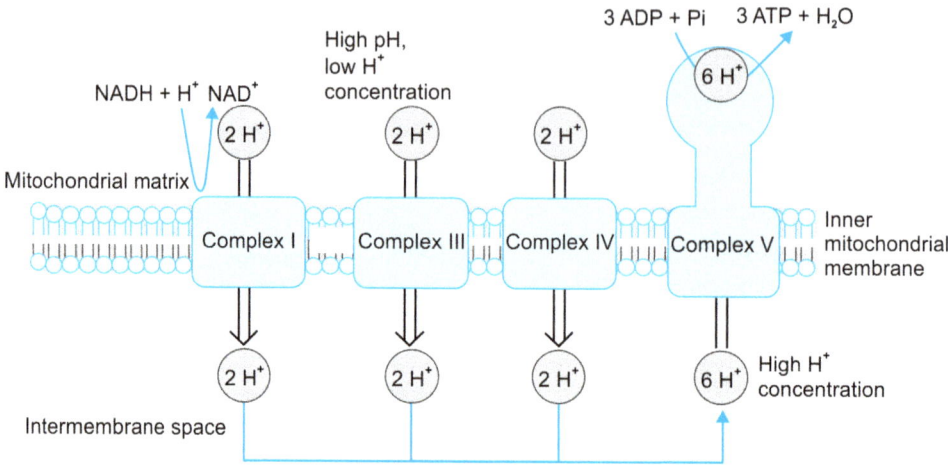

Fig. 14.5: Chemiosmotic hypothesis for oxidative phosphorylation.
(NADH: nicotinamide adenine dinucleotide; ATP: adenosine triphosphate; ADP: adenosine diphosphate; NAD+: nicotinamide adeninedinucleotide)

gradient (with more positive charges on the outside of the membrane than on the inside of the membrane) and a pH gradient (lower pH outside). The energy generated through this proton gradient is more than sufficient to drive ATP synthesis.

Adenosine Triphosphate Synthetase

The ATP synthetase enzyme complex (complex V) synthesizes ATP, utilizing the energy of the proton gradient generated by the ETC. The chemiosmotic hypothesis proposes that after protons have been transferred to the cytosolic side of the inner mitochondrial membrane, they can reenter the mitochondrial matrix by passing through a channel in the ATP synthetase molecule resulting in the synthesis of ATP from ADP and Pi, and at the same time dissipating the pH and electrical gradients.

UNCOUPLERS

The oxidation and phosphorylation proceed simultaneously. There are certain compounds that can uncouple (delink) the electron transport from oxidative phosphorylation. Such compounds increase the permeability of the inner mitochondrial membrane to protons. For example, 2,4-dinitrophenol, a small lipophilic proton carrier molecule, that readily diffuses through the mitochondrial membrane. This uncoupler causes electron transport to proceed at a rapid rate without creating a proton gradient.

The energy produced by the transport of electrons is released as heat rather than being used to synthesize ATP. As a result, ATP synthesis does not occur. The uncouplers allow oxidation of substrates [via NADH or reduced form of flavin adenine dinucleotide (FADH)] without ATP formation.

Other uncouplers are dinitrocresol, pentachlorophenol, trifluorocarbonylcyanide phenylhydrazone, and high-dose aspirin. The thyroxine and long-chain fatty acids act as uncoupler at high concentration.

Significance of Uncoupling

Uncoupling agents also occur naturally. Newborn and hibernating animals contain brown fat. Brown fat mitochondria contain the protein thermogenin, which provides a channel through the inner mitochondrial membrane.

Biological Oxidation

The heat energy released as the protons rush down their concentration gradient through this channel keeps the animal warm.

Oligomycin

Oligomycin antibiotic binds to the stalk of the ATP synthase, closes the H^+ channel, and prevents reentry of protons into the mitochondrial matrix. Due to this, protons get accumulated at higher concentration in the intermediate space. Electron transport ultimately stops because of the difficulty in pumping any more protons against the steep gradients. This indicates that the electron transport and phosphorylation are tightly coupled processes.

SUMMARY

Oxidation-reduction reactions are coupled chemical reactions in which one atom or molecule loses one or more electrons (oxidation), while another atom or molecule gains those electrons (reduction). NADH and FADH resulting from metabolic pathway can be used for reductive biosynthesis. Reducing the potential of mitochondrial NADH is most often used to supply the energy for ATP synthesis by ETC and then via oxidative phosphorylation.

SELF-ASSESSMENT QUESTIONS

1. Briefly discuss how the reactions of the ETC take place?
2. Write the flowchart to show the flow of electrons.
3. List the sites where ATP is synthesized.
4. What is oxidative phosphorylation?
5. Describe the chemiosmotic hypothesis.
6. Lists the inhibitors of electron transport chain and write the site of inhibition.
7. Explain the term "uncouplers" and give any two examples.
8. What is the P:O ratio and write its significance?
9. What is the significance of uncouplers in animals?
10. Describe the action of oligomycin on electron transport chain and oxidative phosphorylation.

MULTIPLE-CHOICE QUESTIONS

1. The site of oxidative phosphorylation is:
   a. Complex I   b. Complex II
   c. Complex IV   d. Complex V
2. P:O ratio:
   a. Refers to the number of ADP utilized for ATP generation for every atom of oxygen consumed
   b. Represents the number of molecules of ATP generated per pair of electrons carried through ETC
   c. For mitochondrial oxidation of NADH is 2
   d. For cytosolic oxidation of FADH is 2
3. Concerning chemiosmotic hypothesis, all of the following statements are true, *except*:
   a. Electron transport is coupled to transport H^+ across the inner mitochondrial membrane
   b. Energy generated through proton gradient is not sufficient to drive ATP synthesis
   c. ATP synthase complex synthesizes ATP, utilizing the energy of the proton gradient
   d. Proton gradient creates low pH outside the mitochondrial membrane
4. The components of ETC are located in the:
   a. Intermediate space of the mitochondrial membrane
   b. Inner mitochondrial membrane
   c. Outer mitochondrial membrane
   d. Cytosolic portion of the cell
5. The inner mitochondrial membrane is not permeable to:
   a. Hydrogen ions   b. Sodium
   c. Potassium   d. Selenium
6. All the following are the sites of ATP synthesis in a respiratory chain, *except*:
   a. Complex I   b. Complex II
   c. Complex III   d. Complex IV
7. 2,4-Dinitrophenol is a:
   a. Uncoupler causes electrons to stop from flowing one complex to other
   b. Inhibitor causes electrons transport at slower speed without creating a proton gradient

c. Uncoupler causes electron transport to proceed at a rapid rate without creating a proton gradient
d. Inhibits the complex IV

8. **All of the following are the uncouplers of oxidative phosphorylation, *except*:**
   a. Dinitrocresol
   b. Carbon tetrachloride
   c. Pentachlorophenol
   d. Trifluorocarbonylcyanide phenylhydrazone

9. **Which of the following applies to the statement, "heat energy released as the protons rush down their concentration gradient through this channel keeps the animal warm"?**
   a. It is a significance inhibition mechanism
   b. It is a significance oxidative phosphorylation
   c. It is a significance of uncoupling mechanism
   d. None of the above

10. **All of the following inhibits the complex II, *except*:**
    a. Amytal
    b. Rotenone
    c. Piericidin
    d. Antimycin

Answers

| 1. d | 2. b | 3. b | 4. b | 5. d |
| 6. b | 7. c | 8. b | 9. c | 10. d |

CHAPTER
15

Mineral Metabolism

OBJECTIVES

At the end of this chapter, students should be able to:
- Understand the daily requirement, functions, and disorders associated with calcium, iron, phosphorous, sodium, potassium, and chloride
- Explain the daily requirement, important functions, and the deficiency manifestations of trace elements such as copper, zinc, selenium, fluoride, iodine, magnesium, and molybdenum.

INTRODUCTION

Minerals are inorganic substances required by the body in small amounts for a variety of functions:
- For the formation of bones and teeth
- Essential constituents of body fluids and tissues
- Components of enzyme systems
- For normal nerve function.

Some minerals are needed in larger amounts than others, e.g. calcium, phosphorus, magnesium, sodium, potassium, and chloride, which are called bulk elements. Others are required in smaller quantities and are sometimes called trace minerals, e.g. iron, zinc, iodine, fluoride, selenium, and copper. Despite being required in smaller amounts, trace minerals are no less important than other minerals.

Minerals are often absorbed more efficiently by the body if supplied in foods rather than as supplements. Also, a diet that is short in one mineral may well be low in others, and so the first step in dealing with this is to review and improve the diet as a whole. Eating a varied diet will help ensure an adequate supply of most minerals for healthy people. This includes:
- Bulk elements (macronutrients)
- Trace elements (micronutrients).

Bulk elements: These are calcium, magnesium, sodium, potassium, phosphorus, sulfur, and chloride. They constitute 60–80% of all inorganic material in the body.

Trace elements: These are required in very small amounts. They are iron, iodine, cobalt, manganese, molybdenum, zinc, lead, selenium, and fluoride.

MACROMINERALS OR BULK ELEMENTS

Calcium

Calcium Content of Body and Blood

- Calcium (Ca^{2+}) is the most abundant mineral and cation of the extracellular fluid (ECF) in the body.
- Calcium element is comprising nearly 2% of the body weight. Human body contains 1,200 g of calcium.
- Major amount (99%) present in bone and teeth as hydroxyapatite and remaining 1% is in blood and soft tissues.
- Calcium level of serum in adult human is 9–11 mg/100 mL.
- Blood calcium present in three different forms:

1. Ionized calcium is the physiologically active form, which constitutes 50% of the total calcium (4.5–5.5 mg%).
2. Protein (albumin) bound form; this is 45% of total level.
3. Calcium complexes with citrate, phosphate, and bicarbonate. This fraction is only 5%.

Sources

Rich sources: Milk and its products
Good sources: Meat, fish, green leafy vegetables, cereals, and pulses.

Recommended Dietary Allowance

- Children: 1.2 g/day
- Adults: 0.8 g/day
- Pregnancy and lactation: 1.2 g/day.

Absorption

Several factors favoring calcium absorption are:
- 1,25-dihydroxyvitamin D_3
- Gastric acidity
- Lactose
- Amino acids and citrate
- Calcium:phosphate ratio of the diet
- Low phosphate level.

The substances decreases absorption are:
- Oxalate and phytates of food
- Fatty acids. All these form insoluble salts with calcium and decreases the absorption.
- Chronic renal failure.

Functions

The functions of calcium are as follows:
- It is required for the formation of bone and teeth; it gives hardness and strength to bone and teeth.
- It is required for blood coagulation process.
- It is required for the contraction of heart and muscle.
- It controls the permeability of the cell membranes.
- It activates pancreatic lipase in the digestion of fats.
- It activates phosphorylase during the breakdown of glycogen.
- It regulates the excitability of nerve fibers.
- It releases hormones, i.e. insulin from storage granules.
- It serves as a second messenger in the action of hormones, i.e. adrenaline.
- Responses of calcium are mediated by interaction with a receptor protein called calmodulin. This cytosolic protein has calcium-binding sites. Calmodulin-calcium complex activates protein kinases, which in turn activate other enzymes and through these, it bring about metabolic effects. In this mechanism, cyclic adenosine monophosphate (cAMP) is also involved. It is required for the formation of calcium paracaseinate (insoluble curd).

Regulation of Serum Calcium Level

The ionic calcium level is maintained by vitamin D and hormones such as parathyroid hormone (PTH), and calcitonin.

Action of vitamin D

The following list shows the action of vitamin D:
- It increases the absorption of calcium (and phosphate) from the small intestine
- It causes removal of calcium from bone (bone resorption).

The mechanism by which 1,25-dihydroxy-vitamin D_3 increases calcium absorption from intestine is detailed below.

The 1,25-dihydroxyvitamin D_3 enters the intestinal cell and binds to a cytoplasmic receptor. The vitamin D_3 receptor complex then moves to the nucleus where it interacts with deoxyribonucleic acid (DNA). This results in the synthesis of messenger ribonucleic acid (mRNA) and this in turn forms a calcium-binding protein. The calcium-binding protein increases the absorption of calcium from intestine.

Mineral Metabolism

Action of PTH on kidney and bone
- The PTH increases the activity of 1-α-hydroxylase in kidney, which increases the synthesis of 1,25-dihydroxyvitamin D_3, and this in turn enhances the absorption of calcium from intestine (**Fig. 15.1**).
- It increases the reabsorption of calcium from glomerular filtrate in kidneys.
- It causes the resorption of calcium from bone. These three actions correct the hypocalcemia and bring it to normal level.
- The PTH also causes excretion of phosphate in urine by inhibiting phosphate reabsorption in kidney.

Action of Calcitonin
Calcitonin is a hormone from "C" cells of thyroid glands. Hypercalcemia stimulates its secretion.

Calcitonin inhibits calcium reabsorption from kidneys and resorption from bone. Thus it corrects hypercalcemia.

Normal value: It ranges from 9 to 10.6 mg/100 mL serum or 4.5–5.4 mEq/L.

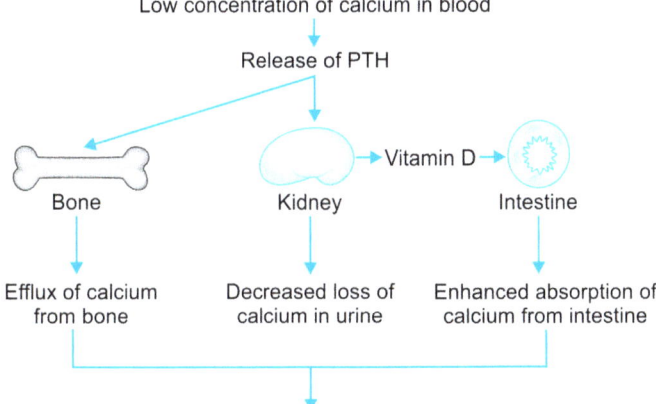

Fig. 15.1: Role of PTH in restoring low plasma calcium to normal.
(PTH: parathyroid hormone)

- Hypo and hypercalcemia (**Tables 15.1 and 15.2**).

Table 15.1: Hypocalcemia.

Causes	Symptoms	Treatment

- Hypoparathyroidism
- Vitamin D deficiency
- Magnesium deficiency
- Eating disorders
- *Chronic renal failure*: The kidney loses its capacity to synthesize 1,25-dihydroxycholecalciferol. Increased PTH secretion in response to hypocalcemia may lead to bone disease, if untreated
- Pseudohypoparathyroidism is a condition associated primarily with resistance to the PTH
	- Convulsions
	- Arrhythmias
	- Tetany and numbness
	- Petechiae
	- *Latent tetany*: Trousseau sign of latent tetany (eliciting carpal spasm by inflating the BP cuff and maintaining the cuff pressure above systolic)
	- Tendon reflexes are hyperactive
	- Life-threatening complications:
	  ➢ Laryngospasm
	  ➢ Cardiac arrhythmias
		Two ampules of intravenous calcium gluconate 10% are given slowly in a period of 10 minutes, or if the hypocalcemia is severe, calcium chloride is given instead

(BP: blood pressure; PTH: parathyroid hormone)

Table 15.2: Hypercalcemia.

Causes	Signs and symptoms	Treatment

• Primary hyperparathyroidism:
  ➢ Solitary parathyroid adenoma
  ➢ Primary parathyroid hyperplasia
  ➢ Parathyroid carcinoma
• Solid tumor with metastasis (e.g. squamous cell carcinoma)
• Hematologic malignancy (multiple myeloma, lymphoma, and leukemia)
• Hypervitaminosis D (vitamin D intoxication)
• Elevated 1,25-(OH)$_2$D (for details refer calcitriol/vitamin D) levels (e.g. sarcoidosis and other granulomatous diseases)
• Renal diseases
• Disorders related to high-bone turnover rates:
  ➢ Hyperthyroidism
  ➢ Prolonged immobilization
  ➢ Paget's disease of the bone
  ➢ Multiple myeloma
	• Stones (renal or biliary)
	• Bones (bone pain)
	• Thrones (sit on throne—polyuria)
	• Fatigue
	• Anorexia
	• Pancreatitis
		• Hydration, increasing salt intake, and forced diuresis
		• Bisphosphonates are pyrophosphate analogs with high affinity for bone, especially areas of high-bone turnover

Phosphorus

Sources

Good sources of phosphorus are as follows:
- Milk
- Meat
- Cereals
- In general, a diet supplying sufficient calcium will supply an adequate amount of phosphorus as well.

Recommended Dietary Allowance

- Adult: 800 mg/day
- Extra allowance is needed for growth and pregnancy.

Phosphorus Content of Body and Blood

- Phosphorus forms 1% of the body weight.
- Whole body contains 700 g of phosphorus; 80% of this is present in bones and teeth as hydroxyapatite.

Functions

The functions of phosphorus are as follows:
- Phosphorus helps in the formation of bone and teeth. Inorganic phosphorus is a major constituent of hydroxyapatite in bone, thereby playing an important part in structural support of the body **(Box 15.1)**.
- Acts as a buffer in blood. Mixture of HPO_4^- and $H_2PO_4^-$ constitutes the phosphate buffer, which plays a role in maintaining the pH of the body fluid.
- Helps in the formation of compounds such as nucleic acids, nucleotides, i.e. adenosine triphosphate (ATP), guanosine triphosphate, and adenosine diphosphate. as organic phosphate esters in glycolysis and other metabolic reactions.
- It is also required in energy metabolism, synthesis of phospholipids, cAMP, phosphoproteins, and coenzymes such as thiamine pyrophosphate.

Normal level: Normal serum inorganic phosphate level:
- Adults: 2.5–4.5 mg%
- Children: 4–6 mg%.
- Hypo and Hyperphoshatemia **(Box 15.1)**

Magnesium

Magnesium (Mg^{2+}) is the major intracellular cation (15 mEq/L) next to potassium. About 70% of total magnesium is in skeletal tissues.

> **Box 15.1: Hypo- and hyperphosphatemia**
>
> **Hypophosphatemia (decreased level of phosphorus)**
> - Rickets
> - Hyperparathyroidism
> - Condition associated with decrease in the reabsorption of phosphate from the glomerular filtrate (Fanconi's syndrome):
>   – In the treatment of diabetes, the effect of insulin is causing the shift of glucose into cells also enhances the transport of phosphate into cells, which may result hypophosphatemia
>   – Clinical symptoms such as muscle pain and weakness with respiratory failure, and decreased myocardial output
>
> **Hyperphosphatema** *(increased phosphate level)*
> - Seen in hypoparathyroidism
> - Hypervitaminosis D
> - Renal failure
>
> Elevated phosphate may cause a decrease in serum calcium concentration. Therefore it may lead to tetany and seizures

The remainder is in muscle, brain, and other tissues.

Sources

The sources of magnesium are as follows:
- Magnesium is abundant in chlorophyll pigment of vegetables.
- Good sources are whole grains.
- Nuts.
- Milk.
- Meat.

Recommended Dietary Allowance

- Adults: 300 mg/day
- Children: 250 mg/day.

Functions

The functions of magnesium are as follows:
- Magnesium is an essential activator of many enzymes especially those involving transfer of phosphate groups from ATP.
- Examples are hexokinase and phosphofructokinase.
- It also activates a number of enzymes such as:
  – Enolase
  – Glucose-6-phosphate dehydrogenase
  – Pyruvate carboxylase
  – Thiokinase
  – Glucose-6-phosphogluconate dehydrogenase.
- Magnesium along with sodium, potassium, and calcium controls neuromuscular irritability.
- It is important constituent of bone.

Deficiency

- Deficiency symptoms bear some resemblance to those seen in hypocalcemia, with muscle twitching, spasms, and tetany.

Sodium

- Sodium (Na^+) is the major cation of the ECF.
- Most of the body's sodium is located in the blood and in the fluid in the space surrounding the cells. Sodium is required by all cells in the body to maintain a normal fluid balance.

Sources

The major sources are table salt, cereals, legumes, egg, carrot, tomato, and milk.
- Average intake from table salt is 5–10 g/day
- Requirement: 5 g/day.

Normal range in blood: Sodium should be 130–145 mEq/L (intracellular Na^+ is 10 mEq/L).

Functions

The functions of sodium are as follows:
- Maintains the osmotic pressure, thus to maintain the volume of blood and blood pressure (BP) (i.e. protection against fluid loss); sodium loss causes blood volume to decrease.
- Regulates the electrolyte and pH balance of the extracellular compartment.
- Controls the electronic potentials of excitable tissues such as nerve and muscle.

- Helps in the active transport of glucose, galactose, and amino acids across intestinal mucosa, and for Na^+/K^+-ATPase.

Average serum sodium level: It should be 142 mEq/L (intracellular sodium is 10 mEq/L).

Osmolality

- Plasma osmolarity/osmolality measures the body's electrolyte–water balance.
- Osmolality is a measure of the osmoles (Osm) of solute per kilogram of solvent (osmol/kg or Osm/kg), and osmolarity is defined as the number of osmoles of solute per liter (L) of solution (osmol/L or Osm/L).
- Osmolality can be measured on an analytical instrument called osmometer.

Clinical relevance

As cell membranes in general are freely permeable to water, the osmolality of the ECF is approximately equal to that of the intracellular fluid (ICF). Therefore plasma osmolality is a guide to intracellular osmolality.

Osmolality of blood increases with dehydration and decreases with overhydration. In normal people, increased osmolality in the blood will stimulate the secretion of antidiuretic hormone (ADH). This will result in increased water reabsorption, more concentrated urine and less concentrated blood plasma. A low serum osmolality will suppress the release of ADH, resulting in decreased water reabsorption and more concentrated plasma.

Osmolality of a serum or plasma sample can be measured directly or it may be calculated serum osmolality. Clinically, the simplest is:

Serum osmolality (mmol/kg) = 2 × serum sodium (mmol/L).

Clinical Use

Serum osmolality is used in two main circumstances—investigation of hyponatremia and identification of an osmolar gap. Urine osmolality is an important test of renal concentrating ability, for identifying disorders of the ADH mechanism and identifying causes of hyper or hyponatremia.

Serum osmolality

Serum osmolality is a useful preliminary investigation for identifying cause of hyponatremia. If a patient with significant hyponatremia (serum sodium <130 mmol/L) has a normal plasma osmolality, the patient may have pseudohyponatremia due to excess lipids or proteins, or the sample may have been collected from a drip arm-containing dextrose. If the patient has an increased osmolality it is likely the patient has reactive hyponatremia due to an excess of solute pulling water out of cells. Examples of this include glucose in diabetes mellitus or hyperglycinemia after transurethral resection of the prostate.

Urine osmolality

Urine osmolality is an important test for the concentrating ability of the kidney. Interpretation of urine osmolality must always be made in the light of the appropriate physiological response to the state of hydration of the patient. The test is useful in the following areas:

- For determining the differential diagnosis of hyper or hyponatremia.
- For identifying syndrome of inappropriate ADH (SIADH) (urine osmolality >200 mmol/kg, urine sodium >20 mmol/L, low serum sodium, patient not dehydrated and no renal, adrenal, thyroid, cardiac or liver disease, or interfering drugs).
- For differentiating prerenal from renal kidney failure (high urine osmolality is consistent with prerenal impairment; in renal damage the urine osmolality is similar to plasma osmolality).
- For identifying and diagnosing diabetes insipidus.

Atrial natriuretic peptide

- Atrial natriuretic peptide (ANP) is a potent vasodilator and a protein secreted by cardiac muscle cells. It is a circulating hormone regulates atrial BP **(Fig. 15.2)**.

Mineral Metabolism

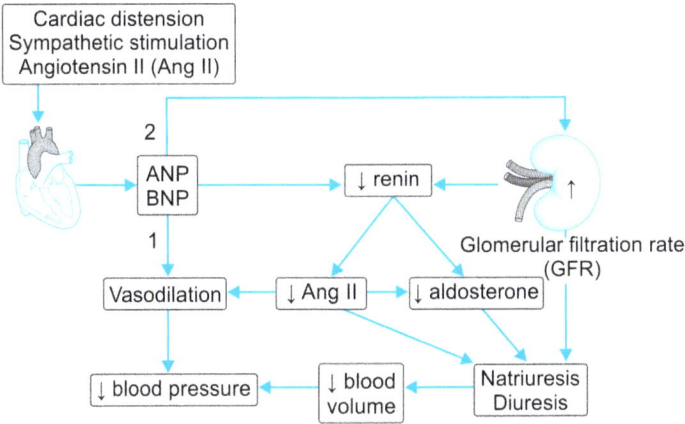

Fig. 15.2: Role of ANP and BNP.
(ANP: atrial natriuretic peptide, BNP: brain natriuretic peptide)

- It controls the body water, Na, K, and fat. This hormone is released by muscle cells of upper chamber of heart when BP elevated.
- It reduces water and sodium and blocks the release of several hormones.
- It is produced, piled up, and secreted by myocytes.
- ANP level usually increases in state of hypertension and excessive of fluids. Human heart secretes ANP and brain natriuretic peptide (BNP).
- Both BNP and ANP levels increase hypertension, secondary hypertensions, and chronic heart failure during heart pacing, chronic renal failure, an acute myocardial infarction determined. These receptors are having their own functions and purposes.
- ANP has four receptors such as renal, vascular, cardiac, and adipose tissues.
- ANP attaches to a specific group of receptors. These receptors are design to cause a reduction in blood volume and reduction in cardiac output, and systematic BP.
- Renal reduces aldosterone secretion by adrenal cortex.
- Renal inhibits the renin secretion. In vascular, it relaxes the vascular smooth muscles in arterioles. Adipose tissues increase the release of fatty acids from adipose tissues.
- The ANP in combination with the BNP helps in reducing the volume of blood as well as the excessive pressure on the blood, which allows keeping everything related to the heart and blood to normal levels. This ensures best control over the blood flow through body as well as a great control over the entire body and its functions.

Deficiency

- The nutritional deficiency is almost highly important.
- On a low-sodium diet, the kidney decreases the excretion of sodium in urine.
- A low blood sodium triggers the kidney to release angiotensin, which causes the adrenal cortex to secrete aldosterone the latter induces the renal tubules to reabsorb sodium from the glomerular filtrate.
- Another mechanism involves the pituitary gland, which secretes ADH. ADH causes the kidneys to conserve water. The retained sodium and water lead to decreased urine production, which 1eventually leads to an increase in blood volume.

Hyponatremia (reduced sodium in the blood) (see Chapter 24).
Hypernatremia (elevated sodium in the blood) (see Chapter 24).
Treatment (see Chapter 24 for the details).

Potassium

- Potassium (K^+) is the most important cation of ICF.
- ICF is the 150 mEq/L.
- ECF potassium concentration: 3.5–5.0 mEq/L.
- ECF potassium is important for its controlling influence upon neuromuscular irritability, cardiac muscle (a proper balance between potassium and calcium is essential for the contraction of heart muscle) and the operation of Na^+/K^+-ATPase (Na^+ pump) against the concentration gradient.
- In cells, there is a significant concentration gradient of sodium and potassium across cell membranes.
- The high intracellular potassium is maintained by an energy requiring extrusion of three sodium out of the cell with replacement by two potassium (**Fig. 15.3**).
- Intracellular potassium is essential for a number of enzyme reactions (such as pyruvate kinase, glycogen synthesis, and protein synthesis) for maintaining osmotic and acid-base balance.
- Nearly all of the total body potassium (98%) are inside cells. For example, there is significant tissue damage, the contents of cells, including potassium, leak out into the extracellular compartment, causing potentially dangerous increases in serum potassium.

Sources
Sources include as whole and skim milk, bananas, tomatoes, oranges, melons, potatoes, sweet potatoes, prunes, raisins, spinach, turnip greens, collard greens, kale, other green leafy vegetables, most peas and beans, and salt substitutes [potassium chloride (KCl)].

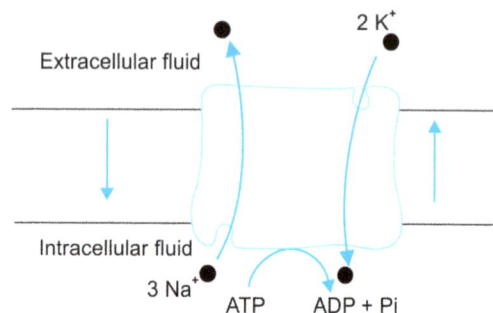

Fig. 15.3: Movement of potassium and sodium across the compartments.
(ATP: adenosine triphosphate; ADP: adenosine diphosphate)

Recommended Dietary Allowance
An average diet provides 4 g K^+/day.
Normal value: Serum level is 3–5.0 mEq/L.

Functions
The functions of potassium are as follows:
- Potassium is the principal cation of ICF.
- It is required for the functioning of nerves, skeletal muscle, and cardiac muscles. Either decreased potassium or increased potassium levels finally cause cardiac arrest.
- It is required as a cofactor in several enzymatic reactions in the body.
- It is involved in the acid-base balance.

Tests
- Serum potassium determination
- Arterial blood gas
- Basic or comprehensive metabolic panel
- Electrocardiogram
- Blood tests to check glucose, magnesium, calcium, sodium, phosphorus, thyroxine, and aldosterone levels.

Hyperkalemia (Box 15.2)
Tests
To gather enough information for diagnosis, the measurement of potassium needs to be repeated, as the elevation can be due to hemolysis in the first sample.

Box 15.2: Hyperkalemia.

- It occurs in Addison's disease and in intravenous infusion of potassium at a rate excess of 25 mmol/h
- Treatment using concentrated potassium solutions.

Causes
- Renal insufficiency (renal failure)
- Medication that interferes with urinary excretion:
  - Angiotensin converting enzyme (ACE) inhibitors and angiotensin receptor blockers
  - Potassium-sparing diuretics (e.g. amiloride and spironolactone)
  - Nonsteroidal anti-inflammatory drugs (NSAIDs) such as ibuprofen, naproxen, or celecoxib
  - The calcineurin inhibitor immunosuppressants cyclosporine and tacrolimus
  - The antibiotic trimethoprim
  - The antiparasitic drug pentamidine
- Mineralocorticoid deficiency or resistance, such as:
  - Addison's disease
  - Aldosterone deficiency
- Excessive intake: Excess intake with salt-substitute, potassium-containing dietary supplements or potassium chloride (KCl) infusion
- Pseudohyperkalemia: Pseudohyperkalemia is a rise in the amount of potassium that occurs due to excessive leakage of potassium from cells, during or after blood is drawn.

Signs and symptoms
Fatigue, weakness, tingling, numbness, paralysis, palpitations, and difficulty in breathing.

Box 15.3: Hypokalemia.

Hypokalemia: Hypokalemia is a metabolic disorder that occurs when the level of potassium in the blood drops too low:
- It is the condition in which serum potassium is reduced
- This condition decreases the heartbeat and interferes with vital muscles such as those involved in respiration.
- Antibiotics: These are penicillin, nafcillin, carbenicillin, gentamicin, amphotericin B, and foscarnet
- Diarrhea, diseases that affect the kidneys' ability to retain potassium
- Diuretic medications, which can cause excess urination
- Eating disorders (such as bulimia)
- Magnesium deficiency
- Sweating and vomiting
- Since aldosterone increases the excretion of potassium or administration of cortisone leads to hypokalemia
- Certain diuretics increase the excretion of potassium. It is therefore important to supplement enough potassium when these diuretics are used
- Alkalosis can cause transient hypokalemia by two mechanisms. First, the alkalosis causes a shift of potassium from the plasma and interstitial fluids into cells; perhaps mediated by stimulation of Na^+, H^+ exchange, and a subsequent activation of Na^+/K^+-ATPase activity. Second, an acute rise of plasma HCO^- concentration (caused by vomiting). For example, it will exceed the capacity of the renal proximal tubule to reabsorb this anion, and potassium will be excreted as an obligate cation partner to the bicarbonate. Metabolic alkalosis is often present in states of volume depletion, so potassium is also lost via aldosterone-mediated mechanisms.

Signs and symptoms
A big drop in the level can be life-threatening. Symptoms include:
- Abnormal heart rhythms (dysrhythmias), especially in people with heart disease, constipation, and fatigue
- Muscle damage (rhabdomyolysis), muscle weakness or spasms, and paralysis (which can include the lungs).

Treatment
- Mild hypokalemia can be treated by taking potassium supplements by mouth. Persons with more severe cases may need to get potassium through a vein (intravenously)
- If diuretics used, doctor may try to keep potassium in the body (such as triamterene and amiloride)

Normal range: As follows:
- In serum: 3.5–5 mEq/L
- In plasma: 3.5–4.5 mEq/L.

Hypokalemia (Box 15.3)

Treatment

Several agents are used to transiently lower K^+ levels. Choice depends on the degree and cause of the hyperkalemia, and other aspects of the patient's condition:
- Serum potassium level above 7 mEq/L and below 2.5 mEq/L is serious, life-threatening, and requires immediate attention.
- Hemolyzed samples are not suitable for electrolyte analysis because of the release of potassium from the RBC, which will cause a false increase in the potassium values.

- Urine collection for electrolyte estimation should be made without any preservative.
- Serum, plasma, or urine must be stored at 2–4°C or frozen if the analysis is delayed.

Specimen: Serum, heparinized plasma, sweat, urine, feces, or gastrointestinal fluids are used for the assay.

Chloride

- Chloride (Cl⁻) is the major extracellular anion.
- Serum concentration is 105 mEq/L.

Functions

The functions of chloride are as follows:
- Chloride is involved in maintaining osmotic pressure, proper body hydration, and electric neutrality.
- Chloride ions have important physiological roles:
  - In the central nervous system (CNS), the inhibitory action of glycine and some of the action of gamma-aminobutyric acid rely on the entry of Cl- into specific neurons.
  - The chloride-bicarbonate exchanger biological transport protein relies on the chloride ion to increase the blood's capacity of carbon dioxide, in the form of the bicarbonate ion.
- Dietary chloride is almost completely absorbed by the intestinal tract. It is filtered out by the glomerulus and passively reabsorbed in conjunction with Na⁺ by the proximal tubules. Excess chloride is excreted in urine and through sweating. Excessive sweating stimulates aldosterone secretion, which acts on the sweat glands to conserve Na⁺ and chloride.

Hypochloremia (Box 15.4)

Box 15.4: Hypo- and hyperchloremia.

Hypochloremia (low serum chloride)
Metabolic alkalosis:
- Vomiting and diarrhea

Contd...

Contd...
- Diuretics
- Gastric suction
- Respiratory losses.

Associated with hyponatremia
- Addison's disease
- Salt-losing nephritis
- Syndrome of inappropriate antidiuretic hormone (ADH) secretion
- Renal failure
- Excessive sweating
- Thiazide diuretics
- Burns

Hyperchloremia (high serum chloride)
- Metabolic acidosis
- Dehydration
- Decreased renal blood flow
- Medications-containing ammonium chloride
- Hyperparathyroidism

MICROMINERALS OR TRACE ELEMENTS

Trace elements are present in the body in very small amounts and are essential for certain biochemical processes. They are iron, iodine, cobalt, copper, manganese, molybdenum, zinc, lead, selenium, and fluoride.

Iron

- Iron (Fe) is a trace element, which are present in the body in much smaller amounts.
- Total body iron is about 5 g.

Sources

The sources are liver, meat, egg yolk, vegetables, whole wheat, legumes, cashew nuts, dates, and shell fish.

Functions

The functions of iron are as follows:
- Iron is necessary for the synthesis of certain proteins.
- Iron-containing proteins in the body are of two types:
  1. Heme proteins: Proteins with heme group. Examples are:

- Hemoglobin: This accounts for 70% total body iron.
- Myoglobin: This is the muscle oxygen-binding protein, 5% of total Fe is in this form; both proteins function in the transport of oxygen.
- Catalase and peroxidase: Function of this is in the decomposition of H_2O_2, a toxic compound.
- Cytochrome b, $c1$, c, and $a3$: These take part in respiratory chain.

2. Nonheme proteins: Proteins with nonheme group:
   - Ferritin and hemosiderin: These are iron storage proteins in liver, spleen, and bone marrow; these comprise 15% of body iron.
   - Transferrin: This is the iron transport protein in blood.
   - Aconitase of Krebs TCA cycle.
   - Iron–sulfur proteins: Succinate dehydrogenase is an example; some iron–sulfur proteins function in respiratory chain.

Recommended Dietary Allowance

The amount of iron required each day to compensate for the losses depends on age and sex; it is highest in pregnancy and menstruating females:
- Adult males: 12 mg/day
- Females: 20 mg/day
- Pregnancy and lactation: 40 mg/day.

Iron Absorption

Absorption takes place mainly in duodenum **(Table 15.3)**.

Hydrochloric acid (HCl) of stomach liberates Fe^{3+} from nonheme iron compounds of food. Iron is absorbed as Fe^{2+}.

Mechanism of iron absorption and transport

- Normally, about 5–10% of dietary iron is absorbed by the active transport process in the duodenum **(Fig. 15.4)**.

Table 15.3: Factors influencing iron absorption.

Factors favoring	Factors reducing
Ferrous form	Ferric form
Inorganic iron	Organic iron
Acids—HCl	Alkalis and antacids
Vitamin C	Pancreatic secretions
Iron deficiency	Iron excess
Increased erythropoiesis	Decreased erythropoiesis
Pregnancy	Infection

(HCl: hydrochloric acid)

- Heme of food is absorbed directly from the intestine and nonheme iron is absorbed in the ferrous state (Fe^{2+}) into the mucosal cell as described below. The gastric HCl and organic acids in the diet convert organic ferric compound of the diet into free ferric (Fe^{3+}) ions. These ferric ions are reduced with ascorbic acid and glutathione of food to more soluble ferrous form (Fe^{2+}), which is more readily absorbed than ferric form (Fe^{3+}). In the intestinal mucosa, the iron is either stored in the form of ferritin in the mucosal cells or transported across the mucosal cells to the plasma in the form of transferrin. The mucosal cell storage is dependent on body's iron status.
- After absorption of Fe^{2+} into the intestinal mucosal cell, it is oxidized to Fe^{3+}.
- This combines with intracellular carrier protein.
- This complex either delivers a fixed amount of Fe to mitochondria or transfers some iron to another protein called apoferritin, which binds Fe^{3+} to form ferritin.
- The ferritin is a storage form of iron.
- Some iron binds with plasma α-1-globulin called apotransferrin, to form transferrin. Each molecule of apotransferrin binds two ferric ions. The transferrin is a transport form of iron. As mentioned above the proportions of iron transferred to apoferritin and apotransferrin depend upon the iron status of the person. Iron always transports in the

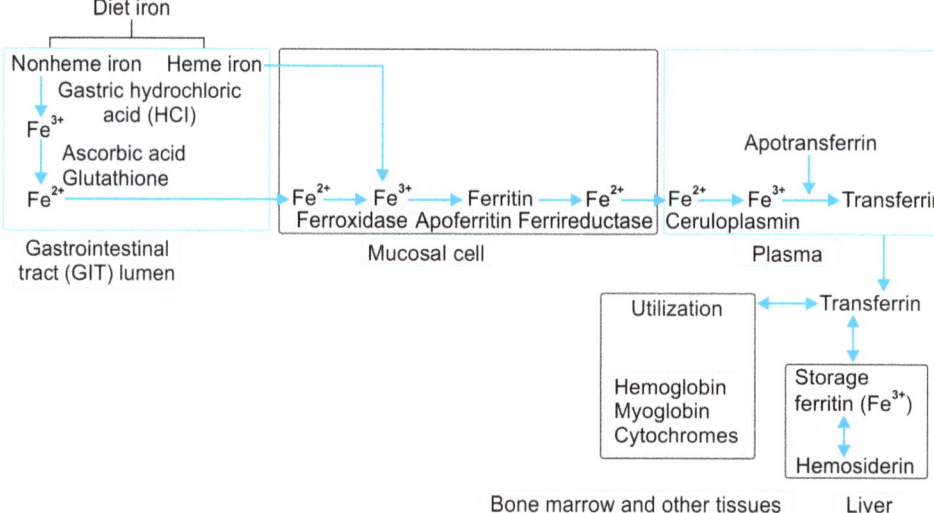

Fig. 15.4: Absorption and transport of dietary iron.

ferric form. The transfer of storage ferritin (Fe^{3+}) to plasma involves reduction of Fe^{3+} to Fe^{2+} in the mucosal cell with the help of ferrireductase. This ferrous enters the plasma and is reoxidized to ferric form by a copper protein, ceruloplasmin or serum ferroxidase, and then this ferric form incorporated into transferrin by combining with apotransferrin.
- In the iron-deficient state, more iron is delivered to apotransferrin and much less to apoferritin.
- In the case of iron overload, more iron is transferred to apoferritin and much less to apotransferrin. Thus entry of iron into the body is regulated at the intestine level.

Ferritin: It is the major storage form of iron and it is readily available for metabolic requirements. The storage occurs in liver, spleen, and bone.

Hemosiderin: In addition to ferritin, iron can also be found in a form of hemosiderin. This hemosiderin is insoluble in aqueous medium and iron is released slowly from this. Normally very little hemosiderin is found in the liver, but the quantity increases during iron overload and it may represent protective role against iron overload.

Serum Content

About 100 mL of blood contains about 300 mg of transferrin, which is capable of carrying 360 µg of Fe, but normally it carries an average of only 100 µg of Fe. In deficiency this level is much less **(Box 15.5)**.

Copper

Sources

The sources of copper are as follows:
- Fish, liver
- Nuts
- Green vegetables
- Milk and cereals are poor sources.

Recommended Dietary Allowance

Adult: 3 mg/day.

Functions

The need for copper (Cu^{2+}) is linked to its functional role in several copper-containing enzymes:
- Ceruloplasmin (also called serum ferroxidase). This copper-containing protein catalyzes the oxidation of Fe^{2+} to Fe^{3+}.

Box 15.5: Iron deficiency and excess.

Iron deficiency
Hypochromic microcytic anemia: RBCs of reduced in size.
Causes are:
- Hemorrhage.
- Malabsorption.
- Hookworm infestation depletes the body iron even if the diet is adequate.
- The pronounced and repeated Fe losses resulting from menstruation, pregnancy, and lactation render women of childbearing age especially vulnerable to depletion of iron stores.
- Anemic patients are found to be pale, tired, and restless and have palpitation, lesions of oral cavity, and spoon-shaped nails.

Iron overload
Hemosiderosis, hemochromatosis, and iron poisoning are the conditions associated with iron overload.
Hemochromatosis: It is an excessive hemosiderin accumulation in tissues such as liver, spleen, and skin caused by an excessive intestinal absorption of iron due to a genetic disorder.
This results in bronze-colored skin, cirrhosis of liver, and damage to pancreas leading to diabetes. This is called bronze diabetes.
Hemosiderosis: It is an excessive accumulation of iron. This may be seen in the Bantu people of Africa, who consume large amount of Fe obtained from their cooking pots made of iron.

Box 15.6: Copper deficiency.

Hypochromic microcytic anemia
Hypochromic microcytic anemia due to copper deficiency in milk-fed infants has been observed. It responds to copper, but not to iron therapy.
Wilson's disease
Wilson's disease or hepatolenticular degeneration is a fatal inherited disease. In this blood copper level decreases.
Menkes syndrome
Menkes syndrome or kinky-hair disease is a rare X-linked recessive disorder. The genetic defect is in absorption of copper from intestine. Both serum copper and ceruloplasmin and liver copper content are reduced. The clinical manifestations are:
- Kinky or twisted brittle hair due to loss of copper catalyzed disulfide bond formation
- Depigmentation of the skin and hair
- Seizures
- Mental retardation
- Lesions of the blood vessels

- Cytochrome oxidase of the respiratory chain contains Fe^{3+} and Cu^{2+}.
- Dopamine—oxidase of catecholamine synthetic pathway.
- Monoamine oxidase and diamine oxidase.
- Cytoplasmic superoxide dismutase contains Cu^{2+} and Zn^{2+}.
- Phosphate hydroxyphenylpyruvate hydroxylase of tyrosine catabolism.
- Lysyl oxidase involved in crosslinking process in the conversion of tropocollagen to collagen.
- Tyrosinase of melanin synthetic pathway is a copper-dependent enzyme.

Absorption and Transport in Blood

About 50% of the average daily dietary copper is absorbed from the stomach and the small intestine. Then transported to the liver bound to albumin and exported to peripheral tissues (90%) bound to ceruloplasmin, and to a lesser extent (10%) to albumin. The route of excretion of copper is through bile **(Box 15.6)**.

Copper Excess

There is an excessive storage of copper in the liver, probably owing to defective synthesis of ceruloplasmin by the liver cells. Besides deposition in liver, copper is also deposited in kidney, brain, and cornea (brown ring called Kayser-Fleischer ring at the margin of cornea). Cirrhosis of liver, neurological disorders, tubular damage, and high urinary copper are also seen. Penicillamine, a copper-chelating agent, is used in its treatment. Excess copper is thus excreted.

Zinc

Sources

The sources of zinc are as follows:
- Meat
- Egg
- Marine fish
- Unmilled cereals

- Legumes corn
- Spinach
- Lettuce.

Recommended Dietary Allowance
- Adults: 10-15 mg/day
- Children: 3-15 mg/day
- Pregnancy and lactation: 20-25 mg/day.

Functions
The functions of zinc are as follows:
- Zn is required as an activator ion for the following enzymes:
  - Carbonic anhydrase
  - Alkaline phosphatase
  - Liver alcohol dehydrogenase
  - Carboxypeptidase A
  - DNA polymerase
  - Cytosolic superoxide dismutase (both Cu^{2+} and Zn^{2+}).
- It is required for the wound healing processes.
- It is a necessary factor in the biosynthesis and integrity of connective tissue.

Deficiency
The deficiency in zinc leads to the following:
- It may cause dwarfism.
- Other deficiency manifestations are hypogonadism.
- Loss of taste sensation.
- Impaired wound healing.
- Acrodermatitis enteropathica: It is an autosomal recessive disorder and its clinical manifestations appear to be related to zinc deficiency. The clinical manifestations of this are chronic diarrhea, alopecia, wasting and thickened ulcerated skin around the body orifices, and extremities.

Manganese

Sources
The sources of manganese are as follows:
- Wheat germs seeds
- Nuts
- Leafy vegetables
- Meat.

Recommended Dietary Allowance
- Adults: 3.5 mg/day
- Children: 0.2 mg/day.

Functions
The functions of manganese are as follows:
- Manganese acts as a cofactor or an activator for several enzymes, such as:
  - Acetyl-CoA carboxylase
  - Mitochondrial superoxide dismutase
  - Arginase
  - 6-phosphate-gluconate dehydrogenase
  - Squalene synthase
  - Isocitrate dehydrogenase
  - Glutamine synthetase
  - Kinases.
- Manganese also functions with vitamin K in the formation of prothrombin.

Manganese Deficiency
In both birds and mammals, the manganese deficiency is characterized by defective growth, bone abnormalities, reproductive dysfunction, and CNS manifestations.

Manganese Excess
The toxicity has been seen in miners as a result of absorption of manganese through respiratory tract after prolonged exposure to manganese dust.

Molybdenum

Sources
The sources of molybdenum are as follows:
- Legumes
- Whole grains
- Milk
- Leafy vegetables
- Organ meat.

Recommended Dietary Allowance
Adults: 0.5 mg/day.

Functions

Molybdenum (Mg^{2+}) is required as a catalytic component of the metalloenzymes such as:
- Xanthine oxidase
- Aldehyde oxidase
- Sulfite oxidase.

Deficiency

It is reported to cause xanthinuria.

Cobalt

Sources

The sources of cobalt are as follows:
- Liver
- Kidney
- Muscle meats
- Oysters
- Clams.

Functions

The functions of cobalt are as follows:
- Cobalt can be found in vitamin B_{12} and its coenzymes.
- Cofactor for glycylglycine dipeptidase of intestinal juice.

Deficiency

A cobalt deficiency is accompanied by all the signs and symptoms of a vitamin B_{12} deficiency. The most important among them is anemia.

Cobalt Toxicity

Polycythemia.

Selenium

Sources

The sources of selenium are as follows:
- Fish
- Whole grain
- Meat
- Liver and kidney.

Recommended Dietary Allowance

Adult: 0.2 mg/day.

Functions

The functions of selenium are as follows:
- Selenium (Se) is an integral component of glutathione peroxidase. This enzyme scavenging the free radicals and protect the cells, and membranes against oxidative damage. Thus it acts as an antioxidant.
- This mineral complements the action of vitamin E.
- It also is a constituent of iodothyronine deiodinase, the enzyme that converts thyroxine to triiodothyronine.

Absorption

The principal dietary forms of selenium selenocysteine and selenomethionine are absorbed from gastrointestinal tract.

Deficiency

Selenium deficiency has been associated in some areas of China with Keshan disease, a cardiomyopathy, which primarily affects children. Symptoms are loss of appetite nausea and congestive heart failure.

Fluoride

Sources

The sources of fluoride are as follows:
- Fish
- Tea
- Drinking water.

Recommended Dietary Allowance

- Adults: 1–2 mg/day
- Drinking water provides fluoride [1 part per million (1 ppm)] fluoride. 2 L water consumed by an individual provides 2 mg fluoride.

Functions

The functions of fluoride are as follows:
- It is a component of a hydroxyapatite.

- Fluoride is needed for bone and teeth formation. The surface layer of enamel contains a higher content of fluoride than deeper layers of enamel or dentine. It strengthens the enamel surface of teeth and renders it resistant to dental carries (decay).

Deficiency

Deficiency of fluoride causes dental caries and osteoporosis.

Fluoride Excess

Excess fluoride causes fluorosis. In this condition, there is mottling of enamel. The mottled enamel is discolored, corroded, and pitted. High concentrations of fluoride inhibit magnesium-requiring enzyme enolase.

Chromium

Sources

The sources of chromium are as follows:
- Brewer's yeast
- Molasses
- Meat products
- Cheese.

Recommended Dietary Allowance

For adults 0.05–20 mg.

Functions

The functions of chromium are as follows:
- Chromium (Cr) functions in the control of glucose and lipid metabolism.
- It acts as cofactor for insulin in increasing glucose utilization and transport of amino acids into cells.
- Organochromium complex is known as the glucose tolerance factor. The researchers showed that it enhances the action of insulin.

Deficiency

Deficiency of chromium may develop the symptoms of glucose intolerance and weight loss.

Chromium Toxicity

- Known to cause inflammation and necrosis of the skin and nasal passages
- Oral ingestion can lead to GI tract and renal damage.

Iodine

- The adult human body contains about 50 mg of iodine.
- The blood plasma contains 4–8 µg of protein bound iodine per 100 mL.

Sources

The sources are seafood, drinking water, iodized table salt, onions, vegetables, etc.

Recommended Dietary Allowance

The dietary allowance should be 150 µg/day.

Functions

The most important role of iodine in the body is in the synthesis of thyroid hormones, triiodothyronine (T3) and tetraiodothyronine (T4), which influence a large number of metabolic functions.

Deficiency Manifestation

A deficiency of iodine in children leads to cretinism and in adults' endemic goiter **Box 15.7**.

Box 15.7: Iodine deficiency.

Cretinism: Severe iodine deficiency in mothers leads to intrauterine or neonatal hypothyroidism results in cretinism in their children, a condition characterized by mental retardation, dwarfism, and slow growth.

Goiter: It is an enlarged thyroid with decreased thyroid hormone production. The iodine deficiency in adults stimulates the proliferation of epithelial cells and resulting in enlargement of the thyroid gland. Normally thyroid gland collects iodine from the blood to synthesize thyroid hormones. In iodine-deficient state, the thyroid gland undergoes compensatory enlargement in order to extract iodine from blood.

Functions of Minerals (Summary) (Table 15.4)

Table 15.4: Functions of minerals.

Minerals	Functions
Sodium	Fluid balance, nerve transmission, and muscle contraction
Chloride	Fluid balance and stomach acid production
Potassium	Fluid balance, nerve transmission, and muscle contraction
Calcium	Bone and teeth health maintenance, nerve transmission, muscle contraction, and blood clotting
Phosphorous	Bone and teeth health maintenance and acid-base balance
Magnesium	Protein production, nerve transmission, and muscle contraction
Sulfur	Protein synthesis
Iron	Carries oxygen and helps in energy production
Zinc	Protein and DNA production, wound healing, growth, and immune system function
Iodine	Thyroid hormone production, growth, and metabolism
Selenium	Antioxidant
Copper	Coenzyme and iron metabolism
Manganese	Coenzyme
Fluoride	Bone and teeth health maintenance, tooth decay prevention
Chromium	Assists insulin in glucose metabolism
Molybdenum	Coenzyme

SUMMARY

Minerals are the essential chemical elements required for living organism and they are classified into bulk and trace elements. Bulk elements are seven in number such as calcium, magnesium, sodium, potassium, phosphorus, sulfur, and chloride. They constitute 60–80% of all inorganic material in the body. Trace elements are those, which are required in very small amounts. They are nine in number such as iron, iodine, cobalt, manganese, molybdenum, zinc, lead, selenium, and fluoride. The deficiency of these minerals results in various disorders. For example, hypocalcemia may lead to numbness and bone disorders, iodine deficiency results in goiter, fluoride deficiency causes dental decay, and iron deficiency results in anemia.

SELF-ASSESSMENT QUESTIONS

Long-Answer Questions

1. Write a note on the requirement and functions of calcium.
2. What are the factors, which favor iron absorption?
3. Add a note on the absorption and transport of iron.
4. Name the heme and nonheme proteins, which contain iron.
5. Mention the functions of phosphorus.
6. Name any four enzymes, which need magnesium as an activator ion.
7. Which trace element deficiency leads to Wilson's disease?
8. Mention the important source of fluoride. What is fluorosis?
9. What are the sources for copper?

10. What are trace elements and name any four of them?
11. What are the importance of sodium and potassium in the human body?
12. Give the normal values of Na$^+$ and K$^+$.

Short-Answer Questions

1. Explain whether copper is an example of trace or bulk element.
2. Give the normal serum value of calcium.
3. Name the nonheme protein, which contains iron.
4. Which form of iron is absorbed from GI tract?
5. The deficiency of iron leads to what?
6. Name the storage form of iron.
7. Antioxidant property is observed in which trace element?
8. Give an example for copper-containing enzyme.
9. The fluoride deficiency leads to what?
10. Name the major cation of the ECF.
11. What is hyponatremia?
12. Mention the name of the major extracellular anion.

Fill in the Blanks

1. Copper is a/an _____ element.
2. The normal serum value of calcium is _____.
3. The example for nonhemeprotein that contains iron is _____.
4. The form of iron, which absorbed from GI tract is _____.
5. The deficiency of iron leads to _____.
6. Storage form of iron is called _____.
7. Antioxidant property is observed in the trace element is _____.
8. Cytochrome oxidase is a/an _____ containing enzyme.
9. The fluoride deficiency leads to _____.
10. The major cation of the ECF is _____.
11. Hyponatremia means _____.
12. The major extracellular anion is _____.

MULTIPLE-CHOICE QUESTIONS

1. All the following factors affect calcium absorption, *except*:
   a. 1,25-dihydroxyvitamin D$_3$
   b. Gastric acidity
   c. Lactose
   d. Calcium:Magnesium ratio of the diet

2. Oxalates may:
   a. Decrease the calcium absorption
   b. Increase the calcium absorption
   c. Regulate the calcium metabolism
   d. Do not have any effect on calcium

3. Concerning calcium content of the body, one of the following statements is incorrect:
   a. It is the major inorganic element comprising nearly 2% of the body weight
   b. Human body contains 1,200 g of calcium
   c. Major amount (99%) present in bone and teeth
   d. Blood calcium exists only in as ionized form

4. Concerning the functions of calcium, all of the following statements are true, *except*:
   a. It is required for the formation of bone and teeth
   b. It increases the absorption of iron
   c. It is required for blood coagulation process
   d. It activates phosphorylase during the breakdown of glycogen

5. All the following are the symptoms of hypophosphatemia, *except*:
   a. Rickets
   b. Hyperparathyroidism
   c. Fanconi's syndrome
   d. Renal failure

6. Magnesium is the second major:
   a. Intracellular cation
   b. Intracellular anion
   c. Extracellular cation
   d. Extracellular anion

7. All of the following are the functions of sodium, *except*:
   a. It maintains the osmotic pressure
   b. It regulates the electrolyte and pH balance of the extracellular compartment
   c. It controls the movement of ions in muscle
   d. It helps in the active transport of glucose

8. Cushing's disease presents with:
   a. Hypernatremia
   b. Hyperphosphatemia
   c. Hyperphosphatemia
   d. None of the above

9. The major intracellular cation is:
   a. Sodium   b. Magnesium
   c. Calcium   d. Potassium

10. All the following conditions result in hyperkalemia, *except*:
    a. Burns   b. Renal failure
    c. Malnutrition   d. Shock

Mineral Metabolism

11. Major extracellular anion is:
    a. Fluoride
    b. Chloride
    c. Bicarbonate
    d. Selenium
12. All the following are the heme proteins, which contains iron, *except*:
    a. Ferritin
    b. Myoglobin
    c. Catalase
    d. Cytochrome *b*
13. Which of the following does not contain iron?
    a. Transferrin
    b. Succinate dehydrogenase
    c. Aconitase
    d. Hexokinase
14. All of the following favor iron absorption, *except*:
    a. Vitamin C
    b. Ferric iron
    c. Pregnancy
    d. Increased erythropoiesis
15. Concerning iron metabolism, all of the following statements are correct, *except*:
    a. Ferritin is the storage form of iron
    b. Transferring is the transport from of iron
    c. Iron oxidized to Fe^{3+} after absorption
    d. In the case iron overload more iron is transported as transferrin
16. All the following conditions result in iron deficiency, *except*:
    a. Shock
    b. Malabsorption
    c. Hookworm infestation
    d. Hemorrhage
17. Concerning the functions of copper, all of the following statements are true, *except*:
    a. Ceruloplasmin is a copper-containing protein
    b. Glutaminase is a copper-dependent enzyme
    c. Superoxide dismutase is a copper-dependent enzyme
    d. Tyrosinase is a copper-dependent enzyme
18. Acrodermatitis enteropathica results from the deficiency of:
    a. Zinc
    b. Copper
    c. Magnesium
    d. Fluoride
19. Which of the following vitamin has cobalt in its structure?
    a. Vitamin B_6
    b. Vitamin C
    c. Vitamin B_{12}
    d. Vitamin B_1
20. The trace element, which has antioxidant property is?
    a. Fluoride
    b. Selenium
    c. Molybdenum
    d. Manganese
21. Concerning fluoride, one of the following statements is incorrect:
    a. 2 L waters consumed by an individual provides 10 mg of fluoride
    b. It is a component of a hydroxyapatite
    c. Excess fluoride causes fluorosis
    d. Its reduced levels causes to dental carries
22. The blood level of sodium in a normal individual is:
    a. 3.5–5.0 mEq/L
    b. 103 mEq/L
    c. 8–11 mEq/L
    d. 130–145 mEq/L
23. Which of the following causes hypercalcemia?
    a. Sarcoidosis
    b. Primary hyperparathyroidism
    c. Acute pancreatitis
    d. Metastatic bronchial carcinoma
24. With respect to iron metabolism:
    a. The body contains about 40 g of iron
    b. Part of the iron in the body is contained in ferritin
    c. Iron is transported in plasma as ferritin
    d. Hemosiderin is the main form in which iron is stored in tissues
25. Glucose intolerance is the feature of the deficiency of:
    a. Cobalt
    b. Chromium
    c. Selenium
    d. Iodine

Answers

1. d	2. a	3. d	4. b	5. d
6. a	7. c	8. a	9. d	10. c
11. b	12. a	13. d	14. b	15. d
16. a	17. b	18. a	19. c	20. b
21. a	22. d	23. c	24. b	25. b

CHAPTER 16

Vitamins

OBJECTIVES

At the end of this chapter, students should be able to:
- Understand the sources, daily requirement, functions, metabolism, and deficiency manifestation of vitamins A, D, E, and K
- Discuss the sources, functions, and disorders associated with vitamin C
- Explain the sources, requirement, coenzyme forms, functions, and disorders associated with vitamins thiamine, riboflavin, pyridoxine, niacin, biotin, pantothenic acid, folic acid, and B_{12}.

INTRODUCTION

Vitamins are naturally occurring organic substances. Their coenzyme forms are essential in metabolic processes. They serve nearly the same roles in all forms of life. The daily requirement of any vitamin depends on a number of factors and may increase during growth, pregnancy, and lactation. They are essential nutrients and have various roles in the human body. The vitamins are divided into two groups:
1. Fat-soluble vitamins (A, D, E, and K), foods that contain these vitamins will not lose them when cooked.
2. Water-soluble vitamins (B complex) and vitamin C.

FAT-SOLUBLE VITAMINS

Vitamins A, D, E, and K are called fat-soluble vitamins because they dissolve in fat (**Table 16.1**). They are absorbed from the small intestines along with dietary fat. Fat-soluble vitamins are primarily stored in the liver and adipose tissues. With the exception of vitamin K, fat-soluble vitamins are generally excreted more slowly than water-soluble vitamins, and vitamins A and D can accumulate and cause toxic effects in the body.

Vitamin A

- Vitamin A comprises the preformed retinoid and the precursor forms, the provitamin A carotenoid.
- Preformed retinoid is a collective term for retinol, retinal, and retinoic acid all of which are biologically active:

- The provitamin A carotenoids include β-carotene and others, which are converted to retinoids. The retinoids are sensitive to heat, light, and oxidation by air. The β-carotene is relatively more stable.
- Retinoids are converted to retinol in the intestines and transported with dietary fat to the liver, where it is stored. A special transport protein, retinol-binding protein, transports vitamin A from the liver to other tissues. Carotenoids are absorbed intact at a much lower absorption rate than retinol. Of all the carotenoids, β-carotene has the highest potential vitamin A activity. The

active forms of vitamin A have three basic functions:
1. Vision
2. Growth and development of tissues
3. Immunity.

Sources
- Cod liver oil, fish liver oils, animal liver, milk and milk products, and eggs.
- The carotenoid pigments present in carrots, sweet potato, and green leafy vegetables such as spinach and amaranth.
- The yellow pigment, β-carotene present in vegetables is a precursor of vitamin A.
- It has two ionone rings connected by a polyprenoid chain.
- One molecule of β-carotene can theoretically give rise to two molecules of vitamin A, but it may produce only one in biological systems.

Recommended dietary allowance
- Adult: 800–1,000 µg/day (5,000 IU/day)
- Pregnancy and lactation: 1,000–1,200 µg/day (4,000 IU/day)
- Infants and children: 400–600 µg/day (3,000 IU/day).

Physiological role
- Role of vitamin A in vision: Retina of the eye contains two types of cells:
  a. Rod cells (vision in dim light): It has a photosensitive pigment called rhodopsin, which is a conjugated protein made up of opsin and 11-*cis*-retinal (**Fig. 16.1**).
  b. Cone cells (vision in bright light).
- Rhodopsin once exposed to light, it dissociates into all *trans*-retinal and opsin. All *trans*-retinal reduced to all *trans*-retinol in the retina and transported to liver where it is isomerized to 11-*cis*-retinol, then this is transported back to retina then oxidized to 11-*cis*-retinal, which combines with opsin to form rhodopsin.
- Retinoic acid form of vitamin A maintains structural and functional integrity of epithelium.
- Retinol form of vitamin A is required for growth and reproductive function.

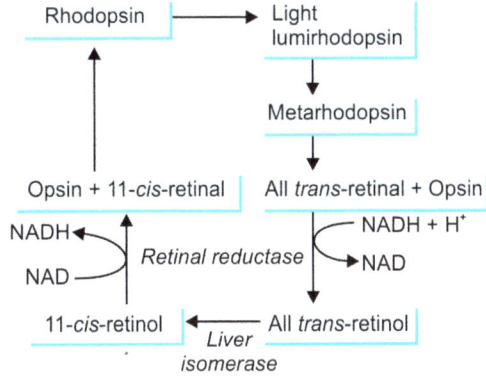

Fig. 16.1: Wald's visual cycle.
(NAD: nicotinamide adenine dinucleotide; NADH: nicotinamide adenine dinucleotide hydrogen)

- Retinol is also known to require for the formation of bone and teeth.

Deficiency
- Night blindness.
- Keratinization of lacrimal glands.
- *Keratomalacia:* Dryness of the cornea; corneal epithelium becomes keratinized and opaque and may become softened, and ulcerated.
- *Follicular keratosis:* Deficiency will affect hair follicles and causes scaly skin.
- *Hypervitaminosis:* It is rare; if occurs, it leads to headache, nausea, vomiting, loss of appetite, and pain in bones.

Vitamin D (Cholecalciferol)

Sources
- D_2 in plants.
- D_3 in fish, egg, and liver.
- Ergosterol vitamin D_2 (ergocalciferol):

Ergocalciferol (D_2)

- Cholesterol→7-dehydrocholesterol and vitamin D_3 (cholecalciferol):

Cholecalciferol (D_3)

- The 7-dehydrocholesterol, an intermediate of a minor pathway of cholesterol synthesis, is available in the epidermis. If the skin is on exposure to sunlight, the 7-dehydrocholesterol can be converted to cholecalciferol.

Recommended dietary allowance
- Children: 10 μg/day (400 IU/day)
- Adults: 5–10 μg/day (400 IU/day)
- Pregnancy and lactation: 10 μg/day (400 IU/day).

Vitamin D_2 or D_3 is not active biologically but converted to active form by hydroxylation.

Regulation of formation of $1,25(OH)_2$ vitamin D_3
- Low plasma calcium level stimulates parathyroid hormone (PTH) secretion; this in turn acts on kidney to secrete 1-α-hydroxylase (**Fig. 16.2**).
- High level of $1,25(OH)_2$ vitamin D_3 inhibits the secretion of 1-α-hydroxylase.
- High plasma calcium level inhibits the activity of 1-α-hydroxylase.
- Low plasma phosphate level also activates the 1-α-hydroxylase, but independent of PTH.
- High plasma phosphate inhibits the activity of 1-α-hydroxylase.
- When calcium level is normal, the production of $1,25(OH)_2$ vitamin D_3 suppressed, which results in the stimulation of 24-hydroxylase, which converts 25-hydroxyvitamin D_3 to $24,25(OH)_2$ vitamin D_3.

Functions
Vitamin D maintains an adequate calcium level by the following mechanisms:
- Increases the absorption of calcium from the intestine on vitamin D_3, enters the intestinal cell, then binds to cytoplasmic receptor. This complex interacts with deoxyribonucleic acid (DNA) in the nucleus results in the synthesis of messenger ribonucleic acid. This in turn forms a calcium-binding protein (CBP) known as calbindin and osteocalcin. This CBP increases the absorption of calcium.
- Reabsorption of calcium and phosphate from the kidney, 1,25-dihydroxycholecalciferol causes the increased reabsorption of calcium and phosphate in the distal convoluted tubule from glomerular filtrate.
- Mobilization of calcium and phosphate from bone. Vitamin D has both anabolic and catabolic role on bone causing removal

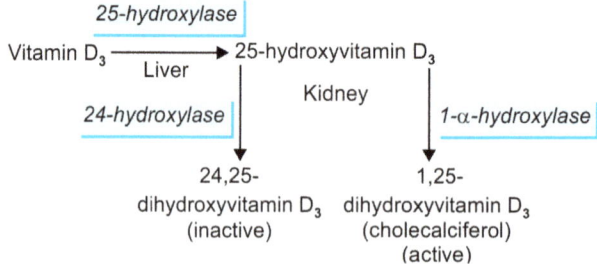

Fig. 16.2: Formation of active vitamin D_3.

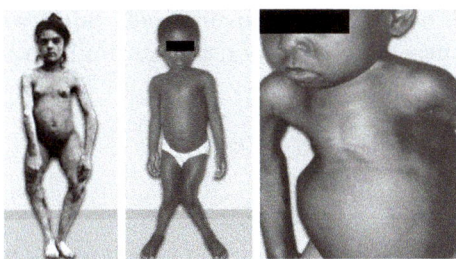

Fig. 16.3: Features of vitamin D_3 deficiency.

of calcium from bone (resorption of bone calcium).

Deficiency
- The deficiency of vitamin D leads to rickets in children
- Signs and symptoms are bowlegs, knock knee, pigeon chest, hypocalcemia, and hypophosphatemia (**Fig. 16.3**)
- Osteomalacia in adults
- Signs and symptoms are soft and pliable bones.

Sources, Recommended Daily Requirement, Metabolism, Biochemical Functions, and Deficiency Manifestations of Vitamin E and K

Vitamin E (Tocopherol)

Sources
- Vegetable oils such as wheat germ oil, corn oil, cottonseed oil, and safflower oil.
- Vitamin E is absorbed from intestine together with dietary lipid. It is delivered to the tissues via chylomicrons. The major site of vitamin E storage is in the adipose tissue.

Recommended dietary allowance
- *Adult male*: 15 mg/day (22 IU/day)
- *Female*: 15 mg/day (22 IU/day)
- *Children*: 10 mg/day (16 IU/day).

Functions
- Potent physiological antioxidant: Vitamin E protects membranes with lipids from oxidative damage.
- Vitamin E, which is present in cell membranes, prevents the destructive nonenzymatic oxidation of polyunsaturated fatty acids by molecular oxygen and it maintains the membrane integrity.
- It protects erythrocytes from hemolysis by oxidizing agent's hydrogen peroxide (H_2O_2).
- It is required for normal reproduction in animals.
- It prevents liver necrosis and muscular dystrophy.
- It protects cellular and subcellular membranes.

Deficiency
- Reproductive failure in animals
- Hemolysis of erythrocytes, which may lead to anemia
- Muscular weakness, fragile red blood cells (RBCs).

Vitamin K

The important forms of vitamin K are:
- Phylloquinone (K_1):

- Menaquinone (K_2):

$n = 4 - 13$

- Menadione (K_3):

  [structure of menadione]

Sources
- Green leafy vegetables (spinach, alfalfa grass, cauliflower, and cabbage).
- Tomato.
- Putrid fish meal.
- It is also synthesized by microorganisms in the intestinal tract.

Functions
- Required for the maintenance of normal concentration of following blood clotting factors:
  - Prothrombin
  - Stable factor
  - Plasma thromboplastin component
  - Stuart–Prower factor.
- Each of these is synthesized in the liver in an inactive form.
- Conversion of inactive to active form involves γ-carboxylation of glutamic acid residues from the N-terminal end. This process creates negative charges and depends on vitamin K:

  Protein–NH   Vitamin K   Protein–NH
  | |
  CHOH–protein ─────────────────────▶ CHOH–protein
  | Carboxylase |
  CH_2 CH_2
  | CO + O |
  CH_2 CH
  | / \
  COOH   COO COO^-
                                            \ /
                                            Ca^{2+}

- The Ca^{2+} and phospholipids bond with negative charges and activate prothrombin to thrombin:

  Fibrinogen ─── Thrombin ───▶ Fibrin

- In the absence of γ-carboxylation, chelation with Ca^{2+} is impaired.
- The vitamin-dependent γ-carboxylation is also necessary for the functional activity of C-reactive protein and osteocalcin. The osteocalcin binds to hydroxyapatite crystals of bone; this binding mainly dependent on the level of γ-carboxylation. The vitamin K helps to retain calcium by this mechanism.
- The vitamin K-dependent carboxylase enzyme requires oxygen, carbon dioxide (CO_2), reduced form of nicotinamide adenine dinucleotide (NAD) phosphate (NADPH) and reduced vitamin K. In this process, the vitamin passes through a cycle (**Fig. 16.4**). For reconversion of vitamin K, reduced lipoamide is necessary. This process is inhibited by a vitamin K antagonist, warfarin and dicoumarol:

  [structures of Dicoumarol and Warfarin]

Recommended dietary allowance
- Intestinal bacteria synthesizes vitamin K.
- Newborn and infancy: 2.0 µg/day.
- Children 60 µg/day.

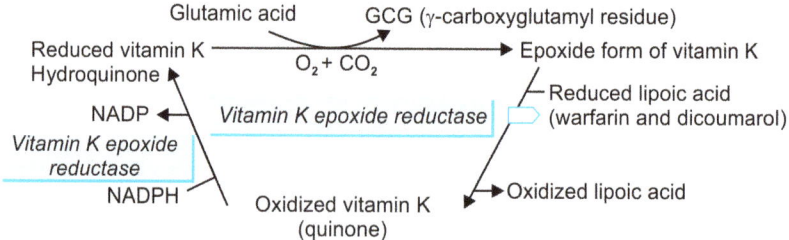

Fig. 16.4: Vitamin K cycle.
(NAD: nicotinamide adenine dinucleotide; NADPH: nicotinamide adenine dinucleotide phosphate)

- Adults: 60–140 µg.
- Pregnancy and lactation: 90 µg/day.

Deficiency
- Normally does not occur.
- The drug therapy (sulfa drugs) inhibits the bacteria, which help in vitamin K synthesis.
- Steatorrhea and pancreatic failure with decreased fat absorption result in vitamin K deficiency.
- If deficiency arises, profuse bleeding and prolonged clotting time are the main symptoms (refer to **Table 16.1**).

WATER-SOLUBLE VITAMINS

Vitamin C (Ascorbic Acid)

- B-complex vitamins and vitamin C are water-soluble vitamins that are not stored in the body and must be replaced each day.
- These vitamins are easily destroyed or washed out during food storage and preparation.
- The B-complex group is found in a variety of foods such as cereal, grains, meat, poultry, eggs, fish, milk, legumes, and fresh vegetables.
- Citrus fruits are good sources of vitamin C.
- Use of heavy doses of vitamins is not recommended (**Table 16.2**).

Sources
- The rich sources are citrus fruits (orange, lemon).
- Tomatoes, strawberries, green vegetables, guava fruit, green pepper.

Recommended dietary allowance
- Adults: 60 mg/day
- Children: 40 mg/day.

Functions
- *Collagen synthesis*: Vitamin C is very important for the *hydroxylation of proline*

Table 16.1: Summary of fat-soluble vitamins.

Vitamins	Sources	Functions	Deficiency	Overconsumption
Vitamin A (retinol, retinoic acid, and retinal)	Liver, fortified milk and dairy products. *Provitamin A:* Carrots, green leafy vegetables, sweet potatoes, apricots	Skin and mucous membrane formation; night vision, bones and teeth development, and β-carotene is an antioxidant and may protect against cancer	Night blindness, Intestinal infections, impaired vision, inflammation of eyes, keratinization of skin and eyes, and blindness in children	Nausea, irritability, growth retardation, enlargement of liver and spleen, loss of hair, bone pain
Vitamin D	*Vitamin D:* Fortified dairy products, fortified margarine, fish oils, egg yolk and synthesized by sunlight action on skin	Promotes hardening of bones and teeth, increases the absorption of calcium	Rickets in children; osteomalacia in adults	Nausea, weight loss, movement of calcium from bones into soft tissues
Vitamin E	Vegetable oil, margarine, butter, green leafy vegetables, wheat germ	Spares the action of vitamins A and prevents damage to cell membranes and antioxidant	Possible anemia in low-birth-weight infants	Nontoxic under normal conditions
Vitamin K	Dark green leafy vegetables, liver; also made by bacteria in the intestine	Helps blood to clot	Excessive bleeding	None reported

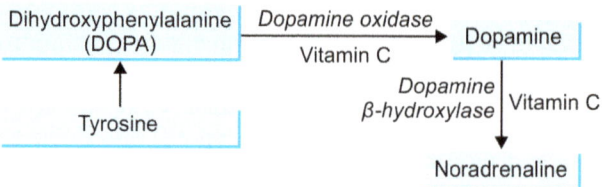

Fig. 16.5: Role of vitamin C.

and lysine residues (via prolyl hydroxylase and lysyl hydroxylase), which are the collagen precursors.
- It helps in the absorption of iron by reducing from ferric (Fe^{3+}) to ferrous (Fe^{2+}) in the stomach.
- It acts as an electron donor for eight different enzymes.
- Reaction between amino groups of protein and nitrites formed in the intestine produces nitrosamines that may cause cancer. So, vitamin C acts as an antioxidant, scavenging the free radicals, and reduces the nitrosamine formation.
- The conversion of dihydroxyphenylalanine to dopamine and dopamine to noradrenaline requires vitamin C as an activator (**Fig. 16.5**).
- The vitamin C in high dose (1 g/day) decreases the severity of cold:

Deficiency
The vitamin C deficiency leads to scurvy (**Fig. 16.6**).

Signs and symptoms are:
- Spongy gums
- Loose teeth
- Fragile blood vessels
- Aching swollen joints

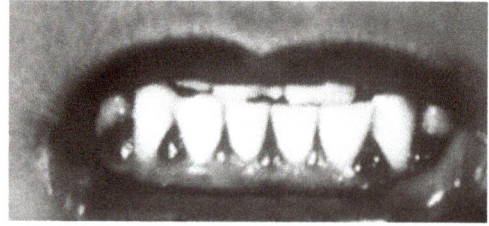

Fig. 16.6: Symptoms of scurvy.

- Anemia
- Delay in wound healing.

B-COMPLEX VITAMINS

Thiamine (B_1)

- It is a sulfur-containing vitamin
- It has thiazole and pyrimidine rings.

Sources
- Whole grains (unpolished rice, wheat)
- Legumes (beans, peas)
- Meat
- Bananas
- Soybeans.

Recommended dietary allowance
- Children: 1.2 mg/day
- Adults: 1.5 mg/day
- Pregnancy and lactation: –2.0 mg/day.

Functions
- The coenzyme form of thiamine is thiamine pyrophosphate (TPP).
- TPP is required as coenzyme for several reactions, which are taking place in the human body.
- Pyruvate dehydrogenase complex:

Pyruvate $\xrightarrow{\text{TPP}}$ Acetyl-CoA

α-ketoglutarate $\xrightarrow[\text{TPP, FAD}]{\alpha\text{-ketoglutarate dehydrogenase complex}}$ Succinyl-CoA

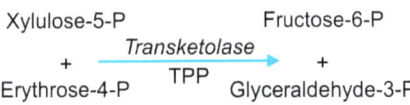

- Thiamine monophosphate and thiamine triphosphate (ThTP) are the other two derivatives of thiamine.
- ThTP was considered as a specific neuroactive form of thiamine. However, recently it was shown that ThTP exists in bacteria, fungi, plants, and animals suggesting a much more general cellular role.

Deficiency
- Caused by alcoholism and malnutrition.
- Thiamine deficiency leads to failure of carbohydrate metabolism, where the TPP is required for many enzymes to catalyze the reactions. This results in the decreased production of ATP and thus impaired cellular functions of central nervous system, heart, and gastrointestinal tract. The overall picture of this vitamin deficiency, including neurological, cardiovascular, and gastrointestinal disorders, is referred to as beriberi. Beriberi is of four types:
  a. Dry beriberi (peripheral neuritis)
  b. Wet beriberi (cardiac manifestation)
  c. Cerebral beriberi (Wernicke-Korsakoff syndrome)
  d. Infantile beriberi.

Difference between Dry Beriberi and Wet Beriberi

Dry Beriberi
- Loss of appetite
- Weight loss
- Muscle wasting
- Peripheral neuritis with numbness
- Tingling sensations in the lower legs and feet (**Fig. 16.7**)
- Ataxic gait.

Wet Beriberi
- With the symptoms of dry beriberi
- Edema
- Foot drop and wrist drop
- Enlargement of heart.

Cerebral Beriberi (Wernicke-Korsakoff Syndrome)

It occurs in alcoholics who consume less food and characterized by intelligence disturbance:
- Ataxia
- Double vision
- Nystagmus (rapid involuntary movement of the eyes)
- If this condition untreated progresses to Korsakoff's psychosis, which is irreversible.

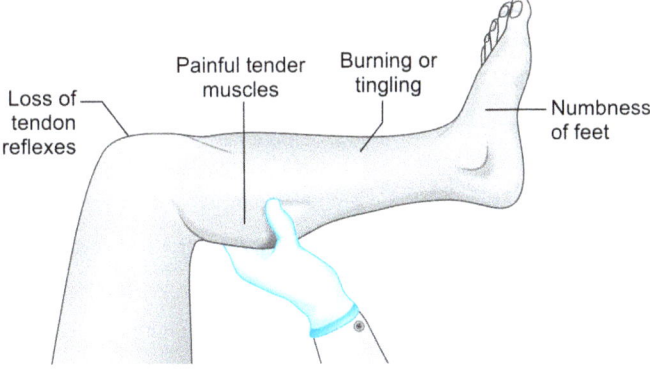

Fig. 16.7: Symptoms of dry beriberi.

Infantile Beriberi

It is due to the low thiamine content of breast milk from a deficient mother and it is characterized by:
- Anorexia
- Tachycardia
- Vomiting
- Convulsions
- Edema.

Thiaminase is present in raw fish and seafood may destroy the thiamine.

Riboflavin (B_2)

Chemistry

Riboflavin has a dimethyl isoalloxazine ring attached to ribitol (the reduced form or ribose). B_2 is stable to heat but is sensitive to light.

Sources

The sources are animal liver, yeast, green leafy vegetables, milk, and eggs.

Recommended Dietary Allowance
- Adults: 2 mg/day
- Children: 1.2 mg/day
- Pregnancy and lactation: 2 mg/day.

Active form of Riboflavin

- The riboflavin has two coenzyme forms—(1) flavin mononucleotide (FMN) and (2) flavin adenine dinucleotide (FAD); both of them are nucleotides.
- Some enzymes have FMN and FAD as their integral part. Such enzymes are called flavoproteins.

Functions of flavin mononucleotide and flavin adenine dinucleotide

They take part in oxidation reactions:

Flavin mononucleotide is required for:
- L-Amino acid oxidase
- Cytochrome c reductase.

Flavin adenine dinucleotide is required as coenzyme for:
- Succinate dehydrogenase
- Pyruvate dehydrogenase complex
- α-Ketoglutarate dehydrogenase complex
- Xanthine oxidase.

Deficiency results in:
- Malabsorption
- Malnutrition
- Anorexia
- Chronic alcoholism.

Ariboflavinosis

A medical condition caused by deficiency of riboflavin (**Fig. 16.8**). It is often associated with

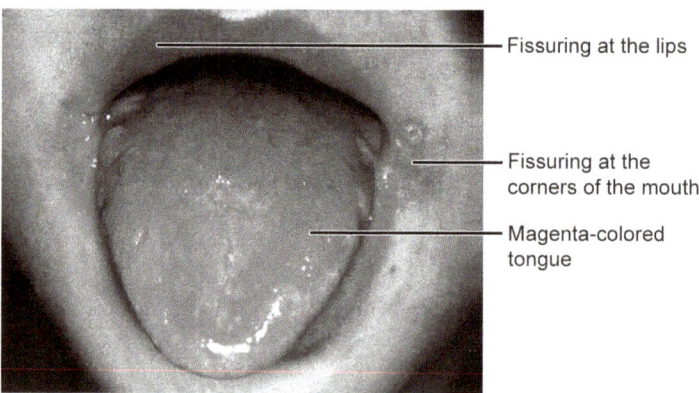

Fig. 16.8: Signs and symptoms of ariboflavinosis.

protein energy malnutrition and alcoholism. Ariboflavinosis is characterized by:
- Glossitis (magenta-colored tongue)
- Cheilosis (fissuring of the lips)
- Fissuring at the corners of mouth
- Seborrheic dermatitis and corneal vascularization are the symptoms of riboflavin deficiency.

Niacin (Nicotinic Acid or B_3)

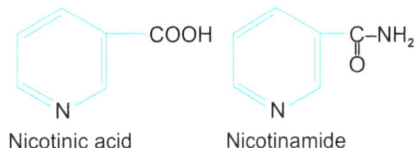

Nicotinic acid   Nicotinamide

Niacin is also known as nicotinic acid. The amide form of niacin is nicotinamide. Both of these have equal biological activities. The compounds have pyridine ring. The niacin is stable in nature.

Sources
The major sources are lean meats (liver), legumes, peanuts (groundnuts), green vegetables, and whole grains.

Amino acid tryptophan can be converted to the coenzyme NAD.

About 60 mg of tryptophan yields 1 mg of niacin.

Milk and eggs are low in niacin, but are rich in tryptophan.

Recommended dietary allowance
- Adults: 16–20 mg/day
- Children: 9–16 mg/day
- Infants: 5–8 mg/day.

Coenzyme forms
The active forms of niacin are:
- NAD.
- NADPH.
- They take part mainly in oxidation reactions of our body.
- The NAD is required as a coenzyme for pyruvate dehydrogenase complex and α-ketoglutarate dehydrogenase complex to mediate the reactions.
- The NADPH is required for glucose-6-phosphate dehydrogenase and 6-phosphate gluconate dehydrogenase-mediated reactions.

Deficiency
- The deficiency of niacin leads to a condition called pellagra (**Fig. 16.9**).

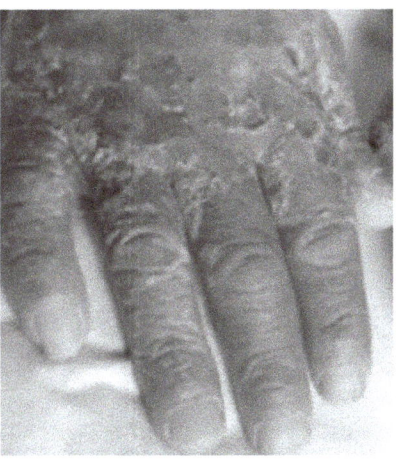

Fig. 16.9: Pellagra.

- It involves skin, gastrointestinal tract, and central nervous system.
- Its symptoms are called three-dimensional symptoms, diarrhea, dermatitis, and dementia (disturbances of CNS) and if untreated is followed by death.
- Fate of these vitamins when given in large doses: Nicotinic acid and nicotinamide are converted to their corresponding N-methyl derivatives before they are excreted in urine. This is an example of detoxification by *trans*-methylation.

Pyridoxine (B_6)

Chemistry
- Pyridoxine, pyridoxal, and pyridoxamine (all are active).
- They have a pyridine ring.
- Pyridoxine is heat stable but decomposes in the light or in alkaline solutions.

Sources
The sources are whole grains, poultry fish, potatoes, organ meats, eggs, and legumes.

Recommended dietary allowance
- Adults: 2.2 mg/day
- Children: 1.2 mg/day
- Infants: 3 mg/day.

Active form of pyridoxine
The coenzyme form of pyridoxine is pyridoxal phosphate (PLP), which is active. The PLP is required as coenzyme in the reactions involved amino acid metabolism for the enzymes such as:
- Transaminases
- Decarboxylases
- Kynureninase
- Cystathionine α-synthase
- Cystathionine gamma-lyase and aminolevulinic acid (ALA) synthase.

Enzymes such as serine hydroxymethyltransferase and phosphorylase contain PLP, but role of PLP in their action is not known.

Deficiency
The deficiency leads to:
- Hypochromic microcytic anemia.
- Glossitis.
- Pigmented scaly dermatitis similar to pellagra.
- Numbness and tingling sensations in the extremities.
- Irritability, depression, and convulsive seizures.
- Tuberculous patients who are on long-term therapy with antituberculosis drug isonicotinic acid hydrazide (INH) suffer from B_6 deficiency. This drug has a structure similar to B_6 and antagonizes the action of B_6. Hence, along with INH, they have to be given large doses of B_6 as antagonists (deoxypyridoxine, methoxypyridoxine):

- The deficiency occurs also in women taking oral contraceptives.

Pyridoxine is used in the treatment of seizures, Down syndrome, autism (psychiatric disorder of childhood), and premenstrual syndrome.

Biotin (B_7)

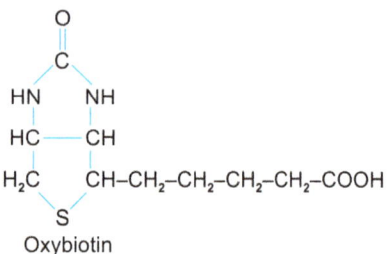
Oxybiotin

Sulfur-containing vitamin consists of two fused rings, one is imidazole and the other is thiophane, and an attached valeric acid side chain.

Sources
The sources are egg yolk, organ meats (liver and kidney), milk, legumes, and nuts.

Recommended dietary allowance
Adults: 0.3 mg/day.

Functions
- The intestinal bacteria also synthesize biotin to some extent.
- *The coenzyme form:* Biotin itself acts as coenzyme.
- It functions as a coenzyme in the reactions involving fixation of CO_2:

$$Pyruvate \xrightarrow[H_2O + CO_2 \text{ biotin}]{Pyruvate\ carboxylase} Oxalocetate$$

$$Propionyl\text{-}CoA \xrightarrow[CO_2 \text{ bioton}]{Propionyl\text{-}CoA\ carboxylase} d\text{-methyl malonyl-CoA}$$

$$Acetyl\text{-}CoA + CO_2 + ATP \xrightarrow[Biotin]{Acetyl\text{-}CoA\ carboxylase} Malonyl\text{-}CoA + ADP + Pi$$

Deoxypyridoxine   Methoxypyridoxine

- **Antivitamin:** Avidin, a glycoprotein present in raw egg white when fed to animals can produce biotin deficiency. Since, avidin causes egg-white-injury, biotin is called anti-egg-white-injury factor. Avidin, being protein, on heating it will be denatured and loses its biotin-binding activity.
- **Antagonists:** Desthiobiotin and oxybiotin:

$$\text{Desthiobiotin}$$

```
        O
        ‖
        C
      /   \
     NH    NH
     |     |
    H₂C — CH—(CH₂)₄COOH
```
Desthiobiotin

```
        O
        ‖
        C
      /   \
     NH    NH
     |     |
     C     C
    H|    H|
    CH₂   CH—(CH₂)₄COOH
      \  /
       O
```
Oxybiotin

Deficiency and symptoms
It is rare, and experimental animals show the symptoms such as anorexia, depression, insomnia, muscle pain, and dermatitis.

Pantothenic Acid (B₅)
Consists of a dihydroxy dimethyl butyric acid joined to α-alanine by a peptide bond:

```
      Pantoic acid        β-alanine
    ⎯⎯⎯⎯⎯⎯⎯⎯⎯⎯⎯⎯    ⎯⎯⎯⎯⎯⎯⎯⎯⎯⎯
       CH₃OH O  H                O
        |  |  ‖  |                ‖
 HO–CH₂–C–CH–C–N–CH₂–CH₂–C–OH
        |
       CH₃
```

Sources
The major sources are eggs, animal liver, meat, milk, vegetables, and grains.

Recommended dietary allowance
- Adults: 5–10 mg/day
- Children: 4–5 mg/day
- Infants: 1–2 mg/day.

Functions
- Active form is the coenzyme (CoA-SH) form.
- Its reactive group is sulfhydryl group (–SH).
- CoA-SH is required for:

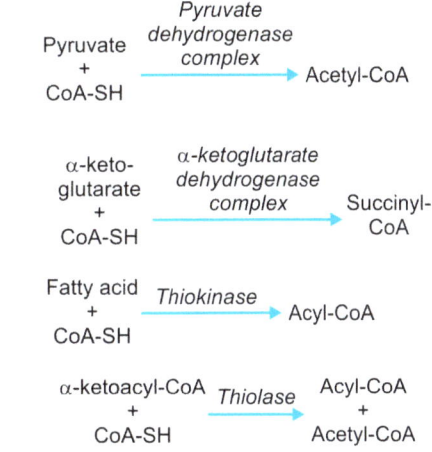

- Detoxification of benzoic acid.
- Synthesis of bile salts.

Deficiency
It is rare. When it is produced experimentally, it has the symptoms, fatigue, sleep disorders, weakness, abdominal cramp, and a burning sensation of the feet.

Folic Acid
Composed of pteridine ring attached to *para*-aminobenzoic acid and conjugated with glutamic acid residues:

Sources
The sources are fresh green vegetables, liver, whole grains, meat, and legumes.

Recommended dietary allowance
- Children: 300 μg/day
- Adults: 400 μg/day
- Pregnancy and lactation: 800 μg/day.

Functions
- The coenzyme form of folic acid is tetrahydrofolic acid (THF/FH_4), which is the active form.
- It is formed from folic acid (**Fig. 16.10**).
- The THF is a carrier of single carbon and it is involved in single carbon transfer reactions.
- The single carbon may be in the form of formyl (–CHO).
- Combined role of vitamin B_{12} and folate in the synthesis of methionine:

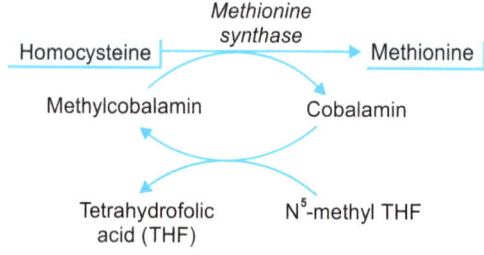

Deficiency
- Megaloblastic anemia
- Growth failure.

The deficiency of folate leads to impairment of the methionine synthase reaction due to which purine ring synthesis is impaired. The impaired synthesis of DNA prevents cell division and formation of the nucleus of new RBCs. Megaloblasts are formed instead of normoblast. These megaloblasts are accumulated in the bone marrow and lead to megaloblastic anemia.

Causes: Low dietary intake, malabsorption syndrome, during pregnancy.

Formiminoglutamic acid excretion test: In the deficiency of folic acid, the availability of FH_4 is less or totally absent. So, the intermediate of histidine metabolism, formiminoglutamate accumulates in the blood and excreted in the urine. This is one of the tests to detect the megaloblastic anemia to check whether it is due to folic acid or vitamin B_{12} deficiency.

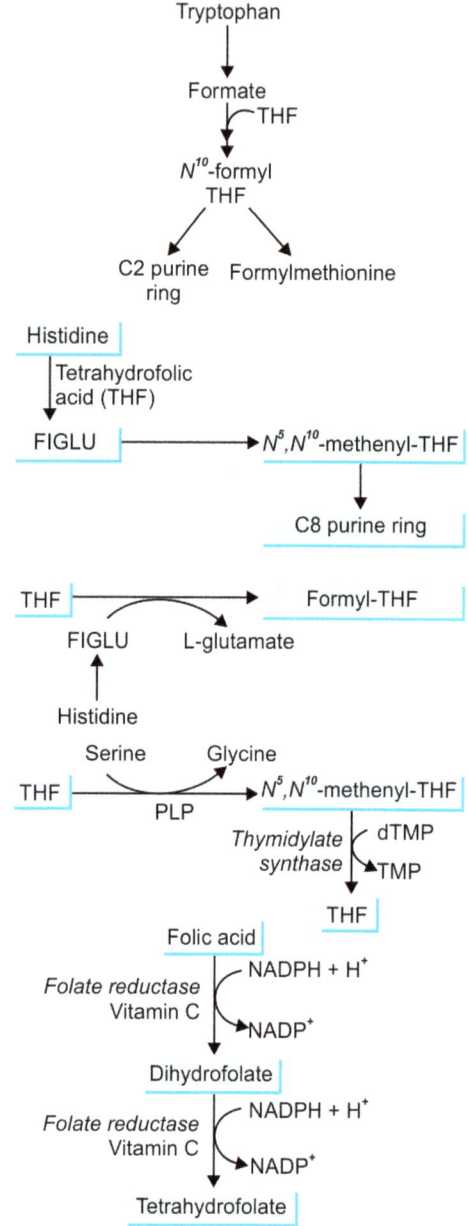

Fig. 16.10: Formation of tetrahydrofolate.
(FIGLU: formiminoglutamic acid; PLP: pyridoxal phosphate; NADPH: nicotinamide adenine dinucleotide phosphate; NADP: nicotinamide adenine dinucleotide phosphate)

Vitamin B$_{12}$ (Cobalamin)

Cobalamin has a corrin ring linked to cobalt atom held in the center of the corrin ring by four coordination bonds with the nitrogen of the pyrrole groups. The remaining coordination bonds of the cobalt are linked with the nitrogen of dimethylbenzimidazole nucleotide and sixth bond is linked either methyl or 5′-deoxyadenosyl or hydroxyl group to form methylcobalamin, adenosylcobalamin, or hydroxocobalamin, respectively.

Sources
The sources are liver, meat, fish, eggs, and milk.

Human beings get small amount of vitamin B$_{12}$ from their intestinal flora.

Recommended dietary allowance
- Children: 2 µg/day
- Adults: 3 µg/day
- Pregnancy and lactation: 4 µg/day.

Functions
- Methylcobalamin and 5′-deoxyadenosylcobalamin are the two active forms of vitamin B$_{12}$.
- Absorption: A glycoprotein is the castle's intrinsic factor and vitamin B$_{12}$ is called extrinsic factor.

Vitamin B$_{12}$ of food binds to intrinsic factor in the stomach, this complex moves to ileum, there it bind to specific receptors. Then the B$_{12}$ is transported to mucosal cell and then to blood, and carried by B$_{12}$-binding proteins. The coenzyme form of vitamin B$_{12}$ is 5′-deoxyadenosylcobalamin.

Vitamin B$_{12}$ along with folic acid is required for the development of RBCs beyond megaloblastic stage.

It acts as coenzyme for the mutase enzyme, which converts methylmalonyl-CoA into succinyl-CoA.

Methylcobalamin is required in the conversion of homocysteine to methionine.

It is involved in the conversion of ribonucleotides to deoxyribonucleotide.

Deficiency
The common cause of deficiency is malabsorption. Pernicious anemia is caused by a deficiency of intrinsic factor, which leads to impaired absorption of cobalamin:
- Megaloblastic anemia
- Glossitis and inflammation of mouth
- Methylmalonic aciduria.

Folate trap: Deficiency of this vitamin produces megaloblastic anemia due to its role in folate metabolism. During the many transformations of folate from one form to another, a proportion gets accidentally converted to N^5-methyl-THF, an inactive metabolite. This is called "folate trap," since there is no way for active N^5, N^{10}-methyl-THF to be regenerated except through a reaction for which a form of vitamin B$_{12}$, methyl-B$_{12}$, is a cofactor. Deficiency of B$_{12}$ then produces a situation where more and more folate is trapped in an inactive form with no biochemical means of escape. The end result is failure to synthesize adequate DNA (see **Table 16.2**).

Table 16.2: Summary of water-soluble vitamins.

Sources	Functions	Deficiency symptoms	Overconsumption symptoms	Characteristics
Vitamin C (ascorbic acid)				
Citrus fruits broccoli, strawberries, melon, green pepper, tomatoes, dark green vegetables, potatoes	Formation of collagen, wound healing, maintaining blood vessels, bones, teeth; absorption of iron, production of brain epinephrine and norepinephrine, antioxidant	Bleeding gums, poor wound healing, bruise easily, dry, rough skin, scurvy, sore joints and bones	Nontoxic under normal conditions	
Vitamin B_1 (thiamine)				
Liver, whole grains, enriched grain products, peas, meat, legumes	Helps release energy from foods; promotes normal appetite; important in function of nervous system	Mental confusion, muscle weakness, wasting, edema, impaired growth, beriberi	Not known	Losses depend on cooking method
Vitamin B_2 (riboflavin)				
Liver, milk, dark green vegetables, whole and enriched grain products, eggs	Helps release energy from foods; promotes good vision, healthy skin	Cracks at corners of mouth dermatitis around nose and lips; eyes sensitive to light	Not known	Sensitive to light
Vitamin B_3 niacin (nicotinamide and nicotinic acid)				
Liver, fish, poultry, meat, peanuts, whole and enriched grain products	Energy production from foods, aids digestion, promotes normal appetite, promotes healthy skin, nerves	Skin disorders, diarrhea, weakness, mental confusion, irritability	Abnormal liver function, cramps, nausea, irritability	
Vitamin B_6 (pyridoxine, pyridoxal, and pyridoxamine)				
Pork, meats, whole grains and cereals, legumes, green leafy vegetables	Helps in protein metabolism, absorption; aids in RBC formation; helps body use fats	Skin disorders, dermatitis; cracks at corners of mouth; anemia	Not known	Considerable losses during cooking
Folacin (folic acid)				
Liver, kidney, dark green leafy vegetables, meats, fish, whole grains, fortified grains and cereals, legumes, citrus fruits	Aids in protein metabolism; promotes RBC formation; prevents birth defects of spine, brain; lowers homocysteine levels and thus coronary heart disease risk	Anemia, diarrhea	May mask pernicious anemia	Easily destroyed by storing and cooking

Contd...

Contd...

Vitamin B₁₂ (cobalamin)

Sources	Functions	Deficiency	Requirement	Remarks
Animal foods such as meats, liver, kidney, fish, eggs, milk and milk products, oysters, shellfish	Aids in building of genetic material; aids in development of normal RBCs; maintenance of nervous system	Pernicious anemia, neurological disorders; degeneration of peripheral nerves that may cause numbness, tingling in fingers and toes	Not known	

Vitamin B₅ (pantothenic acid)

Liver, kidney, meats, eggs yolk, whole grains, legumes; also made by intestinal bacteria	Involved in energy production; aids in formation of hormones	Fatigue, nausea, abdominal cramps	Not known	About half of pantothenic acid is lost in the milling of grains

Vitamin B₇ (biotin)

Liver, kidney, egg yolk, milk, most fresh vegetables, also made by intestinal bacteria	Helps release energy from carbohydrates; aids in fast synthesis	Fatigue, loss of appetite, nausea, vomiting, depression	Not known	Most unstable under; heat, drying, storage; very soluble in water

(RBC: red blood cell)

SUMMARY

Vitamins are naturally occurring organic substances. The coenzyme form of B-complex vitamins is essential for many of the metabolic reactions taking place in our body. All the vitamins serve nearly the same roles in all forms of life. The daily requirement of any vitamin depends on a number of factors and may increase during growth, pregnancy, and lactation. The vitamins are divided into fat-soluble vitamins (A, D, E, and K) and water-soluble vitamins (B-complex) and vitamin C. Dietary deficiency of vitamins results in many symptoms. For example, vitamin A deficiency leads to night blindness, D deficiency results in rickets in children, K deficiency result in clotting disorder, C deficiency result in scurvy, and B-complex deficiency results in dermatitis (niacin), magenta-colored tongue (riboflavin), and anemia (folic acid).

SELF-ASSESSMENT QUESTIONS

Essay Questions

1. Briefly discuss the sources and requirement of vitamin A.
2. Discuss the functions and deficiency manifestations of vitamin A.
3. Explain the functions of vitamin and deficiency symptoms of vitamin D
4. Describe the sources and functions of vitamins E and K.
5. Discuss the requirement, sources, functions, and deficiency manifestations of vitamin C.
6. List the B-complex vitamins.
7. State the coenzyme form of thiamine and write the reactions which catalyzes.
8. What is beriberi? Explain briefly.
9. Name the enzymes that are dependent on PLP as coenzyme.
10. Discuss the symptoms of pyridoxine deficiency.
11. Briefly describe the sources, requirement, functions, and deficiency manifestations of niacin.

12. What are the functions of biotin in the body?
13. Mention the coenzyme form for pantothenic acid.
14. Mention the enzymes that need FMN and FAD as coenzymes.
15. Write about the deficiency symptoms of riboflavin.
16. Discuss the sources, functions, and deficiency manifestations of vitamin B_{12}.
17. Discuss the requirement and deficiency diseases of folic acid.
18. What is formiminoglutamic acid (FIGLU) excretion test? and what is its importance?

Short-Answer Questions

1. Which form of vitamin A has a role in vision?
2. Cod liver oil is a rich source for which vitamin?
3. Which vitamin deficiency results in night blindness?
4. Name the two forms of vitamin.
5. In adults and children, deficiency of vitamin D leads to what?
6. The antioxidant property is observed in which vitamin?
7. Name the naturally occurring form of vitamin K.
8. Which vitamin involved in γ-carboxylation of the glutamic acid residues of the inactive clotting factor?
9. Name the important source for vitamins K and E.
10. Which vitamin is responsible for the hydroxylation of prolyl residues?
11. The vitamin C deficiency leads to what type of disorders?
12. Name the coenzyme form of thiamine.
13. Which vitamin deficiency leads to beriberi?
14. Which vitamin deficiency leads to the disease pellagra?
15. Mention the coenzyme form of pyridoxine.
16. Name the two coenzyme forms of niacin.
17. Which vitamin deficiency leads to magenta-colored tongue?
18. Write the requirement of niacin for adults and children.
19. Name the coenzyme forms of riboflavin.
20. Which vitamin is called anti-egg-white-injury factor?
21. CoA-SH is the coenzyme form of which vitamin?
22. Give the requirement of folic acid for pregnant and lactating women.
23. What is the other name for vitamin B_{12}?
24. The folic acid deficiency leads to what type of disorders?
25. Mention the importance of FIGLU excretion test.

Fill in the Blanks

1. _____ form of vitamin A has a role in vision.
2. Cod liver oil is a rich source for vitamin _____.
3. Night blindness is due to the deficiency of _____.
4. The two forms of vitamin D are _____ and _____.
5. The deficiency of vitamin D leads to _____ in adults and _____ in children.
6. The antioxidant property is observed in vitamin _____.
7. Phylloquinone is the naturally occurring form of vitamin _____.
8. The vitamin K is involved in _____ of the glutamic acid residues of the inactive clotting factor.
9. The requirement of vitamin C for children is _____.
10. The hydroxylation of prolyl residues is brought about by vitamin _____.
11. The vitamin C deficiency leads to _____.
12. The coenzyme form of thiamine is called _____.
13. The beriberi is due to the deficiency of _____.
14. The pellagra is due to the deficiency of _____.
15. The coenzyme form of pyridoxine is _____.
16. The coenzyme forms of niacin are _____ and _____.
17. The magenta-colored tongue is due to the deficiency of _____.
18. The requirement of niacin for adults is _____.
19. The coenzyme forms of riboflavin are _____ and _____.
20. Anti-egg-white-injury factor is called _____.
21. CoA-SH is the coenzyme form of _____.
22. The requirement of folic acid for pregnant and lactating women is _____.
23. The vitamin B_{12} is also called _____.
24. The folic acid deficiency leads to _____.
25. The coenzyme form of vitamin B_{12} is _____.

MULTIPLE-CHOICE QUESTIONS

1. All the following are the symptoms of vitamin A deficiency, *except*:
   a. Night blindness
   b. Fragile RBCs
   c. Keratinization of lacrimal glands
   d. Keratomalacia
2. Concerning the vitamin D, all of the following statements are true, *except*:
   a. Low calcium stimulates the 1-hydroxylase
   b. Vitamin D_3 increases the absorption of calcium from the intestine
   c. Its deficiency leads to scurvy
   d. Its deficiency leads to rickets
3. One of the following is not a form of vitamin K:
   a. Phylloquinone   b. Menaquinone
   c. Menadione   d. Ubiquinone
4. Concerning the functions of vitamin E, all of the following statements are correct, *except*:
   a. Antioxidant
   b. Normal reproduction in animals
   c. Helps in vision
   d. Protects cellular membrane
5. Scurvy is the result of:
   a. Deficiency of vitamin A
   b. Deficiency of vitamin C
   c. Deficiency of vitamin D
   d. Deficiency of vitamin E
6. The incorrect statement regarding vitamin B_{12} is:
   a. It is extrinsic factor
   b. Vitamin B_{12} of food binds to intrinsic factor in the stomach
   c. The coenzyme form of vitamin B_{12} is 5'-deoxyadenosylcobalamin
   d. Vitamin B_{12} along with vitamin C is required for the development of RBCs beyond megaloblastic stage
7. The tetrahydrofolic acid (FH_4) does all of the following, *except*:
   a. Carries of single carbon and it is involved in single carbon transfer reactions
   b. Contributes to C-2 purine ring
   c. Contributes to C-8 purine ring
   d. Synthesis of uridine monophosphate (UMP)
8. One of the following enzymes *does not* require coenzyme A (CoA-SH):
   a. Pyruvate dehydrogenase (DH) complex
   b. α-ketoglutarate DH complex
   c. Hexokinase
   d. Thiokinase
9. Deficiency of vitamin B_6 leads to the following, *except*:
   a. Hypochromic microcytic anemia
   b. Glossitis
   c. Pigmented scaly dermatitis similar to pellagra
   d. Megaloblastic anemia
10. Concerning riboflavin, all the following statements are true, *except*:
    a. Has a dimethyl isoalloxazine ring attached to ribitol
    b. Recommended dietary allowance (RDA) for adults is 2 mg/day
    c. Nicotinamide dinucleotide (NAD) is its coenzyme form
    d. Flavin adenine dinucleotide is its coenzyme form
11. One of the following is not dependent on the coenzyme PLP for its activity:
    a. Transaminases
    b. Decarboxylases
    c. Pyruvate dehydrogenase
    d. Aminolevulinic acid synthase
12. All the following statements are correct regarding niacin, *except*:
    a. Nicotinamide adenine dinucleotide is its coenzyme
    b. Flavin adenine dinucleotide is its coenzyme form
    c. Nicotinamide adenine dinucleotide phosphate is its coenzyme form
    d. The deficiency of niacin leads to a condition called pellagra
13. Thiamine is essential for all the following, *except*:
    a. Pyruvate dehydrogenase complex
    b. α-ketoglutarate dehydrogenase complex
    c. Protect against night blindness
    d. Protect against beriberi
14. Concerning warfarin, all of the statements are true, *except*:
    a. Reduces the concentration of vitamin A–dependent clotting factors
    b. Has a half-life of about 36 hours
    c. Crosses the placenta and should be avoided in pregnancy
    d. Doses should be reduced in liver disease
15. All of the following have antioxidant property, *except*:
    a. Vitamin C   b. Vitamin K
    c. Vitamin A   d. Vitamin E

16. Osteoporosis is associated with:
    a. Vitamin E deficiency
    b. Vitamin K deficiency
    c. Prolonged bed rest
    d. Hyperparathyroidism
17. Hemolysis is one of the symptom due to the deficiency of:
    a. Vitamin A
    b. Vitamin B_1
    c. Vitamin K
    d. Vitamin E
18. Reduced RBC transketolase activity indicates the deficiency of:
    a. Vitamin B_1
    b. Vitamin B_6
    c. Vitamin B_{12}
    d. Vitamin E
19. All of the following are vitamin K-dependent clotting factors, *except*:
    a. Prothrombin
    b. Factor XII
    c. Factor VII
    d. Factor X
20. The enzyme, which requires vitamin B_{12} as the coenzyme is:
    a. Isocitrate dehydrogenase
    b. Lactate dehydrogenase
    c. Glucose-6-phosphate dehydrogenase
    d. Homocysteine methyltransferase
21. Which of the following help in blood coagulation?
    a. Heparin
    b. Ethylene diamine tetra acetic acid
    c. Warfarin
    d. Phylloquinone
22. Conversion of ribonucleotides to deoxyribonucleotides by ribonucleotide reductase requires:
    a. Tetrahydrofolate
    b. NADPH
    c. Coenzyme A
    d. Pyridoxal phosphate
23. If a person had glossitis and cheilosis, the physician may suspect a deficiency of:
    a. Niacin
    b. Thiamin
    c. Riboflavin
    d. Pyridoxal phosphate
24. Defective parietal cells would result in malabsorption of which vitamin?
    a. Vitamin C
    b. Vitamin B_2
    c. Vitamin B_{12}
    d. Folic acid

Answers

1. b	2. c	3. d	4. c	5. b
6. d	7. d	8. c	9. d	10. c
11. c	12. b	13. c	14. a	15. b
16. c	17. d	18. a	19. b	20. d
21. d	22. a	23. c	24. c	

CHAPTER 17

Nutrition

OBJECTIVES

At the end of this chapter, students should be able to:
- Understand the importance of macro and micronutrients and disorders associated with their deficiency
- Explain the basal metabolic rate (BMR) and the factors affecting it
- Calculate the calorie requirement for different types of work
- Describe the protein–energy malnutrition (PEM)
- Know the dietary requirement for people with diabetes, cardiovascular disease, and pregnancy.

INTRODUCTION

Nutrition is the processes by which a human body takes in and utilizes various food substances. Nutrients are substances required by the body to perform its basic functions. Most nutrients must be obtained from our food, since the human body does not synthesize or produce them. Nutrients are required for many basic functions: they provide energy, contribute to body structure, and regulate chemical processes in the body. These basic functions allow humans to detect and respond to environmental surroundings, move, excrete wastes, breathe, grow, and reproduce.

Essential nutrients include protein, carbohydrate, fat, vitamins, minerals, and electrolytes. Normally, 85% of daily energy use is from fat and carbohydrates and 15% from protein.

Macro- and Micronutrients

Nutrients that are needed in large amounts are called macronutrients. There are three classes of macronutrients: *carbohydrates, lipids, and proteins*. Macronutrients are carbon-based compounds that can be metabolically processed into cellular energy through changes in their chemical bonds. The chemical energy is converted into cellular energy known as *ATP*, which is utilized by the body to perform different types of work and conduct basic functions.

The amount of energy a person consumes daily comes primarily from the three macronutrients. Food energy is measured in kilocalories. For ease of use, food labels state the amount of energy in food in "calories," meaning that each calorie is actually multiplied by 1,000 to equal a kilocalorie. "Calorie" (with a capital "C") is equivalent to a kilocalorie. Therefore *1 kilocalorie = 1 Calorie–1,000 calories.*

A measurement of energy is done in a bomb calorimeter.

Calorie is the amount of heat taken to raise the temperature of 1 g of water by 1°C.

Food is measured in kilocalories (kcal) "calories" with "C" on nutrition label are in kcal.

Water is also a macronutrient in the sense that the body needs it in large amounts, but unlike the other macronutrients, it does not contain carbon or yield energy.

Nutrients that are needed in smaller amounts are called micronutrients.

Micronutrients are also essential for carrying out bodily functions. Micronutrients include all the *essential minerals* and *vitamins*. There are 16 essential minerals and 13 essential vitamins (refer to Chapters 15 and 16).

In contrast to carbohydrates, lipids, and proteins, micronutrients are not sources of energy (calories) for the body. Instead they play a role as cofactors or components of enzymes (as coenzymes) that facilitate chemical reactions in the body. They are involved in all aspects of body functions from producing energy, to digesting nutrients, to building macromolecules. Micronutrients play many essential roles in the body.

CALORIC VALUES OF MACRONUTRIENTS

Caloric Values of Carbohydrates, Fats, and Proteins

Caloric value is the amount of heat obtained when 1 g of substance is completely oxidized **(Fig. 17.1)**:
Energy = Calorie (cal) in nutrition
- When 1 g of carbohydrate is oxidized in the body, 4 cal are formed.
- When 1 g of protein is oxidized in the body, 4 cal are formed.
- When 1 g of fat is oxidized in the body, 9 cal are formed.

RESPIRATORY QUOTIENT OF FOOD STUFFS

The respiratory quotient (RQ) is the volume of carbon dioxide (CO_2) produced divided by the volume of oxygen (O_2) consumed at the whole body level. Because of inherent chemical differences in the composition of carbohydrates, fats and proteins, different amounts of oxygen are required to completely oxidize carbon, and hydrogen atoms in carbohydrates, fats, and proteins into CO_2 and water. Thus the quantity of CO_2 produced relative to the O_2 consumed will vary depending on the proportional mix of energy nutrients (carbohydrate, fat, protein) metabolized:

$$RQ = \frac{\text{Volume of } CO_2 \text{ produced}}{\text{Volume of } O_2 \text{ utilized}}$$

where,
CO_2 = Carbon dioxide
O_2 = Oxygen
RQ = Respiratory quotient.
RQ = VCO_2/VO_2
Where, VCO_2 = Volume of carbon dioxide, VO_2 = Volume of oxygen.

Carbohydrates

When carbohydrates are completely oxidized, their RQ is:
$C_6H_{12}O_6$ (glucose) + 6 O_2 → 6 CO_2 + 6 H_2O

$$RQ = \frac{VCO_2 \text{ produced}}{VO_2 \text{ utilized}} = \frac{6}{6} = 1$$

Fats

When palmitic acid completely oxidized:
$C_{15}H_{32}COOH$ (palmitic acid) + 23 O_2 → 16 CO_2 + 16 H_2O

$$RQ = \frac{VCO_2 \text{ produced}}{VO_2 \text{ utilized}} = \frac{16}{23} = 0.7$$

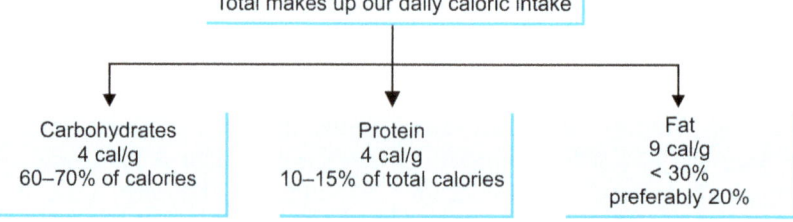

Fig. 17.1: Caloric value of carbohydrates, proteins and fats.

This reaction shows fats have relatively low RQ, since they have low O_2 content.

Proteins

The protein is not completely oxidized to CO_2 and cannot be represented by the formula. For example, the protein albumin is oxidized as follows:

$$C_{72}H_{112}N_2O_{22}S + 77\,O_2 \rightarrow 63\,CO_2 + 38\,H_2O + SO_3 + 9\,CO(NH_2)_2$$

- The respiratory exchange ratio for protein is 0.82 (indirect measurements).
- The RQ of a mixed diet is 0.8.
- The RQ value is important not only in determining the body's rate of energy expenditure, but it also enables the investigator to determine the nutrient mixture being metabolized during rest or exercise.
- The RQ is very helpful in understanding the kind of food, which is predominantly oxidized at any time.

NUTRITIONAL IMPORTANCE OF CARBOHYDRATES, PROTEINS, AND FATS

Carbohydrates

- The cells of nervous system and brain almost exclusively use glucose for energy.
- Simple carbohydrates are monosaccharides (glucose, fructose, and galactose) and disaccharides (maltose, sucrose, and lactose).
- Complex carbohydrates (glycogen, starches, and fiber): Foods rich in complex carbohydrates tend to be low in fat, sugar and can therefore add bulk to meals.
- Glycogen is not a significant food source of carbohydrate. However, the body stores much of its glucose as glycogen.
- Glycogen is released, when the body needs glucose for energy.
- Starch: Plants store starch as human bodies store glycogen and when we eat the plant, our body hydrolyzes the starch to glucose.
- Grains are the richest food source of starch and provide much of the food energy for people all over the world.
- Some examples of starches are rice, corn, rye, barley, and oats.
- Fibers are different from starches in that they cannot be broken down by the digestive system and therefore they provide little or no energy for the body.
- Fiber has been shown to protect against heart disease and diabetes by lowering cholesterol, and glucose levels.
- Fiber has also been shown to help provide a feeling of fullness and promote proper bowel function.
- Some examples of good sources of fiber are bran cereals, okra, butter beans, kidney beans, navy beans, sweet potatoes, and pears.

Proteins

The roles of proteins in the body are many, which are as follows:
- Whenever our body is growing, repairing, or replacing tissue, proteins are involved.
- Proteins form the building blocks of bones, teeth, muscles, skin, and blood.
- In addition, proteins help to regulate fluid balance; act as enzymes, transporters, and some hormones are proteins as well.
- As antibodies, proteins also help with the body's defense against disease.
- Proteins can also be used as a source of energy if needed.

Complete and Incomplete Proteins

- Complete proteins contain all of the essential amino acids needed for growth.
- Essential amino acids must be acquired in the diet; foods derived from animals such as meat, fish, poultry, cheese, eggs, yogurt, and milk generally provide complete proteins.

- Sources: Milk, fish, poultry, cheese, eggs, and yogurt.
- Incomplete proteins are missing one or more essential amino acids needed for growth; these are found in the plant form.
- Sources of incomplete proteins: Vegetables, seeds, nuts, grains, and legumes.
- Complementary proteins: Two or more dietary proteins, whose amino acid compositions complement each other in such a way that the essential amino acids missing from one are supplied by the other. By combining two or more plants proteins; we can consume all of the essential amino acids needed to support growth. We can receive all of the amino acids we need over the course of a day by choosing a variety of grains, legumes, seeds, nuts, and vegetables.

Protein and Weight Gain

- Ideally protein should contribute up to 10–35% of energy intake.
- Protein-rich foods are often higher in fat, which can contribute to weight gain.
- In order to prevent weight gain, choose lean cuts of meat and trim away visible fat from meats, and poultry before cooking.
- Boil or grill meat instead of frying.

Protein and Weight Loss

- It is generally not advisable to use a high-protein diet to lose weight.
- High-protein diets can be effective in weight loss. However, the reason that high-protein diets work is because they increase the feeling of satiety and are lower in calories.
- Eating excess protein may trouble the kidney with extra work. As the kidneys work to eliminate the excess protein, they also excrete a lot of water out of our system.
- While the scale may show a dramatic weight loss, this may not be a real weight loss.
- It is generally wise to consume extra amounts of water if eating extra protein.

Recommended Daily Allowance for Protein

The recommended daily allowance for adults is 0.8 g of protein/kg/body weight/day.
- Infants: 2.4 gm/kg/day
- Children: 1.7 gm/kg/day
- Adults: 0.8-1 gm/kg/day
- Pregnancy: 2 gm/kg/day
- Lactation: 2.5 gm/kg/day.

Fats

- Fat in our body provides us with 60% or our energy needs at rest, it spares protein, insulates our bodies against extreme temperatures, and protects us against shock by providing a cushion for bones, and vital organs.
- Fat also helps to maintain cell membranes and aids in the absorption of vitamins A, D, E, and K.
- As a food ingredient, fat provides flavor, consistency, stability, and satiety.
- *Unsaturated fats:* The most effective dietary strategy in preventing heart disease may be replacing saturated fats in the diet with monounsaturated and polyunsaturated fats:
    - *Sources of monounsaturated fats:* Olive oil, canola oil, peanut oil, and avocados
    - Sources of polyunsaturated fats: Vegetable oils (safflower, sesame, soy, corn, and sunflower), nuts, and seeds.
- *Essential fatty acids:* The body can make all except two linoleic and linolenic acids. These two acids must be supplied by our diet:
    1. *Linoleic acid sources:* Sunflower, safflower, corn, and soybean oils
    2. *Linolenic acid sources:* Soybean, canola oils, walnuts, and salmon.

Saturated Fats and its Risks

Main sources come from animal sources such as whole milk, cream, butter, cheese, and fatty cuts of beef and pork. Coconut, palm and

palm kernel oils, and products containing them (pastries, pies, doughnuts, and cookies) are also sources of saturated fat:
- Saturated fat is implicated in raising low-density lipoprotein (LDL) cholesterol.
- LDL cholesterol raises risk of heart disease.

Trans Fat

The majority of *trans* fats are formed when liquid oils are made into solid fats such as hard margarine. However, it is found naturally in some animal-based foods as well. *Trans* fat is made when hydrogen is added to an unsaturated fat such as vegetable oil, in a process called hydrogenation. Hydrogenation increases the shelf life of the products containing these fats. Found in deep-fried foods, cakes, cookies, margarine, meat, and dairy products. Partially hydrogenated oils are the main dietary source of *trans* fats.

Risks of trans fat: Trans fats, such as saturated fats, can increase the LDL, blood cholesterol levels, and thereby the risk of heart disease.

DIETARY FIBER

Definition: Dietary fiber is a complex mixture of plant materials that are resistant to breakdown (digestion) by the human digestive enzymes.
- There are two major kinds of dietary fiber. Insoluble (cellulose, hemicelluloses, and lignin) found in whole-grain products such as whole-wheat bread. Soluble (gums, mucilages, and pectins) fibers found in fruits, vegetables, dry beans and peas, and some cereals such as oats.
- Insoluble fiber promotes normal elimination by providing bulk for stool formation and thus fastening the passage of the stool through the colon. Insoluble fiber also helps to satisfy appetite by creating a full feeling. Some studies indicate that soluble fibers may play a role in reducing the level of cholesterol in the blood.
- Eating a variety of foods that contain dietary fiber is the best way to get an adequate amount. Healthy individuals who eat a balanced diet rarely need supplements. The list of foods will help you select those that are significant sources of dietary fiber as you follow the dietary guidelines.
- Breads, cereals, other grain products, fruits, vegetables, meat, poultry, fish, and alternatives are the sources.

Importance

Use of Fiber in Irritable Bowel Syndrome

Irritable bowel syndrome (IBS) is one of the most common disorders of the lower digestive tract:
- It creates bothersome symptoms such as altered bowel habits, constipation, diarrhea, or both alternately.
- There may also be bloating, abdominal pain, cramping, and spasm. An attack of IBS can be triggered by emotional tension and anxiety, poor dietary habits, and certain medications.
- Increased amounts of fiber in the diet can help relieve the symptoms of IBS by producing soft, bulky stools.
- This helps to normalize the time it takes for the stool to pass through the colon.
- Liquids help to soften the stool.
- IBS, if left untreated, may lead to diverticulosis of the colon.

Fiber and Colon Polyps/Cancer

Colon cancer is a major health problem and is most common in western cultures:
- Most colon cancer starts out as a colon polyp, a benign mushroom-shaped growth.
- In time it grows and in some people it becomes cancerous.
- Colon cancer is usually always curable, if polyps are removed when found or if surgery is performed at an early stage.

- It is now known that people can inherit the risk of developing colon cancer, but diet may be important too.
- There is a very low rate of colon cancer in residents of countries where grains are unprocessed and retain their fiber.
- The theory is that in the western world, cancer-containing agents (carcinogens) remain in contact with the colon wall for a longer time and in higher concentrations. So, a large bulky stool may act to dilute these carcinogens by moving them through the bowel more quickly.
- Less carcinogenic exposure to the colon may mean fewer colon polyps and less cancer.

Fiber and Diverticulosis

Prolonged, vigorous contraction of the colon, usually in the left lower side, may result in diverticulosis:
- This increases pressure causing small and eventually larger ballooning pockets to form. These pockets usually cause no problems.
- However, sometimes they can become infected (diverticulitis) or even break open (perforate) causing pockets of infection or inflammation of the sac lining the abdomen (peritonitis).
- A high-fiber diet may increase the bulk in the stool and thereby reduce the pressure within the colon.
- The formation of pockets is reduced or possibly even stopped.

Fiber, Cholesterol, and Gas

Insoluble fiber is found in wheat, rye, bran, and other grains:
- Insoluble fiber means it does not dissolve in water.
- It also cannot be used by intestinal-colon bacteria as a food source, so these beneficial bacteria generally do not grow and produce intestinal gas.
- Soluble fiber, on the other hand, does dissolve in water forming a gelatinous substance in the bowel.
- Soluble fiber is found in oatmeal, oat bran, fruit, barley, and legumes.
- Soluble fiber, among its other benefits, seems to bind up cholesterol allowing it to be eliminated with the stool (10–15%).
- The downside of soluble fiber is that it can be metabolized by gas forming bacteria in the colon.
- These bacteria are harmless, but for those who have an intestinal gas or flatus problems are probably best to avoid or carefully test soluble fibers to see, if they are contributing to intestinal gas.
- Whenever possible, both soluble and insoluble fiber should be eaten on a daily basis.

Glycemic Index

The **glycemic index (GI)** is a relative ranking of carbohydrate in foods according to how they affect blood glucose levels.

Foods with a high GI are quickly digested and absorbed, causing a rapid rise in blood sugar. These foods that rank high on the GI scale are often—but not always—high in processed carbohydrates and sugars. Pretzels, for example, have a GI of 83; and a baked potato without the skin clocks in at 98.

Foods with a low GI are digested and absorbed at a slower rate and, subsequently, cause a slower rise in blood sugar levels. These are typically rich in fiber, protein, and/or fat. Examples of these include apples with a GI of 28, Greek-style yogurt at 11, and peanuts at 7. Note that a low GI doesn't mean the food is high in nutrients. We still need to choose healthy foods from all five food groups.

Diets centered on mostly low-GI foods can make it easier to achieve and maintain a healthy weight, since these foods keep us feeling fuller, longer. Low-GI diets also have been shown to improve insulin resistance (IR) and lower glucose, cholesterol, and triglyceride levels in people with type 2 diabetes.

Dietary replacement of saturated fats by carbohydrates with a low GI may be beneficial for weight control.

Several evidences have shown that individuals who followed a low-GI diet over many years were at a significantly lower risk for developing both type 2 diabetes, coronary heart disease, and age-related macular degeneration than others.

Example of calculation of GI for white bread:
- Subject fed 50 g of glucose (i.e. 50 g carbohydrate)
- Blood glucose level after 2 hours is 180 mg/dL
- Subject fed 71 g of bread (i.e. 50 g carbohydrate)
- Blood glucose level after 2 hours is 126 mg/dL
  GI = 100 × (126/180) = 70
- Pregnancy: Women tend to weigh an average of 4-6 lb more after a pregnancy than they did before the pregnancy. This can compound with each pregnancy.

Obesity: People are generally considered **obese** when their body mass index (BMI), a measurement obtained by dividing a person's weight by the square of the person's height, is over 30 kg/m²; the range 25–30 kg/m² is defined as overweight.

Cause: Eating fewer calories than body metabolizes will reduce weight. Therefore the most common **causes** of **obesity** are overeating and physical inactivity. Ultimately, body weight is the result of genetics, metabolism, environment, behavior, and culture.

Sex: Men have more muscle than women, on average. Because muscle burns more calories than other types of tissue, men use more calories than women, even at rest. Thus women are more likely than men to gain weight with the same calorie intake.

Age: People tend to lose muscle and gain fat as they age. Their metabolism also slows somewhat. Both of these lower their calorie requirements.

Diagnostic method: BMI > 30 kg/m².

Complications: Overweight and **obesity** will increase blood pressure. High blood pressure is the leading cause of strokes. Excess weight also increases:
- Heart disease
- Diabetes
- Osteoarthritis (especially knee and hip joint pain, and lower back pain)
- Gout
- Gallstones
- Lung disease
- Insomnia from sleep apnea (snoring)
- Fungal rashes in skin folds
- Colon cancer
- Endometrial cancer
- Depression
- Dementia.

Symptoms: Increased fat.

Treatment: Diet, exercise, medications, and surgery.

METABOLIC RATE/ENERGY EXPENDITURE

Basal and Resting Metabolic Rate

Basal Metabolic Rate

Basal metabolic rate (BMR) is defined as the minimum amount of energy required by the body to maintain life at complete physical and mental rest in the postabsorptive period (12 hours after the intake of last meal).
- BMR includes the energy expended in ventilation, blood circulation, intestinal contraction, the activities of internal organs, and maintenance of thermal equilibrium. Stringent measurement of BMR requires that the subject be in a fasting (minimum of 12 hours), well-rested state having not exercised for the previous 12 hours and being in a supine position within a nonstressful, controlled

environment for a minimum of 30 minutes prior to measurement.
- The BMR is expressed as cal/m² body surface per hour.

Resting Metabolic Rate

Resting metabolic rate (RMR) is the energy expended, while an individual is resting quietly in a supine position. RMR and BMR are sometimes used interchangeably, but there are some small differences.
- RMR includes the thermal effect of substrate metabolism and heightened metabolic activity due to prior physical or mental activity. These factors, collectively known as facultative thermogenesis, may be thought of as components of a person's RMR and are not part of the BMR.

Measurement of Metabolic Rate or Energy Expenditure

Energy expenditure can be measured in two different ways:
1. The determination of energy expenditure by measuring the amount of heat produced over a period of time is called direct calorimetry.
2. The determination of energy expenditure by measuring the amount of CO_2 consumed over a period of time is called indirect calorimetry.

Two procedures of indirect calorimetry are closed-circuit and open-circuit spirometry (Douglas bag).

During metabolic energy transformations, oxygen is consumed and heat is produced. Either of these variables can therefore be used to estimate energy expenditure.

Using the fact that 1 L of oxygen liberates 4.82 kcal of heat energy when a mixture of carbohydrate, fat, and protein is burned in a bomb calorimeter; a highly accurate indirect measure of energy production is possible.

Factors Affecting Basal Metabolic Rate

- *Body surface area*:
  - This is a reflection of height and weight.
  - The greater the body surface area factor, the higher your BMR.
  - Tall, thin people have higher BMRs. If we compare a tall person with a short person of equal weight, then if they both follow a calorie-controlled diet to maintain the weight of the taller person, the shorter person may gain up to 15 lb in a year.
- *Sex*: Males have a higher BMR because of a greater proportion of lean body mass.
- *Body temperature*: Fever, e.g., increases BMR.
- *Hormones*: Thyroid hormones have a stimulatory effect on the metabolism of the body and, therefore, BMR. Thus BMR is raised in hyperthyroidism and reduced in hypothyroidism.
- *Age:* Metabolic rate declines with age. In infants and children BMR is higher, and in adults it is less.
- *Diet*: Starvation or serious abrupt calorie reduction can dramatically reduce BMR (30%). Restrictive low-calorie weight loss diets may cause BMR to drop as much as 20%.
- *Pregnancy/breastfeeding:* These increase the metabolic rate.
- *Environment*: In cold climates, the BMR is higher compared to warm climates.
- *Rapid growth and/or development*: Infancy, growth spurts, healing after illness or injury.
- *Disease states:* The BMR is higher in cardiac failure, leukemias, and hypertension, while it is marginally lowered in Addison's disease.
- *Weight:* The heavier our weight, the higher our BMR, e.g. the metabolic rate of obese women is 25% higher than the metabolic rate of thin women.
- *Exercise*: Physical exercise not only influences body weight by burning calories, it also helps raise our BMR by building extra lean tissue (lean tissue is more metabolically demanding than fat tissue). So we burn more calories even when sleeping.

- Amount of lean body mass: Muscle, liver, brain, kidney—all metabolize at a high rate at rest and have high energy needs when more active.

CALCULATION OF BASAL METABOLIC RATE

The first step in designing a personal nutrition plan for ourselves is to calculate how many calories we burn in a day; our total daily energy expenditure (TDEE). TDEE is the total number of calories that our body expends in 24 hours, including all activities.

METHODS OF DETERMINING CALORIC NEEDS

Quick Method (Based on the Total Body Weight) Equations Based on Basal Metabolic Rate

A much more accurate method for calculating TDEE is to determine BMR using multiple factors, including height, weight, age, and sex, then multiplying the BMR by an activity factor to determine TDEE. BMR is the total number of calories our body requires for normal bodily functions. BMR usually accounts for about two thirds of total TDEE. The BMR may vary dramatically from person to person depending on genetic factors.

Harris–Benedict Formula (Basal Metabolic Rate Based on the Total Body Weight)

The Harris–Benedict equation is a calorie formula using the factors of height, weight, age, and sex to determine BMR. This makes it more accurate than determining calorie needs based on total bodyweight alone. The only variable it does not take into consideration is lean body mass. Therefore this equation will be very accurate in all, but extremely muscular and extremely over fat:

Men: BMR = 66 + (13.7 × weight in kg) + (5 × height in cm) – (6.8 × age in year)

Women: BMR = 655 + (9.6 × weight in kg) + (1.8 × height in cm) – (4.7 × age in year).

Note:
- 1 in. = 2.54 cm
- 1 kg = 2.2 lb.

For example, female, 30 years old, and 5.6 ft. tall (167.6 cm), weighing 120 lb. (54.5 kg):
BMR = 655 + 523 + 302 – 141 = 1,339 cal/day

To determine TDEE from BMR, you simply multiply BMR by the activity multiplier.

Activity Multiplier

- Sedentary = BMR × 1.2 (little or no exercise, desk job)
- Lightly active = BMR × 1.375 (light exercise/sports 1–3 days/week)
- Moderately active = BMR × 1.55 (moderate exercise/sports 3–5 days/week)
- Very active = BMR × 1.725 (hard exercise/sports 6–7 days/week)
- Extra active = BMR × 1.9 (hard daily exercise/sports and physical job or 2 × day training, i.e. marathon and contest).

Examples
- BMR is 1,339 cal/day.
- Activity level is moderately active (work out three to four times per week).
- Activity factor is 1.55.
- TDEE = 1.55 × 1,339 = 2,075 cal/day.

Specific Dynamic Action

Ingestion of food is accompanied by an increased rate of heat production. The extra heat production by the body, over and above the calculated caloric value, when a given food is metabolized by the body, is called specific dynamic action (SDA). Various names for this effect have been suggested, including SDA, specific dynamic effect, heat increment of a feeding, calorigenic effect of foods, and thermogenic effect:
- Imagine that a man requires 1,800 cal/day to maintain his basal metabolic requirement, his heat output may exceed 1,800 cal (by about 180 cal) after eating food. This means that the excess calories

would have to come from his own tissues and maintain his weight, he has to take about 2,000 [1,800 + extra 10% (180)] cal. If he continues with 1,800 cal, he would lose weight.
- The SDA values vary according to the type of food taken. If a person eats 25 g of protein, we expect his heat output is 100 cal (25 × 4 cal, a caloric value of protein). But his actual heat output is 130 cal (a rise of 30%). So the SDA for protein is 30%.
- The SDA value for carbohydrate is 5%. After he consumes 25 g of carbohydrate the heat output is 105 cal instead of 100 cal.
- The SDA value for fat is 12%. After he consumes 11 g fat, the heat output is 112 cal instead of 100 cal (11 × 9 + 12).
- For a mixed diet, the SDA is 10%. This is because of the presence of carbohydrates and fats, which reduces the SDA of protein.
- The significance of SDA of a protein is the maintenance of body temperature in cold climate. The higher SDA for protein indicates that it is not a good source of energy.

Determining Energy Expenditure Using Specific Dynamic Action

Explanation of the calculation of caloric requirement with examples

1. **Calculate the energy requirement of a man (age = 20 years, BMR = 42 cal/m² body surface per hour, and body surface area = 1.7 m²) engaged in light work:**
   The energy demand depends on three important factors:
   - BMR
   - Physical activity
   - Specific dynamic action

   The food provides energy for:
   - Basal metabolism (8 hours)
   - Simple activities: Standing, sitting, walking, dressing, and writing (8 hours)
   - Professional work:
     - Light work
     - Moderate work
     - Heavy work
     - Very heavy work.
   - Other 10% as SDA

   The daily energy requirement is variable, which depends on age, sex, and body size:
   - Sleep basal level (8 hours) BMR × body surface area × 8 hours = 42 × 1.7 × 8 = 571 cal
   - Simple activities (8 hours):
     - At basal level = 571 cal
     - For simple activities at 25 cal/h: Over basal level = 25 × 8 = 200 cal.
   - For professional work (light work):
     - At basal level = 571 cal
     - For professional work at 60 cal/h: Over basal level = 55 × 8 = 440 cal
   - Subtotal = 2,353 cal
   - Extra 10% for SDA = 235 cal
   - Total = 2,588 cal/day.

2. **Calculate the energy requirement of dental student (age = 18 years, BMR = 40 cal/m² body surface per hour, and body surface area = 1.7 m²) engaged in moderate work:**
   - Sleep basal level (8 hours) BMR × body surface area × 8 hours = 40 × 1.7 × 8 = 544 cal
   - Simple activities (8 hours):
     - At basal level = 544 cal
     - For simple activities at 25 cal/h: Over basal level = 25 × 8 = 200 cal.
   - For professional work (light work):
     - At basal level = 544 cal
     - For professional work at 75 cal/h: Over basal level = 75 × 8 = 600 cal
   - Subtotal = 2,432
   - Extra 10% for SDA = 243 cal
   - Total = 2,675 cal/day.

3. **Calculate the energy requirement of a man (age = 25 year, BMR = 40 cal/m² body surface per hour, and body surface area = 1.7 m²) engaged in heavy work:**
   - Sleep basal level (8 hours) BMR × body surface area × 8 hours = 40 × 1.7 × 8 = 544 cal

Nutrition

- Simple activities (8 hours):
  - At basal level = 544 cal
  - For simple activities at 25 cal/h: Over basal level 25 × 8 = 200 cal.
- For professional work (heavy work):
  - At basal level = 544 cal
  - For professional work at 150 cal/h: Over basal level = 75 × 8 = 1,200 cal
  - Subtotal = 3,032
  - Extra 10% for SDA = 303 cal
  - Total = 3,335 cal/day.

From the abovementioned calculations, the reference ranges of caloric requirements of various types of work for an adult per day is as follows:
Light work 2,100–2,600
Moderate work 2,500–3,000
Heavy work 3,000–3,500
Very heavy work 3,500–4,000.

Biological Value of Protein

Biological value (BV) of protein (BVP) is a measurement of protein quality expressing the rate of efficiency with which protein is used for growth. A protein with high BV has all the essential amino acids in the right proportion. The BVP can be calculated by using a formula:

$$BVP = \frac{N\ (intake) - N\ (excretion\ in\ urine\ and\ feces)}{N\ (intake) - N\ (excretion\ in\ feces)} \times 100$$

$$= \frac{N\ (retained)}{N\ (absorbed) - N} \times 100$$

Egg contains the highest quality of food protein known. Based on the essential amino acids it provides, egg protein is second only to mother's milk for human nutrition. On a scale with 100 representing top efficiency, the BVPs in several foods are listed in **Table 17.1**.

Protein from animal sources (meat, fish, dairy products, and egg white) is considered high BVP or a "complete" protein because all nine essential amino acids are present in these proteins. An exception to this rule is collagen-derived gelatin, which lacks in tryptophan.

Table 17.1: Biological values of proteins in several foods.

Protein-rich foods	Values
Whole egg	93.7
Milk	84.5
Fish	76.0
Beef	74.3
Soybeans	72.8
Polished rice	64.0
Wheat, whole	64.0
Corn	60.0
Beans dry	58.0

NITROGEN BALANCE

Nitrogen balance is when a person's daily intake of nitrogen from proteins equals the daily excretion of nitrogen:
- If a person excretes more nitrogen than he or she consumes, then their body will break down muscle tissue to get the nitrogen it needs (negative nitrogen state) and muscle loss occurs.
- If a person consumes more nitrogen than he or she excretes, then that person will be in an anabolic muscle-building state (positive nitrogen state).

BALANCED DIET

A balanced diet includes variety of foods from all five food groups (carbohydrates, proteins, fats, vitamins, and minerals). It should provide enough calories to ensure a desirable weight and should include all the necessary daily nutrients. The healthiest combination for a balanced diet is low fat, low refined carbohydrates, healthy carbohydrates, and moderate protein **(Table 17.2)**. For example, as a general rule:
- About 50% of your calories should come from complex carbohydrates.

Table 17.2: Sample menu.

Breakfast	Lunch	Dinner	Snack
Grapefruit 1/2 Oatmeal 3/4 cup	Vegetable soup 1 cup Hamburger patty 3 oz	*Garden salad:* Lettuce 1, cucumber 1/6, tomato 1/2, bean sprouts 1/6, cup salad dressing 2 tbsp	Bran muffin or one slice bread orange or apple juice 1/2 cup
Raisins 2 tsp	Bun 1	Broiled chicken 3 oz (fat trimmed)	
Whole-wheat toast 2 slices	Tomato 1 small	Brown rice 1/2 cup	
Margarine 2 tsp	Lettuce	Broccoli with cheese sauce 1/2 cup	
Jelly/jam	Baked beans 1/2 cup	Strawberries 1/2 cup with plain low-fat	
Skim milk 1 cup	Apple 1	Skim milk 1 cup	
Coffee 3/4 cup or	Rice 1/2 cup		
Tea 3/4 cup	Yogurt 1/2 cup		
Sample diet may provide			
Calories	2,491	Fat	89 g
Protein	121 g	Sodium	3,585 mg
Carbohydrates	318 g	Fiber	38 g

- About 20% should come from protein.
- About 30% should come from all fat (of this, a maximum of one third may be saturated fat).

ASSESSING NUTRITIONAL STATUS

- The nutritional status of an individual is the result of many interrelated factors.
- It is influenced by food intake, quality, quantity, and physical health.
- The spectrum of nutritional status spread from obesity to malnutrition.

Importance of Nutritional Assessment

Nutritional assessment is required to:
- Develop health-care programs, which meet the community needs, which are defined by the assessment
- Measure the effectiveness of the nutritional programs and intervention once initiated.

Methods of Nutritional Assessment

Nutritional assessment is done by direct and indirect methods.

Direct Method

Direct methods deal with the individual and measure objective criteria and summarized as ABCD:
- **A**nthropometric methods
- **B**iochemical, laboratory methods
- **C**linical methods
- **D**ietary evaluation methods.

Indirect Method

Community health indices reflect nutritional influences. These include:
- Ecological variables including crop production
- Economic factors, e.g. per capita income, population density and social habits

- Vital health statistics particularly infant under-5 mortality and fertility index.

Clinical Assessment Method

- Simplest and most practical method of ascertaining the nutritional status of a group of individuals.
- It utilizes a number of physical signs that are known to be associated with malnutrition and deficiency of vitamins, and micronutrients.
- Good nutritional history should be obtained.
- General clinical examinations, with special attention to organs, such as hair, nails, skin, gums, eyes, muscles tongue, angles of mouth, and thyroid gland.
- Detection of relevant signs helps in establishing the nutritional diagnosis (**Table 17.3**).

Advantages
- Fast and easy to perform
- Inexpensive
- Noninvasive.

Limitations
It may not detect the early stages.

Clinical Signs and Symptoms of Nutritional Deficiency

Clinical signs and symptoms of nutritional deficiency are shown in **Table 17.3**.

Table 17.3: Clinical signs of nutritional deficiency.

Clinical signs	Factors
Hair	
Spare and thin	Due to protein, zinc, or biotin deficiency
Easy to pull out	Protein deficiency
Corkscrew coiled hair	Vitamins C and A deficiency
Mouth	
Glossitis	Riboflavin, niacin, and folic acid deficiency
Angular stomatitis cheilosis and fissured tongue	Riboflavin, pyridoxine, and niacin deficiency
Bleeding and spongy gums	Vitamin C deficiency
Leukoplakia	Vitamins A and B_{12}, folic acid, and niacin deficiency
Sore mouth and tongue	Vitamin B_6, niacin, and iron deficiency
Eyes	
Night blindness and exophthalmia	Vitamin A deficiency
Photophobia, blurring, and conjunctival inflammation	Vitamin A deficiency
Nails	
Spooning (**Fig. 17.2A**)	Iron deficiency
Transverse lines	Protein deficiency
Skin	
Pallor	Folic acid, iron, vitamin B_{12} deficiency
Follicular hyperkeratosis	Vitamins B and C deficiency
Flaking dermatitis	Vitamins B_{12} and A, PEM, zinc, and niacin deficiency
Pigmentation and desquamation	Niacin and protein–energy malnutrition (PEM)
Bruising purpura	Vitamins K and C and folic acid deficiency
Thyroid gland	
Goiter (**Fig. 17.2B**)	Iodine deficiency
Bones and joints	
Rickets (**Fig. 17.2C**)	Vitamin D deficiency

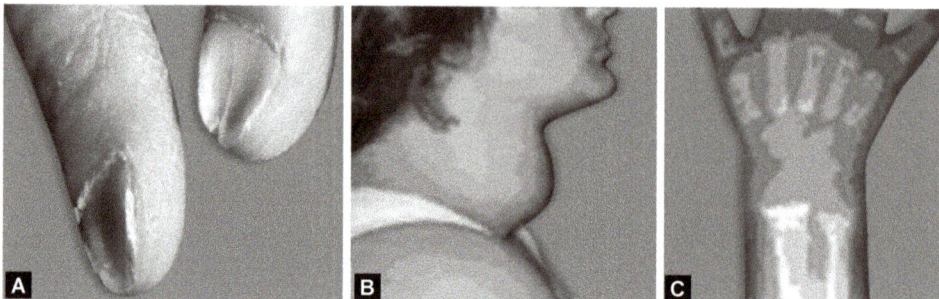

Figs. 17.2A to C: Signs of iron, iodine, and vitamin D deficiency: (A) Spooning of nails; (B) goiter; and (C) rickets.

METHODS AVAILABLE TO MEASURE THE NUTRITIONAL STATUS

Anthropometric Measurements

- Anthropometry is the measurement of body weight and proportions.
- It is an essential part of clinical examination of infants, children, and pregnant woman.
- It is also used to evaluate both under- and overnutrition.
- The measured values reflect the current nutritional status.

Other Anthropometric Measurements

- Mid-upper arm circumference
- Head circumference
- Skinfold thickness
- Head/chest ratio
- Hip/waist ratio.

Anthropometry for Children

Accurate measurement of height and weight is necessary to evaluate the physical growth of the child.

Height/age

- Height of index child compared with the expected weight of a healthy child of the same age.
- Helps in measuring long-term nutritional status or stunting.

Weight/height

Measure of wasting, i.e. appropriate weight for given height.

Mid-upper arm circumference

- Measured half-way between the acromion process of scapula and tip of elbow (ulnar) with arm hanging vertically and forearm supinated
- Provides an estimate of arm muscle area: Reflect skeletal protein reserves-lean body mass useful in monitoring vulnerable groups, especially children.

Head circumference

Useful in children under the age of 3 and is an indicator of nonnutritional abnormalities. Undernutrition must be severe to affect head circumference.

Anthropometry for Adults

Height measurement

The subject stands erect and bare footed on a stadiometer with a movable headpiece is leveled with skull vault, and height is recorded to the nearest 0.5 cm.

Weight measurement

- Use of regularly calibrated electronic or balanced-beam scale is suggested to measure the weight.
- During weight measurement, wearing light clothes without shoes is suggested.
- Read to the nearest 100 g.

Skinfolds

Triceps, biceps, subscapular, and suprailiac—used in combination to obtain body fat **(Fig. 17.3)**.

Nutrition

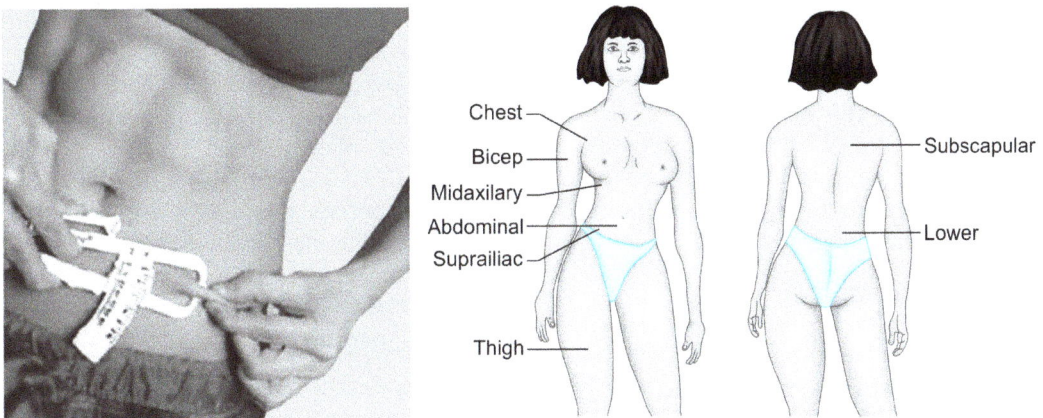

Fig. 17.3: Measurement of skinfolds of abdominal, suprailiac and subscapular region.

Nutritional indices in adults
- The international standard for assessing body size in adults is the BMI.
- BMI is computed using the following formula:
  - $BMI = \dfrac{Weight\ (kg)}{Height\ (m^2)}$ in kg/m²
    - <18.5 = Underweight
    - 18.5–24.9 = Normal weight
    - 25–29.9 = Overweight
    - 30–34.9 = Moderate obese (class 1)
    - 35–39.9 = Severely obese (class 2)
    - ≥40 = Extreme obesity.
  - $BMI = \dfrac{Weight\ (lbs)}{Height\ (m^2)} \times 703$ **(Fig. 17.4)**
    - <18.5 = Underweight
    - 18.5–24.9 = Normal weight
    - 25–29.9 = Overweight
    - 30–34.9 = Moderate obese (class 1)
    - 35–39.9 = Severely obese (class 2)
    - 40 = Extreme obesity (class 3).
3. High BMI (obesity level) is associated with type 2 diabetes and high risk of cardiovascular morbidity and mortality.

Waist/hip ratio
- Waist circumference is measured at the level of the umbilicus to the nearest 0.5 cm.

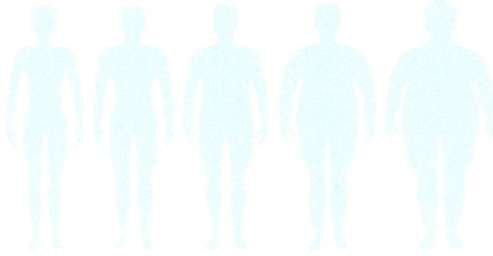

Categories of weight

| Normal BMI 18.5–24.9 | Overweight BMI 25–29.9 | Obese BMI 30–34.9 | Severely obese BMI 35–39.9 | Morbidly obese BMI ≥ 40 |

BMI = weight (kg) / height (m²)

Fig. 17.4: Categories of weight.

- The subject stands erect with relaxed abdominal muscles, arms at the side, and feet together.
- The measurement should be taken at the end of a normal expiration.

Waist circumference
- Waist circumference predicts mortality better than any other anthropometric measurement.
- It has been noted that waist circumference alone can be used to assess obesity and two levels of risks have been identified:

Levels	Males	Females
Level 1	>94 cm	>80 cm
Level 2	>102 cm	>88 cm

- Level 1 is the maximum acceptable waist circumference irrespective of the adult age and there should be no further weight gain.
- Level 2 detects the obesity and requires weight management to reduce the risk of type 2 diabetes and cardiovascular complications.

Hip circumference
- Hip circumference is measured at the point of greatest circumference around hips and buttocks to the nearest 0.5 cm.
- The subject should be standing and the measurer should squat beside patient.
- Both measurements should be taken with a flexible, nonstretchable tape in close contact with the skin, but without indenting the soft tissue.

Interpretation of waist/hip ratio
High-risk waist/hip ratio (WHR is more than 0.80 for females and greater than 0.95 for males, i.e. waist measurement more than 80% of hip measurement for women and 95% for men indicates central obesity and is considered high risk for diabetes and cardiovascular disorders). A WHR below these cutoff levels is considered low risk.

Advantages of Anthropometry
- Simple, noninvasive.
- Equipment is inexpensive, portable.
- Relatively unskilled personnel can perform measurements.
- Methods are reproducible.
- Measures long-term nutritional history.
- Quickly identifies mild-to-moderate malnutrition.
- Measures many variable of nutritional significance such as height, weight, skinfold thickness, head circumference, WHR, and BMI.

Disadvantages of Anthropometry
- Relatively insensitive to short-term nutritional status.
- Cannot identify specific nutrient deficiencies.
- Unable to distinguish disturbances in growth or body composition induced by nutrient deficiencies.
- Measurements: Skinfolds difficult to carry out in obese people.
- Ethnic differences in fat deposition.

Biochemical and Other Laboratory Measurements
- Blood: Accessible, relatively noninvasive reflect recent dietary intakes, but influenced by diet, drugs, infection, and stress.
- Samples collected under controlled and standardized conditions, e.g. hormones, trace elements, processing time, and hemolysis.
- Hemoglobin is the most important test and useful index of the overall state of nutrition. Besides anemia, it also gives idea about protein and trace element nutrition.
- Stool examination: To detect the presence of ova and intestinal parasites.
- Urine examination: Albumin, sugar, and blood.
- Red blood cell vs. white blood cells: Gives idea about long/short-term nutrient status.
- Analysis of hair, nails, and skin for micronutrients [copper (Cu), selenium (Se), zinc (Zn), mercury (Hg), etc.].
- Detection of abnormal amount of metabolites in the urine (creatinine/hydroxyproline ratio).
- Functional tests done to study about the metabolic pathways.

Advantages
- Biochemical measurements are useful in detecting early changes in body metabolism and nutrition before the appearance of overt clinical signs.
- It is precise, accurate, and reproducible.
- Useful to validate data obtained from dietary methods (e.g. comparing salt intake with 24-hour urinary excretion).

Nutrition

Disadvantages
- Expensive
- Time consuming
- Needs trained personal and facilities.

Dietary Assessment

Nutritional intake of humans is assessed by five different methods:
1. 24-hour dietary recall
2. Food frequency questionnaire
3. Dietary history from the beginning
4. Food dairy technique
5. Observed food consumption.

24-Hour Dietary Recall
- A trained interviewer asks the subject to recall all food and drink taken in the previous 24 hours.
- It is quick, easy and depends on short-term memory, but it may not be truly representative of the person's usual intake.

Food Frequency Questionnaire
- The subject is given a list of around 100 food items to indicate his/her intake (frequency and quantity) per day, per week, and per month.
- It is inexpensive, more representative, and easy to use.

Limitations
- Long questionnaire
- Errors with estimating size
- Needs updating with new food commercial food products to keep pace with changing dietary habits.

Dietary History from the Beginning
- Dietary history is an accurate method for assessing the nutritional status.
- The information should be collected by a trained interviewer.
- Details about the usual intake, types, amount, frequency, and timing need to be obtained.
- Cross-checking to verify data is very important.

Food Dairy Technique
- Food intake (types and amounts) should be recorded by the subject at the time of consumption.
- The length of the collection period range between 1 and 7 days.
- It is reliable but difficult to maintain.

Observed Food Consumption
- The most unused method in clinical practice (must for research).
- The meal eaten by the individual is weighed and contents are to be calculated exactly.
- High degree of accuracy but expensive and needs more time and efforts.

Interpretation of Dietary Data

Qualitative method
- Using the food pyramid and the basic food groups method.
- Different nutrients are classified into five groups (fats and oils, bread, cereals, milk products, meat, fish, poultry, vegetables, and fruits).
- Determine the number of serving from each group and compare it with minimum requirement.

Quantitative method
- The amount of energy and specific nutrients in each food consumed can be calculated using food composition tables, and then compare it with the recommended daily intake
- Evaluation by this method is expensive and time consuming, unless computing facilities are available.

NUTRITION-RELATED DISEASES

Megaloblastic Anemia

The deficiency of Vitamin B_{12} and folate (folic acid) causes megaloblastic anemia. The bone marrow produces large and abnormal red cells (megaloblasts).

Symptoms

- People may be weak, short of breath, and pale.
- Nerves may also malfunction.
- Blood tests can detect abnormal cells that indicate vitamin deficiency anemia.

Iron Deficiency Anemia

Iron deficiency anemia is caused by insufficient iron intake and is the major cause of anemia in childhood.

Causes

- Insufficient iron in the diet
- Poor absorption of iron by the body
- Ongoing blood loss, most commonly from menstruation or from gradual blood loss in the intestinal tract
- Periods of rapid growth.

Symptoms

- Fatigue and weakness
- Pale skin and mucous membranes
- Rapid heartbeat or a new heart murmur
- Irritability
- Decreased appetite
- Dizziness or a feeling of being light headed.

Dietary Requirements during Pregnancy and Lactation

The pregnant/lactating woman should eat a wide variety of foods to make sure that her own nutritional needs as well as those of her growing fetus are met.

Approximately 300 extra calories are needed daily to maintain a healthy pregnancy. These calories should come from a balanced diet of protein, fruits, vegetables, and whole grains, with sweets and fats kept to a minimum. A healthy, well-balanced diet during pregnancy can also help to minimize some pregnancy symptoms such as nausea and constipation.

The Academy of Nutrition and Dietetics recommends the following key components of a healthy lifestyle during pregnancy: appropriate weight gain, eating a balanced diet, exercising regularly, and appropriate and timely vitamin and mineral supplementation.

Fluid intake is also an important part of healthy pregnancy nutrition. Women can take in enough fluids by drinking several glasses of water each day, in addition to the fluids in juices and soups. All alcohol should be avoided in pregnancy.

It is better for all women of childbearing age consume 400 µg (0.4 mg) of **folic acid** each day. This folic acid is present in some green leafy vegetables, most berries, nuts, beans, citrus fruits, fortified breakfast cereals, and some vitamin supplements can help reduce the risk for birth defects of the brain and spinal cord (called neural tube defects).

Folic acid is most beneficial during the first 28 days after conception, when most neural tube defects occur. Unfortunately, many women do not realize they are pregnant before 28 days. Therefore folic acid intake should begin prior to conception and continue through pregnancy.

Iron is needed for hemoglobin synthesis, mental function, and providing immunity against diseases.

Deficiency of iron leads to anemia.

Iron deficiency is common particularly in women of reproductive age and children.

Iron deficiency during pregnancy increases maternal mortality and low birth weight infants.

In children, it increases susceptibility to infection and impairs learning ability.

Plant foods such as green leafy vegetables, legumes, and dry fruits contain iron.

Iron is also obtained through meat, fish, and poultry products.

Vitamin C-rich fruits such as gooseberries (amla), guava, and citrus improve iron absorption from plant foods.

Most common consumed plant-based diets provide around 18 mg of iron as against recommended intake of 35 mg/day. Therefore supplementation of iron (100 mg elemental iron, 0.5 mg folic acid) is recommended for 100 days during pregnancy from 16th week onward to meet the demands of pregnancy.

Consume the following during pregnancy:
- Vegetables: Carrots, sweet potatoes, pumpkin, spinach, cooked greens, tomatoes, and red sweet peppers (for vitamin A and potassium).
- Fruits: Cantaloupe, honeydew, mangoes, prunes, bananas, apricots, oranges, and red or pink grapefruit (for potassium).
- Dairy: Fat-free or low-fat yogurt, skim or 1% milk, soymilk (for calcium, potassium, vitamins A and D).
- Grains: Ready-to-eat cereals/cooked cereals (for iron and folic acid).
- Proteins: Beans and peas; nuts and seeds; lean meats; salmon, trout, herring, sardines, and pollock.

Avoid the following during pregnancy:
- Unpasteurized milk and foods made with unpasteurized milk (soft cheeses).
- Hot dogs and luncheon meats (unless they are heated until steaming hot before serving).
- Raw and undercooked seafood, eggs, and meat. Do not eat sushi made with raw fish (cooked sushi is safe).
- Refrigerated pâté and meat spreads.
- Refrigerated smoked seafood.

Nutrient needs during lactation depend primarily on the volume and composition of milk produced and on the mother's initial nutrient needs and nutritional status. Among women exclusively breastfeeding their infants, the energy demands of lactation exceed prepregnancy demands by approximately 640 kcal/day during the first 6 months postpartum compared with 300 kcal/day during the last two trimesters of pregnancy.

CAUSES, SIGNS, AND SYMPTOMS OF DIFFERENT TYPES OF PROTEIN–ENERGY MALNUTRITION

Protein–Calorie Malnutrition and Protein–Energy malnutrition

Protein-calorie malnutrition is present when sufficient energy and/or protein is not available to meet metabolic demands, leading to impairment in normal physiologic processes:
- Kwashiorkor (Protein-calorie malnutrition) is a condition, which develops when there is gross protein deficiency though nonprotein calorie intake may be adequate.
- Marasmus (Protein-energy malnutrition) occurs with deficiency of both protein and calories.

Causes
- Inadequate dietary intake
- Poor quality dietary protein
- Increased metabolic demands
- Increased nutrient losses.

Kwashiorkor

Kwashiorkor is a high mortality deficiency disease known as kwashiorkor meaning red boy. The name comes from the odd reddish orange color of the hair, as well as from the skin rash, characteristic of the disease. Moderate-to-severe growth failure is present in kwashiorkor **(Figs. 17.5A and B)**.

For the first few months of life, the breastfed infant in the developing countries grows at a rate that is comparable to that of well-fed infants, but thereafter symptoms starts occurring of a kwashiorkor child if the nutrition is not adequate.

Symptoms
- The increase in stature and retarded tissue development.
- Poorly developed muscle and lack tone.
- Severe edema.
- Potbelly (protruding of the stomach).

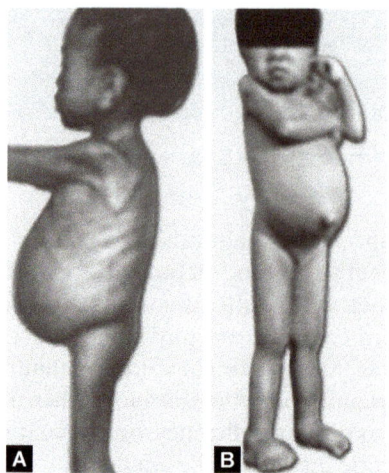

Figs. 17.5A and B: Symptoms of kwashiorkor.

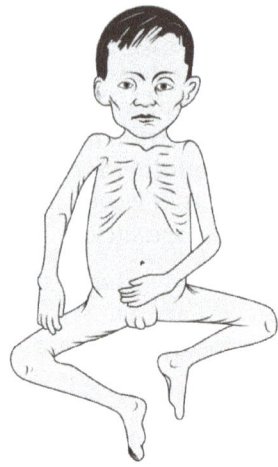

Fig. 17.6: Features of marasmus.

- Swollen legs and face.
- Anorexia and diarrhea are common; poor sanitation is cause of diarrhea.
- Whimpering, but does not cry or scream.
- The child is not interested in or curious about his/her surrounding, but remains seated whenever he/she is put down.

Pathologic and biochemical changes
- Fatty infiltration of the liver.
- Decreased serum levels of triglycerides, phospholipids, and cholesterol.
- Reduced amylase, lipase, and trypsin
- Serum proteins and albumin fractions are markedly reduced.
- Low hemoglobin levels, especially, if parasite infestation is also present.
- Vitamin A levels are usually reduced, which could be a serious complication leading to blindness and death in some children.

Marasmus

Marasmus is a protein-caloric malnutrition caused by a diet deficient in both protein and carbohydrates.

Symptoms
Severe growth failure and emaciation are the most striking characteristics of the marasmic infant (**Fig. 17.6**). Differences between marasmus and kwashiorkor in several important aspects are given in **Table 17.4**.

Obesity
Obesity is a chronic medical condition with excess amount of body fat, or more specifically, a BMI of 30 and above.

Table 17.4: Difference between marasmus and kwashiorkor.

Marasmus	Kwashiorkor
The onset is earlier, usually in the first year of life	Onset is later, after the breastfeeding is stopped
Growth failure is more pronounced	Not very pronounced
There is no edema	Edema present
Blood protein concentration is reduced less markedly	Blood protein concentration is reduced very much
Skin changes are seen less frequently	Red boils and patches are classic symptoms
Liver is not infiltrated with fat	Fatty liver is seen
Recovery is much longer	Recovery period is short

BMI: It is a measurement obtained by dividing a person's weight by the square of the person's height (kg/m^2):

A person with a BMI of 18.5–24.9 has a normal weight.

An adult who has a BMI of 25–29.9 is overweight.

An adult who has a BMI over 30 is obese.

A person with BMI of over 40 is morbidly obese (extreme obesity).

Causes

Obesity is most commonly caused by a combination of excessive food intake, lack of physical activity, genetic susceptibility, social and economic issues, and age.

Complications

Obesity can lead to diabetes, high blood pressure, cardiovascular disease, digestive problems, certain cancers, sleep apnea, and sexual problems.

Prevention

Regular exercise, healthy eating plan, and monitoring the weight.

Role of Gastrointestinal Peptides and Adipokines in Obesity

Ghrelin is produced principally by the stomach and, to a lesser extent, the duodenum.

Endogenous levels of ghrelin increase before meals and decrease after food intake, suggesting its role in both meal initiation and weight gain.

Ghrelin stimulates the brain, which leads to an increase in appetite, and it slows metabolism and decreases the body's ability to burn fat **(Fig. 17.7)**.

Leptin is a **hormone**, made by fat cells, that decreases our **appetite. It** is a mediator

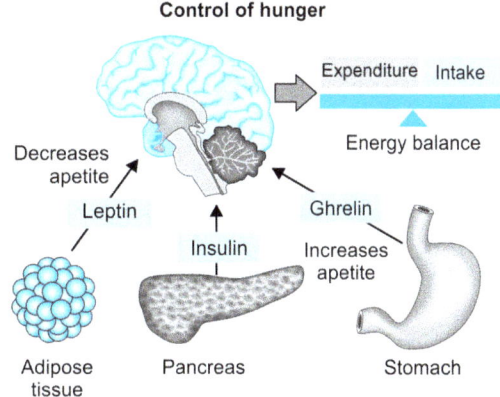

Fig. 17.7: Control of hunger.

of long-term regulation of energy balance, suppressing food intake and thereby inducing weight loss.

LEP gene mutations that **cause** congenital **leptin deficiency lead to** an absence of **leptin**. As a result, the signaling that triggers feelings of satiety **does** not occur, leading to the excessive hunger and **weight gain** associated with this disorder. Congenital **leptin deficiency** is a rare **cause** of **obesity**.

Adiponectin is a protein hormone that modulates a number of metabolic processes, including glucose regulation and fatty acid oxidation.

Adiponectin is secreted from adipose tissue. **It** is a fat-derived hormone that appears to play a crucial **role** in protecting against IR/diabetes and atherosclerosis. Decreased **adiponectin** levels are thought to play a central **role** in the development of type 2 diabetes, **obesity**, and cardiovascular disease in humans

In **obesity** and type 2 diabetes mellitus, alterations in the expression of **adiponectin** and its AdipoRs reduce **adiponectin** sensitivity leading to IR, which in turn aggravates hyperinsulinemia.

SUMMARY

For every physical activity, the human body requires energy and the amount depends on the duration and type of activity. Energy is measured in Calories and is obtained from the body stores or the food we consume. This chapter deals with different components of our diet and their importance to the human body. Carbohydrates, proteins, and fat give 4, 4, and 9 cal, respectively, per gram, when they oxidized. Dietary fiber is another important component of our diet, which plays a major role in protecting humans from diseases. Kwashiorkor and marasmus are the two major types of protein-calorie malnutrition seen in malnourished children.

SELF-ASSESSMENT QUESTIONS

1. Mention the caloric values for proteins, carbohydrates, and fats.
2. What is respiratory quotient and mention its significance?
3. What are complete and incomplete proteins?
4. How do you explain protein and weight gain?
5. Add a note on protein and weight loss.
6. Write the importance of carbohydrates.
7. Briefly discuss the dietary fiber and its importance.
8. What is protein-calorie malnutrition?
9. How do you differentiate kwashiorkor from marasmus?
10. Give the signs and symptoms of kwashiorkor.
11. What is biological value of protein and write the formula to calculate it?
12. Discuss the components of balanced diet.
13. What is specific dynamic action and mention its importance?
14. Define BMR. Mention the factors affecting BMR.
15. Briefly discuss the negative and positive nitrogen balance.
16. Calculate the energy requirement of allied health student (age 18 years, BMR = 40 cal/m^2 body surface per hour, body surface area = 1.7 m^2) engaged in moderate work.
17. What is resting metabolic rate?
18. How do you differentiate soluble fiber from insoluble fiber?

MULTIPLE-CHOICE QUESTIONS

1. **The caloric value for a gram of fat is:**
   a. 9   b. 6
   c. 3   d. 4
2. **The respiratory quotient for carbohydrate is:**
   a. 0.8   b. 1.0
   c. 2.0   d. 0.7
3. **All the following foods give complete proteins, *except*:**
   a. Meat   b. Fish
   c. Legumes   d. Cheese
4. **Concerning fat, one of the following statements is incorrect:**
   a. It provides us 60% our energy needs
   b. It helps to maintain cell membrane structure
   c. It helps in the absorption of vitamins A and D
   d. Protein-rich foods are deficient in fat
5. ***Trans* fat:**
   a. Increases blood glucose
   b. Increases blood LDL
   c. Increases blood high-density lipoprotein (HDL)
   d. Increases blood chylomicron
6. **Concerning the dietary fiber, all the following statements are true, *except*:**
   a. They are resistant to breakdown by the human digestive enzymes
   b. Insoluble fiber promotes normal elimination by providing bulk for stool formation

c. Increased amounts of fiber in the diet is the reason for irritable bowel syndrome
d. Fruits and vegetables are rich in soluble fiber

7. **Concerning BMR, one of the following statements is incorrect:**
   a. It is expressed as cal/m² body surface per hour
   b. Age and sex may affect the BMR
   c. The Harris-Benedict formula may be used to calculate the BMR
   d. Hormones do not affect the BMR

8. **Negative nitrogen balance may results in:**
   a. Unconsciousness
   b. Muscle loss
   c. Liver disorder
   d. Amino acid degradation

9. **All of the following are causes for protein–calorie malnutrition, *except*:**
   a. Increased carbohydrate
   b. Inadequate dietary intake
   c. Poor quality dietary protein
   d. Increased metabolic demands

10. **Which of the following is not a symptom of protein–calorie malnutrition?**
    a. Poorly developed muscle and lack tone
    b. Severe edema
    c. Potbelly
    d. High serum vitamin A

Answers

| 1. a | 2. b | 3. d | 4. b | 5. c |
| 6. d | 7. d | 8. b | 9. a | 10. d |

CHAPTER 18

Chemistry of Nucleic Acid

OBJECTIVES

At the end of this chapter, students should be able to:
- Know about the nucleosides, nucleotides, nucleoside derivatives and their importance
- Explain the structure and function of deoxyribonucleic acid (DNA)
- Understand the types of ribonucleic acid (RNA), including their structure and functions.

INTRODUCTION

- Nucleic acids present in all living cells in combination with proteins to form conjugated protein are called nucleoprotein. The proteins present usually are basic and they are protamines and histones.
- Nucleic acids transfer genetic information from parents to offspring.
- Nucleic acids are polymers of specific nucleotides. The nucleic acids are of two different types:
    a. DNA
    b. RNA.

NUCLEOSIDES AND NUCLEOTIDES

Nucleoside is a combination of either a pyrimidine or purine base and sugar. When nitrogenous bases are coupled to D-ribose or 2-deoxy-D-ribose through a α-*N*-glycosidic bond between the anomeric carbon of the ribose and the N9 of a purine or N1 of a pyrimidine, they are termed "nucleosides."

Nucleotides have a distinctive structure composed of three components covalently bound together.
1. A nitrogen-containing "base"—either a pyrimidine (one ring) or purine (two rings)
2. A 5-carbon sugar—ribose or deoxyribose
3. A phosphate group.

Nucleotides also exist in activated forms containing two or three phosphates, called nucleotide diphosphates or triphosphates. If the sugar in a nucleotide is deoxyribose, the nucleotide is called deoxynucleotide; if the sugar is ribose, the term "ribonucleotide" is used.

Nitrogenous bases of RNA and DNA

The following list shows the information about nitrogenous bases:
- The nitrogenous bases of nucleic acids are from purine and pyrimidine bases.

- There are five major bases found in cells.
- The purine bases are adenine and guanine.
- Pyrimidine bases are thymine, cytosine, and uracil. The common abbreviations used for these five bases are A, G, T, C, and U **(Table 18.1)**.

Purine and Pyrimidine-bases

Table 18.1: Purine and pyrimidine-bases.

Base (X=H) Formula	Nucleoside X=ribose or deoxyribose	Nucleotide X=ribose phosphate
Cytosine (C)	Cytidine	CMP
Uracil (U)	Uridine	UMP
Thymine (T)	Thymidine	TMP
Adenine (A)	Adenosine	AMP
Guanine (G)	Guanosine	GMP

(AMP: adenosine monophosphate; CMP: cytidine monophosphate; GMP: guanosine monophosphate; TMP: thymidine monophosphate; UMP: uridine monophosphate)

Minor or Modified Bases

- In addition to the usual purine and pyrimidine bases, DNA and RNA contain minor or modified bases.
- 5-Methylcytosine-base—modification through methylation process.
- Methyladenine and methylguanine present in mammalian RNAs—methylation process 5-hydroxymethylcytosine, present only in bacteria and viruses (hydroxymethylation process).

Dimethylaminoadenine   7-methylguanine   5-methylcytosine   5-hydroxymethylcytosine

Structure and Function of Nucleotides

The structure and function of nucleotides are as follows:
- Nucleotides are phosphorylated nucleosides. The most common site of phosphorylation of nucleotides found in cells is the hydroxyl group attached to the 5'-carbon of the ribose. The carbon atoms of the ribose present in nucleotides are designated with a prime (') mark to distinguish them from the backbone numbering in the bases.
- Nucleotides can exist in the mono-, di-, or tri-phosphorylated forms. As a class, the nucleotides may be considered one of the most important metabolites of the cell. Nucleotides are found primarily as the monomeric units comprising the major nucleic acids of the cell, RNA and DNA.
- However, they also are required for numerous other important functions within the cell.
- Nucleotides have a variety of roles in cellular metabolism.
    - Serve as energy stores for future use in phosphate transfer reactions. These reactions are predominantly carried out by adenosine triphosphate (ATP) (**Fig. 18.1**).
    - Form a part of several important coenzymes such as nicotinamide adenine dinucleotide, nicotinamide adenine dinucleotide phosphate, flavin adenine dinucleotide, and coenzyme A.
    - Serve as mediators of numerous important cellular processes such as second messengers in signal transduction events. The predominant second messenger is cyclic adenosine monophosphate (cAMP), a cyclic derivative of AMP formed from ATP.
    - Control numerous enzymatic reactions through allosteric effects on enzyme activity.
    - Serve as activated intermediates in numerous biosynthetic reactions. These activated intermediates include S-adenosylmethionine involved in methyl transfer reactions as well as the many sugar coupled nucleotides involved in glycogen and glycoprotein synthesis.
    - They are the constituents of nucleic acids such as DNA and RNA.
- DNA serves as the master copy for most information in the cell.
- RNA is of different types, which act to transform information from DNA to the rest of the cell.
- The primary structure of both DNA and RNA is similar.
- Each consists of the sugar/phosphate backbone to which a nitrogenous base is attached.
- The nucleotides found in cells are derivatives of the heterocyclic highly basic compounds, purine and pyrimidine.

Nucleotides of Adenine

Adenine in combination with sugar and phosphate forms various nucleotides. They are:
- ATP (**Fig. 18.1**)
- Adenosine diphosphate (ADP)

Chemistry of Nucleic Acid

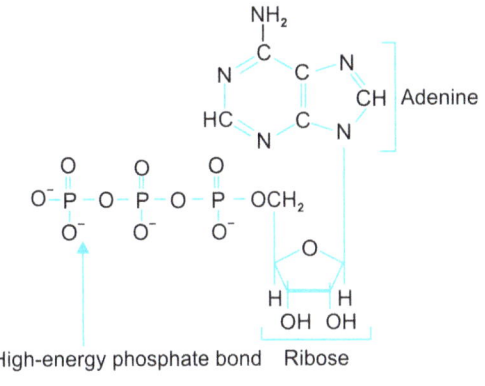

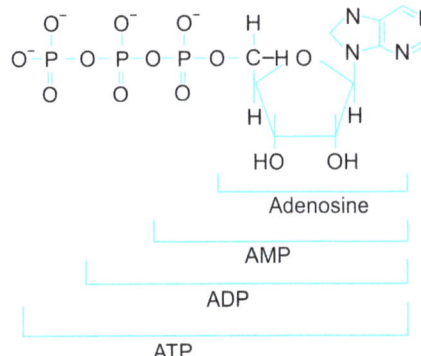

Fig. 18.1: Structure of adenosine triphosphate. (AMP: adenosine monophosphate; ADP: adenosine diphosphate; ATP: adenosine triphosphate)

- cAMP
- Phosphoadenosine phosphosulfate
- S-AMP.
  - ATP serves as main free energy transducer.
  - ATP is the product of oxidative phosphorylation.
  - ADP is the substrate for oxidative phosphorylation.

Formation and Importance of Cyclic Adenosine-3c,5c-Monophosphate

The formation and importance of cAMP are as follows:
- cAMP is formed from ATP by the action of adenylate cyclase. This cAMP is again degraded by phosphodiesterase enzyme.
- cAMP acts as second messenger for many hormones such as calcitonin, human chorionic gonadotropin, follicle-stimulating hormone, glucagon, epinephrine, luteinizing hormone, melanocyte-stimulating hormone, norepinephrine, parathyroid hormone, thyroid-stimulating hormone, and vasopressin.
- cAMP by acting as a second messenger affects many cellular processes such as:
  - Degradation of fat and glycogen.
  - Increasing the secretion of acid by gastric mucosa.
  - It leads to depression of melanin pigment granules.
  - It diminishes the aggregation of platelets cells.

Cytosine Nucleotides

Cytosine Triphosphate

- Cytosine triphosphate is required for the synthesis of phosphoglycerides. CMP-N-acetylneuraminic acid is required for the synthesis of glycoproteins.
- Cytidine diphosphate-choline is required for the synthesis of sphingomyelin.

Nucleotides of Guanine

Guanosine Monophosphate

Following are the nucleotides of guanine:
- Guanosine diphosphate (GDP).
- Deoxyguanosine diphosphate **(Fig 18.2)**
- Guanosine triphosphate (GTP).
- Cyclic guanosine monophosphate (cGMP) and cAMP.
- GDP and GTP participate in the conversion of succinyl-CoA to succinate in citric acid cycle. This reaction is coupled to the substrate level phosphorylation of GDP to GTP.
- Again GTP is involved in the activation of adenylate cyclase.
- GTP acts as an allosteric regulator and energy source for the protein synthesis.

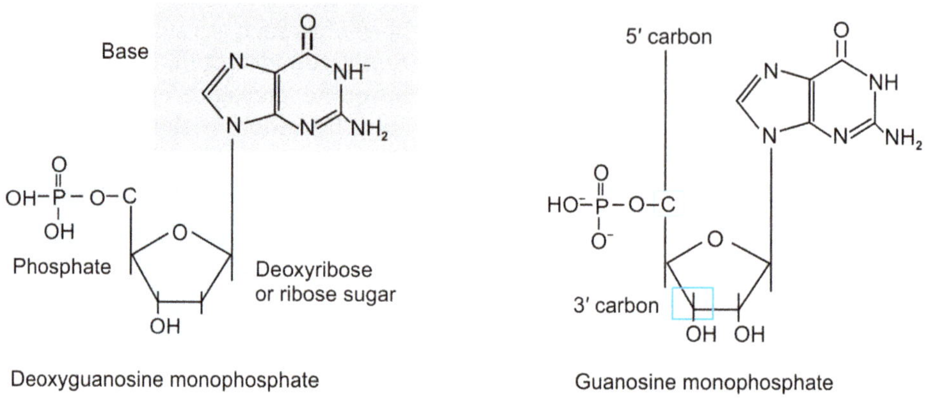

Fig. 18.2: Structure of Guanosine nucleotides.

Cyclic Guanosine Monophosphate

The following list shows the features of cAMP:
- Cyclic guanosine monophosphate is an intracellular second messenger and can act antagonistically to cAMP.
- It is formed from GTP by guanylyl cyclase, which is regulated by hormones, such as atrial natriuretic factor produced in cardiac atrial tissue.
- Nitric oxide, sodium azide, and nitroglycerine act as effectors, increase the activity of guanylyl cyclase, and cause smooth muscle relaxation and vasodilatation.
- cGMP is involved in the relaxation of smooth muscle and vasodilatation.

Uracil Nucleotides

The following list shows about uracil nucleotides:
- Uridine diphosphate (UDP).
- UDP-sugar derivatives act as sugar donors in many metabolic reactions.
- UDP-glucose donates glucose during the synthesis of glycogen.
- UDP-sugar derivatives participate in sugar epimerization such as the interconversion of glucose-1-phosphate and galactose-1-phosphate.
- UDP-glucuronate acts as a glucuronyl donor for conjugation reactions to form glucuronide conjugates of bilirubin.

SYNTHETIC ANALOGS OF NUCLEOTIDES OR ANTIMETABOLITES

Chemically synthesized analogs of purines and pyrimidines, their nucleosides and nucleotides have many therapeutic applications in medicine. An antimetabolite is a chemical with a similar structure to a substance (a metabolite) required for normal biochemical reactions. These are mainly used chemotherapeutically to control cancer or infections.

Synthetic Nucleotide Analogs and their Applications

Synthetic Analogs in Cancer Treatment

Antimetabolites can be used in cancer treatment, as they interfere with DNA production and therefore cell division and the growth of tumors. Antimetabolites act as purine or pyrimidine, which become the building blocks of DNA. They prevent these substances from becoming incorporated into DNA during the S phase of cell cycle, stopping normal development and division.

Chemistry of Nucleic Acid

They also affect RNA synthesis. However, because thymidine is used in DNA, but not in RNA, inhibition of thymidine synthesis via thymidylate synthase selectively inhibits DNA synthesis over RNA synthesis.

Purine Analogs

Azathioprine is the main immunosuppressive cytotoxic substance. It is widely used in transplantations to control rejection reactions. It is nonenzymatically cleaved to 6-mercaptopurine that acts as a purine analog and an inhibitor of DNA synthesis. By preventing the clonal expansion of lymphocytes in the induction phase of the immune response, it affects both the cell and the humoral immunity. It also successfully suppresses autoimmunity.

6-Mercaptopurine

The purine antagonist 6-mercaptopurine has been used as a chemotherapy drug for over 30 years. It is a structural analog of inosine. The drug is usually given orally. When higher doses are required, the drug may be given through an IV. Patients suffering from acute lymphocytic or myelocytic leukemia, lymphoblastic leukemia, and acute myelogenous and myelomonocytic leukemias are often given 6-mercaptopurine in combination with other chemotherapy drugs. In addition to its role in cancer treatment, 6-mercaptopurine is used to treat patients suffering from a variety of inflammatory bowel diseases. The drug is also used to prevent rejection following organ transplants:

6-mercaptopurine

6-Thioguanine

- 6-Thioguanine is a structural analog of guanine.
- It is used to treat acute leukemias and induction of remissions in acute granulocytic leukemias.

6-thioguanine

Fludarabine

- Fludarabine inhibits function of multiple DNA polymerases, DNA primase, DNA ligase I and is S phase specific. Fludarabine is used to treat chronic B-cell lymphocytic leukemia and is administered as an injection.
- Fludarabine is highly effective in treatment of chronic lymphocytic leukemia.
- Fludarabine is a purine analog and can be given both orally and intravenously.
- It inhibits DNA synthesis by interfering with ribonucleotide reductase and DNA polymerase. It is active against both dividing and resting cells.

Fludarabine

Azathioprine

Azathioprine is an immunosuppressant used in organ transplantation, autoimmune disease such as rheumatoid arthritis. It is converted in the body to the active metabolites, 6-mercaptopurine and 6-thioinosinic acid.

Chemistry of Nucleic Acid

Azathioprine

Pyrimidine Analogs

5-Fluorouracil

- 5-Fluorouracil inhibits thymidylate synthase.
- It is a commonly used pyrimidine antagonist. It is a thymine analog.
- Like the other pyrimidine antagonists, 5-fluorouracil (5-FU) is similar in structure to the normal molecule. It functions to inhibit DNA synthesis both by blocking the formation of normal pyrimidine nucleotides via enzyme inhibition and by interfering with DNA synthesis after incorporation into a growing DNA molecule.

5-fluorouracil

Floxuridine

- Floxuridine (FUDR) is most often used in the treatment of colorectal cancer.
- FUDR, an analog of 5-FU is a fluorinated pyrimidine.
- FUDR works because it is broken down by the body into its active form, which is the same as a metabolite of 5-FU.

Floxuridine

Cytosine Arabinoside (Cytarabine)

- Arabinosylcytosine or cytarabine is an antimetabolite that acts as a pyrimidine antagonist.
- In this arabinose replaces ribose.

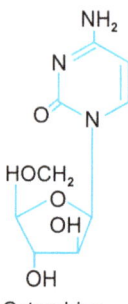
Cytarabine

- It is thought that its activity is primarily interrupting DNA synthesis.
- It is used in the treatment of acute nonlymphocytic leukemia.
- Acute lymphocytic leukemia.
- Chronic myelocytic leukemia.

Azidothymidine

Azidothymidine (AZT) or zidovudine is a structural analog of thymidine used in the treatment of acquired immunodeficiency syndrome. AZT works by inhibiting the action of reverse transcriptase, the enzyme that HIV uses to make a DNA copy of its RNA. The viral double-stranded DNA is subsequently spliced into the DNA of a target cell, where it is called provirus. AZT not only destroys the HIV infection but also delays the progression of the disease and the replication of virus, even at very high doses.

Gemcitabine

Gemcitabine is an antimetabolite that acts as a pyrimidine analog. It is incorporated into a dividing cell's DNA, which causes the cell to undergo apoptosis. Malignancies for which gemcitabine is used include:
- Nonsmall cell lung cancer (in combination with cisplatin)

- Pancreatic cancer (advanced or metastatic)
- Advanced ovarian cancer (in combination with carboplatin.

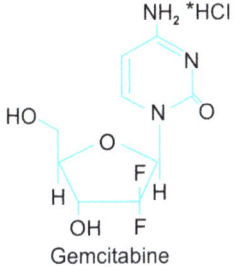
Gemcitabine

THE STRUCTURE OF DNA

- The structure of DNA is illustrated by a right-handed double helix **(Fig. 18.3)**.
- It contains 10 nucleotide pairs per helical turn.
- Each spiral strand, composed of a sugar phosphate backbone and attached bases, is connected to a complementary strand by hydrogen bonding (noncovalent) between paired bases, adenine (A) with thymine (T) and guanine (G) with cytosine (C).

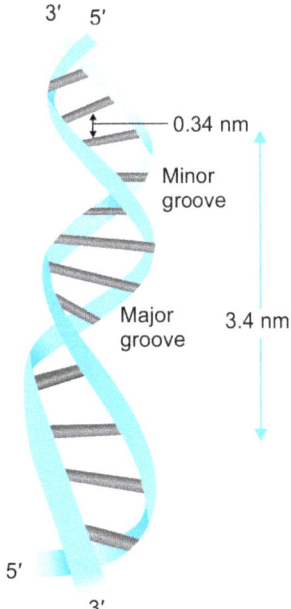

Fig. 18.3: Structure of deoxyribonucleic acid.

- There are four different bases in a DNA molecule:
  1. Adenine (purine)
  2. Cytosine (pyrimidine)
  3. Guanine (purine)
  4. Thymine (pyrimidine).
- The number of purine bases equals the number of pyrimidine bases.
- The number of adenine bases equals the number of thymine bases.
- The number of guanine bases equals the number of cytosine bases.
- Two DNA strands form a helical spiral, winding around a helix axis in a right-handed spiral.
- The two polynucleotide chains run in opposite directions (one in 3′–5′ and the other in 5′–3′).
- Within the double helix, adenine and thymine are connected by two hydrogen bonds (noncovalent) on the opposite strand, while guanine and cytosine are connected by three hydrogen bonds with cytosine on the opposite strand.
- This structure also known as the B form, the helix makes a turn every 3.4 nm and the distance between two neighboring base pairs is 0.34 nm. Hence, there are about 10 pairs per turn.
- The intertwined strands make two grooves of different widths, referred to as the major groove and the minor groove, which may facilitate binding with specific proteins.
- The solution with higher salt concentrations or with alcohol, the DNA structure may change to the A form, which is still right handed, but every 2.3 nm makes a turn and there are 11 base pairs per turn.
- The A form occurs under nonphysiological conditions in dehydrated samples of DNA, while in the cell it may be produced in hybrid pairings of DNA and RNA strands, as well as in enzyme-DNA complexes.
- Segments of DNA, where the bases have been chemically modified by methylation,

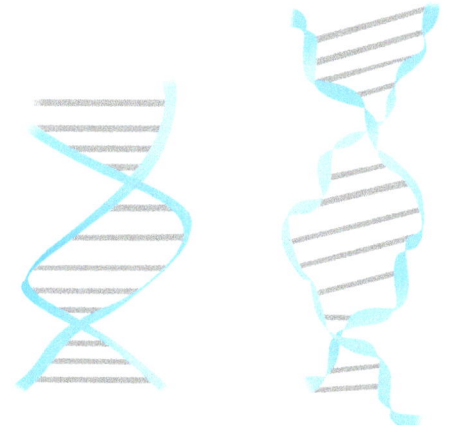

Fig. 18.4: Different forms of DNA (B form and Z form).

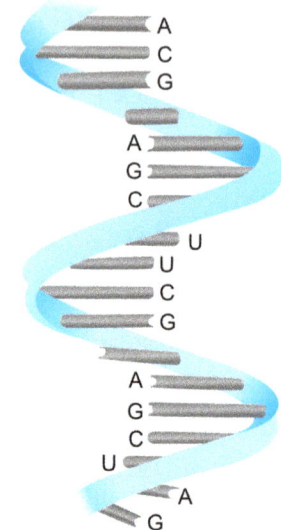

Fig. 18.5: Structure of ribonucleic acid.

may undergo a larger change in conformation and adopt the Z form **(Fig. 18.4)**.
- The structure is called the Z form, because its bases seem to zigzag.
- Z form DNA is left-handed. One turn spans 4.6 nm, comprising 12 base pairs. The DNA molecule with alternating G–C sequences in alcohol or high-salt solution tends to have such structure.
- It is a transient structure, i.e. occasionally induced by biological activity and then quickly disappears.
- It is believed to provide torsional strain relief, while DNA transcription occurs.

Structure and Functions of RNA

RNAs are sugar-phosphate polymers and have nitrogen bases attached to the sugars of the backbone **(Fig. 18.5)** (these features are similar to DNA).
- They differ in composition:
  - The sugar in RNA is ribose and deoxyribose in DNA.
  - The base present in RNA is uracil instead of thymine.
- They also differ in size and structure:
  - RNA molecules are smaller (shorter) than DNA molecules.
  - RNA is single-stranded, not double-stranded like DNA.

- DNA stores only the genetic information in its sequence of nucleotide bases.
- But there are three types of RNA, each with their own function.

TYPES OF RNA

Ribosomal RNAs

Exist outside the nucleus in the cytoplasm of a cell in structures called ribosome. Each ribosome is a complex consisting of about 60% ribosomal RNA (rRNA) and 40% protein. There are four kinds. In eukaryotes, these are:

1. *18S rRNA:* One of these molecules, along with some 30 different protein molecules, is used to make the small subunit of the ribosome.
2. *28S, 5.8S, and 5S rRNA:* One each of these molecules, along with some 45 different proteins, is used to make the large subunit of the ribosome.

The S number given in each type of rRNA reflects the rate at which the molecules sediment in the ultracentrifuge. The larger the number, the larger is the molecule. The

28S, 18S, and 5.8S molecules are produced by the processing of a single primary transcript from a cluster of identical copies of a single gene. The 5S molecules are produced from a different cluster of identical genes.

Messenger RNAs

These are the nucleic acids that "record" information from DNA in the cell nucleus and carry it to the ribosomes and are known as messenger RNA (mRNA).

Transfer RNAs

The function of transfer RNA (tRNA) is to transfer amino acids one by one to protein chains growing at ribosomes **(Fig. 18.6)**. There are some 32 different kinds of tRNA in a typical eukaryotic cell:
- Each is the product of a separate gene.
- The 5′ end starts with a phosphate and guanine.
- They are small (~4S), containing 73–93 nucleotides.
- Many of the bases in the chain pair with each other forming sections of double helix.
- The unpaired regions form three loops.
- Each kind of tRNA carries (at its 3′ end) one of the 20 amino acids (thus most amino acids have more than one tRNA responsible for them).
- First loop from the 5′ end is called D-loop because it contains a minor base dihydrouracil.
- Next to the above loop is an anticodon loop. It contains a sequence of three unpaired bases called anticodon, which is complementary to the three bases (codon) of mRNA.
- Some tRNAs contain an extra arm next to the anticodon small loop.
- Next loop is called $T\psi C$ loop. This contains minor bases such as thymine and pseudouracil.
- Base pairing between the anticodon and the complementary codon on an mRNA

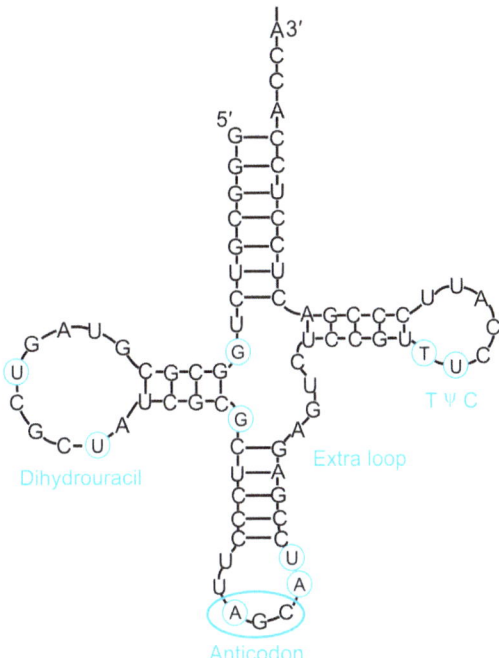

Fig. 18.6: Structure of transfer ribonucleic acid.

molecule brings the correct amino acid into the growing polypeptide chain.
- The 3′ end ends with a sequence C–C–A.

Small Nuclear RNA

DNA transcription of the genes for mRNA, rRNA, and tRNA produces large precursor molecules (primary transcripts) that must be processed within the nucleus to produce the functional molecules for exporting to the cytosol. Some of these processing steps are mediated by small nuclear RNAs.

Small Nucleolar RNA

Small nucleolar RNA within the nucleolus has several functions.

MicroRNA

MicroRNAs are tiny (~22 nucleotides) RNA molecules that appear to regulate the expression of mRNA molecules.

SUMMARY

Nucleic acids present in all living cells in combination with proteins to form conjugated protein are called nucleoprotein. Nucleic acids are polymers of specific nucleotides. The nucleic acids are of two different types such as DNA and RNA. The combination of a base and sugar is called nucleoside (e.g. cytidine, uridine, and adenosine). Nucleosides with phosphate attached are called nucleotides (uridine monophosphate, cytidine monophosphate, adenosine monophosphate, etc.). Nucleotides also exist in activated forms containing two or three phosphates, called nucleotide diphosphates or triphosphates. If the sugar in a nucleotide is deoxyribose, the nucleotide is called deoxynucleotide; if the sugar is ribose, the term "ribonucleotide" is used. The nitrogenous bases of nucleic acids are from purine and pyrimidine bases. The purine bases are adenine and guanine. Pyrimidine bases are thymine, cytosine, and uracil. There are many purine and pyrimidine analogs used in the treatment of various cancers.

SELF-ASSESSMENT QUESTIONS

1. How do you differentiate nucleosides from nucleotides?
2. List the purine and pyrimidine bases present in DNA and RNA.
3. Briefly explain the functions of nucleotides in the human body.
4. Define antimetabolites and briefly explain its role in medicine.
5. List the purine and pyrimidine analogs used in the treatment.
6. Discuss the structural aspects of the DNA.
7. Explain the structure and role of tRNA.
8. Name the different types of RNAs.

MULTIPLE-CHOICE QUESTIONS

1. **In a double-stranded molecule of DNA, the ratio of purines and pyrimidines is:**
   a. Variable
   b. Determined by the base sequence in RNA
   c. Genetically determined
   d. Always 1:1
2. **Which of the following nucleotide bases is not found in RNA?**
   a. Thymine
   b. Adenine
   c. Uracil
   d. Guanine
3. **Which of the following molecules does not form part of DNA?**
   a. Pyrimidine
   b. Deoxyribose
   c. Amino acid
   d. Phosphate
4. **The transcription of DNA to a molecule of messenger RNA occurs:**
   a. On the ribosomes
   b. In the nucleus
   c. Only during cell division
   d. When amino acids are made available by transfer RNA
5. **The process of translation requires the presence of:**
   a. mRNA, tRNA, and ribosomes
   b. mRNA, ribosomes, and RNA polymerase
   c. DNA, mRNA, and RNA polymerase
   d. Free nucleotide bases, amino acids, and ribosomes
6. **Codons are composed of:**
   a. Triplet sequences of nucleotide bases in mRNA
   b. Triplet sequences of nucleotide bases in DNA
   c. Triplet sequences of amino acids in polypeptide chains
   d. Triplet sequences of deoxyribose sugars in DNA
7. **Which of the following best describes the relationships between proteins, DNA, RNA, and genes?**
   a. DNA→Genes→RNA→Proteins
   b. RNA→DNA→Genes→Proteins
   c. Proteins→RNA→DNA→Genes
   d. Genes→RNA→DNA→Proteins

8. The base thymine is always paired with:
   a. Adenine
   b. Guanine
   c. Cytosine
   d. Thymine
9. The sequence of one strand of DNA is 5′ TCGATC 3′. The sequence of the complementary strand would be:
   a. 5′ AGCTAG 3′
   b. 5′ TCGATC 3′
   c. 5′ GCTAGC 3′
   d. 5′ GATCGA 3′
10. The differences between RNA and DNA in the human cell include the following:
    a. RNA is a double helix
    b. RNA contains the sugar ribose and DNA contains deoxyribose
    c. DNA contains the base uracil; RNA does not
    d. There is an RNA polymerase, but no DNA polymerase
11. Purine and pyrimidine bases are bound by hydrogen bonds in the DNA double helix. There are two typical base pair combinations. They include:
    a. Guanine to cytosine
    b. Adenine to guanine
    c. Adenine to thymine
    d. a and c
12. In the DNA double helix shown, the bases are paired by dashed lines, which represent what kind of bonds?
    a. Covalent bonds
    b. Ionic bonds
    c. van der Waals bond
    d. Hydrogen bonds
13. In DNA base pairing, the purine and pyrimidine bases pair up. The following bases pair up with each other in the DNA molecule:
    a. Adenine to thymine and guanine to uracil
    b. Adenine to guanine and thymine to cytosine
    c. Adenine to guanine and cytosine to uracil
    d. Adenine to thymine and guanine to cytosine
14. The following is true regarding ribosomes:
    a. They contain no protein
    b. They contain no RNA
    c. They have two tRNA-binding sites
    d. They are found only on rough endoplasmic reticulum
15. Common lesions found in DNA after exposure to UV light are:
    a. Pyrimidine dimers
    b. Double-strand breaks
    c. Base deletions
    d. Purine dimers

Answers

1. d	2. a	3. c	4. b	5. a
6. a	7. a	8. a	9. d	10. b
11. d	12. d	13. d	14. a	15. a

CHAPTER 19

Nucleic Acid Metabolism

OBJECTIVES

At the end of this chapter, students should be able to:
- Describe the synthesis of purine and pyrimidine nucleotides
- Understand the salvage pathways of purine pyrimidine synthesis
- Explain the catabolism of purine, uric acid, and its importance
- Know about the causes and clinical manifestations of gout and Lesch–Nyhan syndrome.

INTRODUCTION

The synthesis of purine and pyrimidine is essential for the generation of their respective nucleotides.

PURINE METABOLISM

The major site of purine synthesis is liver.

Biosynthesis of Purine

- Synthesis of the purine nucleotides begins with phosphoribosyl pyrophosphate (PRPP) and leads to the first fully formed nucleotide, inosine 5′-monophosphate (IMP) (**Fig. 19.1**).
- The synthesis of IMP requires five moles of adenosine triphosphate (ATP), two moles of glutamine, one mole of glycine, one mole of CO_2, one mole of aspartate, and two moles of formate.
- The formyl moieties are carried on tetrahydrofolate (THF) in the form of N^5, N^{10}-methenyl THF and N^{10}-formyl THF.

IMP represents a branch point for purine biosynthesis, because it can be converted into either adenosine monophosphate (AMP) or guanosine monophosphate (GMP) through two distinct reaction pathways (**Fig. 19.2**).

Regulation of Purine Nucleotide Synthesis

- The rate-limiting steps in purine biosynthesis occur at the first two steps of the pathway.
- The synthesis of PRPP by PRPP synthetase is feedback inhibited by purine-5′-nucleotides such as AMP and GMP.
- GMP also inhibits PRPP amidotransferase.
- Additionally, purine biosynthesis is regulated in the branch pathways from IMP to AMP and GMP.
- The accumulation of excess ATP leads to accelerated synthesis of GMP and excess guanosine triphosphate (GTP) leads to accelerated synthesis of AMP.

Purine Salvage Pathway

Salvage of Purine Nucleotides

- The synthesis of nucleotides from the purine bases and purine nucleosides takes place in a series of steps known as the salvage pathways.
- The free purine bases such as adenine, guanine, and hypoxanthine can be reconverted to their corresponding nucleotides by phosphoribosylation. Two

Nucleic Acid Metabolism

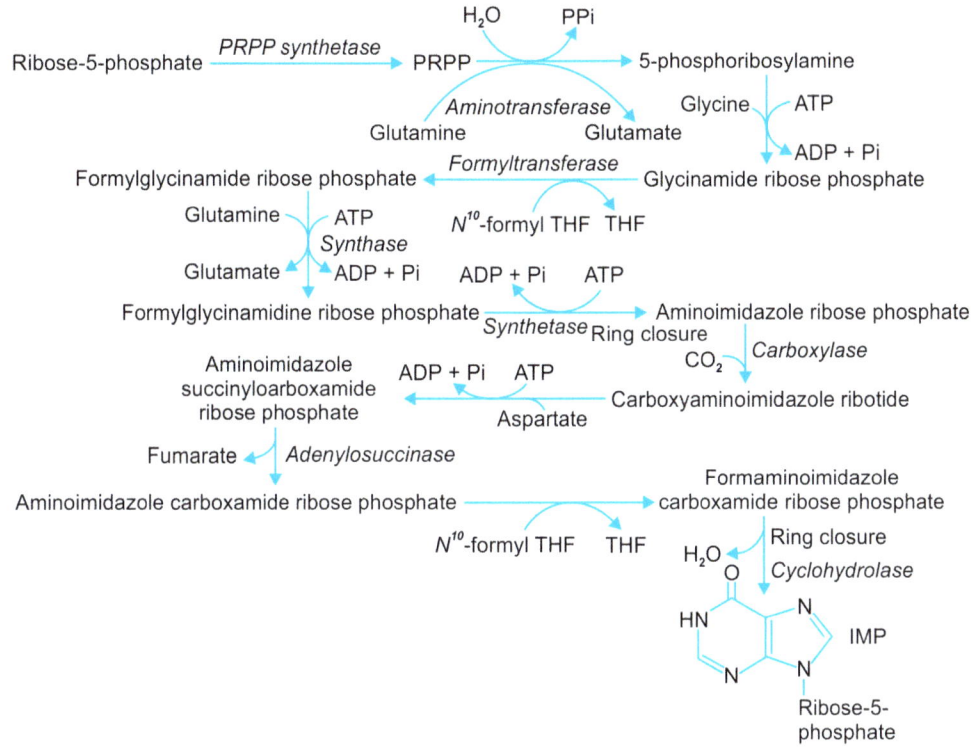

Fig. 19.1: Synthesis of inosine monophosphate.
(THF: tetrahydrofolate; ATP: adenosine triphosphate; ADP: adenosine diphosphate; PRPP: phosphoribosyl pyrophosphate)

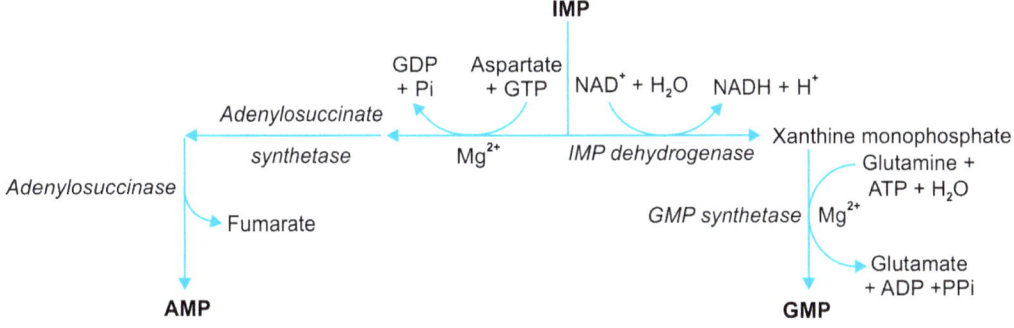

Fig. 19.2: Formation of AMP and GMP.
(AMP: adenosine monophosphate; GMP: guanosine monophosphate; ATP: adenosine triphosphate; ADP: adenosine diphosphate; NAD: nicotinamide adenine dinucleotide; GMP: guanosine monophosphate; GTP: guanosine triphosphate; GDP: guanosine diphosphate)

key transferase enzymes involved in the salvage of purines are:
1. Adenine phosphoribosyltransferase
2. Hypoxanthine-guanine phosphoribosyltransferase.

Adenine + PRPP $\xrightarrow{APRT}$ AMP + PPi

Hypoxanthine + PRPP $\xrightarrow{HGPRT}$ IMP + PPi

Guanine + PRPP $\longleftarrow$ GMP + PPi

- Purine nucleotide phosphorylases can also contribute to the salvage of the bases through a reversal of the catabolism pathways. However, this pathway is less significant than those catalyzed by the phosphoribosyl transferases.
- The synthesis of AMP from IMP and the salvage of IMP via AMP catabolism have the net effect of deaminating aspartate to fumarate. This process has been termed "purine nucleotide cycle."

This cycle is very important in muscle cells. Increases in muscle activity create a demand for an increase in the TCA cycle, in order to generate more nicotinamide adenine dinucleotide (NADH) for the production of ATP. However, muscle lacks most of the enzymes of the major anaplerotic reactions. Muscle replenishes TCA cycle intermediates in the form of fumarate generated by the purine nucleotide cycle.

Catabolism of Purine Nucleotides

Catabolism of the purine nucleotides leads finally to the production of uric acid. Uric acid is insoluble and is excreted in the urine as sodium urate crystals **(Fig. 19.3)**.

Cases

A 65-year-old man with a preference for red meat in his diet awakes one night with a throbbing ache in his big toe. His condition can be treated by a drug that inhibits:
a. Xanthine oxidase
b. PRPP synthetase
c. Amidotransferase
d. Orotate phosphoribosyltransferase

Answer is a

A medical condition characterized by megaloblastic anemia and high levels of orotic acid in the blood can be treated by administering:
a. Cytosine
b. Folic acid
c. Allopurinol
d. Uridine

Answer is d

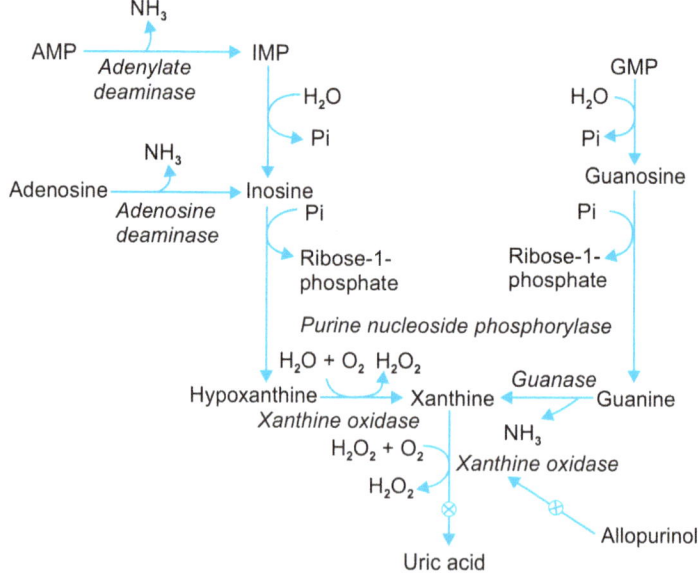

Fig. 19.3: Catabolism of purine nucleotides.
(GMP: guanosine monophosphate; IMP: inosine 5′-monophosphate; AMP: adenosine monophosphate)

Inhibitors of Purine Nucleotide Synthesis

- Azaserine and diazo-norleucine are the synthetic analogs of glutamine. They inhibit the steps of purine synthesis where glutamine reacts.
- Aminopterin and amethopterin resemble folic acid, and they inhibit the reactions of purine synthesis where THF (coenzyme of folic acid) is required.
- Sulfonamides have the similar structure like *para*-aminobenzoic acid, portion of folic acid. So, they inhibit the purine synthesis in bacteria where PABA is required.
- 6-mercaptopurine is similar to adenine and it inhibits the synthesis of AMP and GMP from IMP at steps where the conversion of adenylosuccinate to AMP and IMP to xanthine monophosphate takes place.

Causes and Symptoms of Gout, Lesch–Nyhan Syndrome, and Severe Combined Immunodeficiency Disease

Clinical Significance of Purine Synthesis

- The abnormal catabolism of purines leads to some clinical problems in humans. The clinical consequences of abnormal purine metabolism ranges from mild to severe and even fatal disorders.
- Clinical manifestations of abnormal purine catabolism arise from the insolubility of the catabolic intermediate and uric acid.

Gout

Excess accumulation of uric acid leads to **hyperuricemia** and this condition is commonly called as **gout.**

This results from the precipitation of sodium urate crystals in the synovial fluid of the joints, leading to severe inflammation and arthritis.

Gout may arise as result of excess purine or of a partial deficiency in the salvage enzyme and HGPRT.

Gout can be treated by administering the antimetabolite, **allopurinol**. Allopurinol is a structural analog of hypoxanthine that inhibits xanthine oxidase.

Lesch–Nyhan syndrome

- *Cause:* Loss of a functional *HGPRT* gene.
- The disorder is inherited as a sex-linked trait.
- Patients with this defect exhibit not only severe symptoms of gout but also a severe malfunction of the nervous system.

In the most serious cases, patients resort to self-mutilation. Death usually occurs within the age of 20 years.

Severe combined immunodeficiency disease

- *Cause:* Deficiency of enzyme adenosine deaminase (ADA), which converts adenosine to inosine in the catabolism of the purines.
- This deficiency selectively leads to a destruction of B and T lymphocytes, the cells that mount immune responses.
- In the absence of ADA, deoxyadenosine is phosphorylated to yield levels of dATP that are 50-fold higher than normal. The levels are especially high in lymphocytes, which have abundant amounts of the salvage enzymes, including nucleoside kinases. High concentrations of dATP inhibit ribonucleotide reductase thereby preventing other dNTPs from being produced. The net effect is to inhibit DNA synthesis. Since, lymphocytes must be able to proliferate dramatically in response to antigenic challenge, the inability to synthesize DNA seriously impairs the immune responses and the disease is usually fatal in infancy unless special protective measures are taken.
- A less severe immunodeficiency results, when there is a lack of purine nucleoside phosphorylase and another purine-degradative enzyme.

Von Gierke disease

A glycogen storage disease also leads to excessive uric acid production.

- *Cause:* Deficiency in glucose-6-phosphatase activity. The increased availability of glucose-6-phosphate increases the rate of entry through the pentose phosphate pathway, generating elevated level of ribose-5-phosphate and consequently PRPP. The increases in PRPP then result in excess purine biosynthesis.

Clinical Significance of Adenosine Deaminase

The ADA test is not a diagnostic test, but it may be used along with other tests such as pleural fluid analysis, acid-fast bacillus smear and culture, and tuberculosis (TB) molecular testing to help determine whether a person has a *Mycobacterium tuberculosis* infection (TB). Some studies also showed the elevation of serum ADA levels in TB patients.

PYRIMIDINE METABOLISM

Biosynthesis of Pyrimidine Nucleotides

The biosynthesis of pyrimidine nucleotides is as follows:
- Uracil, cytosine and thymine are the pyrimidine bases.
- Uridine monophosphate (UMP), cytidine monophosphate (CMP), and thymidine monophosphate (TMP) are the nucleotide forms.
- UMP is the first synthesized nucleotide **(Fig. 19.4)**. The first completed base is derived from 1 mole of glutamine, 1 mole of ATP and 1 mole of CO_2, and 1 mole of aspartate. An additional mole of glutamine and ATP are required in the conversion of UTP to CTP.
4. From UMP, CMP, and TMP are synthesized **(Fig. 19.5)**.

Regulation of Pyrimidine Nucleotide Biosynthesis

The regulation of pyrimidine nucleotide biosynthesis is as follows:
- The regulation of pyrimidine synthesis occurs mainly at the step which is catalyzed by **carbamoylphosphate synthetase II**.
- The **carbamoylphosphate synthetase** activity is termed **carbamoyl phosphate synthetase II** (CPS-II) as opposed to CPS-I, which is involved in the urea cycle.
- Aspartate transcarbamoylase and CPS-II, is localized to the cytoplasm and prefers glutamine as a substrate.
- CPS-I of the urea cycle is localized in the mitochondria and utilizes ammonia
- The CPS-II domain is activated by ATP and PRPP. Inhibited by uridine diphosphate (UDP), UTP, and CTP.

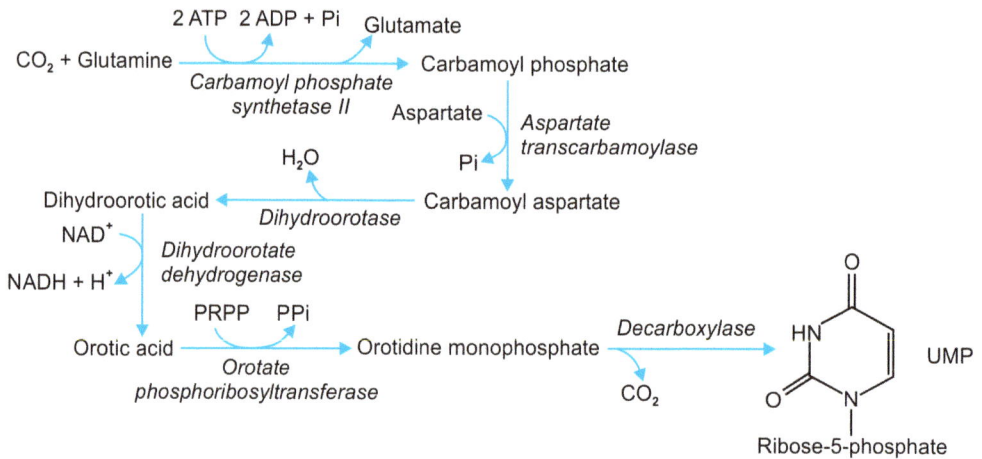

Fig. 19.4: Synthesis of UMP.
(UMP: uridine monophosphate; ATP: adenosine triphosphate; ADP: adenosine diphosphate; UMP: uridine monophosphate; NAD: nicotinamide adenine dinucleotide; PRPP: phosphoribosyl pyrophosphate)

Nucleic Acid Metabolism

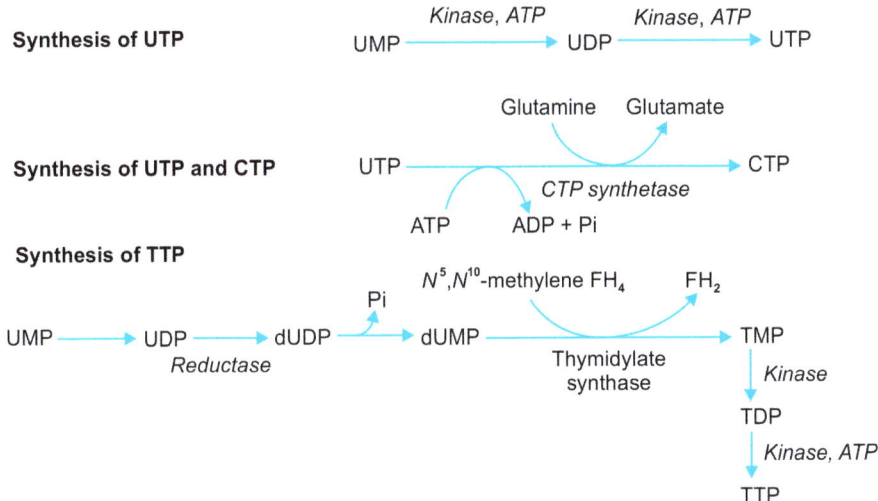

Fig. 19.5: Synthesis of pyrimidine nucleotides.
(UMP: uridine monophosphate; ATP: adenosine triphosphate; ADP: adenosine diphosphate; CTP: cytosine triphosphate; UDP: uridine diphosphate; UTP: Uridine triphosphate; TDP: thymidine triphsphate; TTP: thymidine triphosphate)

Catabolism of Pyrimidines

Pyrimidines undergo ring cleavage and the usual end products of catabolism are β-amino acids plus ammonia, and carbon dioxide. Pyrimidines from nucleic acids or the energy pool are acted upon by nucleotidases and pyrimidine nucleoside phosphorylase to yield the free bases. The four amino groups of both cytosine and 5-methylcytosine are released as ammonia **(Fig. 19.6)**.

They must first be reduced by nicotinamide adenine dinucleotide phosphate (NADPH) for the cleavage of rings. Atoms 2 and 3 of both rings are released as ammonia and carbon dioxide. The rest of the ring is left as a β-amino acid. β-Aminoisobutyrate from thymine or 5-methylcytosine is largely excreted. β-Alanine from cytosine or uracil may either be excreted or incorporated into the brain and muscle dipeptides, carnosine (β-Ala-His) or anserine (β-Ala-methyl-His).

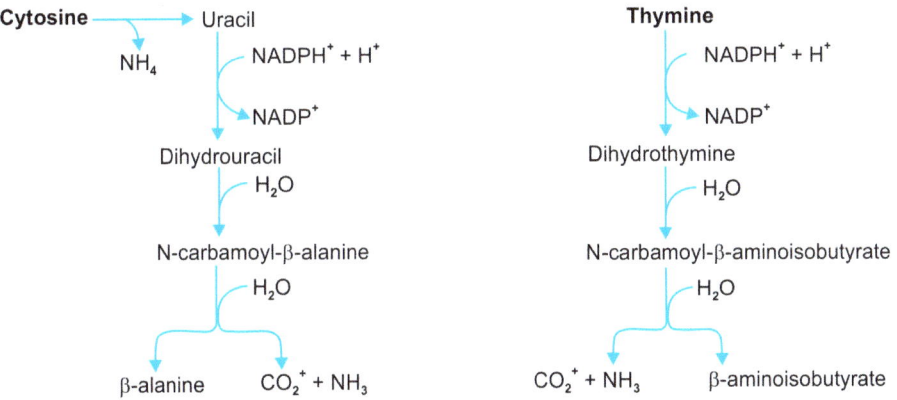

Fig. 19.6: Catabolism of pyrimidine.
(NADPH: nicotinamide adenine dinucleotide phosphate)

Clinical Significance of Pyrimidine Metabolism

As the products of pyrimidine catabolism are soluble, few disorders result from excess levels of their synthesis or catabolism. Two inherited disorders affecting pyrimidine biosynthesis are the result of deficiencies in the bifunctional enzyme catalyzing the last two steps of UMP synthesis, orotate phosphoribosyltransferase (OPRT) and orotidine monophosphate (OMP) decarboxylase. These deficiencies result in orotic aciduria that causes retarded growth and severe anemia caused by hypochromic erythrocytes, and megaloblastic bone marrow. Leukopenia is also common in orotic acidurias. The disorders can be treated with uridine and/or cytidine, which lead to increased UMP production via the action of nucleoside kinases. The UMP then inhibits CPS-II, thus attenuating orotic acid production.

Orotic Aciduria Type I

Defective enzyme: OPRT and OMP decarboxylase.

Symptoms: Retarded growth, severe anemia and leukopenia.

Orotic Aciduria Type II

Defective enzyme: OMP decarboxylase.

Symptoms: Retarded growth, severe anemia and leukopenia.

Orotic Aciduria with no Hematologic Features

Defective enzyme: Urea cycle enzyme and ornithine transcarbamylase.

Symptoms: Increased mitochondrial component exits and augments pyrimidine biosynthesis; hepatic encephalopathy.

Drug-induced Orotic Aciduria

Defective enzyme: OMP decarboxylase.

Cause: Allopurinol and 6-azauridine treatments cause orotic acidurias without a hematologic component; their catabolic by-products inhibit OMP decarboxylase.

β-Aminoisobutyric Aciduria

Defective enzyme: Transaminase, which affects the functions of urea cycle during deamination of α-amino acids to α-keto acids.

Symptoms: Benign.

SUMMARY

This chapter mainly explains the synthesis of purine nucleotides such as IMP, AMP, and GMP. The first reaction in the synthesis of IMP synthesis starts with ribose 5-phosphate and the enzyme is PRPP synthetase. Later AMP and GMP are formed from IMP. The free purine bases adenine, guanine, and hypoxanthine can be reconverted to their corresponding nucleotides by phosphoribosylation and this process is called purine salvage pathway. The catabolism of purine nucleotides results in uric acid. Disturbance in the purine nucleotide metabolism results in Lesch–Nyhan syndrome and the main cause for this is loss of a functional *HGPRT* gene. The UMP, CMP, and TMP are the pyrimidine nucleotides.

SELF-ASSESSMENT QUESTIONS

1. Briefly describe the synthesis of AMP and GMP.
2. Explain the purine salvage pathway.
3. List and state the action of inhibitors of purine nucleotide synthesis.
4. State the causes and symptoms for the following disorders:
    a. Gout
    b. Lesch–Nyhan syndrome
    c. Severe combined immunodeficiency disease
    d. Orotic aciduria type I.

5. Briefly explain the formation of UTP and TPP.
6. Describe the regulation of purine and pyrimidine nucleotide biosynthesis.

MULTIPLE-CHOICE QUESTIONS

1. **Precursors for de novo purine synthesis include all of the following:**
   a. Ribose 5-phosphate, CO_2, and NH_3
   b. Ribose 5-phosphate, ADP, and NH_3
   c. Ribulose 5-phosphate, CO_2, and ADP
   d. Ribulose 5-phosphate, CO_2, and NH_3

2. **Orotic acidurias can develop when the drug allopurinol is administered because:**
   a. It causes an overproduction of carbamoyl phosphate
   b. Products of its breakdown inhibit OMP decarboxylase
   c. It allosterically inhibits orotate phosphoribosyltransferase
   d. Products of its breakdown inhibit PRPP synthase

3. **One of the end products of pyrimidine degradation is:**
   a. β-Valine
   b. α-Alanine
   c. γ-Aminobutyrate
   d. Carbon dioxide

4. **Defects in one of the following enzymes can result in Lesch–Nyhan syndrome:**
   a. Hypoxanthine-guanine phosphoribosyltransferase
   b. Adenosine deaminase
   c. Adenine phosphoribosyltransferase
   d. Xanthine oxidase

5. **The major determinant of the overall rate of de novo synthesis of purines is the concentration of:**
   a. 5-Phosphoribosyl-1-pyrophosphate
   b. Glycinamide ribosyl-5-phosphate
   c. 5-Phospho-β-D-ribosylamine
   d. Formylglycinamide ribosyl 5-phosphate

6. **Orotic aciduria type I reflects a deficiency of the enzyme:**
   a. Dihydroorotate dehydrogenase
   b. Dihydroorotase
   c. Orotate phosphoribosyltransferase and orotidylate decarboxylase
   d. Carbamoyl phosphate synthetase

7. **All of the following enzymes are unique to purine nucleotide synthesis, *except*:**
   a. PRPP synthetase
   b. PRPP glutamyl amidotransferase
   c. Adenylosuccinate synthetase
   d. IMP dehydrogenase

8. **The two nitrogen atoms of pyrimidine nucleotides are contributed by:**
   a. Glutamine and carbamoyl phosphate
   b. Aspartate and carbamoyl phosphate
   c. Glutamate and NH_3
   d. Glutamine and NH_3

9. **Phosphoribosyl pyrophosphate (PRPP) glutamyl amidotransferase, the first enzyme uniquely committed to purine synthesis, is inhibited by:**
   a. AMP
   b. IMP
   c. XMP
   d. CMP

10. **In man, a major catabolic product of pyrimidine is:**
    a. Urea
    b. Uric acid
    c. Guanine
    d. β-Alanine

11. **Orotic aciduria type II reflects a deficiency of the enzyme:**
    a. Orotate phosphoribosyltransferase
    b. Orotidylate decarboxylase
    c. Dihydroorotase
    d. Dihydroorotate dehydrogenase

12. **In the synthesis of purine nucleotides, the N atom at position 7 and the carbon atoms at positions 4 and 5 are contributed by:**
    a. Glutamine
    b. Alanine
    c. Glycine
    d. Aspartate

13. **Some anticancer drugs act by blocking the action of the following enzyme:**
    a. Orotidylate decarboxylase
    b. Dihydroorotate dehydrogenase
    c. Dihydrofolate reductase
    d. Xanthine oxidase

14. **In de novo pyrimidine synthesis, UMP is formed by the catalytic action of:**
    a. Orotidylate decarboxylase
    b. Orotate phosphoribosyltransferase
    c. Aspartate transcarbamoylase
    d. Dihydroorotate dehydrogenase

15. **Precursors of pyrimidine de novo synthesis include:**
    a. Aspartame, glutamate, and carbonate
    b. Aspartate, glutamine, and carbonate

c. Aspartame, histamine, and carbamoylate
d. Aspartate, histamine, and carbamoylate

16. **Gout can be treated by the actions of allopurinol on:**
    a. Hypoxanthine-guanine phosphoribosyl-transferase
    b. Dihydroorotase
    c. PRPP synthase
    d. Xanthine oxidase

17. **Orotic acidurias can develop when the drug allopurinol is administered because:**
    a. It allosterically inhibits orotate phosphoribosyltransferase
    b. It causes an overproduction of carbamoyl phosphate
    c. Products of its breakdown inhibit OMP decarboxylase
    d. Products of its breakdown inhibit PRPP synthase

18. **The enzyme glutamine PRPP amidotransferase is allosterically inhibited by:**
    a. AMP, GMP, and UMP
    b. AMP, GMP, and IMP
    c. IMP and UMP only
    d. AMP and GMP only

19. **Lesch–Nyhan syndrome can result from a deficiency in hypoxanthine-guanine phosphoribosyl transferase (HG-PRTase) and a resultant builds up in:**
    a. Urea   b. Adenosine
    c. Guanosine   d. Uric acid

20. **Which of the following compounds is a general inhibitor of deoxyribonucleotide biosynthesis?**
    a. dATP   b. ATP
    c. dTTP   d. UDP

Answers

1. a	2. b	3. d	4. a	5. a
6. c	7. a	8. b	9. a	10. d
11. b	12. c	13. c	14. a	15. b
16. d	17. c	18. b	19. d	20. a

CHAPTER 20

Molecular Biology

OBJECTIVES

At the end of this chapter, the students should be able to:
- Describe the structure of deoxyribonucleic acid (DNA) and different types of ribonucleic acid (RNA), including their important functions
- Explain the process of replication, transcription, and translation and their inhibitors
- Discuss the different types of mutation
- Explain the polymerase chain reaction (PCR) and recombinant DNA (rDNA) technology, including their importance.

INTRODUCTION

Molecular biology is a topic in which we discuss about the structure of DNA and RNA along with their important functions. DNA has a structure of right-handed double helix made up of adenine, guanine, cytosine, and thymine. DNA transfers the information from parents to offspring. Messenger RNA (mRNA) carries the message and transfer RNA (tRNA) transfers the message to protein-synthesizing machinery. Ribosomal RNA (rRNA) serves as machinery for the protein synthesis.

Deoxyribonucleic acid serves as the master copy for most information in the cell. RNA is of different types, which act to transform information from DNA to the rest of the cell.

DEOXYRIBONUCLEIC ACID

Structure and Function

The structure and function of DNA are as follows:

- The DNA has a right-handed double-helix structure **(Fig. 20.1)**.
- It contains 10 nucleotide pairs per helical turn.
- Each spiral strand composed of a sugar-phosphate backbone and attached bases and is connected to a complementary strand by hydrogen bonding (noncovalent) between paired bases, adenine (A) with thymine (T) and guanine (G) with cytosine (C).
- There are four different bases in a DNA molecule:
  1. Adenine (purine)
  2. Cytosine (pyrimidine)

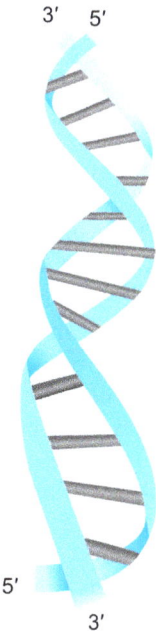

Fig. 20.1: Structure of deoxyribonucleic acid.

3. Guanine (purine)
4. Thymine (pyrimidine).
- The number of purine bases equals the number of pyrimidine bases.
- The number of adenine bases equals the number of thymine bases.
- The number of guanine bases equals the number of cytosine bases.
- Two DNA strands form a helical spiral, winding around a helix axis in a right-handed spiral.
- The two polynucleotide chains run in opposite directions.

Within the double helix, adenine and thymine are connected by two hydrogen bonds (noncovalent) on the opposite strand, while guanine and cytosine are connected by three hydrogen bonds on the opposite strand (refer to Chapter 18 for detailed information about structure of DNA).

Reasons of base pairing
- Replication of DNA requires noncovalent strand separation.
- Stability of DNA is delicate because of phosphates on outside, which are very acidic, and repulsion between phosphates tends to destabilize DNA.
- Uniform structure, identical shape, and size of base pairs are formed.

Three processes of transferring genetic information
1. *Replication:* This is the process by which an identical copy of DNA is made. Replication occurs every time a cell divides, so that information can be preserved and transferred to offspring.
2. *Transcription:* This is the process by which the genetic messages contained in DNA are "read" or transcribed. The product of transcription known as the mRNA leaves the cell nucleus and carries the message to the sites of protein synthesis.
3. *Translation:* This is the process by which the genetic messages carried by mRNA are decoded and used to build proteins.

GENOMICS

Genomics is the study of whole genomes, including the complete set of genes, their nucleotide sequence and organization, and their interactions within a species and with other species.

The DNA sequencing technology results in advances in genomics. Information technology has led to Google Maps that enable us to get detailed information about locations around the globe, genomic information is used to create similar maps of the DNA of different organisms.

Genome mapping is the process of finding the location of genes on each chromosome. The maps that are created are comparable to the maps that we use to navigate streets. A genetic map is an illustration that lists genes and their location on a chromosome. Genetic maps provide the big picture and use genetic markers.

PROTEOMICS AND ITS APPLICATIONS

Proteomics

It is the large-scale study of proteins. Proteins are vital parts of living organisms, with many functions. The **proteome** is the entire set of proteins that is produced or modified by an organism or system.

After genomics and transcriptomics, proteomics is the next step in the study of biological systems. It is more complicated than genomics because an organism's genome is more or less constant, whereas proteomes differ from cell to cell and from time to time.

Practical Applications of Proteomics

The major development to come from the study of human genes and proteins has been the identification of potential new drugs for the treatment of disease. This relies on genome and proteome information to identify proteins associated with a disease, which computer software can then use as targets for new drugs. For example, if a certain protein is implicated in a disease, its 3D structure provides the information to design drugs to interfere with the action of the protein. A molecule that fits the active site of an enzyme, but cannot be released by the enzyme, inactivates the enzyme. This is the basis of new drug-discovery tools, which aim to find new drugs to inactivate proteins involved in disease. As genetic differences among individuals are found, researchers expect to use these techniques to develop personalized drugs that are more effective for the individual.

DIFFERENCE BETWEEN GENOMICS AND PROTEOMICS

Genomics is the study of the genes in an organism and proteomics is the study of the all the proteins in a cell. Proteomics studies are more beneficial because proteins are the functional molecules in cells and represent actual conditions.

METABOLOMICS

Metabolomics is the systematic study of the small molecular metabolites in a cell, tissue, biofluid, or cell culture media that are the tangible result of cellular processes or responses to an environmental stress.

The metabolome represents the complete set of metabolites in a biological cell, tissue, organ, or organism, which are the end products of cellular processes.

The most common techniques used in metabolomics for data acquisition are nuclear magnetic resonance spectroscopy and mass spectrometry, applied in combination to extract from samples as much information as possible.

REPLICATION

The following list shows the process of replication including the functions of each enzyme:
- Replication is a process of duplication of DNA molecules **(Table 20.1)**.
- *Purpose:* DNA makes up the chromosomes. Before a cell divides, it needs to double the number of chromosomes, i.e. the DNA is duplicated. It occurs during the S (synthesis) phase of the cell cycle.
- Replication begins with a partial unwinding of the double-helix DNA at an area known as the replication fork **(Fig. 20.2)**:

Replication

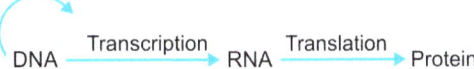

- This unwinding is accomplished by an enzyme known as DNA helicase. This unwound section seen as a "bubble" and is, thus, known as a replication bubble.
- As the two DNA strands separate and the bases are exposed, the enzyme DNA polymerase moves into position at the point where synthesis will begin.

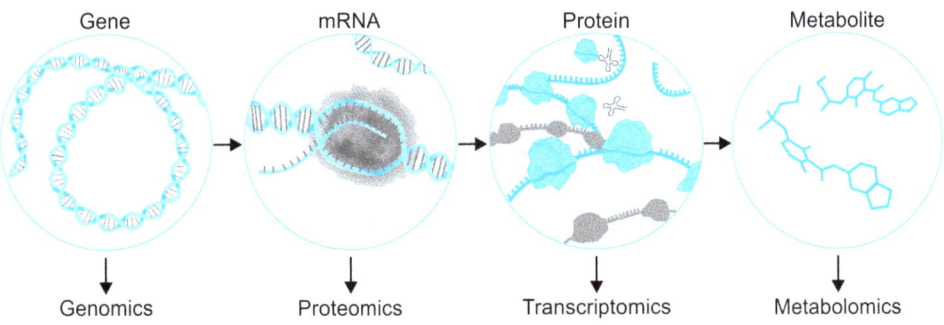

Molecular Biology

Table 20.1: Summary of enzymes and terms involved in replication.

Components of replications	Functions
Helicase	Unwinds or unzips DNA helix
RNA primase	Adds a short RNA primer to start replication
DNA polymerase III	Binds to RNA primer and adds new DNA nucleotides to new strand in 5'–3' direction
DNA ligase	Bonds Okazaki fragments to the lagging strand
DNA polymerase I	Removes RNA primer and replaces it with DNA nucleotides
Replication fork	Section of DNA double-strand opened immediately behind the helicase
Leading strand	Section of DNA that is being synthesized continuously toward the replication fork
Lagging strand	Section of DNA being synthesized away from the replication fork and synthesized as Okazaki fragments
Okazaki fragments	Small sections of new DNA on lagging strand
Mutation	Mistakes in genetic code, but small mutations are naturally removed by enzymes as replication progresses
rRNA primer	Sequence of about 10 RNA nucleotides placed at the 5' end of the new DNA strand

(DNA: deoxyribonucleic acid; RNA: ribonucleic acid; rRNA: ribosomal RNA)

- The start point for DNA polymerase is a short segment of RNA known as RNA primer. The very term "primer" is indicative of its role, which is to "prime" or start DNA synthesis at certain points. The primer is "laid down" complementary to the DNA template by an enzyme known as RNA polymerase or primase.
- The DNA polymerase adds nucleotides one by one in an exactly complementary manner, A to T and G to C.
- DNA polymerase is described as being "template dependent," in which it will read the sequence of bases on the template strand and then synthesize the complementary strand.
- The template strand is read in the 3'–5' direction. The new DNA strand (complementary) synthesized in the 5'–3' direction.
- Both strands of a DNA molecule are antiparallel in direction.
- DNA polymerase catalyzes the formation of the hydrogen bonds between each arriving nucleotide and the nucleotides on the template strand.
- DNA polymerase also catalyzes the reaction between the 5' phosphate on an incoming nucleotide and the free 3' OH on the growing polynucleotide (phosphodiester bond). As a result, the new DNA strands

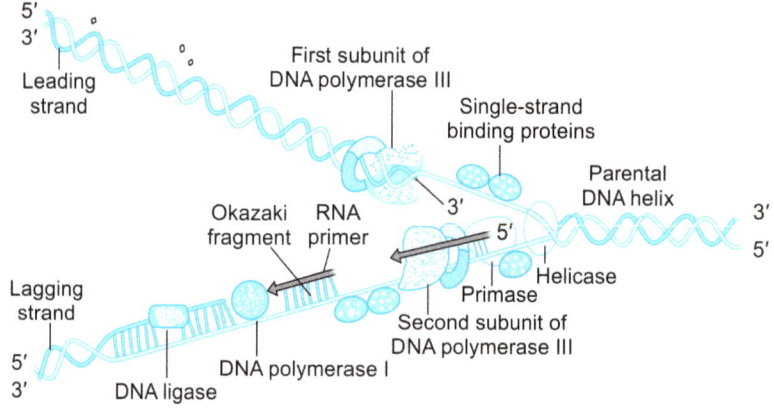

Fig. 20.2: Replication process in eukaryotes.

can grow only in the 5′–3′ direction and strand growth must begin at the 3′ end of the template.
- The original DNA strands are complementary and run antiparallel; only one new strand can begin at the 3′ end of the template DNA and grow continuously as the point of replication (the replication fork) moves along the template DNA. The other strand must grow in the opposite direction because it is complementary, not identical to the template strand. The result of this side discontinuous replication is the production of a series of short sections of new DNA called *Okazaki* fragments.
- New strand of short segments is made into a continuous strand; the sections are joined by the action of an enzyme called DNA ligase, which ligates the pieces together by forming the missing phosphodiester bonds.
- The last step is for an enzyme to come along and remove the existing RNA primers and then fill in the gaps with DNA. This is the job of yet another type of DNA polymerase, which has the ability to chew up the primers and replace them with the deoxynucleotides that make up DNA:

- Since each new strand is complementary to its old template strand, two identical new copies of the DNA double helix are produced during replication.
- In each new helix, one strand is the old template and the other is newly synthesized, a result described by saying that the replication is semiconservative (**Fig. 20.3**).
- Conservative replication leaves original DNA molecule and generate a completely new molecule.
- Dispersive replication would produce two DNA molecules with sections of both old and new DNA interspersed along each strand.
- Semiconservative replication would produce molecules with both old and new DNA, but each molecule would be composed of one old strand and one new one.

TELOMERE AND TELOMERASE

Telomere and its Importance

A telomere is a region of repetitive nucleotide sequences at each end of a chromosome, which protects the end of the chromosome from deterioration or from fusion with neighboring chromosomes (**Fig. 20.4**). Telomeres also play an important role in making sure that our DNA gets copied properly when cells divide.

During chromosome replication, the enzymes that duplicate DNA cannot continue their duplication all the way to the end of a chromosome, so in each duplication the end of the chromosome is shortened (this is because the synthesis of Okazaki fragments requires RNA primers attaching ahead on the lagging strand).

The shortening of telomeres is directly linked to the aging of living organisms. Telomere shortening can also cause other health complications, including cardiovascular and neurological conditions.

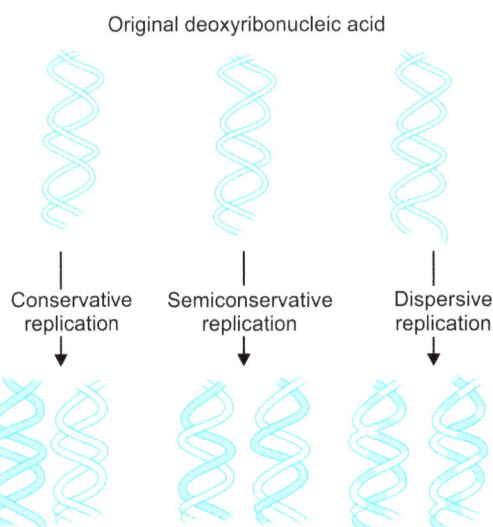

Fig. 20.3: Types of replication.

Telomerase and its Importance

Telomerase is the enzyme responsible for lengthening telomeres by addition of guanine-rich repetitive sequences. The activity of **telomerase** is exhibited in gametes and stem and tumor cells. A study on mice suggested that premature ageing can be reversed by reactivating an enzyme that protects the tips of chromosomes.

When cell begins to become cancerous, it divides more often, and its telomeres become very short. The cell may die if its telomeres get too short. Often times, these cells escape death by making more telomerase enzyme, which prevents the telomeres from getting even shorter.

The regulation of telomerase activity in human cells plays a significant role in the development of cancer. Telomerase is tightly repressed in the vast majority of normal human somatic cells but becomes activated during cellular immortalization and in cancers **(Fig. 20.4)**.

DEOXYRIBONUCLEIC ACID REPAIR

Process of DNA Repair

Deoxyribonucleic acid repair is a collection of processes by which a cell identifies and corrects damage to the DNA molecules that encode its genome.

In human cells, both normal metabolic activities and environmental factors (radiation) can cause DNA damage, resulting in millions of individual molecular lesions per cell per day.

Many of these lesions cause structural damage to the DNA molecule and can alter or eliminate the ability of the cell to transcribe the gene that the affected DNA encodes.

Other lesions induce harmful mutations in the cell's genome, which affect the survival of its daughter cells after it undergoes mitosis. As a result, the DNA repair process is constantly active as it responds to damage in the DNA structure. When normal DNA repair processes stops functioning and cellular apoptosis does not occur, irreparable DNA damage may occur, including double-strand breaks and DNA cross-linkages. This can eventually lead to malignant tumors, or cancer.

The rate of DNA repair is dependent on many factors, including the cell type, the age of the cell, and the extracellular environment. A cell that has accumulated a large amount of DNA damage, or one that no longer effectively repairs damage happened to its DNA, can enter one of three possible states:

1. An irreversible state of dormancy (senescence)
2. Apoptosis or programmed cell death (cell suicide)
3. Unregulated cell division, which can lead to the formation of a tumor that is cancerous.

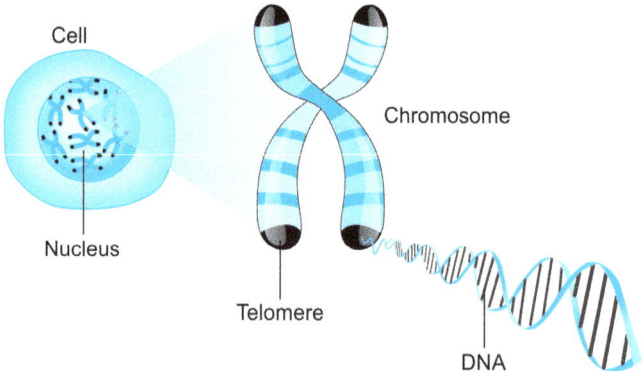

Fig. 20.4: Telomere.

There are three major DNA repairing mechanisms:
1. **Base excision**
2. **Nucleotide excision**
3. **Mismatch repair**.

The DNA repair enzymes recognize and correct physical damage in DNA, caused by exposure to radiation, ultraviolet (UV) light or reactive oxygen species produced from normal metabolic byproducts.

The correction of these DNA damages increases loss of genetic information, generation of double-strand breaks, and DNA cross-linkages.

Deoxyribonucleic acid damaging agents are widely used in oncology to treat both hematological and solid cancers. Some most common used modalities include ionizing radiation, platinum drugs (cisplatin, oxaliplatin, and carboplatin), cyclophosphamide, chlorambucil, and temozolomide.

Deoxyribonucleic acid damage can be subdivided into two main types:
1. The replication of damaged DNA before cell division can lead to the incorporation of wrong bases opposite damaged ones. Daughter cells that inherit these wrong bases carry mutations from which the original DNA sequence is unrecoverable.
2. There are many types of damage to DNA due to endogenous cellular processes:
   - Oxidation of bases and generation of DNA strand interruptions from reactive oxygen species.
   - Alkylation of bases (usually methylation), such as formation of 7-methylguanosine, 1-methyladenine, 6-O-methylguanine.
   - Hydrolysis of bases, such as deamination, depurination, and depyrimidination.
   - Mismatch of bases, due to errors in DNA replication, in which the wrong DNA base is inserted into place in a newly forming DNA strand, or a DNA base is skipped over or mistakenly inserted.
   - Mono-adduct damage cause by change in single nitrogenous base of DNA.

Diseases Associated with DNA Repair

Deoxyribonucleic acid repair defects are seen in nearly all of the diseases described as accelerated aging disease, in which various tissues, organs, or systems of the human body age prematurely.
- Human disorders with accelerated aging
- Ataxia–telangiectasia (AT)
- Bloom syndrome
- Cockayne syndrome
- Fanconi anemia (FA)
- Progeria (Hutchinson-Gilford progeria syndrome)
- Rothmund-Thomson syndrome
- Trichothiodystrophy
- Werner syndrome (WS)
- Xeroderma pigmentosum (XP).

Ataxia–telangiectasia (AT or A-T) (or ataxia–telangiectasia syndrome or Louis-Bar syndrome): It is a rare, neurodegenerative, autosomal recessive disorder causing severe disability. Ataxia refers to poor coordination and telangiectasia to small dilated blood vessels, both of which are hallmarks of the disease.

Ataxia–telangiectasia impairs certain areas of the brain, including the cerebellum, causing difficulty with movement and coordination. It weakens the immune system, causing a predisposition to infection. It prevents repair of broken DNA, increasing the risk of cancer.

Symptoms of this AT first appear in early childhood when children begin to sit or walk.

Bloom syndrome: It is a rare autosomal recessive disorder characterized by short stature, predisposition to the development of cancer, and genomic instability. It is caused by mutations in the *BLM* gene, which is a member of the RecQ DNA helicase family.

It is a member of a class of clinical entities that are characterized by chromosomal instability, genomic instability, or both and by cancer predisposition.

Fanconi anemia: It is a rare genetic disease resulting in impaired response to DNA damage. Majority of the affected people develop cancer, most often acute myelogenous leukemia, and 90% develop bone marrow failure (the inability to produce blood cells) by age 40. About 60-75% of people have congenital defects, commonly short stature, abnormalities of the skin, arms, head, eyes, kidneys, and ears, and developmental disabilities. Around 75% of people have some form of endocrine problems, with varying degrees of severity.

Fanconi anemia is the result of a genetic defect in a cluster of proteins responsible for DNA repair via homologous recombination.

Werner syndrome (or adult progeria): It is a rare, autosomal recessive disorder, which is characterized by the appearance of premature aging.

Xeroderma pigmentosum: It is a genetic disorder in which there is a decreased ability to repair DNA damage, which is caused by UV light.

Symptoms may include a severe sunburn after only a few minutes in the sun, freckling in sun exposed areas, dry skin, and changes in skin pigmentation. Nervous system problems, such as hearing loss, poor coordination, loss of intellectual function, and seizures, may also occur. Complications include a high risk of skin cancer, with about half having skin cancer by age 10 without preventive efforts, and cataracts. There may be high chances of developing brain cancers.

It is an autosomal recessive disorder, with at least nine specific mutations able to result in the condition. Normally, the damage to DNA which occurs in skin cells from exposure to UV light is repaired by nucleotide excision repair. In people with XP, this damage is not repaired. As more abnormalities form in DNA, cells malfunction and eventually become cancerous or die. Diagnosis is suspected based on symptoms and confirmed by genetic testing.

MUTATION

Mutation and its Different Types

- A mutation is a permanent change in the DNA sequence of a gene. Mutations in a gene's DNA sequence can alter the amino acid sequence of the protein encoded by the gene.
- Humans acquire some changes to their DNA during the course of their lives. These changes occur in a number of ways. Sometimes there are simple copying errors that are introduced when DNA replicates itself. Other changes are introduced as a result of DNA damage through environmental agents such as sunlight and radiation. Human body cells have built in mechanisms that can identify and repair most of the changes that occur during DNA replication or from environmental damage. Some of these changes occur in cells of the body, such as in skin cells as a result of sun exposure, but they are not transferred to children. But other errors can occur in the DNA of cells that produce the eggs and sperm. These are called germline mutations and can be passed from parent to child. If a child inherits a germline mutation from their parents, all cell in their body will have this error in their DNA.

Frameshift Mutation

Frameshift type of mutation occurs when the addition or loss of DNA bases changes a gene's reading frame. A reading frame consists of groups of three bases that each code for one amino acid. A frameshift mutation shifts the grouping of these bases and changes the code for amino acids. The resulting protein is usually nonfunctional. Insertions, deletions, and duplications can all be frameshift mutations. The earlier in the sequence, the deletion or insertion occurs, the more altered the protein produced is insertion or deletions involving one or two base pairs can have devastating consequences to the gene because translation of the gene is "frameshifted." The mRNA is translated in new groups of three nucleotides and the protein specified by these new codons will be of no use.

Frameshifts often create new termination codons and thus generate nonsense mutations. Perhaps that is just as well as the protein would probably be too garbled anyway to be useful to the cell. Insertion or deletions of three nucleotides or multiples of three may be less serious because they preserve the reading frame. However, a number of inherited human disorders are caused by the insertion of many copies of the same triplet of nucleotides. Huntington's disease and the Fragile X syndrome are examples of such trinucleotide repeat diseases.

There are several types of gene mutations. These include:
- Translocation
- Duplication
- Deletion
- Insertion
- Inversion
- Substitution.

Translocation

- Translocations are the transfer of a piece of one chromosome to a nonhomologous chromosome. Translocations are often reciprocal, i.e. the two nonhomologous swap segments **(Fig. 20.5)**.

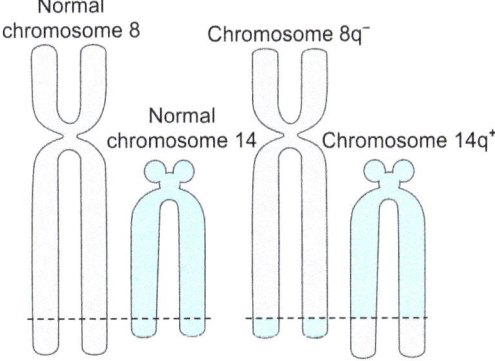

Fig. 20.5: Translocation at the chromosomal level.

- Translocations can alter the phenotype in several ways:
  - The break may occur within a gene destroying its function.
  - Translocated genes may come under the influence of different promoters and enhancers so that their expression is altered. The translocations in Burkitt's lymphoma are an example.
  - The breakpoint may occur within a gene creating a hybrid gene. This may be transcribed and translated into a protein with an N-terminal of one normal cell protein coupled to the C-terminal of another. The Philadelphia chromosome found so often in the leukemic cells of patients with chronic myelogenous leukemia (CML) is the result of a translocation, which produces a compound gene (Bcr-Abl).

Duplication

- Duplication is the repetitive occurrence of a base nucleotide or nucleotides due to a gene mutation as shown:

IAIBICIDIEIFIGI   IAIBICIDICIDIEIFIGI
(DNA molecule)   →   (duplication has occurred)

- Duplications are a doubling of a section of the genome. During meiosis, crossing over between sister's chromatids that are out of alignment can produce one chromatid with a duplicated gene and the other having two genes with deletions. **Figure 20.6** shows unequal crossing over created a second copy of a gene needed for the synthesis of the steroid hormone aldosterone.
- However, this new gene carries inappropriate promoters at its 5′ end (acquired from the 11-β-hydroxylase gene) that cause it to be expressed more strongly than the normal gene. The mutant gene is dominant, i.e. all members of one family who inherited at least one chromosome carrying this duplication suffered from

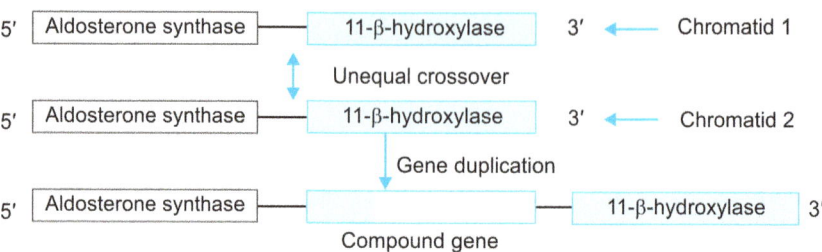

Fig. 20.6: Duplication of enzyme.

high blood pressure and were prone to early death from stroke.
- Gene duplication has also been implicated in many neurological disorders.
- Gene duplication has occurred repeatedly during the evolution of eukaryotes, which can be beneficial.
- Overtime, the duplicates can acquire different functions:
  - The proteins they encode can take on different functions.
  - Changes in the regulatory sequences of the genes (promoters and enhancers) may cause the same protein to be expressed at different times and/or in different tissues.

Deletion

Deletion is the removal of a base nucleotide or several nucleotides as shown:

IAIBICIDIEIFIGI   IAIBIEIFIGI
(DNA ⟶ (deletion
molecule)   has occurred)

Insertion is the addition of a base nucleotide into a sequence of nucleotides known as a polynucleotide chain:

UACUAUGCU   UACUAGUGCU
(DNA ⟶ (insertion
molecule)   has occurred)

Collectively, insertions and deletions are known as indels. These indels cause frameshift mutation. Frameshift mutation result in the formation of abnormally long or abnormally short polynucleotides. This can therefore alter the shape and function of the protein, rendering it useless.

Inversion

Inversion is also a gene mutation that causes a section of nucleotides to be arranged in reverse. For example:

IAIBICIDIEIFIGI ⟶ IAIBIEIDICIFIGI

Substitution

Substitution is the replacement of a base nucleotide by another base nucleotide. There are three types of substitution:
- *Silent mutation:* These cause no change to protein structure or function. For example:

  UAU ⟶ UAC
  Tyrosine (Tyr)   Try

  They may occur in a noncoding region (outside of a gene or within an intron) or they may occur within an exon in a manner that does not alter the final amino acid sequence.
- *Missense mutation:* This type of mutation may cause structural and functional change. For example:

  UAU ⟶ UCU
  Tyr   Serine
- *Nonsense mutation:* This type of mutation results in the premature termination of polypeptide chains. For example:

  UAU ⟶ UCU
  Tyr   -Serine

*Note: Stop codons are UAA, UAG, or UGA.

Nucleotide Repeat Diseases

Fragile X Syndrome

Several disorders in humans are caused by the inheritance of genes that have undergone insertions of a string of three or four nucleotides repeated over and over. A locus on the human X chromosome contains such a stretch of nucleotides in which the triplet CGG is repeated (CGGCGGCGGCGG, etc.). The number of CGGs may be as few as 5 or as many as 50 without causing a harmful phenotype (these repeated nucleotides are in a noncoding region of the gene). Even up to 100 repeats cause no harm.

However, these longer repeats have a tendency to grow longer still from one generation to the next. This causes a constriction in the X chromosome, which makes it quite fragile. Males who inherit such a chromosome (only from their mothers) show a number of harmful phenotypic effects, including mental retardation. Females who inherit a fragile X (from their mothers) are only mildly affected.

Huntington's Disease

In **Huntington's disease,** the repeated trinucleotide is CAG, which adds a string of glutamine (Gln) to the encoded protein (called huntingtin). The abnormal protein increases the level of the p53 protein in brain cells causing their death by apoptosis.

Muscular Dystrophy

Some forms of muscular dystrophy that appear in adults are caused by tri- or tetranucleotide, e.g. (CTG)n and (CCTG)n, repeats where n may run into the thousands. The huge RNA transcripts that result interfere with the alternative splicing of other transcripts in the nucleus.

Duchenne muscular dystrophy (DMD) is a lethal, X-linked recessive disease affecting approximately 1 in 3,300 live male births. The disease becomes symptomatic in early childhood. Inability to walk occurs by the end of the first decade and death usually occurs by the second decade. Nearly all patients show the complete absence of the protein dystrophin, which is abundant in skeletal and cardiac muscle. The dystrophin gene (or *DMD* gene), located at Xp21, is approximately 2,300 kb in size, making it one of the largest known genes of any species. It contains 24 regions of 109 amino acids that are similar, but not identical repeats of each other. In women, the similarity of these sequences can lead to the misalignment of homologous material at meiotic synapsis. In association with a recombination event, this misalignment gives rise to frameshift mutations, leading to an untranslatable mRNA. This series of events occurs at an extremely high rate of about 1 in 10,000.

Effect of Mutation on Health and Development

To function correctly, each cell depends on thousands of proteins to do their jobs in the right places at the right times. Sometimes, gene mutations prevent one or more of these proteins from working properly. By changing a gene's instructions for making a protein, a mutation can cause the protein to malfunction or to be missing entirely. When a mutation alters a protein that plays a critical role in the body, it can disrupt normal development or cause a medical condition. A condition caused by mutations in one or more genes is called genetic disorder.

In some cases, gene mutations are so severe that they prevent an embryo from surviving until birth. These changes occur in genes that are essential for development and often disrupt the development of an embryo in its earliest stages. Because these mutations have very serious effects, they are incompatible with life.

RIBONUCLEIC ACID

Structure of RNA

Describe the RNA under the following headings: (1) different types and their

Molecular Biology

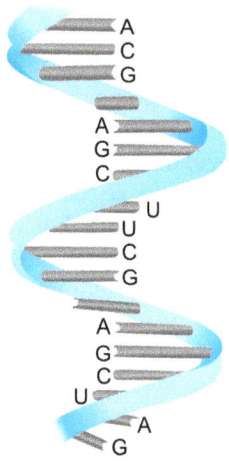

Fig. 20.7: Structure of ribonucleic acid.

individual functions and (2) structure of tRNA (Fig. 20.7).

Refer to Chapter 18, Chemistry of Nucleic Acid, for details.

Types

There are three types of RNA, each with their own function:

1. *rRNA:* Exist outside the nucleus in the cytoplasm of a cell in structures called ribosome.
2. *mRNA:* These are the nucleic acids that "record" information from DNA in the cell nucleus and carry it to the ribosomes and are known as mRNA.
3. *tRNA:* The function of tRNA is to transfer amino acids one by one to protein chains growing at ribosomes (**Fig. 20.8**).

TRANSCRIPTION

The following list shows the process of transcription through which mRNA is synthesized:

- The process of converting the information contained in a DNA segment into proteins

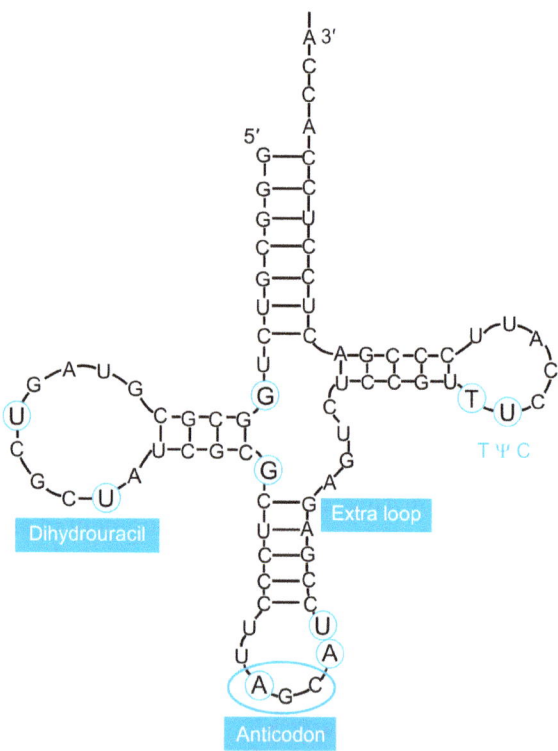

Fig. 20.8: Structure of tRNA.
(tRNA: transfer ribonucleic acid)

begins with the synthesis of mRNA molecules (**Fig. 20.9**).

- Each protein in the human body is synthesized from a different mRNA that has been transcribed from a specific gene on DNA.
- mRNA is synthesized in the cell nucleus by transcription of DNA:
  a. A small section of the DNA double helix unwinds and the bases on the two strands are exposed (refer to **Figs. 20.10 and 20.11**).
  b. RNA nucleotides line up in the proper order by hydrogen bonding to their complementary bases on DNA; the nucleotides are joined together by a DNA-dependent RNA polymerase enzyme and mRNA results.
  c. Only one of the two DNA strands is transcribed into mRNA.
  d. The DNA strand that is transcribed is called template strand (also known as the antisense strand) and its complement is called informational strand (also called coding or sense strand).
  e. The starting point of a gene is marked by a certain base sequence, which is called promoter site. These sites are recognized by a factor called sigma. The sigma factor recognizes the promoter sites and conveys the message to DNA-dependent RNA polymerase where to begin transcription.
  f. Once the RNA polymerase has been directed to the start point of the gene

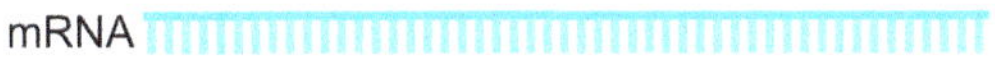

mRNA

Fig 20.9: mRNA molecule.

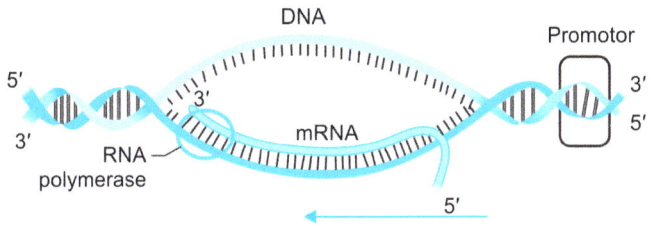

Fig. 20.10: Transcription.

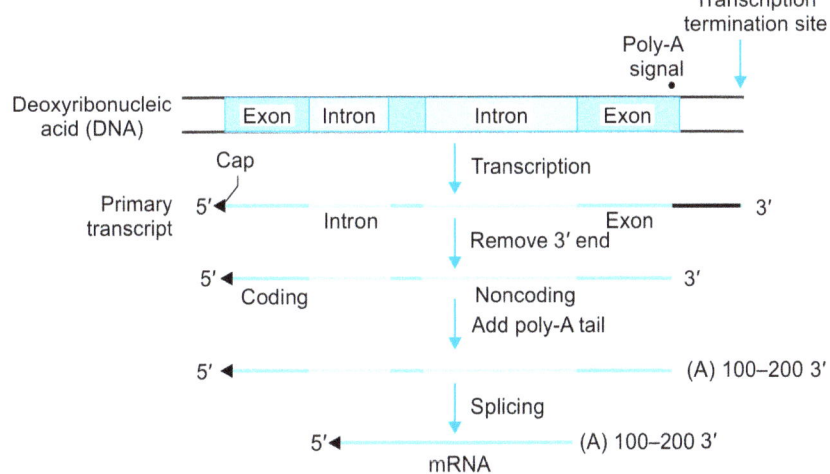

Fig. 20.11: Synthesis of mRNA.
(mRNA: messenger ribonucleic acid)

by sigma, the sigma factor is released and the RNA polymerase carries out the process of transcription.

g. Another factor called "Rho" aids in terminating the process of transcription. When the end of the gene is near, the Rho factor binds to the mRNA and interacts with the RNA polymerase. The interaction of Rho with the RNA polymerase causes the enzyme to "fall off" the DNA.

The newly synthesized mRNA travels out of the nucleus to the cytoplasm where protein synthesis (translation) takes place.

GENETIC CODE

The code consists of at least three bases, according to astronomer George Gamow. To code for the 20 essential amino acids, a genetic code must consist of at least a three base set (triplet) of the four bases. If one considers the possibilities of arranging four things three at a time (4 × 4 × 4), we get 64 possible code words, or codons (a three base sequence on the mRNA that codes for either a specific amino acid or a control word).

TRANSLATION

Process of Translation and Significance of Post-translational Modification in Synthesizing Final Product of Protein

- The translation is a process by which the genetic information transferred from DNA to mRNA in the form of bases is expressed to produce a sequence of amino acids in a protein.
- It occurs in cytoplasm. The machinery for making proteins is the ribosome.
- There are many ribosomes in the cytoplasm of a cell and all the ribosomes are made of a small, and a large subunit. These two subunits open up allowing the mRNA message to slide through. Once the mRNA message is in place and protein synthesis is ready to begin, the two subunits close again so that the mRNA is now in between the two subunits.
- The tRNA comes next, which is responsible for bringing in the proper amino acids. Now the mRNA is held within the two subunits of the ribosome and is relatively immobile. The amino acids are floating free in the cytoplasm.
- The tRNA molecule reads the code from the mRNA and brings the corresponding amino acid into place.
- Every tRNA molecule has its own set of three bases, which is called anticodon. This anti-codon is complementary to mRNA codons. The other "end" of the tRNA molecule has an "acceptor" site where the tRNA-specific amino acid will bind. Even though there are only 20 amino acids that exist, there are actually 64 possible tRNA molecules, i.e.: 4 × 4 × 4 = 64 possible combinations.
- 61 code for specific amino acids and three codes for chain termination as a result of pairing up with "stop codons," signaling the end of the mRNA message.
- UAA, UAG, and UGA are the stop codons.
- AUG is the methionine initiation codon.
- The anticodon on tRNA is complementary to the codon on mRNA. A set of three nucleotide bases on an mRNA molecule are called codon.
- Protein synthesis may be disrupted at different levels by the inhibition of specific enzymes involved **(Table 20.2)**.

Steps of Protein Synthesis

Activation of Amino Acids

The aminoacyl-tRNA synthetase is the enzyme responsible for the activation of each amino acid. The enzyme is specific for the amino acid and the corresponding tRNA.

Initiation

- The mRNA binds to the 40S ribosome (30S in bacteria) in the presence of initiation factor 3 (IF-3) to form a complex I.

Molecular Biology

Table 20.2: Inhibitors of protein synthesis.

Inhibitors	Actions
Mitomycin C and novobiocin	Inhibit cell division and DNA polymerase
Rifampicin and actinomycin D	Inhibit RNA polymerase
Adriamycin HCl	Inhibits DNA and RNA synthesis by forming complexes with DNA translation
Chloramphenicol	Inhibits prokaryotic peptidyl transferase
Streptomycin	Inhibits prokaryotic peptide chain initiation, also induces mRNA misreading
Tetracycline	Inhibits prokaryotic aminoacyl-tRNA binding to the ribosome small subunit
Neomycin	Inhibits prokaryotic peptide chain initiation and also induces mRNA misreading
Erythromycin	Similar in activity to streptomycin and inhibits prokaryotic translocation through the ribosome large subunit
Puromycin	Resembles an aminoacyl-tRNA and interferes with peptide transfer resulting in premature termination in both prokaryotes and eukaryotes

(DNA: deoxyribonucleic acid; HCl: hydrochloride; mRNA: messenger RNA; RNA: ribonucleic acid; tRNA: transfer RNA)

- Then the methionyl tRNA binds with guanosine triphosphate (GTP) in the presence of IF-2 to form a complex II **(Fig. 20.12)**.

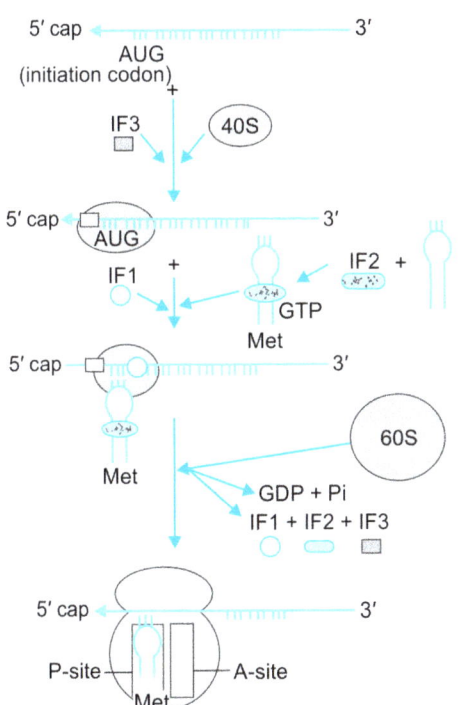

Fig. 20.12: Initiation.
(IF: initiation factor; Met: methionine; GDP: guanosine diphosphate; GTP: guanosine triphosphate)

- The complex I interacts with complex II in the presence of IF-1 to form a complex III.
- The anticodon of tRNA binds with the initiation codon AUG. Anticodon of each amino acyl-tRNA recognizes its codon in mRNA.
- In eukaryotes, initiator tRNA carries methionine (Met). Bacteria use a modified Met designated formylmethionine (fMet).
- Once the IFs is released, the 60S ribosome (50S in bacteria) attaches to the complex III and GTP provides energy by hydrolyzing to guanosine diphosphate (GDP) and inorganic phosphate.
- The complete ribosome (80S) is ready with attached mRNA. At this step, the ribosome has two sites called P-site (peptidyl) and A-site (aminoacyl).
- At this point, the P-site contains methionyl-RNA and A-site is vacant.

Inhibitors of Protein Synthesis

Elongation

- An aminoacyl-tRNA able to base pair with the next codon on the mRNA arrives at the A-site associated with an elongation factor, EF-1 (EF-Tu in bacteria) and GTP (as the energy source) **(Fig. 20.13)**.

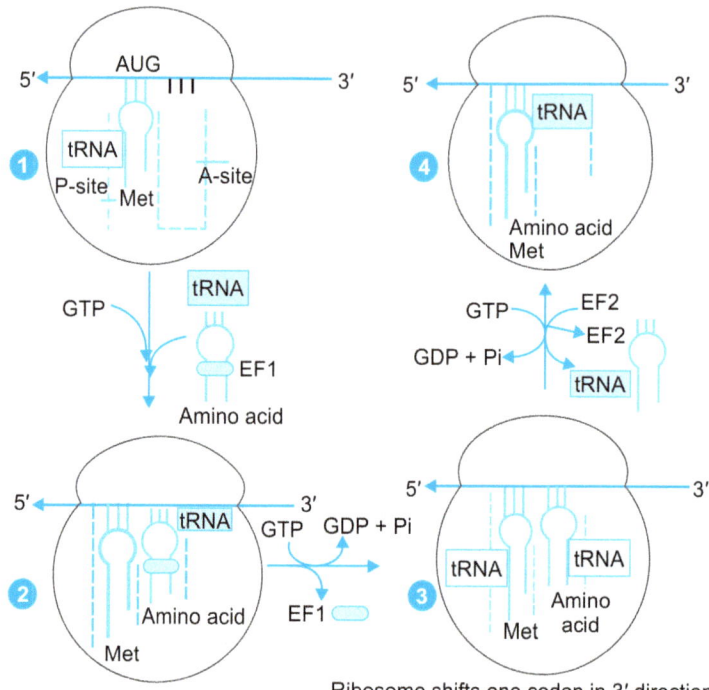

Fig. 20.13: Elongation.
(GDP: guanosine diphosphate; GTP: guanosine triphosphate; EF: elongation factor)

- Preceding amino acid (Met at the start of translation) is covalently linked to the incoming amino acid with a peptide bond. This special type of bond is formed by the enzyme peptidase.
- Initiator tRNA is released from the P-site.
- The tRNA with the two amino acids on it is now sitting on the P-site. The ribosome slides down three bases (one codon on the mRNA) exposing a new A-site by the action of a translocase. The next appropriate tRNA molecule "lands" bringing its amino acid right next to the tRNA holding the two amino acids. At this point, the process repeats itself.
- The ribosome slides down another codon and the procedure repeats itself until the termination event occurs.
- This last step is promoted by another protein elongation factor, EF-2 (EF-G in bacteria) and the energy of another molecule of GTP.

Termination

- The end of translation occurs when the ribosome reaches one of the stop codons (UAA, UAG, and UGA). There are no tRNA molecules with anticodons for stop codons **(Fig. 20.14)**.
- However, a protein release factor recognizes these codons when they arrive at the A-site.
- Binding of this protein releases the polypeptide from the ribosome.
- The ribosome splits into its subunits, which can later be reassembled for another round of protein synthesis.

Post-translational Modification of Proteins

- Proteins undergo proteolytic cleavage following translation. The simplest form of this is the removal of the initiation methionine.

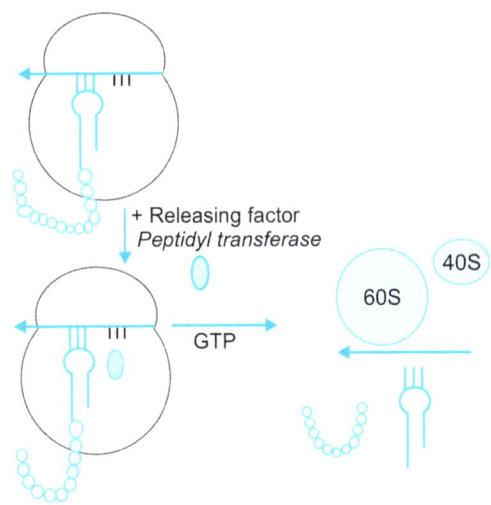

Fig. 20.14: Termination.
(GTP: guanosine triphosphate; EF: elongation factor)

- Many proteins are synthesized as inactive precursors that are activated under proper physiological conditions by limited proteolysis.
- Inactive precursor proteins that are activated by removal of polypeptides are termed "proproteins."
- Best example of post-translational processing of a preproprotein is insulin. Since insulin is secreted from the pancreas it has a prepeptide. Following cleavage of the 24 amino acid signal peptide, the protein folds into proinsulin. This proinsulin is further cleaved yielding active insulin, which is composed of two peptide chains linked together through disulfide bonds.
- Enzymes are synthesized as inactive precursors called zymogens. Zymogens are activated by proteolytic cleavage such as is the situation for several proteins of the blood clotting cascade.

Carbohydrate Linkage to Protein

Attachment of sugars in O-linked glycoproteins occurs post-translationally in the Golgi apparatus. Sugars used for glycoprotein synthesis (both N-linked and O-linked) are activated by coupling to nucleotides. Glucose and N-acetylglucosamine are coupled to UDP and mannose is coupled to GDP.

Acylation

Many proteins are modified at their N-terminal following synthesis. In most cases, the initiator methionine is hydrolyzed and an acetyl group is added to the new N-terminal amino acid. Acetyl-CoA is the acetyl donor for these reactions.

Methylation

Post-translational methylation occurs at lysine residues in some proteins such as calmodulin and cytochrome c. The activated methyl donor is S-adenosylmethionine.

Phosphorylation

- Post-translational phosphorylation is one of the most common protein modifications that occur in animal cells. The vast majority of phosphorylation occurs as a mechanism to regulate the biological activity of a protein and as such is transient (phosphate is added and later removed).
- Physiologically relevant examples are the phosphorylation that occurs in glycogen synthase and glycogen phosphorylase in hepatocytes in response to glucagon release from the pancreas. Phosphorylation of synthase inhibits its activity, whereas, the activity of phosphorylase is increased. These two events lead to increased hepatic glucose delivery to the blood.
- The enzymes that phosphorylate proteins are termed "kinases" and those that remove phosphates are termed "phosphatases." Protein kinases catalyze reactions of the following type:

$$\text{ATP} + \text{Protein} \longleftrightarrow \text{Phosphoprotein} + \text{ADP}$$

Sulfation

Sulfate modification of proteins occurs at tyrosine residues such as in fibrinogen and in some secreted proteins (e.g. gastrin). The universal sulfate donor is 3'-phosphoadenosine 5'-phosphosulfate.

Vitamin C-dependent Modifications

- Modifications of proteins that depend upon vitamin C as a cofactor include proline, lysine hydroxylations, and carboxy (C)-terminal amidation. The hydroxylating enzymes are identified as prolyl hydroxylase and lysyl hydroxylase. The donor of the amide for C-terminal amidation is glycine.
- The most important hydroxylated proteins are the collagen. Several peptide hormones such as oxytocin and vasopressin have C-terminal amidation.

Vitamin K-dependent Modifications

Vitamin K is a cofactor in the carboxylation of glutamic acid residues. The result of this type of reaction is the formation of a ▯-carboxyglutamate referred to as a Gla residue.

Intron and Exon Gene

The **exon** and **introns** are sequences in a protein-coding **gene** region of a double-stranded DNA (dsDNA) molecule that are expressed as proteins, or intervening sequences not so expressed.

An exon is any part of a gene that will encode a part of the final mature RNA produced by that gene after introns have been removed by RNA splicing. The term "exon" refers to both the DNA sequence within a gene and to the corresponding sequence in RNA transcripts.

Main Difference between Introns and Exons

Exons are coding areas, whereas **introns** are noncoding areas.

An **exon** is termed a nucleic acid sequence, which is represented in the RNA molecule.

Introns are termed nucleotide sequences seen within the genes, which are removed through RNA splicing for generating a mature RNA molecule.

Reason for Removal of Introns

Introns are the intervening sequences that are removed from a gene before the RNA product is made. Introns and exons alternate with each other along the length of a gene. Introns are usually considered noncoding regions (they don't code for any enzymes or structural proteins).

Cistron

A cistron is the nucleotide sequence that carries the information required by the production of the polypeptide sequence of a protein. Therefore it resembles the coding sequence of a gene, which codes for a single protein.

Difference between Gene and Cistron

A gene is a nucleotide sequence responsible for the synthesis of an RNA molecule, whereas a cistron is a nucleotide sequence responsible for the synthesis of a polypeptide sequence of a functional protein.

Expression of Genes

For a cell to function properly, necessary proteins must be synthesized at the proper time. All cells control or regulate the synthesis of proteins from information encoded in their DNA. The process of turning on a gene to produce RNA and protein is called **gene expression**.

Gene Regulation

Process of Prokaryotic Cells Regulating Gene Expression

Prokaryotic cells can only regulate gene expression by controlling the amount of transcription.

It therefore became possible to control gene expression by regulating transcription in the nucleus, and also by controlling the RNA levels and protein translation present outside the nucleus.

Gene regulation is the term used to describe any mechanism used by a cell to increase or decrease the production of specific gene products (protein or RNA). Cells can modify their gene expression patterns to trigger developmental pathways, respond to environmental stimuli, or adapt to new food sources.

Prokaryotic and Eukaryotic Gene Regulation

Prokaryotic organisms are single-celled organisms that lack a cell nucleus, and their DNA therefore floats freely in the cell cytoplasm. To synthesize a protein, the processes of transcription and translation occur almost simultaneously. When the resulting protein is no longer needed, transcription stops. The primary method to control type of protein and amount of each protein is expressed in a prokaryotic cell is the regulation of DNA transcription **(Fig. 20.15)**. All of the subsequent steps occur automatically. When more protein is required, more transcription occurs. Therefore, in prokaryotic cells, the control of gene expression is mostly at the transcriptional level.

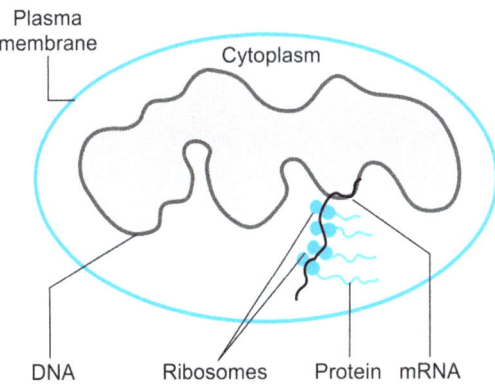

Fig. 20.15: Prokaryotic cell gene regulation.

Bacteria have a simple general mechanism for coordinating the regulation of genes that encode products involved in a set of related processes. The gene cluster and promoter, plus additional sequences that function together in regulation are called an operon.

The lactose operon (*lac* operon)

The lactose operon of *Escherichia coli* encodes the enzyme β-galactosidase, which hydrolyzes lactose into galactose and glucose. The *lac* operon of *E. coli* has three structural genes required for metabolism of lactose, a disaccharide found at high levels in milk:

1. lacZ encodes the enzyme beta-galactosidase, which cleaves lactose into glucose and galactose
2. lacY encodes permease, a membrane protein for facilitated diffusion of lactose into the cell
3. lacA encodes transacetylase, an enzyme that modifies lactose.

An mRNA encoding all three proteins is transcribed at high levels only when lactose is present, and glucose is absent.

Negative regulation by the repressor—in the absence of lactose, the lac repressor protein, encoded by the *lacI* gene with a separate promoter that is always active, binds to the operator sequence in the DNA. The **operator sequence** is a type of DNA regulatory element. Repressor protein bound to the Operator prevents RNA polymerase from initiating transcription.

When lactose is present, an inducer molecule derived from lactose binds allosterically to the repressor and causes the repressor to leave the operator site. RNA polymerase is then free to initiate transcription, if it successfully binds to the *lac* promoter.

Positive regulation by catabolite activator protein (CAP)—glucose is the preferred substrate for energy metabolism. When glucose is present, cells transcribe the *lac* operon only at very low levels, so the cells

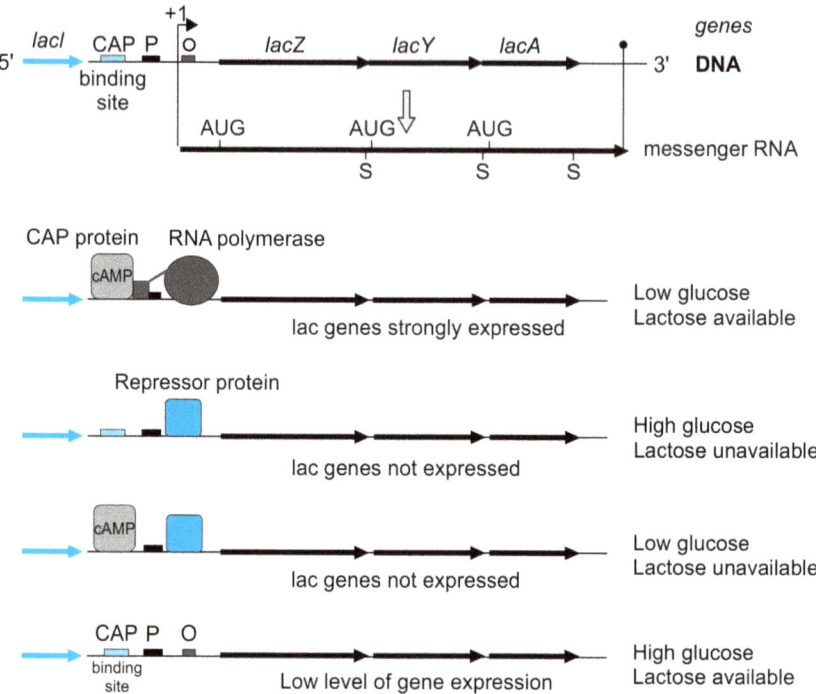

Fig. 20. 16: *Escherichia coli lac* operon: dual positive and negative regulation.

obtain most of their energy from glucose metabolism. RNA polymerase by itself binds rather poorly to the *lac* promoter **(Fig. 20.16)**.

Glucose starvation causes a rise in the level of cyclic adenosine monophosphate (cAMP), an intracellular alarm signal. cAMP binds to the CAP.

The CAP+cAMP complex binds to the CAP-binding site near the *lac* promoter and recruits RNA polymerase to the promoter.

High-level transcription of the lac operon requires both that CAP+cAMP be bound to the CAP-binding site, and that repressor is absent from the operator. These conditions normally occur only in the absence of glucose and presence of lactose.

The *lac* operon in *E. coli* is a classic example of a prokaryotic operon, which is subject to both positive and negative regulation. Positive regulation and negative regulation are universal themes for gene regulation in both prokaryotes and eukaryotes.

Gene Regulation in Eukaryotic Cells

Eukaryotic cells have intracellular organelles that add to their complexity. In eukaryotic cells, the DNA is contained inside the cell's nucleus and there it is transcribed into RNA. The newly synthesized RNA is then transported out of the nucleus into the cytoplasm, where ribosomes translate the RNA into protein. The processes of transcription and translation are physically separated by the nuclear membrane; transcription occurs only within the nucleus, and translation occurs only outside the nucleus in the cytoplasm. The regulation of gene expression can occur at all stages of the process **(Fig. 20.17)**. Regulation may occur when the DNA is uncoiled and loosened from nucleosomes to bind transcription factors (**epigenetic** level), when the RNA is transcribed (**transcriptional** level), when the RNA is processed and exported to the cytoplasm after it is transcribed (**post-transcriptional** level), when the RNA is translated into protein

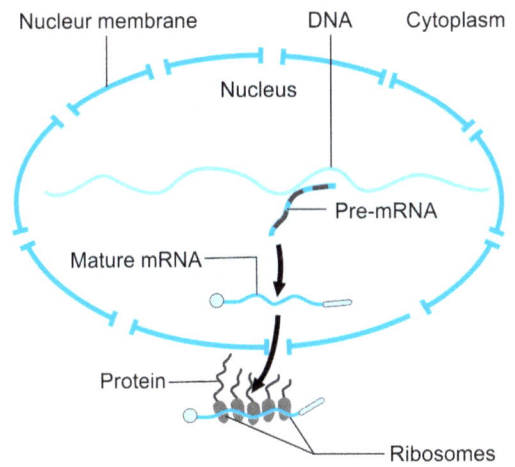

Fig. 20.17: Eukaryotic cell gene regulation.

Table 20.3: Differences in the regulation of gene expression of prokaryotic and eukaryotic organisms.

Prokaryotic organisms	Eukaryotic organisms
No nucleus	Contains nucleus
DNA is located in the cytoplasm	DNA is confined to the nuclear compartment
RNA transcription and protein formation occur almost simultaneously	RNA transcription occurs prior to protein formation, and it takes place in the nucleus. Translation of RNA to protein occurs in the cytoplasm
Gene expression is regulated primarily at the transcriptional level	Gene expression is regulated at many levels (epigenetic, transcriptional, nuclear shuttling, posttranscriptional, translational, and post-translational)

(translational level), or after the protein has been made (**post-translational** level) (**Table 20.3**).

Role of Enhancers, Repressors, and DNA Regulatory Elements

Gene Expression in Eukaryotes by Enhancers, Repressors, and DNA Regulatory Elements

Repressors: Gene expression in eukaryotic cells is **regulated** by repressors as well as by transcriptional activators. A **repressor** is a DNA- or RNA-binding protein that inhibits the expression of one or more genes by binding to the operator or associated silencers. A DNA-binding repressor blocks the attachment of RNA polymerase to the promoter, thus preventing transcription of the genes into mRNA. An RNA-binding repressor binds to the mRNA and prevents translation of the mRNA into protein. This blocking of expression is called **repression**.

Enhancers: An enhancer is a DNA sequence that promotes transcription. Each enhancer is made up of short DNA sequences called distal control elements. Activators bound to the distal control elements interact with mediator proteins and transcription factors.

An **enhancer** is a sequence of DNA that functions to enhance transcription. A **promoter** is a sequence of DNA that initiates the process of transcription. A **promoter** has to be close to the gene that is being transcribed, while an **enhancer** does not need to be close to the gene of interest (**Fig. 20.18**).

Similarities between Prokaryotes and Eukaryotes: Promoters and Regulatory Elements

Promoters are sites in the DNA where RNA polymerase binds to initiate transcription. Promoters also contain, or have near them, binding sites for **transcription factors**, which are DNA-binding proteins that can either help recruit, or repel, RNA polymerase. A **regulatory element** is a DNA sequence that certain transcription factors recognize and bind to in order to recruit or repel RNA polymerase. The promoter along with nearby transcription factor-binding elements regulates gene transcription.

Regulatory elements can be used for either **positive** or **negative** transcriptional control. When a gene is subject to positive transcriptional control, the binding of a specific transcription factor to the regulatory element promotes transcription. When a gene is subject to negative transcriptional control,

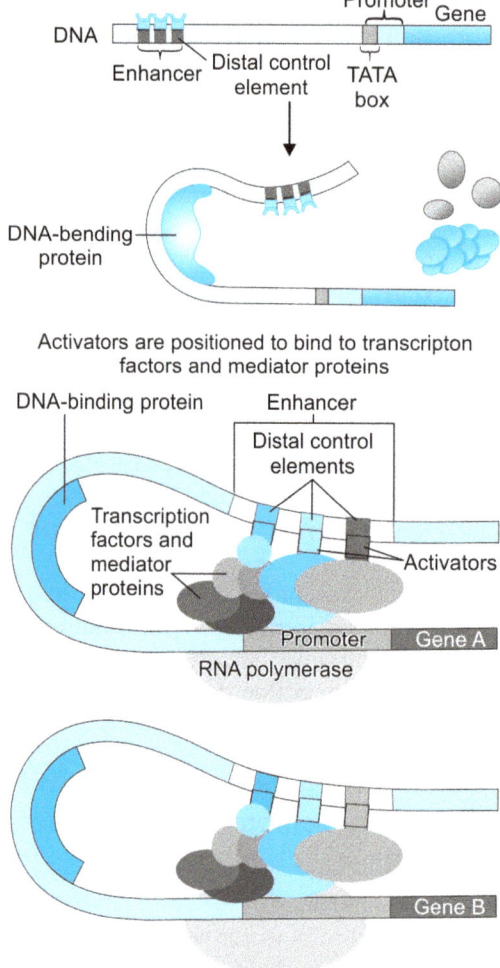

Fig. 20.18: Role of enhancers and promoters.
(TATA box: TATA box is a DNA sequence that indicates where a genetic sequence can be read and decoded)

the binding of a specific transcription factor to a regulator element represses transcription. A single gene can be subject to both positive and negative transcriptional control by different transcription factors, creating multiple layers of regulation.

Gene Amplification

Gene amplification is an increase in the number of copies of a gene without a proportional increase in other genes (either by natural process or artificial). This can result from duplication of a region of DNA that contains a **gene** through errors in DNA replication and repair machinery as well as through fortuitous capture by selfish genetic elements.

There may also be an increase in the RNA and protein made from that gene. Gene amplification is common in cancer cells, and some amplified genes may cause cancer cells to grow or become resistant to anticancer drugs.

Polymerase chain reaction (PCR) is a method widely used in molecular biology to make many copies of a specific DNA segment. Using PCR, copies of DNA sequences are exponentially amplified to generate thousands to millions of more copies of that particular DNA segment.

Artificial DNA Amplification

In research or diagnosis, DNA amplification can be conducted through methods such as:
- PCR, an easy, cheap, and reliable way to repeatedly replicate a focused segment of DNA by polymerizing nucleotides.
- Ligase chain reaction (LCR), a method that amplifies the nucleic acid used as the probe. For each of the two DNA strands, two partial probes are ligated to form the actual one; thus LCR uses two enzymes: a DNA polymerase (used for initial template amplification and then inactivated) and a thermostable DNA ligase.
- Transcription-mediated amplification, an isothermal, single-tube nucleic acid amplification system utilizing two enzymes, RNA polymerase and reverse transcriptase.

Natural DNA Amplification

Deoxyribonucleic acid replication is a natural form of copying DNA with the amount of genes remaining constant. However, the amount of DNA or the number of genes can also increase within an organism through gene duplication, a major mechanism through which new genetic material is generated during molecular evolution.

Gene Rearrangement

In genetics, a chromosomal **rearrangement** is a mutation that is a type of chromosome abnormality involving a change in the structure of the native chromosome. Such changes may involve several different classes of events, such as deletions, duplications, inversions, and translocations. Usually, these events are caused by a breakage in the DNA double helices at two different locations, followed by a rejoining of the broken ends to produce a new chromosomal arrangement of genes, different from the gene order of the chromosomes before they were broken.

Some chromosomal regions are more prone to rearrangement than others and thus are the source of genetic diseases and cancer. This instability is usually due to the propensity of these regions to misalign during DNA repair, exacerbated by defects of the appearance of replication proteins that ubiquitously affect the integrity of the genome.

Ribonucleic acid Processing

In the appropriate cell type and at the correct developmental stage, RNA polymerase transcribes an RNA copy of a gene, the primary transcript. Processing events include protection of both ends of the transcript and removal of intervening nonprotein-coding regions.

It produces a "final draft" of the mRNA before translation gets under way. RNA splicing is the removal of introns and joining of exons in eukaryotic mRNA. It also occurs in tRNA and rRNA. Splicing is accomplished with the help of spliceosomes, which remove introns from the genes in RNA.

Eukaryotic mRNA precursors are processed by 5' capping, 3' cleavage and polyadenylation, and RNA splicing to remove introns before being transported to the cytoplasm where they are translated by ribosomes.

After transcription, eukaryotic pre-mRNAs must undergo several processing steps before they can be translated. Eukaryotic and prokaryotic tRNAs and rRNAs also undergo processing before they can function as components in the protein-synthesizing machinery.

Ribonucleic acid Editing and mRNA Stability

Ribonucleic acid editing is a molecular process through which some cells can make discrete changes to specific nucleotide sequences within an RNA molecule after it has been generated by RNA polymerase. RNA editing may include the insertion, deletion, and base substitution of nucleotides within the RNA molecule (**Fig. 20.19**). RNA editing has been observed in some tRNA, rRNA, mRNA, or miRNA molecules of eukaryotes and their viruses, archaea, and prokaryotes. RNA editing occurs in the cell nucleus and cytosol, as well as within mitochondria and plastids.

mRNA stability: The regulation of mRNA decay is a major control point in gene expression. The stability of a particular mRNA is controlled by specific interactions between its structural elements and RNA-binding proteins that can be general or mRNA-specific. mRNA concentration is a key determinant of stability. In addition to modification of transcription,

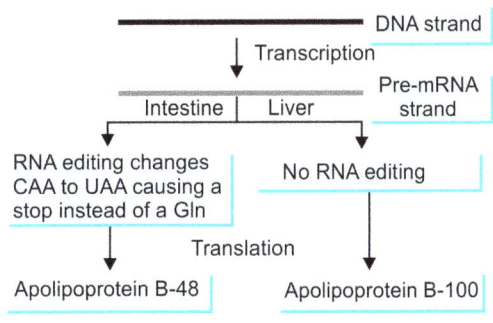

Fig. 20.19: Ribonucleic acid editing.

the regulation of mRNA stability is a key mechanism in regulating gene expression.

More than increasing mRNA stability, the promoter strength can be tuned to increase the gene expression by producing more quantities of the mRNA. The strength is based on efficient promoter recognition and rapid binding of the DNA polymerase.

RECOMBINANT DNA

Role of Recombinant DNA Technology in Creating the New DNA

rDNA is a form of artificial DNA that is created by combining two or more sequences that would not normally occur:

1. The first step in the development of rDNA technology was the characterization of restriction endonucleases enzymes that cleave DNA at specific sequences.
2. These enzymes were identified in bacteria, where they apparently provide a defense against the entry of foreign DNA into the cell.
3. Bacteria have a variety of restriction endonucleases that cleave DNA at more than a hundred distinct recognition sites, each of which consists of a specific sequence of four to eight base pairs.
4. Since restriction endonucleases digest DNA at specific sequences, they can be used to cleave a DNA molecule-at unique sites.

For example, the restriction endonuclease EcoRI recognizes the six base pair sequence GAATTC. This sequence is present at five sites in DNA of the bacteriophage λ, so EcoRI digests λ DNA into six fragments ranging from 3.6 to 21.2 kb long (1 kilobase or kb = 1,000 base pairs). These fragments can be separated depending on the size by gel electrophoresis.

Production of Recombinant DNA Molecules

- The basic strategy in molecular cloning is to insert a DNA fragment of interest into a DNA molecule (vector) that is capable of independent replication in a host cell (**Fig. 20.20**).
- The recombinant molecule or molecular clone obtained composed of the DNA insert linked to vector DNA sequences.
- Large quantities of the inserted DNA can be obtained if the recombinant molecule is allowed to replicate in an appropriate host.
- For example, fragments of human DNA can be cloned in bacteriophage λ vectors. These recombinant molecules can then be introduced into *E. coli*, where they replicate efficiently to yield millions of progeny phages containing the human DNA insert. The DNA of these phages can then be isolated, yielding large quantities of recombinant molecules containing a single fragment of human DNA. Whereas this fragment might represent one part in 100,000 of human genomic DNA, it represents approximately one part in 10 after being cloned in the one vector. Moreover, the fragment can be easily isolated from the rest of the vector DNA by restriction endonuclease digestion and gel electrophoresis, allowing a pure fragment of human DNA to be analyzed and further manipulated.
- The DNA fragments used to create recombinant molecules are usually generated by digestion with restriction endonucleases. Many of these enzymes cleave their recognition sequences at staggered sites, leaving cohesive single-stranded tails that can associate with each other by complementary base pairing. The association between such paired complementary ends can be established permanently by treatment with DNA ligase. Thus two different fragments of DNA, i.e. from human DNA insert and a DNA vector prepared by digestion with the same restriction endonuclease can be readily joined to create an rDNA molecule (refer to **Fig. 20.19**).

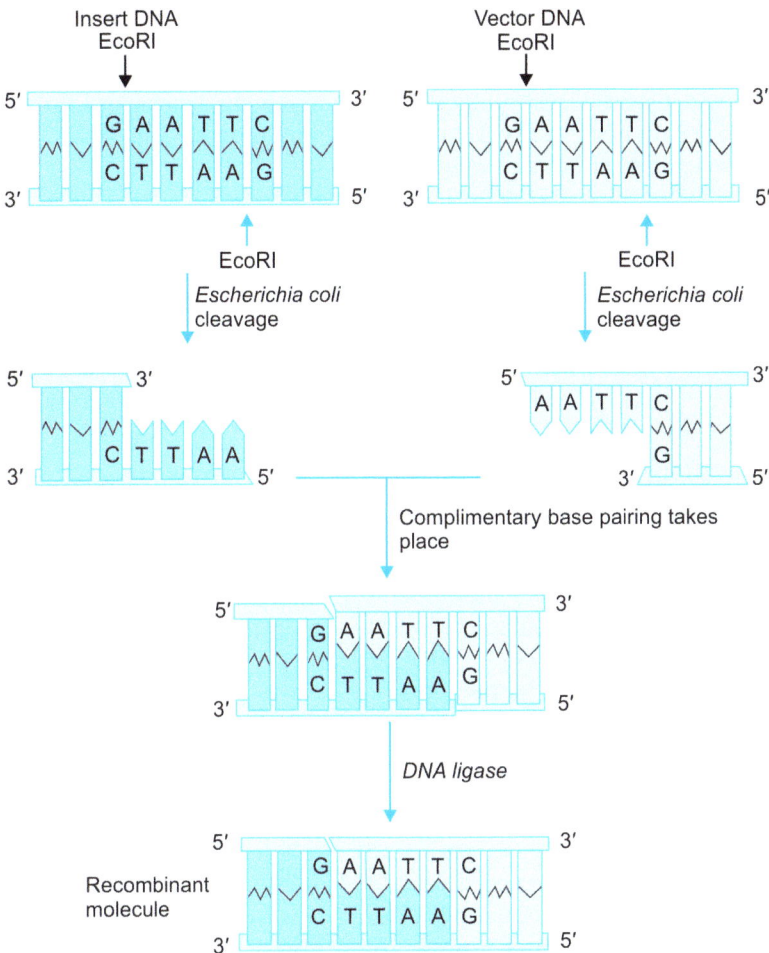

Fig. 20.20: Formation of recombinant DNA.

- Plasmid vectors allow easier manipulation of cloned DNA sequences than do phage vectors.
- Plasmids are small circular DNA molecules that can replicate independently without being associated with chromosomal DNA in bacteria.
- The required thing on the plasmid DNA is an origin of replication (ORI) the DNA sequence that signals the host cell DNA polymerase to replicate the DNA molecule.
- Plasmid vectors carry genes that confer resistance to antibiotics (ampicillin), so bacteria carrying the plasmids can be selected.
- Plasmid vectors usually consist of only 2–4 kb of DNA, in contrast to the 30–45 kb of phage DNA present in one vector, facilitating the analysis of an inserted DNA fragment.
- To be cloned into a plasmid vector, a fragment of the insert DNA is ligated to an appropriate restriction site in the vector and the recombinant molecule is used to transform E. coli.
- Antibiotic-resistant colonies, which contain plasmid DNA, are selected.

- Plasmid-containing bacteria can then be grown in large quantities and their DNA extracted.
- The small circular plasmid DNA molecules of which there are often hundreds of copies per cell can be separated from the bacterial chromosomal DNA; the result is purified plasmid DNA that is suitable for analysis of the cloned insert.

POLYMERASE CHAIN REACTION

PCR: Process and its Applications

The amplification of DNA by the PCR is as follows:
- The PCR is a technique widely used in molecular biology. It derives its name from one of its key components, a DNA polymerase used to amplify a piece of DNA by in vitro enzymatic replication.
- Molecular cloning allows individual DNA fragments to be propagated in bacteria and isolated in large amounts.
- An alternative method for isolating large amounts of a single DNA molecule is the PCR, developed by Kary Mullis (1988). The number of DNA molecules increases exponentially, doubling with each round of replication, so a substantial quantity of DNA can be obtained from a small number of initial template copies.
- For example, a single DNA molecule amplified through 30 cycles of replication would theoretically yield 230 progeny molecules. Single DNA molecules can thus be amplified to yield readily detectable quantities of DNA that can be isolated by molecular cloning or further analyzed directly by restriction endonuclease digestion or nucleotide sequencing.
- The starting material can be either a cloned DNA fragment or a mixture of DNA molecules. For example, total DNA from human cells. A specific region of DNA can be amplified from such a mixture, provided that the nucleotide sequence surrounding the region is known so that primers can be designed to initiate DNA synthesis at the desired point. Such primers are usually chemically synthesized oligonucleotides containing 15-20 bases of DNA.

Initialization

Initialization step consists of heating the reaction to a temperature of 94-96°C (or 98°C, if extremely thermostable polymerases are used), which is held for 1-9 minutes. It is required only for DNA polymerases that need heat activation by hot-start PCR.

Denaturation Step

Two primers are used to initiate DNA synthesis in opposite directions from complementary DNA (cDNA) strands. The reaction is started by heating the template DNA to a high temperature of 95°C, so that the two strands separate.

Annealing

In annealing step, the temperature is lowered to 50-65°C for 20-40 seconds to allow the primers to pair with their complementary sequences on the template strands.

Extension and Elongation

The DNA polymerases used in these reactions are heat-stable enzymes (Taq polymerase) from bacteria such as *Thermus aquaticus*, which lives in hot springs at temperatures of about 75°C. These polymerases are stable even at the high temperatures are used to separate the strands of dsDNA, so the PCR amplification can be performed rapidly and automatically. RNA sequences can also be amplified by this method if reverse transcriptase is used to synthesize a cDNA copy prior to PCR amplification (**Fig. 20.21**).

To check whether the PCR generated the anticipated DNA fragment (also sometimes referred to as the amplimer or amplicon), agarose gel electrophoresis is employed for

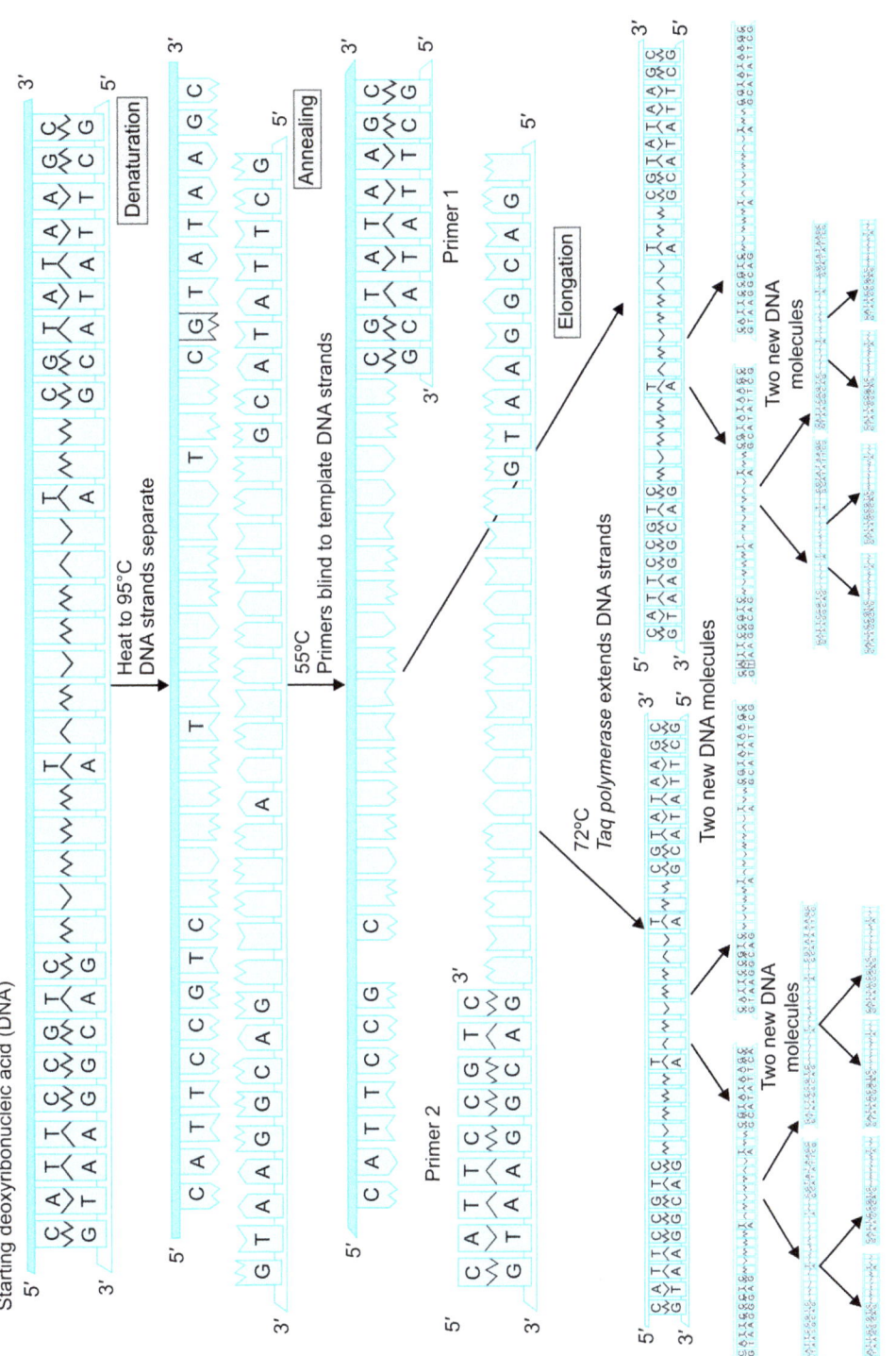

Fig. 20.21: Polymerase chain reaction.

size separation of the PCR products. The size(s) of PCR products is determined by comparison with a DNA ladder (a molecular weight marker), which contains DNA fragments of known size, run on the gel alongside the PCR products.

SOUTHERN, NORTHERN, AND WESTERN BLOTTING AND THEIR APPLICATIONS

Southern Blotting

A Southern blot is a method routinely used in molecular biology for detection of a specific DNA sequence in DNA samples. Southern blotting combines transfer of electrophoresis-separated DNA fragments to a filter membrane and subsequent fragment detection by probe hybridization. Southern blotting was named after Edward M Southern, who developed this procedure in the 1970s. Southern blotting is designed to locate a particular sequence of DNA within a complex mixture. For example, Southern blotting could be used to locate a particular gene within an entire genome. The amount of DNA needed for this technique is dependent on the size and specific activity of the probe.

Procedure

- Digest the DNA with an appropriate restriction enzyme.
- Run the digest on an agarose gel.
- *Denaturing of the DNA:* Soak it in about 0.5 M sodium hydroxide (NaOH), which would separate dsDNA into single-stranded DNA (ssDNA). Only ssDNA can transfer. A depurination step is optional. Fragments greater than 15 kb are hard to transfer to the blotting membrane. Depurination with 0.2 M HCl for 15 minutes takes the purines out, cutting the DNA into smaller fragments. Neutralize the acid after this step or the base after the prior step, if there is no depurination.
- Transfer the denatured DNA to the membrane:
  a. A nitrocellulose membrane is used, although nylon or a positively charged nylon membrane may be used. Nitrocellulose typically has a binding capacity of about 100 µg/cm, while nylon has a binding capacity of about 500 µg/cm. Transfer is usually done by capillary action, which will bind ssDNA. Use a vacuum blot apparatus instead of capillary action. In this procedure, a vacuum sucks SSD through the membrane. After the transfer of DNA to the membrane, treat it with UV light. This cross-links the DNA to the membrane (**Fig. 20.22**).
- Probe the membrane with labeled ssDNA. This is also known as hybridization. This process relies on the ssDNA hybridizing (annealing) to the DNA on the membrane due to the binding of complementary strands. Probing is often done with 32P-labeled adenosine triphosphate (ATP), biotin/streptavidin or a bioluminescent probe. A prehybridization step is required before hybridization to block nonspecific sites to avoid single-stranded probe binding just anywhere on the membrane. To hybridize, use the same buffer as for prehybridization, but add specific probe.
- Visualize radioactively labeled target sequence. If radiolabeled 32P probe is used, then visualize by autoradiograph. Biotin/streptavidin detection is done by colorimetric methods and bioluminescent visualization uses luminescence.

32P-labeled adenosine triphosphate

Treat the dsDNA fragment with a limiting amount of DNase, which causes double-stranded nicks in DNA. Add 32P, deoxy-ATP and other deoxynucleotide triphosphates to DNA polymerase I, which has 5'–3' polymerase activity and 5'–3' exonuclease activity.

Nick translation occurs and as the nick is translated down the DNA strand, the polymerase activity continues to nick, while

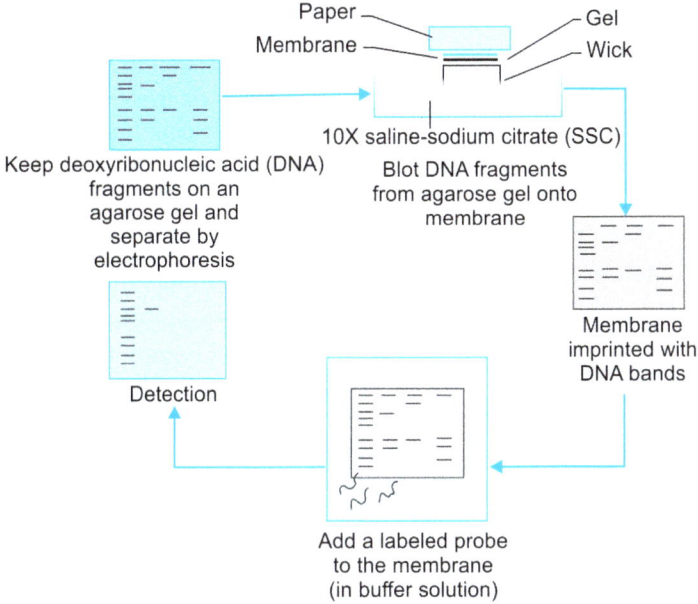

Fig. 20.22: Southern blotting.

the exonuclease activity continues to fill in the nick. As this happens, 32P becomes incorporated into and thus labels the DNA. Heat the DNA to make it single stranded, then immediately place it on ice to keep the two strands from reannealing to each other.

Prehybridization
To prehybridize, add nonspecific ssDNA. Sonicated salmon sperm DNA is commonly used. Add 20x saline-sodium citrate, Denhardt's solution [ficol and polyvinylpyrrolidone (PVP), which are large molecules to take up space and generate more contact; and bovine serum albumin, a nonspecific protein], sodium dodecyl sulfate (SDS), and formamide.

Northern Blotting

- Northern blotting is a technique used in molecular biology research to study gene expression by detection of RNA (or isolated mRNA) in a sample.
- In the 1970s, Southern EM developed a method for locating a particular sequence of DNA within a complex mixture. This technique came to be known as Southern blotting.
- A similar method for locating a sequence of RNA is known as its Northern blotting. It is also known as northern hybridization or RNA hybridization.
- The procedure for and theory behind Northern blotting is almost identical to that of Southern blotting, except RNA is used instead of DNA.

Western Blotting

The Western blot is a widely used analytical technique used to detect specific proteins in a sample of tissue homogenate or extract.

This method is, however, dependent on the use of a high-quality antibody directed against a desired protein. It can produce at least a small portion of the protein from a cloned DNA fragment and use this antibody as a probe to detect the protein of interest. Western blotting gives an idea of how much protein has accumulated in cells.

Procedure

- Separate the proteins using SDS-polyacrylamide gel electrophoresis (SDS-PAGE). This separates the proteins by size.
- Place a nitrocellulose membrane on the gel and, using electrophoresis, drive the protein bands onto the nitrocellulose membrane. Negative charge to be on the side of the gel and the positive charge to be on the side of the nitrocellulose membrane to drive the negatively charged proteins over to the positively charged nitrocellulose membrane. This gives nitrocellulose membrane that is imprinted with the same protein bands as the gel. The proteins binding are better to nitrocellulose at a low pH.
- Incubate the nitrocellulose membrane with a primary antibody. The primary antibody, which is the specific antibody, sticks to protein and forms an antibody-protein complex with the protein of interest.
- Incubate the nitrocellulose membrane with a secondary antibody. This antibody should be an antibody-enzyme conjugate. The secondary antibody should be an antibody against the primary antibody. This means the secondary antibody will "stick" to the primary antibody, just like the primary antibody "stuck" to the protein. The conjugated enzyme is there to allow visualizing all of this.
- To see the enzyme action, we need to incubate it in a reaction mix that is specific for the enzyme. If everything processed properly, we are able to see the bands wherever there is a protein-primary antibody-secondary antibody-enzyme complex.
- Put an X-ray film on the gel to detect a flash of light, which is given off by the enzyme. The reaction usually runs out in about an hour.

Making a primary antibody
- Run the protein on an SDS–PAGE gel.
- Stain the gel with KCl. The KCl forms a precipitate with the SDS. Since the area with the protein has a low concentration of SDS, the area with the protein will not show a precipitate. This will allow seeing the protein band as a clear band against a milky white precipitate on the rest of the gel (**Fig. 20.23**).
- Carefully cut out the band and soak it in 1 mL phosphate-buffered saline buffer.
- Crush it and make an emulsion with 1 mL Freund's complete adjuvant (which is an oily substance).
- The complete adjuvant contains mycobacteria (an immune stimulant) to increase the immune response.
- Inject this subscapular into a rabbit. This is first inoculation. Only use the complete adjuvant for the first inoculation. Never inject a rabbit with complete adjuvant more than one time.
- Rest the rabbit for one month and then repeat the process using an incomplete adjuvant.
- Bleed the rabbit and this is rabbit antisera.
- To get primary antibody, dilute the rabbit antisera in aka carnation nonfat dry instant

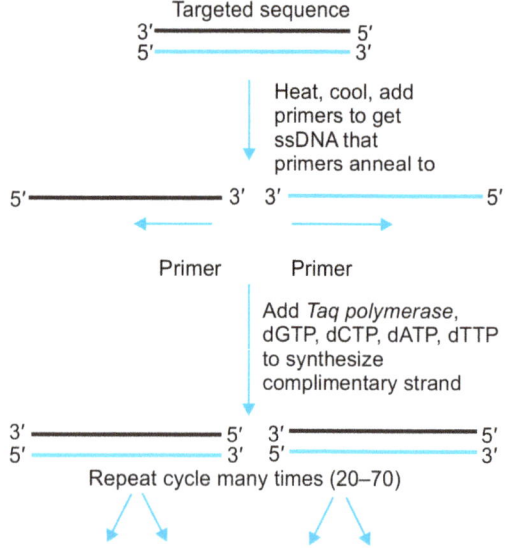

Fig. 20.23: Making a primary antibody.

milk and apply it to your nitrocellulose blot. Make sure to dilute 1:500 to 1:100, less dilution will give background binding.

Secondary antibody
Secondary antibody is much easier than the procedure for the primary antibody. Grab a catalog and look for a goat anti-rabbit antibody conjugated to horseradish peroxidase.

RESTRICTION ENZYMES

Restriction enzymes, also known as restriction endonucleases, are enzymes that cut a DNA molecule at a particular place. They are essential tools for rDNA technology. The enzyme "scans" a DNA molecule, looking for a particular sequence, usually of four to six nucleotides. Once it finds this recognition sequence, it stops and cuts the strands. This is known as enzyme digestion. On dsDNA, the recognition sequence is on both strands but runs in opposite directions. This allows the enzyme to cut both strands. Sometimes the cut is blunt, sometimes uneven with dangling nucleotides on one of the two strands. This uneven cut is known as sticky ends:

Example for a blunt end
- 5' NNNNNNNATT AATNNNNNNNNNN 3'
- 3' NNNNNNNTAA TTANNNNNNNNNN 5'.

Example for a sticky end
- 5' NNNNNNNNNNNNNG AATTCNNNNNNN 3'
- 3' NNTTAA NNNNNNNNNNNNNNNNN 5'.

Most plasmids used for recombinant technology have recognition sequences for a number of restriction enzymes. This allows a scientist to choose from a number of places to cut the plasmid with a restriction enzyme. Ligation enzymes can then be used to sort of paste in new genomic sequences. These mutated, or recombined, plasmids can then be grown up in bacterial cells and used for a number of purposes, including the addition of genes to mammalian genomes.

Most enzymes come in glycerol solution as a storage buffer, but enzymes do not work well in the presence of high glycerol concentration. Be sure to dilute the glycerol content down to less than 5% to ensure proper enzymatic activity. Problems with enzyme activity can occur under the following conditions:
- High glycerol concentration.
- Enzyme-to-DNA ratio is too high.
- pH is too high.
- Organic solvents, particularly ethanol, interfere with your DNA.

Some other helpful tips for working with enzymes include:
- *Wear gloves:* This protects you as well as protecting your sample from contamination from you.
- Keep the enzymes cold.
- Do not reuse tips.
- Contamination will ruin your experiment.

PLASMID

A plasmid is an independent, circular, self-replicating DNA molecule that carries only a few genes. The number of plasmids in a cell generally remains constant from generation to generation. Plasmids are autonomous molecules and exist in cells as extrachromosomal genomes, although some plasmids can be inserted into a bacterial chromosome, where they become a permanent part of the bacterial genome. It is here that they provide great functionality in molecular science (**Fig. 20.24**).

Plasmids are easy to manipulate and isolate using bacteria. They can be integrated into mammalian genomes, thereby conferring to mammalian cells whatever genetic functionality they carry. Thus this gives you the ability to introduce genes into a given organism by using bacteria to amplify the hybrid genes that are created in vitro. This tiny, but mighty, plasmid molecule is the basis of rDNA technology.

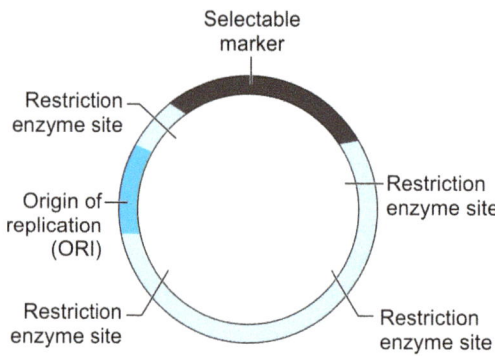

Fig. 20.24: Plasmid.

There are two categories of plasmids. Stringent plasmids replicate only when the chromosome replicates. This is good if you are working with a protein that is lethal to the cell. Relaxed plasmids replicate on their own. This gives you a higher ratio of plasmids to chromosome.

Manipulation of Plasmids

- Mutate those using restriction enzymes, ligation enzymes, and PCR. Mutagenesis is easily accomplished by using restriction enzymes to cut out portions of one genome and insert them into a plasmid. PCR can also be used to facilitate mutagenesis. Plasmids are mapped out indicating the locations of their origins of replication and restriction enzyme sites.
- Select those using genetic markers. Some bacteria are antibiotic resistant. While this is a serious health problem, it is a godsend to molecular scientists. The gene that confers antibiotic resistance can be added (ligated) to the gene you are inserting into the plasmid. So, every plasmid that contains your target gene will not be killed by antibiotics. After you transfect your bacterial cells with your engineered plasmid (the one with the target gene and the antibiotic-resistant marker), you incubate them in a nutrient broth that also contains antibiotic (usually ampicillin). Any cells that were not transfected (this means they do not have your target gene in them) are killed by the antibiotic. The ones that do have the gene also have the antibiotic-resistant gene and therefore survive the selection process.
3. Isolate them (such as with alkaline lysis).
4. Transform them into cells where they become vectors to transport foreign genes into a recipient organism.

Plasmid Requirements for Recombination

Some minimum requirements for plasmids that are useful for recombination techniques are:
- *ORI*: They must be able to replicate themselves or they are of no practical use as a vector.
- *Selectable marker*: They must have a marker so you can select for cells that have your plasmids.
- Restriction enzyme sites in nonessential regions. The plasmid should not be cut at some necessary regions such as the ORI.

In addition to these necessary requirements, there are some factors that make plasmids either more useful or easier to work with:
- *Small*: If they are small, they are easier to isolate, handle, and transform.
- *Multiple restriction enzyme sites*: More sites give you greater flexibility in cloning, perhaps even allowing for directional cloning.
- *Multiple ORIs*: It is important to note that two genes must have different ORIs if they are going to be inserted in the same plasmid.

RESTRICTION FRAGMENT LENGTH POLYMORPHISM

Restriction Fragment Length Polymorphism and its Applications

- Restriction fragment length polymorphism (RFLP) is a difference in homologous

DNA sequences that can be detected by the presence of fragments of different lengths after digestion of the DNA samples in question with specific restriction endonucleases.
- RELP, as a molecular marker, is specific to a single clone/restriction enzyme combination.
- The RFLP probe is a labeled DNA sequence that hybridizes with one or more fragments of the digested DNA sample after they were separated by gel electrophoresis, thus revealing a unique blotting pattern characteristic to a specific genotype at a specific locus. Short, single- or low-copy genomic DNA or cDNA clones are typically used as RFLP probes.

Applications

- The frequencies of particular RFLP alleles may differ for different human subpopulations. This possibility engendered much discussion about the validity of using RFLP analysis for forensic purposes.
- The RFLPs are molecular markers used in creating genetic maps of chromosomes.
- They have many other uses. In forensics, they are used to test whether a tissue sample left at a crime scene (blood, skin, sperm, etc.) could have come from the suspect. In plant and animal breeding, they can reveal, which backcross progeny most resemble the desired parent. RFLPs are used to settle cases where biological parentage is at issue. They are used as starting points for chromosome walks.
4. The RFLPs are used in plant genetic analysis. Note that an RFLP is specified by a hybridization probe and a restriction enzyme.

DEOXYRIBONUCLEIC ACID LIBRARIES

- A DNA library (refer to **Fig. 20.25A**) is a collection of clones of DNA designed so that there is a high probability of finding any particular piece of the source DNA in the collection. When each clone has been placed in a precise physical location relative to others (such as in wells of microtiter plates), the library is said to be ordered.
- DNA libraries can be made (refer to **Fig. 20.25B**) using highly efficient cloning vectors such as lambda phages, cosmids, P1 phages, and bacterial or yeast artificial chromosomes. When the DNA is simply ligated to the vector and packaged in the phage particles, the library is said to be unamplified. An amplified library is one in which the original DNA's have subsequently been increased by replication in bacteria.
- The DNA cloned in libraries (refer to **Fig. 20.25C**) depends on the purposes of the investigators.
- Genomic libraries are made from total nuclear DNA of an organism. In making these libraries, it is important to cut the DNA into cloneable size pieces as randomly as possible. Shearing or partial digestion

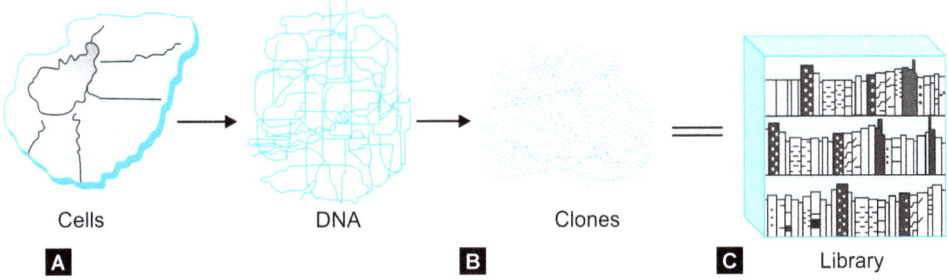

Figs. 20.25A to C: Libraries.

with a frequently cutting restriction endonuclease is often used.
5. Chromosome-specific libraries are made from the DNA of purified isolated chromosomes.
6. cDNA libraries are made from the mRNA populations of particular tissues. There are liver, heart, leaf, root, etc. cDNA libraries.
7. cDNA libraries may be normalized. Normalization eliminates many copies of highly abundant cDNAs. It can be achieved by incubating denatured double-stranded cDNAs to intermediate Cot values in hybridization reactions.
8. cDNA libraries are often expression libraries in which clone construction is such that part or all of the encoded protein is expressed in bacteria harboring the cloned DNA. Such expression is needed in screening libraries using antibodies or enzyme activities (**Fig. 20.25A to C**).

SUMMARY

Deoxyribonucleic acid serves as the master copy for most information in the cell. The RNA is of different types (mRNA, tRNA, and rRNA), which act to transform information from DNA to the rest of the cell. The mRNA acts as a messenger to transfer the message from DNA, tRNA transform the information from DNA and rRNA acts as the machinery for protein synthesis. The bases present in a DNA molecule are adenine, cytosine, guanine, and thymine. The transfer of genetic information takes place in three processes such as replication (process by which an identical copy of DNA is made), transcription (process by which the genetic messages contained in DNA are "read" or transcribed), and translation (process by which the genetic messages carried by mRNA are decoded and used to build proteins). DNA polymerase is the main enzyme of replication. This chapter also deals with recombinant DNA technology; polymerase chain reaction; Southern, Northern, and Western blotting techniques; plasmids; and libraries. The recombinant DNA is the formation of new strand of DNA by combining two or more different strands of DNA. A mutation is a permanent change in the DNA sequence of a gene. Mutations in a gene's DNA sequence can alter the amino acid sequence of the protein encoded by the gene. There are many types of mutation such as frameshift mutation, missense mutation, neutral mutation, nonsense mutation, point mutation, and silent mutation.

SELF-ASSESSMENT QUESTIONS

1. List the purine and pyrimidine bases normally found in DNA and RNA.
2. Briefly explain the structure of DNA.
3. Mention the three mechanisms for transferring genetic information.
4. Explain the process of replication.
5. Explain the conservative and semiconservative replication.
6. List the enzymes of replication.
7. Briefly explain the structure of tRNA.
8. List the functions of different types of RNAs.
9. What is genetic code and mention the initiation and termination codons?
10. Describe the process of translation.
11. List the various post-translational modifications takes place once the translation ends.
12. State the inhibitors of replication, transcription, and translation with their targeted action.
13. What is PCR and state the importance of it?
14. Explain the Southern blotting.
15. List the significance of RELP.
16. What is plasmid and mention its uses?
17. Explain "DNA libraries."

MULTIPLE-CHOICE QUESTIONS

1. **The following molecules are involved in unwinding DNA:**
   a. DNA gyrase   b. DNA helicase
   c. DNA unwindase   d. a and b

2. A strand of DNA or RNA that is synthesized from a DNA template strand is called ___ strand.
   a. Complimentary
   b. Adjacent
   c. Partner
   d. Template
3. Because DNA strands are only made in the 5'–3' direction, the lagging strand has shorter pieces of DNA called:
   a. Leading fragment
   b. Continuous fragment
   c. Okazaki fragment
   d. Primer fragment
4. Number of possible groups of three bases to code for amino acids is:
   a. 20   b. 16
   c. 64   d. 50
5. To get protein synthesis started, the mRNA must have:
   a. A start codon
   b. An Shine-Dalgarno (S–D) sequence
   c. An activator protein
   d. a and b
6. The first amino acid in a newly formed protein is:
   a. Met   b. fMet
   c. MetLife   d. fAla
7. Which type of genetic analysis method can detect the presence of a gene but is not useful for single base pair changes?
   a. Sequencing
   b. Western blot analysis
   c. Southern blot analysis
   d. Cytogenetics
8. Which of the following abnormal base pairings might be found in "wobble" codon–anticodon binding?
   a. Adenosine-uracil
   b. Guanine-uracil
   c. Cytosine-inosine
   d. Guanine-thymine
9. Which of the following statements about the 3' poly (A) tail of mRNA is false?
   a. It helps to align eukaryotic mRNA on the ribosome during translation
   b. It is added to the primary transcript in the nucleus
   c. It is not essential for protein synthesis
   d. It helps contribute to the stability and life span of the mRNA
10. Which of the following proteins is not essential in the synthesis of eukaryotic proteins from DNA templates?
    a. RNA polymerase I
    b. TATA-binding protein (TBP)
    c. Aminoacyl-tRNA synthetases
    d. Transcription factor IID (TFIID)
11. DNA is inherited from:
    a. Paternal only
    b. Maternal only
    c. Both paternal and maternal
    d. The offspring's own DNA
12. Which of the following is true about G-protein signaling?
    a. During activation of G-protein, subunit of the G-protein dissociates from the activated G-protein to activate adenylyl cyclase
    b. During activation of G-protein, the active a-subunit is terminated by the hydrolysis of the bound GTP caused by GTPase
    c. Testosterone can bind to the cell membrane receptor to activate G-protein
    d. The ratio of G-protein coupled receptor to G-protein is 1:1
13. Polyploidy refers to:
    a. Extra copies of a gene adjacent to each other on a chromosome
    b. An individual with complete extra sets of chromosomes
    c. A chromosome, which has replicated, but not divided
    d. Multiple ribosomes present on a single mRNA
14. A gene showing codominance:
    a. Has both alleles independently expressed in the heterozygote
    b. Has one allele dominant to the other
    c. Has alleles tightly linked on the same chromosome
    d. Has alleles expressed at the same time in development
15. Which component of transcribed RNA in eukaryotes is present in the initial transcript but is removed before translation occurs?
    a. Intron
    b. 3' poly (A) tail
    c. Ribosome-binding site
    d. 5' cap
16. Choose the correct statement about the genetic code:

a. Includes 60 codons for amino acids and three stop codons
  b. Not universal; not same in most genetic systems
  c. Six bases per codon
  d. Some amino acids are coded by multiple codons
17. **DNA ligase is:**
  a. An enzyme that joins fragments in normal DNA replication
  b. An enzyme involved in protein synthesis
  c. An enzyme of bacterial origin, which cuts DNA at defined base sequences
  d. An enzyme that facilitates transcription of specific genes
18. **Replication of DNA:**
  a. Takes place in a conservative manner
  b. Takes place in a dispersive manner
  c. Takes place in a "semiconservative" manner
  d. Takes place only in the 3'-5' direction
19. **A duplication is:**
  a. With new genes adjacent to each other
  b. An extra copy of the genes on part of a chromosome
  c. A reversal of order of genes on a chromosome
  d. An extra set of chromosomes in an organism
20. **Mutation in a codon leads to the substitution of one amino acid with another is:**
  a. Nonsense mutation
  b. Missense mutation
  c. Frameshift mutation
  d. Promoter mutation
21. **Zinc finger proteins and helix-turn helix proteins are:**
  a. Types of DNA-binding proteins
  b. Involved in the control of translation
  c. Components of ribosomes
  d. Part of the hemoglobin in blood cells
22. **Transcriptional activator proteins:**
  a. Transcribe a messenger off a DNA template
  b. Bind to ribosomes to activate the production of specific proteins
  c. Are produced during an infection of bacteria by a phage
  d. Bind regions near a eukaryotic gene and allow an RNA polymerase to transcribe a gene
23. **A homeotic mutation is one which:**
  a. Is present in only one form in an individual
  b. Substitutes one body part for another in development
  c. Results in development of a tumor
  d. Is wild type at one temperature and abnormal at another
24. **The RFLP analysis is a technique that:**
  a. Is used to determine whether a gene is transcribed in specific cells
  b. Uses hybridization to detect specific DNA restriction fragments in genomic DNA
  c. Measures the transfer frequency of genes during conjugation
  d. Is used to detect genetic variation at the protein level
25. **Plasmid vectors for cloning:**
  a. Grow within bacteria and are present in bacterial colonies on an agar plate
  b. Can accommodate inserts of over 100 kb
  c. Include centromeres to allow propagation in yeast
  d. Burst bacteria and form plaques on a "lawn" of bacteria
26. **The PCR is a technique that:**
  a. Was used to demonstrate DNA as the genetic material
  b. Uses short DNA primers and a thermostable DNA polymerase to replicate specific DNA sequences in vitro
  c. Measures the ribosome transfer rate during translation
  d. Detects the level of polymerases involved in replication
27. **Large quantities of useful products can be produced through genetic engineering involving:**
  a. Bacteria containing recombinant plasmids
  b. Transgenic plants
  c. Mammals producing substances in their milk
  d. All of the above
28. **The "sticky ends" generated by restriction enzymes allow:**
  a. Selection for plasmids lacking antibiotic resistance
  b. Easy identification of plasmids, which carry an insert
  c. Replication of transfer RNA within the bacterial cell
  d. Pieces of DNA from different sources to hybridize to each other and to be joined together

29. Most new mutations appear to be:
    a. Neutral or deleterious
    b. Present in homozygotes rather than heterozygotes
    c. Detectable using allozyme studies (protein electrophoresis)
    d. Present within pericentric inversions
30. All mitochondrial genomes analyzed to date are:
    a. Circular
    b. Linear
    c. <50 kb in size
    d. None of the above
31. Plasmids are molecules that:
    a. Are linear
    b. Are circular
    c. Are present in all bacteria
    d. Contain essential genes
32. Operons:
    a. Are characteristic for eukaryotic genomes
    b. Contain more than one gene
    c. Contain more than one promoter
    d. Contain always similar genes
33. Most genes are transcribed into:
    a. tRNAs
    b. mRNAs
    c. Ribosomal RNAs
    d. Small nuclear RNAs
34. Beta-sheets are stabilized by:
    a. Hydrophobic bonds
    b. Ionic bonds
    c. Hydrogen bonds
    d. Covalent bonds
35. Restriction endonucleases:
    a. Are located in the nucleus
    b. Degrade DNA completely
    c. Bind to DNA
    d. Were discovered in the 1980s
36. PCR is used for:
    a. Digesting DNA
    b. Copying plasmids
    c. Amplifying DNA
    d. Amplifying proteins
37. DNA polymerases:
    a. Join DNA fragments
    b. Replicate RNA
    c. Synthesize DNA in 5′-3′ direction
    d. Require ATP
38. Genome markers:
    a. Must occur as multiple alleles
    b. Must be repeat DNA sequences
    c. Can be any unique DNA sequence
    d. Are only used in genetic maps
39. Physical mapping:
    a. Requires large numbers of organisms
    b. Is always based on optical methods
    c. Can use DNA fragment libraries
    d. Uses polymorphic restriction sites
40. An RNA polymerase does the following:
    a. Joins together aligned RNA nucleotides during RNA synthesis
    b. Breaks down RNA into individual nucleotides
    c. Joins amino acids together that are bound to tRNA during protein synthesis
    d. Converts guanine to cytosine
41. Transcription is:
    a. The synthesis of protein in the cytoplasm from separate amino acids
    b. The synthesis of RNA in the nucleus from a DNA template
    c. The addition of sugars to proteins in glycoprotein synthesis
    d. The synthesis of enzymes from DNA template
42. Which of the following causes a gene mutation with decreased protein production?
    a. Missense
    b. Nonsense
    c. Point mutation
    d. None of the above
43. A 40-year-old man has Duke's C adenocarcinoma of the colon. There is a strong family history of colon cancer in the absence of polyps. What is the most likely genetic basis?
    a. Mismatch repair genes
    b. Ras
    c. Deletion in colon cancer
    d. *APC* gene
44. A boy with Duchenne muscular dystrophy (DMD) was born to parents with no family history of the disease. The most likely explanation for this occurrence is:
    a. A CGG expansion that resulted in the disruption of the promoter of the dystrophin gene
    b. Infidelity
    c. A point mutation in the dystrophin gene
    d. A recombination event in the dystrophin gene that gave rise to a frameshift mutation leading to an untranslatable mRNA

45. Which of the following(s) is/are found in genetic algorithms?
    i. Evolution
    ii. Selection
    iii. Reproduction
    iv. Mutation
    a. i and ii only
    b. i, ii, and iv only
    c. ii, iii, and iv only
    d. All of the above

Answers

1. d	2. a	3. c	4. c	5. d
6. b	7. c	8. b	9. c	10. a
11. b	12. b	13. b	14. a	15. a
16. d	17. a	18. c	19. d	20. b
21. a	22. d	23. b	24. b	25. a
26. b	27. d	28. d	29. a	30. d
31. b	32. b	33. b	34. c	35. c
36. c	37. c	38. c	39. c	40. a
41. b	42. b	43. d	44. d	45. d

CHAPTER 21

Organ Function Tests

OBJECTIVES
At the end of this chapter, students should be able to:
- Explain the functions performed by liver, kidney, thyroid, and adrenal gland
- Know about the list of biochemical tests performing to diagnose liver, kidney, thyroid, and adrenal disorders.

LIVER FUNCTION TESTS

Introduction
- Liver plays a major role in storing blood (acts as a reservoir of blood).
- The parenchymal cells of the liver are related to the breakdown of hemoglobin to bilirubin and the removal of pigments.
- It plays a central role in the metabolism:
  - Carbohydrates (glycogenesis, glycogenolysis, gluconeogenesis, and alcohol metabolism)
  - Proteins (transamination, oxidative deamination of amino acids, urea synthesis, and protein synthesis)
  - Lipids
  - Hormones
  - Vitamins
  - Bilirubin
  - Bile acids.
- The hepatobiliary tree represents hepatic cells and biliary tract cells **(Fig. 21.1).**
- Inflammation of the hepatic cells results in elevation of alanine aminotransferase or alanine transaminase (ALT), aspartate aminotransferase or aspartate transaminase (AST), and possibly the bilirubin.
- Inflammation of the biliary tract cells results predominantly in an elevation of the alkaline phosphatase (ALP).
- In liver disease, there are crossover between purely biliary disease and hepatocellular disease.
- To interpret these, the physician will look at the entire picture of the hepatocellular and biliary tract disease to determine which one is the primary abnormality.

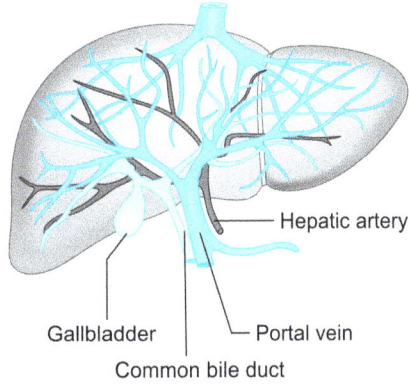

Fig. 21.1: Hepatobiliary tree representing hepatic cells and biliary tract cells.

Indications of Liver Function Test
- Liver function tests (LFTs) are useful in the differential diagnosis of jaundice.
- Detection of liver diseases.
- Assessment of severity and progress of liver disease.

Basic Processes in Liver Diseases

- *Liver cell damage:* This may vary from areas of local damage to destruction of most of the liver cells leading to liver failure.
  Causes: Acute hepatitis may be viral and chronic hepatitis is due to the continuing action of infective or toxic agents or that associated with autoimmune response.
- *Cirrhosis:* Destruction of hepatic cells.
- *Biliary tract involvement:* It is associated with obstruction to bile flow (cholestasis) and may present as obstructive jaundice.

There are two types of obstruction:
- *Intrahepatic cholestasis:* Mainly arises with liver cell destruction
  Causes: Viral hepatitis, use of steroids (during pregnancy or in the case of woman taking oral contraceptives)
- Extrahepatic cholestasis
  Causes: Gallstone in the common bile duct, carcinoma of the pancreas, and cirrhosis of the bile duct.

The LFTs are considered under the following categories:
- Tests, which indicate the liver cell damage, are:
  - AST
  - ALT.
- Tests indicating biliary tract involvement are:
  - ALP
  - Gamma-glutamyl transferase (GGT)
  - 5'-nucleotidase.
- Tests indicating impaired function are:
  - Serum proteins
  - Bilirubin.

Total Protein (Albumin and Globulin)

Albumin

The following list shows the information about albumin:
- Albumin is the major protein present within the blood.
- The liver synthesizes albumin.
- It represents a major synthetic protein and is a marker for the ability of the liver to synthesize proteins.
- It is one of the proteins synthesized by the liver. However, since it is easy to measure, it represents a reliable and inexpensive laboratory test for physicians to assess the degree of liver damage present in the particular patient. Albumin level goes down when liver gets severely damaged.
- Malnutrition can also cause low albumin with no associated liver disease.

Serum Total Protein Estimation

- Albumin estimation
- Globulin estimation.

Methods: The serum proteins are estimated by differential precipitation of albumin and globulin fraction:
- Biuret method
- Albumin by dye-binding method.

Serum Protein Electrophoresis

- This is an evaluation of the types of proteins present in serum.
- With an electrophoresis, major proteins can be separated and this results in four major types of proteins:
  1. Albumin
  2. α-globulins
  3. β-globulins
  4. γ-globulins.
- *Normal range:*
  - Total protein: 5.0–7.5 g/dL
  - Albumin: 3.5–4.5 g/dL
  - Globulin: 2–3 g/dL
  - γ-globulin: 0.5–1.5 g/dL.

Prothrombin Time

- Liver synthesizes clotting factors such as prothrombin, fibrinogen, factors V, VII, and X.
- The prothrombin time is prolonged in the cases of hepatocellular damage. The ability of the parenchymal cells to synthesize clotting factors is impaired.

Jaundice

The following list shows the information about jaundice:
- Jaundice comes from French word "jaune," which means yellow.
- Normal serum bilirubin is around 1.2 mg/100 mL.
- Whenever the level exceeds more than the normal range, it diffuses into the tissues and the skin and sclera of the eye turns yellow. This condition is called jaundice (icterus).
- The yellowish coloration is caused by an excess amount of bilirubin in the skin. Bilirubin is a yellowish-red pigment.
- Normally, small amounts of bilirubin are found in everyone's blood.
- When too much bilirubin is made, the excess is dumped into the bloodstream and is deposited in tissues for temporary storage.
- Jaundice in the infant appears first in the face and upper body and progresses downward toward the toes.

Formation and Metabolism of Bilirubin (Fig. 21.2)

Normal Values
- Total bilirubin = 0.2–1.0 mg%
- Direct bilirubin = 0–0.2 mg%
- Indirect bilirubin = 0–0.8 mg%.

There are three different types of jaundice:
1. Hemolytic jaundice
2. Hepatic jaundice
3. Obstructive or posthepatic jaundice.

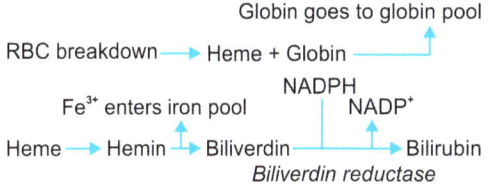

Fig. 21.2: Formation of bilirubin.

Causes and biochemical findings of different types of jaundice are given in **Table 21.1**.

van den Bergh's Reaction

Direct van den Bergh's Test
The conjugated water-soluble bilirubin when treated with diazo reagent [sodium nitrate ($NaNO_3$) + sulfanilic acid] gives red color immediately. This is called direct van den Bergh's test. The bilirubin reacting directly is also called direct bilirubin.

Indirect van den Bergh's Test
The water-insoluble unconjugated bilirubin gives a positive van den Bergh's test only if methanol is added to the serum. This is indirect van den Bergh's test. This is also called indirect bilirubin.

Urobilinogen in Urine and Feces
- The presence of urobilinogen in a test sample can be shown by a test based on the production of red color when urobilinogen reacts with Ehrlich's aldehyde reagent.
- In hemolytic jaundice, there is increased formation of bilirubin, excretion into the intestine through the bile; therefore there will be increased formation of urobilinogen in the intestine and increased level in the urine and feces.

Serum Enzymes in Liver Disease

The assay of serum enzymes is very useful in the differential diagnosis and monitoring of various hepatobiliary disorders.
- Enzymes, which are normally present inside the hepatocytes, released into the blood when there is hepatocellular damage—markers for hepatocellular damage (viral hepatitis, cirrhosis of the liver).
- Enzymes, which are primarily membrane bound (plasma membrane or side of hepatocytes)—markers for cholestasis.

Table 21.1: Causes and biochemical findings of different types of jaundice.

Features	Prehepatic/hemolytic	Hepatic	Posthepatic Obstructive
Causes	Abnormal red cells, antibodies, abnormal hemoglobin	Viral hepatitis, toxic hepatitis, intrahepatic cholestasis of bile duct, drugs and toxins	Extrahepatic cholestasis, gallstones, tumor of bile duct, carcinoma of pancreas
Blood			
Unconjugated bilirubin	Present (++)	Present (++)	Normal
Conjugated bilirubin	Normal	Increases in early phase and later decreases	Present (++)
Urine			
Urine bile salt (Hay's test)	Absent	Absent	Present
Conjugated bilirubin (Fouchet's test)	Absent	Present	Present
Urobilinogen (Ehrlich's test)	Present (+++)	Increases in early phase	Absent
Feces			
Urobilins	Present (++)	In intrahepatic cholestasis decreases	Clay colored
Serum enzymes			
ALP	Normal	Moderately increased	Increased markedly
Alanine aminotransferase or ALT	Normal	Increased markedly	Moderately increased
Aspartate aminotransferase or AST	Normal	Increased markedly	Moderately increased
GGT	Normal	Moderately increased	Increased markedly

(ALP: alkaline phosphatase; ALT: alanine transaminase; AST: aspartate transaminase; GGT: gamma-glutamyl transpeptidase)

Serum Transaminases: Aspartate Transaminase and Alanine Transaminase

- The ALT is specific for liver.
- Its level increases more than the normal in liver diseases (viral hepatitis, cirrhosis of the liver).
- But AST is not specific to liver, its level varies in other forms of tissue damage such as myocardial infarction, muscle necrosis, and renal disorders.

Alkaline Phosphatase

- The serum ALP estimation is the most widely used biochemical test to put in evidence for cholestasis of intrahepatic or extrahepatic origin.
- Normal level = 4–13 kA U or 40–140 IU/L.
- Increase in serum level of ALP from liver is a very sensitive indicator of cholestasis.
- Increased ALP level in cholestasis may be due to two features:
  a. Regurgitation of ALP from bile to blood
  b. Increased synthesis from the cells lining the biliary canaliculi.

Gamma-glutamyl Transferase Estimation

- The GGT enzyme catalyzes the transfer of γ-glutamyl group from glutamyl peptides to another peptide or an amino acid.

- It is a marker of cholestasis.
- The GGT level increases both in liver disease and in cholestasis but is very high in cholestasis.
- It is also considered as a marker enzyme in the patients of cirrhosis in chronic alcoholics. Normal value is 10–30 U/L.

Different Types of Viral Hepatitis

Different types of hepatitis are as follows:
- Hepatitis A caused by hepatitis A virus (HAV)
  Markers: HAV antigen (Ag), HAV antibody (Ab), and HAV immunoglobulin M (IgM)
- Hepatitis B caused by hepatitis B virus (HBV)
  Markers: HBV deoxyribonucleic acid, hepatitis B surface antigen (HBsAg), hepatitis B e-antigen (HBeAg), hepatitis B core antigen, antibody to HBsAg (anti-HBs), antibody to HBeAg (anti-HBe), HBc IgM, and HBc immunoglobulin G (IgG)
- Hepatitis C caused by hepatitis C virus (HCV)
  Markers: HCV ribonucleic acid (RNA) qualitative, HCV RNA quantitative, and anti-HCV
- Hepatitis D caused by hepatitis delta virus (HDV)
  Markers: HDV Ag, HDV RNA (polymerase chain reaction), HDV IgG, HDV IgM, and HDV total (IgG + IgM)
- Hepatitis E caused by hepatitis E virus (HEV)
  Markers: HEV Ag, HEV IgG, HEV IgM, and HEV Ab (total).

RENAL FUNCTION TESTS

- Kidneys are the very important and vital organs.
- They perform many important functions to regulate the internal environment of the human body.
- They are the main regulators of all the substances of body fluids and responsible for maintaining homeostasis.

Functions of Kidney

The functional unit of a kidney is nephron (**Fig. 21.3**). Kidney has five important functions:
1. Urine formation
2. Regulation of fluid and electrolyte balance
3. Regulation of acid–base balance
4. Hormonal function
5. Excretion of nonprotein nitrogen (NPN) substances.

Kidney function tests are grouped under two headings:
1. The tests measuring glomerular filtration rate (GFR)
2. Creatinine clearance test.

It is the volume of plasma completely cleared off creatinine, which is excreted in the urine:

$$\text{Creatinine clearance} = \frac{U \times V}{P} \text{ or } \frac{U \times V \times 1.73/A}{P}$$

where

U = urine creatinine
P = plasma creatinine
1.73 = generally accepted body surface area
A = body surface area of the patient under investigation.

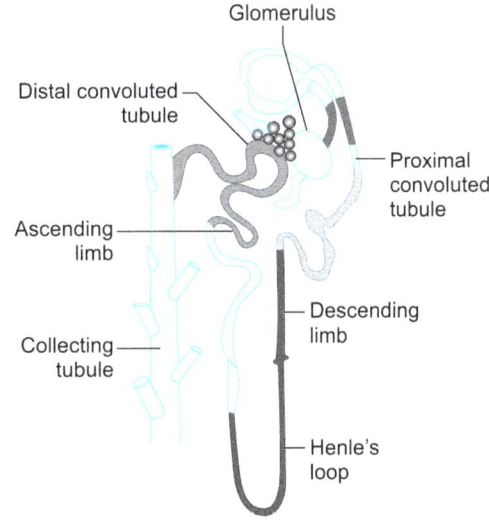

Fig. 21.3: Structure of nephron.

- The creatinine clearance is very convenient to measure GFR.
- It is fulfilling all the requirement of the substance, which is ideal for measuring GFR.
- The amount of creatinine produced is relatively constant and also it is not affected by the dietary intake.

Normal Values

- Male: 105 + 20 mL/min
- Female: 95 + 20 mL/min.

Clinical Significance

Abnormal results are lower than normal GFR measurements and they indicate:
- Acute tubular necrosis
- Congestive heart failure
- Dehydration
- Glomerulonephritis
- Shock
- Acute nephrotic syndrome
- Acute and chronic renal failure.

Study of Elimination of Nonprotein Nitrogen Substances

Study of elimination of NPN substances: Tests measuring the retention of NPN substances in serum such as determination of urea, uric acid, creatinine, amino acids, and ammonia.

Urea

- Urea constitutes about 45% of NPN substances.
- Study of their elimination can be done with blood and urine.
- One of the methods available for the determination of urea is diacetyl monoxime method.

Normal Values

Serum/plasma urea:
- 15–45 mg/dL
- 2.49–7.47 mmol/dL
- Blood urea nitrogen: 7–21 mg/dL.

Clinical Significance

Causes for urea increase are:
- *Prerenal causes:*
  - Cardiac decompensation
  - Water depletion due to decreased intake or excessive loss
  - Increased protein breakdown.
- Renal causes are acute glomerulonephritis (AGN):
  - Chronic nephritis
  - Polycystic kidney
  - Nephrosclerosis
  - Tubular necrosis.
- *Postrenal causes:* Any obstruction to urine flow (stone, tumor, and enlarged prostate).

Normal Value

The normal value of urea is 15–35 mg%.

Creatinine

- Creatinine is a breakdown product of creatine, which is an important part of muscle.
- The most important source of energy inside cells is the adenosine triphosphate (ATP) molecule, with its high-energy phosphate bonds.
- When one of these bonds is broken, energy is released and ATP becomes adenosine diphosphate (ADP).
- Creatine phosphate represents a backup energy source for ATP because it can quickly reconvert ADP back to ATP.
- Over time, the creatine molecule gradually degrades to creatinine.
- It is a waste product, i.e. it cannot be used by cells for any constructive purpose.
- The daily production of creatine and subsequently creatinine depends on muscle mass, which fluctuates little in most normal people over long periods of time.
- It is excreted from the body entirely by the kidneys.

- With normal kidney function, the serum creatinine level should remain constant and normal.

Normal Value
- 0.8–1.4 mg/dL
- Normal value ranges may vary slightly among different laboratories.

Clinical Significance
- Higher than normal levels may indicate:
  - Nephrotic syndrome
  - Chronic glomerulonephritis
  - Acute tubular necrosis
  - Dehydration
  - Diabetic nephropathy
  - Reduced renal blood flow
  - Pyelonephritis
  - Renal failure
  - Urinary tract obstruction.
- Lower than normal levels may indicate:
  - Muscular dystrophy (late stage)
  - Myasthenia gravis.

Uric Acid

Normal Value
The normal value of uric acid is 2.5–7 mg%.

Clinical Significance
Value increases in:
- Renal failure
- Acute gout
- Pneumonia
- Sepsis
- Leukemia
- Polycythemia vera
- Anemia.
  Value decreases in acromegaly.

Tests Measuring Tubular Function
- Excretory function test
- Tests to measure the concentrating and diluting ability are:
  - Specific gravity determination
  - Osmolality determination.

Calcium and Phosphorus
In chronic renal failure, there is impaired excretion of phosphate and progressive hyperphosphatemia occurs. This results in the decreased plasma calcium concentration giving rise to secondary hyperparathyroidism.

Determination of Amino Acids
- Amino acids are a part of NPN.
- Their determination is helpful only in some congenital renal disorders.
- If there is defect in reabsorption, more amino acid will appear in the urine, this condition is called aminoaciduria, e.g. cystinuria and homocystinuria.

Aminoaciduria
Aminoaciduria may be two types:
1. Primary aminoaciduria is due to an inherited enzyme deficiency, this is also called inborn error of metabolism. The defect is located in the pathway by which amino acid is metabolized or in the renal tubular system by which the amino acid is absorbed.
2. Secondary aminoaciduria may be due to disease of the liver or renal tubular dysfunction, or protein energy malnutrition. In both the conditions, metabolites of amino acids accumulated in the blood are excreted in the urine. There are several tests to detect these amino acids and their metabolites in the urine.

Pathological Conditions of the Kidney

Acute Glomerulonephritis
Acute glomerulonephritis is an acute inflammation of the glomeruli, which results in:
- Oliguria
- Hematuria
- Proteinuria

- Anemia
- Increased blood urea and creatinine
- Decreased GFR.

The presence of red blood cells (RBCs) in the urine is an insufficient evidence for AGN as the appearance of blood may be from urinary tract.

Nephrotic Syndrome

- Nephrotic syndrome is a clinical entity characterized by massive proteinuria, edema, hypoalbuminemia, hyperlipidemia, and lipiduria.
- The syndrome has multiple causes.
- Increased membrane permeability leads to massive proteinuria (mainly albumin loss). There will be reduction in plasma osmotic pressure and the fluid movement from vascular to interstitial space that leads to edema.

Tubular Disease

- Proximal renal tubular acidosis [reduced proximal tubular bicarbonate (HCO_3) reabsorption]
- *Distal renal tubular acidosis:* There is an inability of tubular cells to create and maintain the usual pH difference between tubular and blood.

Urinary Tract Infection

- Infection may occur in the bladder (cystitis) or it may involve the kidneys.
- Diagnosis is made by the presence of bacterial concentration of more than 1 lakh colonies/mL of urine.

THYROID FUNCTION TESTS

The function of the thyroid gland is to take iodine found in many foods and convert it into thyroid hormones, i.e. thyroxine (T4) and triiodothyronine (T3).

Thyroid cells are the only cells in the body, which can absorb iodine. These cells combine iodine and the amino acid tyrosine to make T3 and T4. Then the T3 and T4 are released into the bloodstream and are transported throughout the body where they control metabolism. Most of the cells in the body depend upon thyroid hormones for regulation of their metabolism:

- The hypothalamus, pituitary gland, and the thyroid all play a part in the feedback and regulatory mechanisms involved in the production of T4 and T3 from the thyroid gland.
- Thyroid-releasing hormone (TRH) is secreted by the hypothalamus and stimulates the production of the polypeptide thyroid-stimulating hormone (TSH) from the anterior pituitary.
- The TSH then stimulates the production and release of T4 and T3 from the thyroid.
- Once released, T4 and T3 then exert a negative feedback mechanism on TSH production.
- T4 is the main hormone produced by the thyroid.
- T3 is mainly produced by peripheral conversion of T4.
- T3 and T4 both act via nuclear receptors to increase cell metabolism.
- The normal thyroid gland produces about 80% T4 and about 20% T3; however, T3 possesses about four times the hormone "strength" than T4.
- The 70–80% of T3 and T4 are transported in plasma by a thyroid-binding globulin (TBG), a plasma protein.
- The remaining 20–30% of T3 and T4 are transported by T4-binding prealbumin and albumin.
- Only the unbound or "free" portion [free T3 and T4 (FT3 and FT4)] is active.
- It is the free portion of the thyroid hormones, which is the true determinant of the thyroid status of the patient.
- The evaluation of the thyroid status is not a simple procedure because it does not depend mainly on the measurement of circulating thyroid hormones.

- The one or more factors may be abnormal and they are:
  - The TBG concentration and its degree of saturation with T3 and T4
  - Concentration of FT3 and FT4
  - The state of the hypothalamus and anterior pituitary with their respective outputs of TRH and TSH
  - The response of pituitary to TRH and response of the thyroid gland.

Thyroid disease is common, presents with many nonspecific symptoms, so it needs to be considered in many differentials, and once diagnosed, it needs to be regularly monitored for therapy. As a consequence, TFTs are the most commonly used endocrine test. Therefore laboratory investigations of thyroid functions are useful in distinguishing patients with euthyroidism from those with hyperthyroidism and hypothyroidism.

Common Thyroid Problems

The common thyroid problems are as follows:
- *Goiters:* A thyroid goiter is an enlargement of the thyroid gland. Goiters are often removed because of cosmetic reasons or more commonly because they compress other vital structures of the neck, including the trachea and the esophagus making breathing and swallowing difficult. Sometimes goiters actually grow into the chest, where they can cause trouble as well.
- *Thyroid cancer:* It is a fairly common malignancy; however, the vast majorities have excellent long-term survival.
- *Solitary thyroid nodules:* There are several characteristics of solitary nodules of the thyroid, which make them suspicious for malignancy. Although as many as 50% of the population will have a nodule somewhere in their thyroid, the overwhelming majority of these are benign. Occasionally, thyroid nodules can take on characteristics of malignancy and require either a needle biopsy or surgical excision.
- *Hyperthyroidism:* It means too much thyroid hormone. Current methods used for treating a hyperthyroid patient are radioactive iodine, antithyroid drugs, or surgery. Each method has advantages and disadvantages and is selected for individual patients.
- *Hypothyroidism:* It means too little thyroid hormone and is a common problem. In fact, hypothyroidism is often present for a number of years before it is recognized and treated. Hypothyroidism can even be associated with pregnancy.
- *Thyroiditis:* It is an inflammatory process ongoing within the thyroid gland. Thyroiditis can present with a number of symptoms such as fever and pain, but it can also present as subtle findings of hypo- or hyperthyroidism.

Tests for Thyroid Function

The thyroid function tests are grouped into two types:
1. The in vitro tests are:
   - Total serum T3 and T4
   - Free serum T3 and T4
   - Blood TBG
   - Resin uptake test
   - Serum TSH
   - Thyroid autoantibodies.
2. In vivo tests are:
   - Thyroid iodine uptake
   - TRH stimulation test
   - TSH stimulation test.

Total Serum T3 and T4 Determination by Immunoassay (Radioimmunoassay or Enzyme-linked Immunosorbent Assay) and Chemiluminescence Method

Immunoassay and chemiluminescence method are direct measurements of the total T3 and T4 in the blood. The serum T4 assays are more reliable than T3, because it is the major secretory product of thyroid gland.

The majority of the T3 comes from peripheral deiodination of T4. This test mainly helps to rule out hyperthyroidism and hypothyroidism. Radioimmunoassay (RIA) or enzyme-linked immunosorbent assay is the choice.

Normal range
- T4 = 5–12.5 µg/dL
- T3 = 80–180 ng/dL
- TSH = 0.27–4.20 microIU/mL.

Clinical significance
- Value increased in hyperthyroidism and decreased in hypothyroidism.
- The values also decreased in when TBG concentration goes down due to loss in urine and liver disease.

Free T3 and T4 Determination

This is a measure of circulatory T4 and T3 that exists in the free form in the blood. The free thyroid hormone concentration is independent of changes in the concentration and affinity of thyroid-binding proteins and provides more reliable means of diagnosing thyroid dysfunction than measurement of total T3 and T4 hormones.

Normal values
- FT4 = 10–27 pmol/L
- FT3 = 3–9 pmol/L.

Clinical significance
Value increased in hyperthyroidism and thyrotoxicosis and decreased in hypothyroidism.

Hyperthyroidism

Hyperthyroidism occurs as a consequence of excessive thyroid hormone activity. Common causes include thyroiditis, Graves' disease, and toxic nodular goiter.

Diagnosis

- The initial laboratory investigation with a possible diagnosis of hyperthyroidism should be a sensitive serum TSH assay, which will show reduced circulating levels of TSH.
- Low serum TSH is not specific for hyperthyroidism. It may also occur with "nonthyroidal illness" or with the use of some commonly prescribed drugs.
- Patients who have a low TSH may then go on to have further investigations such as (Table 21.2):
  a. *FT4 and FT3 assays:* A subnormal TSH should trigger the measurement of FT4. If this is not elevated, FT3 should be measured to identify cases of T3-thyrotoxicosis.

Table 21.2: Differentiating causes of reduced thyroid-stimulating hormone (TSH) or raised free thyroxine (FT4) or triiodothyronine (FT3).

Conditions	TSH	FT4	FT3	Other investigations
Graves' disease	Reduced ++	Usually raised	Usually raised	*Thyroid scan:* Diffuse isotope uptake; thyroid peroxidase antibodies
Toxic multinodular goiter	Reduced	Raised or normal	Raised or normal	*Thyroid scan:* Functioning nodule with suppression of other tissue
Thyroiditis	Reduced Increased	Increased	Increased	*Thyroid scan:* Low radioiodine uptake thyroglobulin level, markedly raised ESR; often raised
Pregnancy	Normal	Raised total T4 Normal FT4	Raised total T3 Normal FT3	Positive pregnancy test
Thyroxine-induced hyperthyroidism	Reduced	Raised	Raised or normal	*Thyroid scan:* Low radioiodine uptake, thyroglobulin levels absent

(ESR: erythrocyte sedimentation rate)

b. Thyroid autoantibodies, e.g. thyroid peroxidase antibodies and TSH receptor antibodies.
c. *Radioactive iodine uptake:* Thyroid scanning with either iodine-131 (most frequent) or ^{99m}Tc helps to determine cause of hypothyroidism, e.g. diffuse pattern of uptake in Graves' disease compared to one or more "hot" nodules in toxic nodular hyperthyroidism.

Hypothyroidism

- Primary hypothyroidism occurs as a result of undersecretion of thyroid hormone from the thyroid gland.
- Causes include Hashimoto's thyroiditis, irradiation, and drugs such as lithium.

Secondary hypothyroidism may occur as a result of damage or disease of the pituitary or hypothalamus.

Diagnosis

- To diagnose primary hypothyroidism, it is needed to measure both TSH and FT4. Where TSH is more than 10 mU/L and FT4 below reference range, the diagnosis is overt primary hypothyroidism and the patient needs treatment with thyroid replacement therapy.
- Secondary hypothyroidism is suggested by low within or mildly elevated TSH combined with a low FT4. Differentiating this from nonthyroidal illness can be difficult; and clinical history, FT3, and sometimes anterior pituitary hormone tests are necessary.

3. Additional diagnostic tests may include:
   - Thyroid autoantibodies—antithyroid peroxidase and antithyroglobulin antibodies
   - Thyroid scan.

Subclinical Disease

Subclinical thyroid disease is common in American population. Diagnosis is based solely on test results and when to treat subclinical disease is contentious.

Subclinical Hyperthyroidism

- Is diagnosed by low serum TSH, normal FT4 and FT3, in the absence of nonthyroidal illness or relevant drug therapy **(Table 21.3)**.
- May increase risk of developing atrial fibrillation and cardiovascular disease (CVD).
- The TFTs should be repeated at 3–6 months or earlier if elderly, or if patient has preexisting CVD, to determine whether full-blown hyperthyroidism has developed or if the subclinical picture has persisted.

Subclinical Hypothyroidism

- Occurs where TSH is above reference range with a normal FT4.
- Diagnosis should be confirmed with repeat TFTs after 3–6 months.
- Where TSH is less than 10 mU/L, there is no consistent evidence of association with symptoms, hyperlipidemias, or increased risk of CVD. Above this level, there is more evidence of progression to overt thyroid disease and worsening hyperlipidemia.

Table 21.3: Differentiating causes of raised thyroid-stimulating hormone (TSH) or raised free thyroxine (FT4) or triiodothyronine (FT3).

Conditions	TSH	FT4	FT3	Other investigations
Chronic thyroiditis	Normal or raised	Normal or reduced	Normal or reduced	Thyroid nodules occur relatively frequently with this condition and have a 5% risk of malignancy
Hashimoto's thyroiditis	Usually raised	Normal or reduced	Normal or reduced	High titers of autoantibodies in 95%
Sick euthyroid syndrome	Normal or low	Reduced	Normal or reduced	Autoantibodies not present

- Thyroxin therapy is not recommended unless TSH more than 10 mU/L or, below this, if patients are pregnant, have a goiter, or are trying to conceive.

Thyroid-binding Globulin

- Most of the thyroid hormones in the blood are attached to a protein called TBG. If there is an excess or deficiency of this protein, it alters the T4 or T3 measurement but does not affect the action of the hormone. If a patient appears to have normal thyroid function, but an unexplained high or low T4, or T3, it may be due to an increase or decrease of TBG. Direct measurement of TBG can be done and will explain the abnormal value. Excess TBG or low levels of TBG are found in some families as a hereditary trait. These people are frequently misdiagnosed as being hyperthyroid or hypothyroid, but they have no thyroid problem and need no treatment.
- *Normal value:* 12–28 µg/mL.
- TBG value increased in hypothyroidism, pregnancy, and estrogen therapy.
- TBG value decreased in hyperthyroidism, nephrotic syndrome, and liver disease.

Measurement of Pituitary Production of Thyroid-stimulating Hormone

- Pituitary production of TSH is measured by a method referred to as RIA.
- Normally, low levels (<5 U) of TSH are sufficient to keep the normal thyroid gland functioning properly.
- When the thyroid gland becomes inefficient such as in early hypothyroidism, the TSH becomes elevated even though the T4 and T3 may still be within the "normal" range.
- This rise in TSH represents the pituitary glands' response to a drop in circulating thyroid hormone; it is usually the first indication of thyroid gland failure. Since TSH is normally low when the thyroid gland is functioning properly, the failure of TSH to rise when circulating thyroid hormones are low is an indication of impaired pituitary function.
- The new "sensitive" TSH test will show very low levels of TSH when the thyroid is overactive (as a normal response of the pituitary to try to decrease thyroid stimulation). Interpretations of the TSH level depend upon the level of thyroid hormone; therefore the TSH is usually used in combination with other thyroid tests such as the T4 RIA and T3 RIA.

Thyroid-releasing Hormone Test

- In normal people, TSH secretion from the pituitary can be increased by giving a shot containing TRH.
- A baseline TSH of five or less usually goes up to 10–20 after giving an injection of TRH. Patients with too much thyroid hormone (T4 or T3) will not show a rise in TSH when given TRH.
- This "TRH test" is presently the most sensitive test in detecting early hyperthyroidism. Patients who show too much response to TRH (TSH rises greater than 40) may be suffering from hypothyroidism.
- This test is also used in cancer patients who are taking thyroid replacement to see if they are on sufficient medication. It is sometimes used to measure if the pituitary gland is functioning.
- The new "sensitive" TSH test (above) has eliminated the necessity of performing a TRH test in most clinical situations.

Thyroid Iodine Uptake Scan

A means of measuring thyroid function is to measure how much iodine is taken up by the thyroid gland. Remember, cells of the thyroid normally absorb iodine from our bloodstream (obtained from foods we eat) and use it to make thyroid hormone. Hypothyroid patients usually take up too little iodine, while hyperthyroid patients take up too much iodine. The test is performed by giving a dose of radioactive iodine on an empty stomach. The iodine is concentrated in the thyroid gland or excreted in the urine over the next few hours. The amount of iodine that goes into the thyroid gland can be measured by a "thyroid uptake." At other times, the gland will concentrate iodine normally, but it will be unable to convert the iodine into thyroid hormone; therefore interpretation of the iodine uptake is usually done in conjunction with blood tests.

Thyroid Scan

Taking a "picture" of how well the thyroid gland is functioning requires giving a radioisotope to the patient and letting the thyroid gland concentrate the isotope. Therefore it is usually done at the same time that the iodine uptake test is performed. Although other isotopes such as technetium will be concentrated by the thyroid gland; these isotopes will not measure iodine uptake, which is what we really want to know because the production of thyroid hormone is dependent upon absorbing iodine. All scans are now done with radioactive iodine. Pregnant women should not have thyroid scans performed because the iodine can cause development troubles within the baby's thyroid gland.

ADRENAL GLAND

The adrenal gland comprises cortex and medulla.

Cortex has again three zones (**Fig. 21.4**):
1. Zona glomerulosa → produces mineralocorticoids.
2. Zona fasciculata → produces glucocorticoids.
3. Zona reticularis → secretes sex steroids such as androgens and estrogens.

Assessment of Glucocorticoid Secretion

The plasma or serum cortisol level determination is one of the methods for assessing the secretion of glucocorticoids.

Normal value
- 8–26 µg/dL at am (250–850 nmol/L)
- 5–18 µg/dL at pm (110–390 nmol/L).

Control of cortisol secretion

Cortisol and other glucocorticoids are secreted in response to a single stimulator: adrenocorticotropic hormone (ACTH) from the anterior pituitary. ACTH is itself secreted under control of the hypothalamic peptide corticotropin-releasing hormone (CRH). The central nervous system is thus the commander and chief of glucocorticoid responses, providing an excellent example of

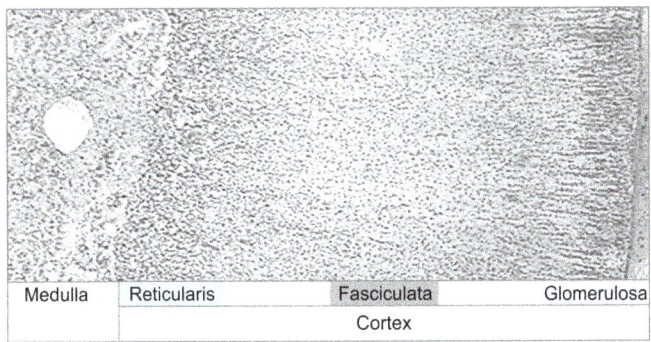

Fig. 21.4: Histology of adrenal gland.

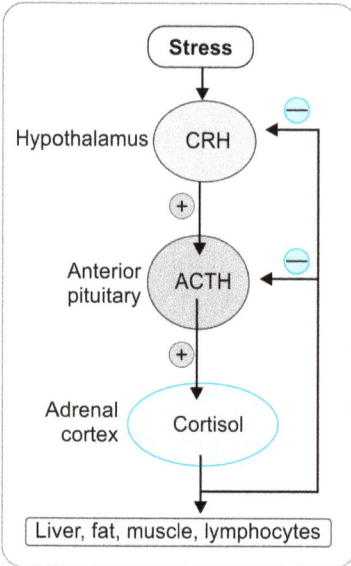

Fig. 21.5: Synthesis of cortisol.
(CRH: corticotropin-releasing hormone; ACTH: adrenocorticotropic hormone)

close integration between the nervous and endocrine systems **(Fig. 21.5)**.

PATHOPHYSIOLOGY

Addison's Disease (Adrenal Insufficiency)

Addison's disease is a rare endocrine or hormonal disorder that occurs in all age groups.

In this condition, the adrenal gland reduces insufficient amounts of steroid hormones (glucocorticoids and often mineralocorticoids).

The disease is also called adrenal insufficiency, or hypocortisolism.

Causes

- Failure to produce adequate levels of cortisol can occur for different reasons. The problem may be due to a disorder of the adrenal glands themselves (primary adrenal insufficiency):
  - Destruction of the adrenal glands by infection
  - Their destruction by an autoimmune attack.
- Inadequate secretion of ACTH by the pituitary gland (secondary adrenal insufficiency).

Adrenocorticotropic Hormone Stimulation Test

This is the most specific test for diagnosing Addison's disease. In this test, blood cortisol, urine cortisol, or both are measured before and after a synthetic form of ACTH is given by injection. In the so-called short, or rapid, ACTH test, measurement of cortisol in blood is repeated 30–60 minutes after an intravenous ACTH injection. The normal response after an injection of ACTH is a rise in blood and urine cortisol levels. Patients with either form of adrenal insufficiency respond poorly or do not respond at all.

Cushing's Syndrome

Cushing's syndrome is a hormonal disorder caused by prolonged exposure of the body's tissues to high levels of the hormone cortisol.

In Cushing's syndrome, the level of adrenal hormones, especially of the glucocorticoids (cortisol), is too high.

Causes

- Excessive production of ACTH by the anterior lobe of the pituitary.
- Excessive production of adrenal hormones themselves (e.g. because of a tumor).
- *Ectopic ACTH syndrome:* Some benign or malignant tumors that arise outside the pituitary can produce ACTH. This condition is known as ectopic ACTH syndrome. Lung tumors cause over 50% of these cases.
- As a result of glucocorticoid therapy for some other disorder such as rheumatoid

arthritis or decreased glucocorticoid hormone synthesis.

Symptoms

- Hyperglycemia.
- High blood pressure.
- Severe protein catabolism results in thinning of skin, muscle wasting, osteoporosis, and negative nitrogen balance.
- There is a peculiar redistribution of fat in trunks.
- Moon face.
- Central obesity and typical buffalo hump.
- Resistant to infection and inflammatory response is impaired.
- Facial hair growth.

24-hour Urinary Free Cortisol Level

This is the most specific diagnostic test. The patient's urine is collected over a 24-hour period and tested for the amount of cortisol. If the cortisol level is higher than 50–100 µg a day for an adult suggests Cushing's syndrome. The normal range may vary from lab to lab depending on the techniques they use.

Dexamethasone Suppression Test

This test is used to distinguish patients with excess production of ACTH due to pituitary adenomas from those with ectopic ACTH-producing tumors. Patients are given dexamethasone, a synthetic glucocorticoid, by mouth every 6 hours for 4 days. For the first 2 days, low doses of dexamethasone are given, and for the last 2 days, higher doses are given. 24-hour urine sample collections are made before dexamethasone is administered on each day of the test. Since cortisol and other glucocorticoids signal the pituitary to lower secretion of ACTH, the normal response after taking dexamethasone is a drop in blood and urine cortisol levels. Different responses of cortisol to dexamethasone are obtained depending on whether the cause of Cushing's syndrome is a pituitary adenoma or an ectopic ACTH-producing tumor.

The dexamethasone suppression test can produce false-positive results in patients with depression, alcohol abuse, high estrogen levels, acute illness, and stress. Conversely, drugs such as phenytoin and phenobarbital may cause false-negative results in response to dexamethasone suppression. For this reason, patients are usually advised by their physicians to stop taking these drugs at least 1 week before the test.

Corticotropin-releasing Hormone Stimulation Test

This test helps to distinguish between patients with pituitary adenomas and those with ectopic ACTH syndrome or cortisol-secreting adrenal tumors. Patients are given an injection of CRH, the CRH, which causes the pituitary to secrete ACTH. Patients with pituitary adenomas usually experience a rise in blood levels of ACTH and cortisol. This response is rarely seen in patients with ectopic ACTH syndrome and practically never in patients with cortisol-secreting adrenal tumors.

Mineralocorticoids

- **It is a steroid hormone and mainly derived from the cholesterol.**
- The mineralocorticoids get their name from their effect on mineral metabolism. The most important of them is the steroid **aldosterone**.
- Aldosterone acts on the kidney promoting the reabsorption of sodium ions (Na^+) into the blood.
- Water follows the salt and this helps maintain normal blood pressure.
- Aldosterone also acts on sweat glands to reduce the loss of sodium in perspiration.
- It acts on taste cells to increase the sensitivity of the taste buds to sources of sodium.

- The secretion of aldosterone is stimulated by:
  - A drop in the level of sodium ions in the blood
  - A rise in the level of potassium ions in the blood
  - Angiotensin II
  - ACTH.

Primary Aldosteronism or Cohn's Syndrome

- Results from an aldosterone-secreting tumor, which leads to elevated levels of plasma aldosterone.
- The plasma pH in this condition increases because of hypokalemic alkalosis and the plasma osmolality also increases.

Adrenal Medulla

Secretes

- Dopamine
- Adrenaline (epinephrine)
- Noradrenaline (norepinephrine).

Functions

- The adrenal medulla consists of masses of neurons that are part of the sympathetic branch of the autonomic nervous system.
- Instead of releasing their neurotransmitters at a synapse, these neurons release them into the blood. Thus although part of the nervous system, the adrenal medulla functions as an endocrine gland.

SUMMARY

This chapter deals with the liver function, renal function, and thyroid function tests. Liver plays a major role in the metabolism. There is no single test to detect the abnormality of the liver because of the variety of the functions performed by the liver. Therefore there are group of tests available to detect the abnormality of the liver. Detection of total protein, albumin, aspartate transaminase, alanine transaminase, bilirubin, and GGT helps in the diagnosis of liver diseases and to diagnose the jaundice. Renal function tests performed to detect the diseases of the kidney. The kidneys perform many important functions to regulate the internal environment of the human body. It is the main regulator of all the substances of body fluids and responsible for maintaining homeostasis. The major functions of the kidney are urine formation, regulation of fluid and electrolyte balance, regulation of acid-base balance, hormonal function, and excretion of nonprotein nitrogen substances. The serum urea and creatinine determination help to detect the abnormal function of the kidneys. Thyroid function tests help to diagnose the thyroid disorders. Thyroid gland secretes T3 and T4 upon stimulation by thyroid-stimulating hormone. The reduced level of thyroid hormones is called hypothyroidism (goiter, Hashimoto's thyroiditis). The high level of thyroid hormones (hyperthyroidism) is seen in Graves' disease, thyroiditis, and toxic multinodular goiter. Thyroid iodine uptake scan will be done to measure how much iodine is taken up by the thyroid gland. Adrenal gland comprises medulla and cortex. The cortex has three regions such as zona glomerulosa that secretes mineralocorticoids (aldosterone), zona fasciculata that secretes glucocorticoids, and zona reticularis that secretes sex steroids. Adrenal medulla secretes dopamine, epinephrine, and norepinephrine. There are several tests done to detect the functions of adrenal gland, e.g. adrenocorticotropic hormone stimulation and dexamethasone suppression test. Elevated level of glucocorticoids results in Cushing's syndrome, whereas reduced level leads to Addison's disease.

SELF-ASSESSMENT QUESTIONS

1. List the tests under LFT panel.
2. What are the indications of LFT?
3. What are the functions performed by the liver?
4. Name the tests related to protein metabolism.
5. Give the normal values for:
   a. Total protein
   b. Albumin
   c. Alanine transaminase
   d. Aspartate transaminase
   e. Total bilirubin
   f. Direct bilirubin.
6. Write the flow chart to show the formation of bilirubin from the RBC.
7. What are the steps involved during the bilirubin excretion?
8. Mention the conditions in which bilirubin metabolism and excretion are disturbed.
9. Define jaundice.
10. What are the different types of jaundice?
11. Write the biochemical findings of any two types of jaundice.
12. What is direct and indirect van den Bergh's test?
13. Which test is used to find the bilirubin in the urine? Write its procedure.
14. Why bile salts sink to the bottom of the solution if it is present in the urine?
15. Which enzymes are considered as marker enzymes for hepatocellular damage?
16. Mention the enzymes, which are used as marker enzymes to detect the cholestasis.
17. How many isoenzyme forms of ALP are there?
18. Give the normal value of ALP.
19. Name the functions performed by the kidney.
20. List the tests under renal function test (RFT).
21. Define creatinine clearance.
22. Give the formula to calculate creatinine clearance.
23. Give the procedure for performing creatinine clearance.
24. Why creatinine is selected for measuring GFR?
25. Mention the conditions in which creatinine clearance decreases.
26. Write the normal values for the following:
    a. Urea
    b. Creatinine
    c. Uric acid
27. Mention the causes in which urea level decreases.
28. Write short notes on:
    a. Nephrotic syndrome
    b. Glomerulonephritis
29. Which tests are used to identify the amino acids?
30. Give the normal creatinine clearance value.

MULTIPLE-CHOICE QUESTIONS

1. **Which of the following enzyme elevated in obstructive jaundice?**
   a. AST
   b. ALP
   c. ALT
   d. LDH
2. **The electrophoresis of serum from liver cirrhosis shows:**
   a. Beta-gamma bridging
   b. Presence of M band
   c. Increased alpha-2 globulin and decreased albumin
   d. Increased albumin and decreased alpha-1 globulin
3. **All the following are the tests used to detect renal function, *except*:**
   a. Uric acid determination
   b. Urea determination
   c. Creatinine determination
   a. Bilirubin determination
4. **Which of the following is *incorrect* concerning renal failure?**
   a. The AST elevated
   b. The serum creatinine elevated
   c. Hyperphosphatemia seen
   d. The serum protein decreased
5. **Which of following is a best marker enzyme for alcoholic cirrhosis?**
   a. ALP
   b. AST
   c. GGT
   d. ALT
6. **Concerning nephrotic syndrome:**
   a. It is characterized by edema
   b. Patient loses globulin in the urine
   c. Patient serum will show very high protein
   d. Patient does not show any symptoms
7. **Which of the following will be elevated in liver disease?**
   a. ALP
   b. Lipase
   c. Amylase
   d. AST
8. **All the following are the symptoms of hyperthyroidism, *except*:**
   a. Rapid heart rate
   b. Inability to sleep
   c. Weight loss
   d. Sensitivity to cold

9. Which of the following is *not* a Biochemical finding of primary hypothyroidism?
   a. Reduced TSH
   b. Reduced T3
   c. Reduced T4
   d. Increased TSH
10. Which of the following elevated in the neonatal jaundice?
    a. Indirect bilirubin
    b. Direct bilirubin
    c. ALP
    d. AST

Answers

1. b   2. a   3. c   4. a   5. c
6. a   7. d   8. d   9. a   10. a

CASE STUDIES

1. A 30-year-old man was admitted to a hospital following episodes of nausea, vomiting, and abdominal pain. Upon examination it was discovered that his kidneys were slightly enlarged. Then the physician requested his blood investigation. Following results were obtained from the clinical biochemistry laboratory:

Fasting blood sugar	85 mg/dL
Blood urea	80 mg/dL
Creatinine	6.0 mg/dL
Uric acid	7.0 mg%
Serum osmolality	380 mOsm/kg
Inorganic phosphorous	3.5 mg%
Potassium	6.0 mEq/L

   1. What is the most likely diagnosis?
   2. How would you make a definite diagnosis?
   3. Can the diagnosis made using the NPN substance values?

2. A 12-year-old female child was brought to the hospital with symptoms of vomiting, anorexia, and a sign of swollen face. The pediatrician admitted the child and after physical examination requested for blood and urine tests.
   Results of laboratory test are as follows:

Laboratory test	Result
Total serum protein	5.0 g/dL
Albumin	2.5 g/dL
Globulins	3.0 g/dL
Urine osmolality	1,200 mOsm/kg H_2O
Urine albumin	Very high

   a. What is the probable diagnosis to be done with the available laboratory results?
   b. How would you make a definite diagnosis?
   c. What is the pathophysiology of this disorder?

3. A 70-year-old man who lived alone was discovered by his friend in a drowsy, confused state. On admission he was extremely dirty and his tongue was dry. Immediately he was given some saline through intravenously. After some time, the doctor requested for blood tests that revealed the following results:

Sodium	141 mEq/L (normal)
Potassium	5.7 mEq/L (elevated)
Chloride	107 mEq/L (elevated)
Creatinine clearance	80 mL/min (reduced)
Urea	70 mg/dL (elevated)
Creatinine	4.0 mg/dL

   a. What is the likely cause of her symptoms?
   b. What is the likely diagnosis?
   c. How would you make a definite diagnosis?

4. An 8-year-old child was brought to the clinic by his parents. They explained that the child is not eating properly and complaining weakness. The physician examined and noticed swelling especially in face and extremities. He requested for RFT and LFT.

Serum bilirubin	1.2 mg%
Direct bilirubin	0.2 mg%
Indirect bilirubin	1.0 mg%
AST	25 U/L
ALT	20 U/L
Alkaline phosphatase	40 U/L
Total protein	4.5 g/dL
Albumin	2.0 g/dL
Globulin	2.5 g/dL
Urea	30 mg%
Creatinine	2.0 mg%
Urinary protein	10 g/L

   a. What diagnosis was made depending on the following blood results? Explain with specific reasons.
   b. What was the reason for swelling in face and extremities?

5. A 50-year-old Mr Joseph was brought to the hospital with the symptoms of pain in the flanks, anorexia (loss of appetite for food), and severe vomiting. The physician admitted him to the ward and examined him thoroughly. Physician asked the nurse

to send his blood sample for sugar and RFT and urine sample for microalbumin. Results of laboratory test are as follows:

Fasting blood sugar	200 mg/dL
Urea	70 mg/dL
Creatinine	10.0 mg/dL
Microalbumin	140 mg/L

a. What probable diagnosis can be made using the above mentioned laboratory results?
b. What is basis for the diagnosis made? Explain with reasons.
c. Why microalbumin was high in urine sample?

6. Mr Joseph visited the physician with several health problems and he explained him that he is feeling tiredness and burning sensation at the feet and above the stomach. He also explained that he is passing urine very frequently. The physician examined him and requested his blood and urine test. The lab results showed the following results:

TSH	3.0 mIU/mL
T3	1.5 ng/mL
T4	6.0 µg/dL
FBS	400 mg/dL
Urea	20 mg/dL
Creatinine	1.0 mg/dL
AST	25 U/L
ALT	20 U/L
Alkaline phosphatase	40 U/L
Total protein	7.5 g/dL
Blood pH	7.0
Plasma HCO_3^-	17 mEq/L
Benedict's test	Brick red color
Urine ketone bodies	Positive

a. What is the diagnosis made by physician with the above results available?
b. How did he explain about the case to his year-3 medical students in clinic?

7. Steve, a 40-year-old man, was admitted to the hospital with the symptoms of anorexia (loss of appetite) vomiting, and diarrhea. He mentioned to the physician that his urine was dark in color and passed the light stools. Serum and blood analysis which was requested revealed the following results:

Serum bilirubin	5.0 mg%
Direct bilirubin	3.6 mg%
Indirect bilirubin	1.4 mg%
AST	55 U/L
ALT	80 U/L
Alkaline phosphatase	100 U/L
Protein	7.5 g/dL
Albumin	4.5 g/dL
Urine bile pigments	Negative
Urine bile salts	Negative
Urobilinogen	Trace
Feces	Normal color

a. What diagnosis can be made with the available lab results?
b. Give specific reasons for elevated bilirubin and transaminase enzymes.
c. Why does the protein value remain normal?

8. Mr Suresh, a 40-year-old man who travels lot and recently visited two countries. After a month of his return, he started getting the symptoms of dark urine, abdominal swelling, pruritus (itching), complaining loss of appetite, unexplained weight loss or gain, and abdominal pain. His wife took him to doctor. The physician examined him and noticed swelling in liver below the ribs. Then he requested for blood test. The laboratory revealed the following results:

Serum bilirubin	10.0 mg%
Direct bilirubin	5.2 mg%
Indirect bilirubin	4.8 mg%
AST	200 U/L
ALT	800 U/L
Alkaline phosphatase	170 U/L
HBS Ag	Positive
Prothrombin time	Delayed

a. What diagnosis made using the above lab results?
b. Explain with reasons for your diagnosis and symptoms mentioned.

9. Mrs Sumathi was admitted at Gynecology ward, where she delivered a baby after 3 days. The neonatologist examined the baby and noticed the yellowish skin and sclera of the eye. He asked house officer to put the baby in phototherapy treatment. He also requested him to send the blood sample to lab. The laboratory results appear as follows:

Serum bilirubin	8.0 mg%
Direct bilirubin	0.2 mg%
Indirect bilirubin	4.8 mg%
AST	25 U/L
ALT	28 U/L

a. What type of jaundice the baby has?
b. Why was phototherapy suggested?

10. Mr Mahesh was admitted to the adult priority care ward with symptoms of anorexia and

abdominal pain. His wife took him to the doctor. The physician examined him and noticed yellowish discoloration of the skin and sclera of the eye. Then he requested for blood and urine test. The laboratory revealed the following results:

Serum bilirubin	12 mg%
Direct bilirubin	11.6 mg%
Indirect bilirubin	0.4 mg%
AST	55 U/L
ALT	60 U/L
Alkaline phosphatase	300 U/L
Urine bile pigments	++
Urine bile salts	++
Urobilinogen	Negative
Feces—stercobilinogen	Negative

a. What diagnosis would be made using the lab results?
b. Explain with reasons for the above mentioned symptoms.

11. Mr David, a 40-year-old man, who travels lot had recently visited two countries. After a month of his return, he started getting the symptoms of dark urine, abdominal swelling, pruritus (itching), complaining loss of appetite, unexplained weight loss or gain, and abdominal pain. He rushed to physician and requested laboratory tests revealed the following results:

Serum bilirubin	10.0 mg%	Elevated
Direct bilirubin	5.2 mg%	Elevated
Indirect bilirubin	4.8 mg%	Elevated
AST	200 U/L	Elevated
ALT	800 U/L	Elevated
Alkaline phosphatase	170 U/L	Elevated
HBS Ag	Positive	Negative

Urea	20 mg/dL	Normal
Creatinine	0.8 mg/dL	Normal
Blood sugar	80 mg/dL	Normal

a. Which tubes were used for collecting blood for analyzing the above parameters?
b. What diagnosis can be made using the above lab results?
c. What could be the cause for his elevated bilirubin and enzymes?
d. Explain with reasons for your diagnosis and symptoms mentioned.

12. A 30-year-old man reported in the emergency ward with complaints of abdominal pain, muscle cramps, and urinary discomfort. His requested laboratory tests revealed the following results:

Urea	100 mg/dL	Increased
Creatinine	12 mg/dL	Increased
Na^+	200 mEq/L	Increased
K^+	6.5 mEq/L	Increased
Chloride	120 mEq/L	Increased
Phosphorous	6.0 mEq/L	Increased
Serum bilirubin	1.0 mg%	Normal
Direct bilirubin	0.2 mg%	Normal
Indirect bilirubin	0.8 mg%	Normal
AST	30 U/L	Normal
ALT	25 U/L	Normal
Alkaline phosphatase	80 U/L	Normal

a. What could be the cause for elevated RFT and electrolytes?
b. List the preanalytical variable that could lead to elevated sodium.
c. Why red-top tube is preferred for sample collection for electrolyte analysis?
d. Which hormone helps to maintain fluid balance? Explain.

CHAPTER 22

Extracellular Matrix

OBJECTIVES

At the end of this chapter, students should be able to:
- Understand the composition and functions of collagen, elastin, fibrillin, fibronectin, and laminin
- Be able to know about the role of extracellular matrix (ECM) in health and disease.

INTRODUCTION

Extracellular matrix is a complex structural entity surrounding and supporting cells that are found within mammalian tissues. It is often referred to as the connective tissue.

BIOMOLECULES IN EXTRACELLULAR MATRIX

The ECM contains three major classes of biomolecules:
1. *Structural proteins:* Collagen, fibrillin, and elastin
2. *Specialized proteins:* Fibrillin, fibronectin, and laminin
3. *Proteoglycans:* Composed of a protein core attached with long chains of repeating disaccharide units termed "glycosaminoglycans (GAGs)" forming extremely complex high-molecular-weight components of the ECM.

COLLAGEN

Collagen is the main protein of connective tissue in animals and the most abundant protein in mammals, making up about 25% of the total protein:
- It is the major protein comprising the ECM.
- It is one of the long, fibrous structural proteins.
- Its functions are quite different from those of globular proteins such as enzymes.
- It is tough and inextensible, with great tensile strength.
- It is the main component of cartilage, ligaments, and tendons.
- It is the main protein component of bone and teeth.
- Along with soft keratin, it is responsible for skin strength and elasticity, and its degradation leads to wrinkles that accompany aging.
- It strengthens blood vessels and plays a role in tissue development.
- It is present in the cornea and lens of the eye in crystalline form.
- It is also used in cosmetic surgery, e.g. lip enhancement.

Types of Collagen

Collagen occurs in many places throughout the body and occurs in different types, which include the following:

Type I collagen: This is the most abundant collagen of the human body. It has triple helical structure. The mature collagen type I contains approximately 1,000 amino acids. Each α-chain is twisted into a left-handed helix of three residues per turn. Three α-chains are wound into a right-handed superhelix, forming a rod-like molecule 1.4 nm in diameter and about 300 nm long. It is present in scar tissue (the end product when tissue heals by repair). It is found in tendons and the organic part of bone.

Type II collagen: Articular cartilage.

Type III collagen: This is the collagen of granulation tissue and is produced quickly by young fibroblasts before the tougher type I collagen is synthesized.

Type IV collagen: The best well-characterized example of collagen discontinuous triple helices is an important component of basement membrane. It occurs in basal lamina and eye lens.

Type V collagen: Most interstitial tissue, associated with type I.

Type VI collagen: Most interstitial tissue, associated with type I.

Type VII collagen: Epithelium.

Type VIII collagen: Some endothelial cells.

Type IX collagen: Cartilage, associated with type II.

Type X collagen: Hypertrophic and mineralizing cartilage.

Type XI collagen: Cartilage.

Type XII collagen: Interacts with types I and III.

Type XIII collagen: Interacts with types I and II.

There are 27 types of collagen in total. Types I, II, and III are the most abundant and form fibrils of similar structure. Type IV collagen forms a two-dimensional reticulum and is a major component of the basal lamina. Collagens are predominantly synthesized by fibroblasts, but epithelial cells also synthesize these proteins.

Structure

Lateral interactions of triple helices of collagens result in the formation of fibrils roughly 50 nm diameter. The packing of collagen is such that adjacent molecules are displaced approximately one fourth of their length (67 nm). This staggered array produces a striated effect that can be seen in the electron microscope **(Fig. 22.1)**:

- Collagen is synthesized on ribosomes in a precursor form, i.e. preprocollagen, which contains a leader sequence that directs the polypeptide chain into the lumen of the endoplasmic reticulum.
- As it enters the endoplasmic reticulum, this leader sequence is enzymatically removed and becomes procollagen.
- Type I procollagen contains an additional 150 amino acids at the N-terminus and 250 at the C-terminus. These prodomains are globular and form multiple intrachain disulfide bonds.
- The disulfides stabilize the proprotein allowing the triple helical section to form. Collagen fibers begin to assemble in the endoplasmic reticulum and Golgi complexes.
- Specific proline residues are hydroxylated by prolyl 4-hydroxylase and prolyl 3-hydroxylase. Specific lysine residues also are hydroxylated by lysyl hydroxylase. Both hydroxylases are dependent upon vitamin C as cofactor.

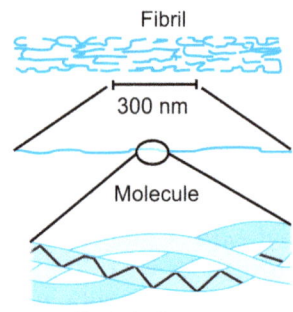

Fig. 22.1: Structure of collagen.
(Gly: glycine)

Table 22.1: Diseases result from abnormalities in the synthesis of collagen.

Syndrome/Disease	Feature	Effects
Ehlers–Danlos IV	Decrease in type III	Arterial, intestinal and uterine rupture, bruised skin
Ehlers–Danlos V	Decreased cross-linking	Skin and joint hyperextensibility
Ehlers–Danlos VI	Decreased hydroxylysine	Poor wound healing, musculoskeletal deformities, skin and joint hyperextensibility
Ehlers–Danlos VII	N-terminal propeptide not removed	Easily bruised skin, hip dislocations, hyperextensibility
Osteogenesis imperfecta	Decrease in type I	Blue sclera, bone deformities
Scurvy	Decreased hydroxyproline	Poor wound healing, deficient growth, capillary weakness

- O-linked glycosylation also occurs during Golgi transit. The processed procollagens are secreted into the extracellular space where extracellular enzymes remove the prodomains.
- The collagen molecules then polymerize to form collagen fibrils. The oxidation of certain lysine residues by the extracellular enzyme lysyl oxidase forms reactive aldehydes.
- These reactive aldehydes form specific cross-links between two chains thereby, stabilizing the staggered array of the collagens in the fibril.
- Methyl violet, trichrome, or van Gieson are the stains used to stain the collagen in tissue samples.
- Diseases due to abnormalities in the collagen synthesis **(Table 22.1)**.

ELASTIN

- Elastin is a connective tissue protein, i.e. responsible for extensibility and elastic recoil in tissues.
- It is present in large amounts in lungs, large arterial blood vessels, and some elastic ligaments.
- It is also present in skin, ear cartilage, and other tissues in smaller amounts.
- It is synthesized as a soluble monomer called tropoelastin.
- Some of the proline residues of tropoelastin are hydroxylated to hydroxyproline by prolyl hydroxylase. After secretion from the cell, certain lysyl residues of the tropoelastin are oxidatively deaminated to aldehydes by lysyl oxidase. The cross-links formed in elastin are the desmosines, which result from the condensation of three of these lysine-derived aldehydes with an unmodified lysine to form a tetrafunctional cross-link. The cross-linked extracellular elastin is highly insoluble and stable with low turnover rate.
- It exhibits a variety of random coil conformations, which permit the elastin to stretch and recoil during its physiological functions.
- It does not contain hydroxylysine.
- It is not synthesized in proform like collagen.
- It does not contain repeat "Gly–X–Y" sequences, triple helical structure.
- The deletions of elastin gene have been found in majority of the subjects with Williams's syndrome. It is a disorder affecting connective tissue and central nervous system.

FIBRILLIN

Fibrillin is a glycoprotein "a structural component of microfibril," 10–12 nm fibers found in tissues. It is secreted into the ECM by fibroblasts and incorporated into the insoluble microfibrils. It is found in the zonular fibers of the lens, associated with the elastin fibers in the aorta.

Marfan's syndrome: Inherited autosomal dominant trait disorder affecting connective tissue. It affects the eyes, skeletal system, and cardiovascular system (dilation of the ascending aorta).

FIBRONECTIN

- Fibronectin is a first well-characterized adhesive protein.
- It has multiple domains, each with specific binding sites for other matrix macromolecules and for receptors on the surface of cells.
- At least six tightly folded domains were identified each with a high affinity for a different substrate such as heparan sulfate, collagen (separate domains for types I, II, and III), fibrin, and cell surface receptors.
- They are dimers of two similar peptides. Each chain is 60–70 nm long and 2–3 nm thick.
- The role of fibronectin is to attach cells to a variety of ECMs.
- It attaches cells to all matrices except type IV that involves laminin as the adhesive molecule.
- Approximately about 20 different fibronectin chains have been identified that arise by alternative ribonucleic acid splicing of the primary transcript from a single fibronectin gene.

LAMININ

- All basal laminae contain a common set of proteins and GAGs. These are type IV collagen, heparan sulfate proteoglycans, entactin, and laminin. The basal lamina is often referred to as the type IV matrix.
- Each of the components of the basal lamina is synthesized by the cells that rest upon it. Laminin anchors cell surfaces to the basal lamina **(Fig. 22.2)**.

Like fibronectin it has multiple domains to bind cell surface receptors, heparin sulfate, and collagen. It has three chains bound together to form a crucifix-shaped structure.

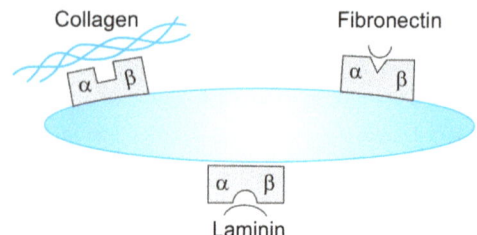

Fig. 22.2: Cell interacting through receptors with collagen, fibronectin, and laminin present in ECM.
(ECM: extracellular matrix)

GLYCOSAMINOGLYCANS

- GAGs are the abundant heteropolysaccharides found in the body **(Table 22.2)**.
- These are long-unbranched polysaccharides with repeating disaccharide unit.
- The disaccharide units contain either of two modified sugars such as *N*-acetylgalactosamine or *N*-acetylglucosamine and an uronic acid such as glucuronate or iduronate.
- These are highly negatively charged molecules, with extended conformation that imparts high viscosity to the solution.
- These are located primarily on the surface of cells or in the ECM.
- The viscous and low compressibility nature of GAGs makes them ideal for a lubricating fluid in the joints. At the same time, their rigidity provides structural integrity to cells and provides passageways between cells, allowing for cell migration.

The specific GAGs are hyaluronic acid, dermatan sulfate, chondroitin sulfate, heparin, heparan sulfate, and keratan sulfate I and II.

Functions of Glycosaminoglycans

Hyaluronic Acid

- Hyaluronic acid is in high concentration in embryonic tissues.
- It plays an important role in permitting cell migration and during morphogenesis, and wound healing.
- It contributes high compressibility to cartilage.

Table 22.2: Composition and location of glycosaminoglycans.

Glycosaminoglycan	Composition and linkage	Location
Hyaluronic acid	N-acetylglucosamine, glucuronic acid and β-1,3 linkage	Synovial fluid of joints, vitreous humor of eye, umbilical cord, and skin
Chondroitin sulfate	N-acetylgalactosamine, glucuronic acid and β-1,3 linkage	Cartilage, bone, and cornea
Dermatan sulfate	N-acetylgalactosamine, iduronic acid or glucuronic acid and β-1,3 linkage	Skin, blood vessels, and heart valves
Keratan sulfate I	N-acetylgalactosamine, galactose and β-1,4 linkage	Cornea
Keratan sulfate II	N-acetylgalactosamine, galactose and β-1,4 linkage	Loose connective tissue
Heparin	N-acetylglucosamine, iduronic acid or glucuronic acid and β-1,4 linkage; G1cN are sulfated	Blood anticoagulant, liver, lungs, and mast cells
Heparan sulfate	N-acetylglucosamine, glucuronic acid and β-1,4 linkage; few N-sulfates	Basement membrane and cell surfaces

Chondroitin Sulfate

Located inside certain neurons and may provide exoskeletal structure.

Dermatan Sulfate

Dermatan sulfate present in cornea. They lie between collagen fibrils and play a role in corneal transparency. In sclera, it may play a role in maintaining the overall shape of the eye.

Keratan Sulfate

Keratan sulfate present in cornea and cartilage. They lie between collagen fibrils and play a role in corneal transparency.

Heparin

- Important anticoagulant binds with factors IX and XI.
- Free heparin complexes with and activates antithrombin III, which in turn inhibits all the serine proteases of the coagulation cascade. This phenomenon has been clinically exploited in the use of heparin injection for anticoagulation therapies.
- Binds with lipoprotein lipase of capillary walls, causing the release of this enzyme into the circulation.

Heparan Sulfate

- Acts as receptors and may participate in the mediation of cell growth and cell communication.
- Several genetically inherited diseases, e.g. the lysosomal storage diseases, result from defects in the lysosomal enzymes responsible for the metabolism of complex membrane-associated GAGs.
- These specific diseases, termed "mucopolysaccharidoses," lead to an accumulation of GAGs within cells **(Table 22.3)**.
- There are at least 14 known types of lysosomal storage diseases that affect GAG catabolism; some of the more commonly encountered. For example, Hurler's syndrome, Hunter's syndrome, Sanfilippo's syndrome, Maroteaux-Lamy syndrome, and Morquio syndrome.
- All of these disorders, except Hunter's syndrome, are inherited in an autosomal recessive manner.

PROTEOGLYCANS

- Proteoglycans are proteins that contain covalently linked GAGs. The proteins linked to GAGs are called core proteins.

Table 22.3: Disorders of glycosaminoglycan (GAG) metabolism.

Type	Enzyme defect	Affected GAG	Symptoms
MPS IH (Hurler's syndrome)	α-L-Iduronidase	Dermatan sulfate, heparan sulfate	Corneal clouding, dysostosis multiplex, organomegaly, heart disease, mental retardation
MPS IS (Scheie's syndrome)	α-L-Iduronidase	Dermatan sulfate, heparan sulfate	Corneal clouding, aortic valve disease, joint stiffening
MPS IH/S (Hurler–Scheie syndrome)	α-L-Iduronidase	Dermatan sulfate, heparan sulfate	Intermediate between IH and IS
MPS II (Hunter's syndrome)	L-Iduronate sulfatase	Dermatan sulfate, heparan sulfate	Mild and severe forms, only X-linked MPS, dysostosis multiplex, organomegaly, facial and physical deformities, no corneal clouding, mental retardation, death before 15 except in mild form then survival to 20–60
MPS IIIA (Sanfilippo's A syndrome)	Heparan N-sulfatase	Heparan sulfate	Profound mental deterioration; hyperactivity; skin, brain, lungs, heart, and skeletal muscle are affected in all four types of MPS III
MPS IIIB (Sanfilippo's B syndrome)	α-N-acetyl-D-glucosaminidase	Heparan sulfate	Phenotype similar to IIIA
MPS IIIC (Sanfilippo's C syndrome)	N-acetylglucosaminidase acetyltransferase	Heparan sulfate	Phenotype similar to IIIA
MPS IIID (Sanfilippo's D syndrome)	N-acetylglucosamine-6-sulfatase	Heparan sulfate	Phenotype similar to IIIA
Morquio's A syndrome	Galactosamine-6-sulfatase	Keratan sulfate, chondroitin-6-sulfate	
Morquio's B syndrome	α-Galactosidase	Keratan sulfate	

(MPS: mucopolysaccharidoses)

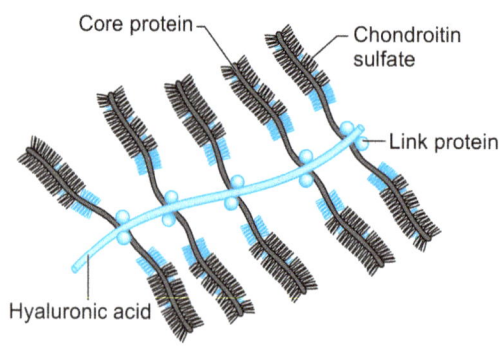

Fig. 22.3: Structure of proteoglycan.

The amount of carbohydrate in a proteoglycan is usually greater than that found in a glycoprotein (about 95% of its weight) **(Fig. 22.3)**.

- The aggrecan, major type found in cartilage. Its structure resembles a bottle brush. It contains a long strand of hyaluronic acid to which link proteins are attached and these interact with core protein molecules from which other GAGs project.
- The linkage of GAGs to the protein core involves a specific trisaccharide composed of two galactose and a xylulose residue (GAG-Gal-Xyl-O-CH_2-protein) **(Fig. 22.4)**.
- The trisaccharide linker is coupled to the protein core through an O-glycosidic bond to S-residue in the protein. Some forms of keratan sulfates are linked to the protein core through N-asparaginyl bond.

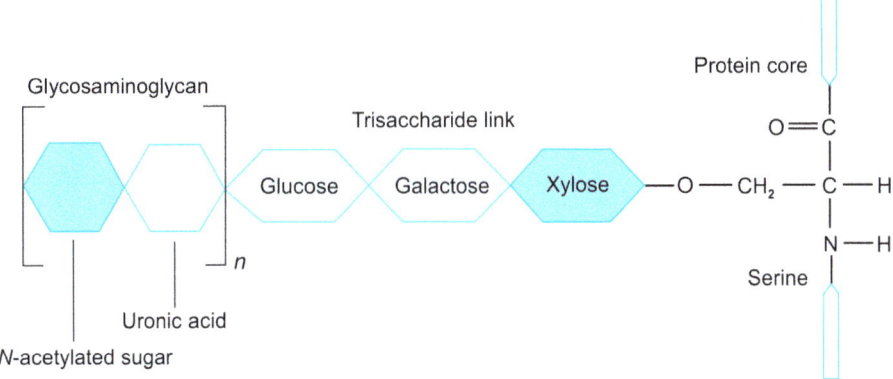

Fig. 22.4: Structure of GAG linkage to protein in proteoglycans.
(GAG: glycosaminoglycan)

- It is found in all tissues of the body, mainly in the ECM or ground substance.
- Therefore they act as structural components of the ECM.
- They have specific interactions with collagen, elastin, fibronectin, laminin, and growth factors such as transforming growth factor alpha.
- Act as polyions, bind polycations and cations.
- The long extended nature of the polysaccharide chains of GAGs and their ability to gel makes proteoglycan to act as sieves, restricting the passage of large molecules into the ECM and allowing free diffusion of small molecules.

SUMMARY

Extracellular matrix is a complex structural entity surrounding and supporting cells that are found within mammalian tissues and often referred to as the connective tissue. The ECM contains three major classes of biomolecules such as structural proteins (collagen, fibrillin, and elastin), specialized proteins (fibrillin, fibronectin, and laminin), and proteoglycans (composed of a protein core attached with long chains of repeating disaccharide units termed "GAGs"). Collagen is the main protein of connective tissue in animals and the most abundant protein in mammals. There are 27 types of collagen in total. GAGs are the abundant heteropolysaccharides found in the body and are long-unbranched polysaccharides with repeating disaccharide unit.

SELF-ASSESSMENT QUESTIONS

Essay Questions

1. Explain the reason of collagen being the important tissue of human body.
2. What is the main biochemical composition of collagen? Mention the enzyme and coenzyme catalyzing its synthesis.
3. Give the features and biochemical defect of scurvy.
4. Describe the various sources of ATP in muscle.
5. Outline the diagnostic uses of creatine phosphokinase.
6. Differentiate proteoglycans from mucopolysaccharides.
7. List the chemical composition and site of occurrence for hyaluronic acid, chondroitin

sulfate, dermatan sulfate, and keratan sulfate.
8. Mention the defective enzyme and clinical symptoms of Hurler's syndrome.
9. Explain how Ca^{2+} regulates skeletal muscle contraction.

MULTIPLE-CHOICE QUESTIONS

1. **Collagen is the:**
   a. Major protein of the extracellular fluid
   b. Main protein of connective tissue in animals
   c. Minor protein comprising the ECM
   d. Nonfibrous protein
2. **Proteoglycans contain:**
   a. A lipid core attached to protein
   b. Carbohydrate attached to fatty acid and glycerol
   c. Polyunsaturated fatty acid attached to a disaccharide unit
   d. A protein core attached to repeating disaccharide units
3. **Concerning laminin, all of the following statements are true, *except*:**
   a. It anchors cell surfaces to the basal lamina
   b. It has three chains wound together to form a crucifix-shaped structure
   c. It is tough and inextensible, with great tensile strength
   d. It has multiple domains to bind cell surface receptors
4. **Hurler's syndrome results from reduced levels of:**
   a. Glucosaminidase
   b. Sulfatase
   c. Acetyltransferase
   d. L-Iduronidase
5. **The composition of hyaluronic acid is:**
   a. Glucuronic acid and *N*-acetylgalactosamine
   b. Glucuronic acid and *N*-acetylglucosamine
   c. Galactose and *N*-acetylgalactosamine
   d. Iduronic acid and *N*-acetylglucosamine
6. **Heparin:**
   a. Is an excellent lubricator and shock absorber
   b. Has glucuronic acid and galactosamine
   c. Is highly sulfated
   d. Is found in the synovial fluid of joints
7. **In the structure shown below:**
   a. A represents chondroitin sulfate

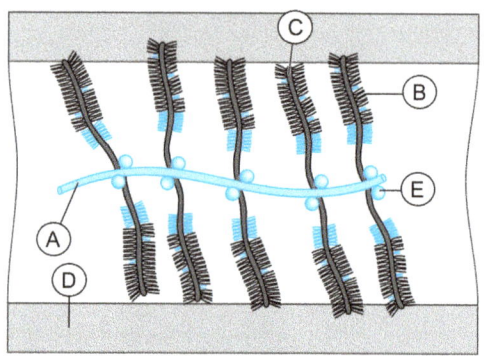

   b. B represents hyaluronic acid
   c. C represents link protein
   d. D represents collagen

8. **Concerning fibronectin:**
   a. It is the first collagen to be well characterized
   b. It has single domain
   c. It is a dimer with similar peptides
   d. It attaches cells to all matrices except type IV
9. **Collagen synthesis depends on:**
   a. Hydroxylysine and vitamin K
   b. Glycine and fluoride
   c. Epinephrine and vitamin C
   d. Hydroxyproline and vitamin C
10. **Heparin is:**
    a. Composed of glucuronic acid and *N*-acetyl-glucosamine
    b. Nonsulfated
    c. Absent in liver
    d. Found in synovial fluid
11. **Hurler's syndrome presents with:**
    a. Organomegaly and dwarfism
    b. Bruised skin and magenta-colored tongue
    c. Profuse bleeding and delayed clotting time
    d. Skeletal and smooth muscle disorder
12. **Type III collagen is produced by:**
    a. Fibroblasts after type I collagen formation
    b. Young fibroblasts before tougher type I collagen is synthesized
    c. Fibroblasts after the type IV collagen formation
    d. Fibroblasts quickly after the tougher type collagen IX is synthesized
13. **Fibronectin:**
    a. Contains six tightly folded domains
    b. Does not attach cells to matrices
    c. Attaches type IV collagen to matrices
    d. Is a well-characterized adhesive protein

14. The high viscosity and low compressibility of GAGs make them ideal for:
    a. Binding tightly to bones
    b. Hardening bones and teeth
    c. Lubricating the joints
    d. Attaching ligaments to bone
15. Chondroitin sulfate consists of:
    a. Glucuronic acid and N-acetylgalactosamine
    b. Glucuronic acid and N-acetylglucosamine
    c. Iduronic acid and N-acetylgalactosamine
    d. Iduronic acid and galactosamine
16. Concerning the proteoglycan shown below:

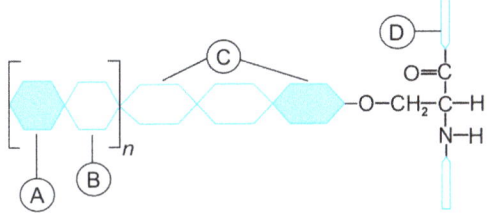

    a. A represents N-acetylated sugar
    b. B represents galactose
    c. D represents the glycoprotein
    d. C represents tryptophan rings
17. The most abundant collagen in the human body is type:
    a. II
    b. I
    c. IV
    d. V
18. Determination of hydroxyproline levels may be used to estimate the tissue levels of:
    a. Collagen
    b. Fibronectin
    c. Hyaluronic acid
    d. Myosin
19. Concerning collagen:
    a. It is the minor glycoprotein found in bone
    b. Its degradation leads to wrinkles that accompany aging
    c. It gives strength to ligaments
    d. It is used in the treatment of ulcers
20. The disorder that results from the defect in collagen synthesis is:
    a. Sanfilippo's A
    b. Ehlers–Danlos V
    c. Comprises monomers with a length of 70 nm
    d. Has at least 20 peptide chains
21. The cofactor essential for hydroxylation of proline is:
    a. Pantothenic acid
    b. Vitamin B_{12}
    c. Vitamin C
    d. Folic acid
22. Concerning glycosaminoglycans:
    a. They are long-branched polysaccharides
    b. The disaccharide units contain N-acetyl-galactosamine and N-acetylglucosamine
    c. They are located primarily on the surface of cells and the ECM
    d. They are positively charged molecules
23. Concerning the hyaluronic acid, one of the following statements is false. It:
    a. Is composed of glucuronic acid and N-acetylglucosamine
    b. Is found in synovial fluid
    c. Is found in the vitreous humor
    d. Contains α-1,6 linkage
24. Keratan sulfate contains:
    a. Galactose and N-acetylglucosamine
    b. Glucuronic acid and galactosamine
    c. Glucuronic 2-sulfate and N-acetylglucosamine
    d. Galactose and N-acetylgalactosamine

Answers

1. b	2. d	3. c	4. d	5. b
6. c	7. d	8. d	9. d	10. a
11. a	12. b	13. c	14. c	15. a
16. a	17. b	18. a	19. b	20. b
21. c	22. c	23. c	24. d	

CHAPTER 23

Biochemistry of Muscle Structure and Function

OBJECTIVES
At the end of this chapter, students should be able to:
- Understand about the types and structure of muscles and the muscle fiber
- Explain their role of muscles and their fibers in various conditions.

INTRODUCTION

Muscles in the human body have biochemical specialization, which makes them to perform many physiological functions. Animals use muscles to convert the chemical energy of adenosine triphosphate (ATP) into mechanical work.

TYPES OF MUSCLES

Three different kinds of muscles are found in vertebrate animals.

Heart Muscle (Cardiac Muscle)

Heart muscle makes up the wall of the heart; throughout life, it contracts some 70 times per minute pumping about 5 L of blood each minute.

Smooth Muscle

Smooth muscle is found in the walls of all the hollow organs of the body (except the heart). Its contraction reduces the size of these structures. Its other functions are to:
- Regulate the flow of blood in the arteries
- Move food along through gastrointestinal tract
- Expel urine from urinary bladder
- Send babies out into the world from the uterus
- Regulate the flow of air through the lungs.

The contraction of smooth muscle is generally not under voluntary control.

Skeletal Muscle

Skeletal muscle is attached to the skeleton; it is also called striated muscle. The contraction of skeletal muscle is under voluntary control.

Muscle Fiber

Skeletal muscle is made up of thousands of cylindrical muscle fibers often running all the way from origin to insertion. The fibers are bound together by connective tissue through which run blood vessels and nerves. Each muscle fiber contains:
- An array of myofibrils that are stacked lengthwise and run the entire length of the fiber
- Mitochondria
- An extensive smooth endoplasmic reticulum
- Many nuclei.

The multiple nuclei arise from the fact that each muscle fiber develops from the fusion of many cells (myoblasts).

A muscle fiber is not a single cell; its parts are often given special names such as:
- Sarcolemma for plasma membrane
- Sarcoplasmic reticulum (SR) for endoplasmic reticulum
- Sarcosome for mitochondrion

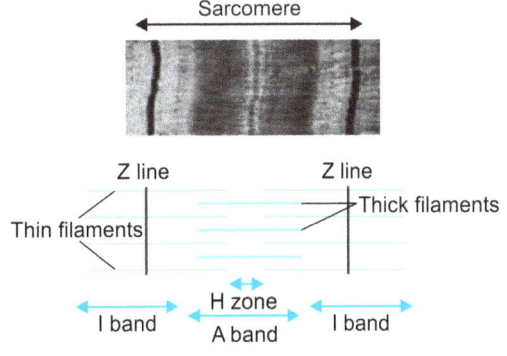

Fig. 23.1: Structure of sarcomere.

- Sarcoplasm for cytoplasm.

The striated appearance of the muscle fiber is created by a pattern of alternating dark A bands and light I bands **(Fig. 23.1)**:
- The A bands are bisected by the H zone.
- The I bands are bisected by the Z line.
- Each fiber is composed of myofibrils and each myofibril is made up of arrays of parallel filaments, which is a series of repeating structural units called sarcomeres.
- Sarcomeres are composed of thick (myosin) and thin (actin) filaments **(Fig. 23.2)**.

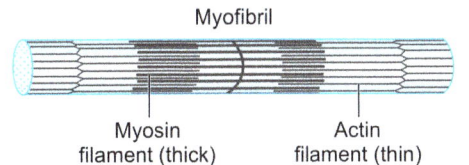

Fig. 23.2: Structure showing thick and thin filaments.

Thick Filament
- The thick filaments have a diameter of about 15 nm.
- These are composed of numerous protein strands, which are called myosin filaments.
- Each myosin filament is composed of a two twisted strands called heavy chains and two other, but each different pairs of twisted strands called light chains. These light chains are found in the myosin heads **(Fig. 23.3)**.
- Myosin filament is flexible at the point of the myosin head and the stacking of the myosin molecules leaves the myosin heads protruding from the filament at ~60°. This spacing maximizes chances for interaction with actin-binding sites.
- Myosin ATPase is found in the myosin heads.
- Another structural element, titin, connects the ends of the myosin filaments to the Z disks.
- The M region, centered in the middle of the myosin filaments and cross-links with other myosin, serves as structural support for the sarcomeres; a part of the M region contains creatine phosphokinase (CPK).

Thin Filament

- The thin filaments have a diameter of about 5 nm.
- Actin exists as a polymer of repeating globular proteins called G-actin.
- Two actin filaments are twisted into a single-stranded filament. These strands are anchored at one end to the Z disk.

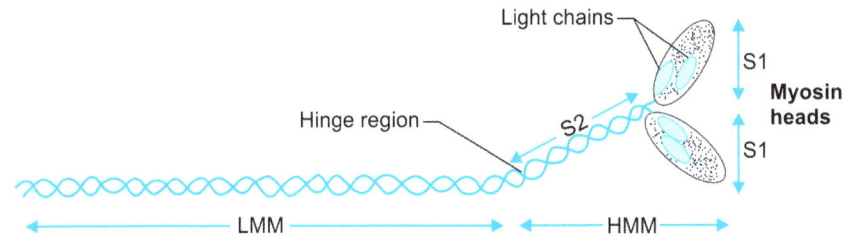

Fig. 23.3: Thick filament.
(HMM: heavy meromyosin; LMM: light meromyosin)

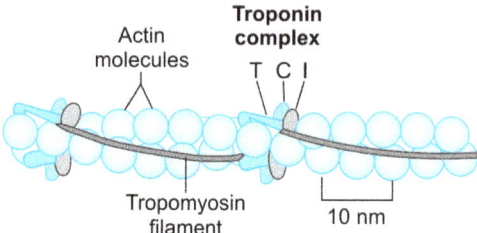

Fig. 23.4: Relationship between actin, troponin, and tropomyosin filaments.

- An adenosine diphosphate (ADP) molecule on each G-actin molecule is thought to be the active or binding site on the actin filament.
- Lying in the groove formed by the actin filaments is a series of rod-shaped protein molecules called tropomyosin. Each tropomyosin molecule is six to seven G-actin molecules in length.
- Bound to the end of each tropomyosin is a third protein called troponin **(Fig. 23.4)**.
- Troponin consists as three small bound protein molecules—the troponin I (TnI), troponin T (TnT), and troponin C (TnC). One molecule is bound to the actin filament, one to the tropomyosin and the third is available to bind with calcium ions (Ca^{2+}). The calcium-mediated contraction of striated muscle (fast and slow skeletal and cardiac muscles) is regulated by the troponin complex; contraction of smooth muscle is regulated by calmodulin.

The cross-sectional view of the myosin and actin filaments is shown in **Fig. 23.5**. The actin filaments (smaller dots) are positioned every 60°, so that they are aligned with the myosin heads that protrude from the myosin filaments (larger dots). Thus six actin filaments surround each myosin filament, moreover active sites from an actin filament are available to three different myosin filaments **(Table 23.1)**.

ACTIVATION OF SKELETAL MUSCLE

The contraction of skeletal muscle is controlled by the nervous system. Skeletal muscle differs from smooth and cardiac muscle. Both cardiac and smooth muscle can contract without being stimulated by the nervous system.

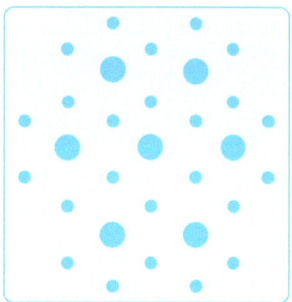

Fig. 23.5: Cross-sectional view of myosin and actin filaments.

Neuromuscular Junction

Nerve impulses traveling down the motor neurons of the sensory-somatic branch of the nervous system cause the skeletal muscle fibers at which they terminate to contract. The junction between the terminal of a motor neuron and a muscle fiber is called the neuromuscular junction (NMJ). It is simply one kind of synapse. The terminals of motor axons contain thousands of vesicles filled with acetylcholine (ACh).

When a nerve impulse (action potential) reaches the axon terminal, hundreds of these vesicles discharge their ACh onto a specialized area of postsynaptic membrane on the fiber. This area contains a cluster of *trans*-membrane channels that are opened by ACh and let sodium ions (Na^+) diffuse in.

The interior of a resting muscle fiber has a resting potential of about –95 mV. The influx of Na^+ reduces the charge, creating an end plate potential (EPP). If the EPP reaches the threshold voltage (approximately –50 mV), Na^+ flow in with a rush and an action potential is created in the fiber. The action potential sweeps down the length of the fiber just as it does in an axon.

Table 23.1: Some skeletal muscle proteins and their functions.

Component	Function
Actin	• Major component of the thin filaments • Important cytoskeletal protein in nonmuscle cells • Six human isoforms are known
α-actinin	Cross-link actin at the Z disks
CapZ	Caps the plus ends of actin filaments at the Z disk
Caldesmon	Thin filament regulation in smooth muscle
Desmin	• Intermediate filaments protein • The muscle form links together adjacent myofibrils at the Z disk
Dystrophin	• Anchors some actin filaments to the sarcolemma • Defective or absent in muscular dystrophies
Myosin	Adult fast skeletal muscle heavy chains
Nebulin	Actin-binding protein
Titin	• Elastic element • Links thick filaments to Z lines • Titin is the largest protein in the human genome
Tropomyosin	Thin filament component, seven repeats, each with a major and a minor actin-binding site
Tropomodulin	Caps the minus ends of thin filaments
Troponin C	• Cardiac and slow-twitch skeletal muscle • Fast-twitch skeletal muscle • Binds calcium and troponin T
Troponin I	• Slow-twitch skeletal • Fast-twitch skeletal • Cardiac muscle • Binds to actin and troponin T • Inhibits the actin-myosin interaction unless calcium is bound to troponin C
Troponin T	• Slow skeletal • Cardiac • Fast skeletal • Binds to tropomyosin, troponin I and troponin C
Vinculin	Binds to α-actinin

No visible change occurs in the muscle fiber during the action potential. This period is called the latent period, lasts from 3 to 10 milliseconds. Before the latent period is over:
- The enzyme acetylcholinesterase breaks down the ACh in the NMJ:
  - The Na^+ channels close.
  - The field is cleared for the arrival of another nerve impulse.
- The resting potential of the fiber is restored by an outflow of potassium ions.

Sliding Filament Model

Each molecule of myosin in the thick filaments contains a globular subunit called the myosin head. The myosin heads have binding sites for the actin molecules in the thin filaments and ATP.

Activation of the muscle fiber causes the myosin heads to bind to actin. An allosteric change occurs, which draws the thin filament a short distance (~10 nm) past the thick filament. Then the linkages break (for which

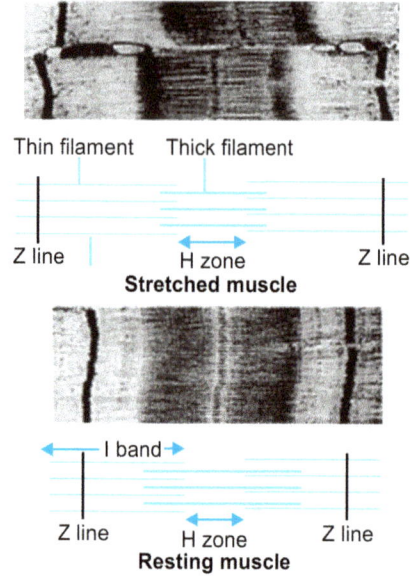

Fig. 23.6: Sliding filament model.

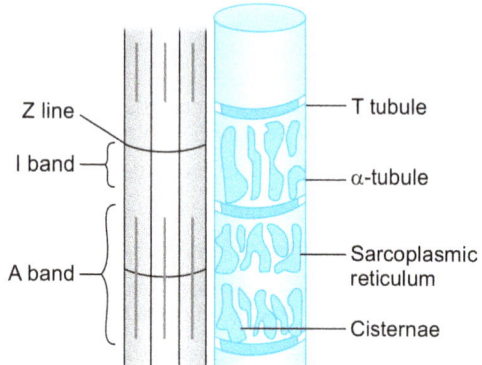

Fig. 23.7: Sarcotubular system.

ATP is needed) and reform farther along the thin filament to repeat the process. As a result, the filaments are pulled past each other in a ratchet-like action **(Fig. 23.6)**. There is no shortening, thickening, or folding of the individual filaments. Electron microscopy supports this model. As a muscle contracts:
- The Z lines come closer together.
- The width of the I bands decreases.
- The width of the H zones decreases, but there is no change in the width of the A band.

Conversely, as a muscle is stretched, the width of the I bands and H zones increases, but there is still no change in the width of the A band.

Coupling Excitation to Contraction

Calcium ions (Ca^{2+}) link action potentials in a muscle fiber to contraction:
- In resting muscle fibers, Ca^{2+} are stored in endoplasmic (sarcoplasmic) reticulum.
- Spaced along the plasma membrane (sarcolemma) of the muscle fiber are inpocketings of the membrane that form tubules of the "T system". These tubules plunge repeatedly into the interior of the fiber.
- The tubules of the T system terminate near the calcium-filled sacs of the SR **(Fig. 23.7)**.
- Each action potential created at the NMJ sweeps quickly along the sarcolemma and is carried into the T system.
- The arrival of the action potential at the ends of the T system triggers the release of Ca^{2+} from tubules.
- The Ca^{2+} diffuse among the thick and thin filaments, where they bind to troponin on the thin filaments.
- This turns on the interaction between actin and myosin and the sarcomere contracts.
- Because of the speed of the action potential, the action potential arrives virtually simultaneously at the ends of all the tubules of the T system, ensuring that all sarcomeres contract in unison.
- When the process is over, the Ca is pumped back into the SR using a Ca^{2+} ATPase.

Fueling Muscle Contraction

Adenosine triphosphate is the immediate source of energy for muscle contraction. Although, a muscle fiber contains only enough ATP to power a few twitches, its ATP "pool" is replenished as needed. There are three sources of high-energy phosphate to keep the ATP pool in balance **(Fig. 23.8)**:
1. Creatine phosphate

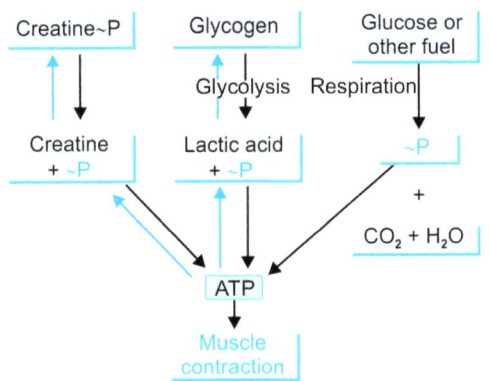

Fig. 23.8: Energy sources for muscle contraction.

2. Glycogen
3. Cellular respiration in the mitochondria of the fibers.

Creatine Phosphate

The phosphate group in creatine phosphate is attached by a "high-energy" bond like that in ATP. Creatine phosphate derives its high-energy phosphate from ATP and can donate it back to ADP to form ATP:

Creatine phosphate + ADP ↔ Creatine + ATP

The pool of creatine phosphate in the fiber is about 10 times larger than that of ATP and thus serves as a modest reservoir of ATP.

Glycogen

Skeletal muscle fibers contain about 1% glycogen. The muscle fiber can break down this glycogen by glycogenolysis producing glucose-1-phosphate. This enters the glycolytic pathway to generate two molecules of ATP for each pair of lactic acid molecules produced; not much, but enough to keep the muscle functioning if it fails to receive sufficient oxygen to meet its ATP needs by respiration. However, this source is limited and the muscle eventually depends on cellular respiration.

Cellular Respiration

Cellular respiration is required not only to meet the ATP needs of a muscle engaged in prolonged activity but also afterward to enable the body to resynthesize glycogen from the lactic acid produced earlier.

TYPE I VERSUS TYPE II FIBERS

Two different types of muscle fiber can be found in most skeletal muscles. The "type I" and "type II" fibers differ in their structure and biochemistry **(Table 23.2)**.

- Most skeletal muscles contain some mixture of "type I" and "type II" fibers, but a single motor unit always contains one type or the other, never both.
- The ratio of "type I" and "type II" fibers can be changed by endurance training (producing more type I fibers).
- The skeletal muscle is rich in glycogen located in granules close to the I bands.
- The release of glucose from glycogen is dependent on muscle glycogen that in turn is dependent on muscle glycogen phosphorylase, which can be activated by Ca^{2+}, epinephrine, and adenosine monophosphate (AMP).

Table 23.2: Difference between type I and type II muscle fibers.

Type I fibers	Type II fibers
Loaded with mitochondria	Few mitochondria
Low in glycogen	Rich in glycogen
Depend on cellular respiration for ATP production	Depend on glycolysis for ATP production
Resistant to fatigue	Fatigue easily
Rich in myoglobin and hence red in color	Low in myoglobin, hence whitish in color
Activated by small diameter, thus slow-conducting motor neurons	Activated by large diameter, thus fast-conducting motor neurons
Also known as "slow-twitch" fibers	Also known as "fast-twitch" fibers
Dominant in muscles that depend on tonus, e.g. those responsible for posture	Dominant in muscles used for rapid movement

(ATP: adenosine triphosphate)

- Synthesis of ATP through oxidative phosphorylation depends on oxygen.
- Because of the heme group, muscles-containing myoglobin is red, whereas muscles with less or no myoglobin are white.
- Glucose derived from the blood glucose or endogenous glycogen and fatty acids derived from triglyceride of adipose tissue are the main substances used for aerobic metabolism in muscle.

Energy for Sprinter

A sprinter uses creatine phosphate and anaerobic glycolysis to make ATP. In this case, the type II fibers are used predominantly. The major sources of energy in the athlete during 100 m race are creatine phosphate (4–5 seconds) and then anaerobic glycolysis, using stored glycogen of muscle as glucose source. In the beginning, the muscle glycogen phosphorylase is activated by Ca^{2+} and then by epinephrine, and AMP. Phosphofructokinase-1 is also activated by AMP, inorganic phosphate (Pi), and ammonia (NH_3) to increase the glycolysis.

Marathon Runner

In marathon, the "type I" fibers are used and aerobic metabolism is the principal source of ATP. The major fuel sources are blood glucose and free fatty acids, which are derived from the breakdown of triglycerides of adipose tissue that is stimulated by the epinephrine. The liver glycogen is broken down to maintain the blood glucose. Muscle glycogen is also a source during this marathon, but it is gradually degraded more in marathon than sprint. The blood glucose will supply the muscle with energy during a marathon for 4 minutes, but the glycogen of liver will supply energy for 18 minutes. Glycogen of muscle and triglyceride of adipose tissue supply the muscle with energy during a marathon for 70 and 3,500 minutes, respectively. The oxidation of both glucose and fatty acids is very important for energy contribution in the marathon.

CARDIAC MUSCLE

Cardiac or heart muscle resembles skeletal muscle in some ways. It is striated and each cell contains sarcomeres with sliding filaments of actin and myosin. However, cardiac muscle has a number of unique features that reflect its function of pumping blood:
- The myofibrils of each cell and cardiac muscle are made of single cells; each with a single nucleus is branched.
- The branches interlock with those of adjacent fibers by adherens junctions; these strong junctions enable the heart to contract forcefully without ripping the fibers apart.
- Cardiac muscle has a much richer supply of mitochondria than skeletal muscle; this reflects its greater dependence on cellular respiration for ATP.
- Cardiac muscle has little glycogen and gets little benefit from glycolysis when the supply of oxygen is limited.

Catecholamine hormones such as adrenalin are released during frightening or stressful situations. They increase the force and frequency of cardiac contractions by binding to beta-1 receptors, which are protein molecules protruding from the outer surface of the cardiac sarcolemma. These activate G-proteins within the membrane, which in turn activate the enzyme adenylyl cyclase on the inner surface of the sarcolemma. Adenylyl cyclase produces cyclic AMP (cAMP), which is an important second messenger controlling numerous intracellular activities. The cAMP activates protein kinase A, which phosphorylates many intracellular enzymes, temporarily modifying their properties.

Cardiac muscle contains muscarinic ACh receptors. These are also linked to adenylyl cyclase and to a K^+ channel in the cardiac sarcolemma. ACh reduces the levels of cAMP

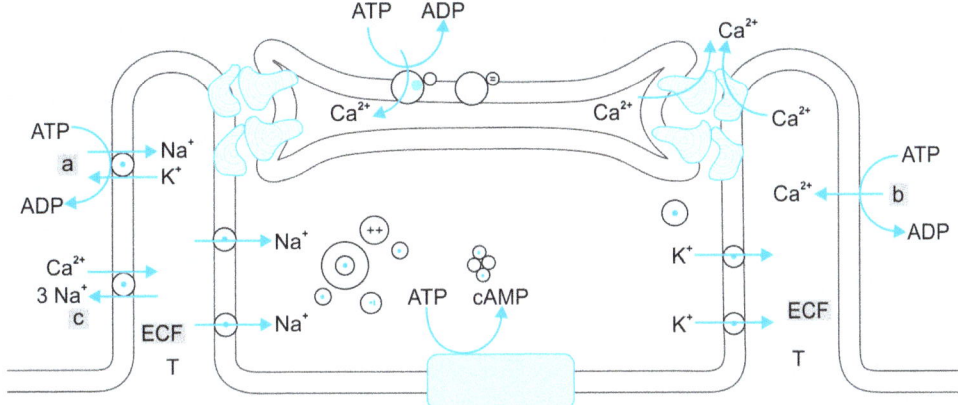

Fig. 23.9: Changes during cardiac muscle contraction.
(ECF: extracellular fluid ; ATP: adenosine triphosphate; ADP: adenosine diphosphate)

and increases K currents, promoting slower, less forceful beats **(Fig. 23.9)**. Depending on the type of smooth muscle, catecholamines may produce either contraction or relaxation. This relaxation is apparently mediated by the cAMP-dependent phosphorylation and inactivation of the enzyme myosin light chain kinase (MLCK), which plays a central role in smooth muscle contraction. Vascular smooth muscle redistributes the blood supply during exercise and visceral smooth muscle empties the gut in stressful or frightening situations. In contrast to all this, the force of contraction in voluntary muscle is unaffected by circulating hormones.

Control of Cardiac Contraction

The control of cardiac muscle contraction is shown in **Fig. 23.9**.
- The sodium–potassium adenosine triphosphatase (Na^+/K^+-ATPase) or sodium pump:
  - Works continuously, using the energy from ATP to maintain a high K^+ concentration inside the cells and a high Na^+ concentration in the extracellular fluid (ECF). The cell membrane (sarcolemma) is usually more permeable to K^+ than to Na^+ and this gives rise to a membrane potential of about 80 mV (inside negative) in relaxed muscle. The Ca^{2+} are also removed from the cytosol into the ECF by an ATP-driven calcium pump.
  - In all tissues, cardiac muscle possesses an additional sodium–calcium exchange protein.
  - This export system is driven by the preexisting Na^+ gradient. The calcium concentration inside resting cells is low but rises sharply during contractions.
- Contraction in cardiac muscle is triggered by a wave of membrane depolarization, which spreads from neighboring cells. The change in electric field activates voltage-gated Na channels in the sarcolemma, each of which allows a few hundred positively charged Na^+ to enter the negatively charged cytosol, further reducing the cardiac membrane potential until the whole sarcolemma is depolarized.
- The Na channel undergoes a second conformational change, as a result of which these channels close spontaneously after a few milliseconds in all excitable tissues. In cardiac muscle, but not skeletal muscle, slower voltage-gated Ca channels, probably identical with dihydropyridine receptors, take over and maintain a positive inward current for several hundred milliseconds

during the plateau phase of the cardiac action potential.
- Dihydropyridine drugs (e.g. nifedipine) inhibit calcium entry into heart and reduce blood pressure. About 10% of the calcium needed to activate cardiac contraction enters during each beat from the ECF. This is often described as "trigger Ca". The remainder is released from the SR through a channel known as the ryanodine receptor. Ryanodine receptors are widely distributed in the body and are present in nonmuscle tissues such as brain. Different tissues have their own specific isoenzymes.
- Calcium ions from both sources bind to the regulatory protein TnC located in the thin filaments, leading to a change in filament shape. This allows flexible head groups from the protein myosin in the thick filaments to interact with the protein actin in the thin filaments. A change in myosin conformation causes the thick and thin filaments to slide against each other and hydrolyze ATP, which provides the energy for contraction. Movement and ATP hydrolysis continue until the Ca^{2+} are removed from the cytosol at the end of each contraction. Most of the Ca^{2+} are returned to the SR by calcium pump, but about 10% leave the cell via proteins. The Ca^{2+} is stored within the SR loosely bound to a protein, calsequestrin.
- In cardiac muscle, circulating hormones such as catecholamines and glucagon bind to specific receptors on the outer surface of the sarcolemma, changing their shape. This change is communicated via G-proteins within the sarcolemma to adenylyl cyclase bound to the internal face of the sarcolemma. Several G-proteins are known, some activators, others inhibitory. The steady-state concentration of cAMP depends on the balance between synthesis and degradation. The cAMP in turn controls the activity of cAMP-dependent protein kinase. This enzyme phosphorylates several of the proteins involved in the contraction process and temporarily alters their properties, until a protein phosphatase restores the status by removing the phosphate group.
- The Na^+ pump is activated by phosphorylation, which allows it to handle the increased ion traffic across the sarcolemma when cardiac work output rises.
- The dihydropyridine receptor is activated by phosphorylation, increasing the Ca entry into the cells. The ryanodine receptor (6) is also activated, increasing the rate of Ca release from the SR. The TnI component in the thin filaments is phosphorylated and this reduces Ca binding to the neighboring TnC.
- A small protein called phospholamban associated with the SR Ca^{2+} pump is phosphorylated and this accelerates calcium uptake by the SR pump.
- The enzymes triglyceride lipase and glycogen phosphorylase are activated by phosphorylation.
- Skeletal muscle can contract in the absence of extracellular Ca and skeletal SR shows depolarization-induced Ca release. In contrast to this, cardiac SR needs external "trigger Ca" to enter the cells via the dihydropyridine receptors during the plateau phase of each action potential to initiate Ca-induced Ca release. Dihydropyridine receptors are also present in some smooth muscles. They are blocked by the important drugs verapamil and nifedipine, which reduce the force of cardiac contraction, while maintaining an adequate cardiac output by relaxing vascular smooth muscle and reducing the peripheral vascular resistance.

SMOOTH MUSCLE

Smooth muscle is made up of single, spindle-shaped cells. It gets its name because no striations are visible in them. Smooth muscle cell contains thick (myosin) and thin (actin) filaments that slide against each other to produce contraction of the cell. The thick and thin filaments are anchored near the plasma membrane (with the help of intermediate filaments).

Smooth muscle does not depend on motor neurons to be stimulated. However, motor neurons reach smooth muscle and can stimulate it or relax it depending on the neurotransmitter they release, e.g. noradrenaline or nitric oxide (NO).

Contraction of Smooth Muscle

Smooth muscle can also be made to contract:
- By other substances released in the vicinity (paracrine stimulation):
  - For example, release of histamine causes contraction of the smooth muscle lining our air passages (triggering an attack of asthma).
- By hormones circulating in the blood:
  - For example, oxytocin reaching the uterus stimulates it to contract to begin childbirth.

The contraction of smooth muscle tends to be slower than that of striated muscle. Many types of smooth muscle require external Ca in order to contract and have nifedipine-sensitive Ca^{2+} channels very similar to the dihydropyridine receptors observed in cardiac muscle.

Troponin is absent from smooth muscles and their actin regulatory system differs considerably from the thin filament regulatory system found in striated muscles. Caldesmon is a smooth muscle protein that binds reversibly to the actin/tropomyosin filaments and blocks the actomyosin ATPase activity. Caldesmon can be sequestered away from the actin by two separate Ca-dependent methods:
- By phosphorylation using protein kinase C.
- By binding calcium and calmodulin to form a caldesmon–calcium–calmodulin complex that is unable to bind to actin.

- In contrast to this, troponin is a permanent feature of striated muscle thin filaments and never dissociates from the actin.

The myosin regulatory system is much more important in smooth muscles than in striated muscle. The enzyme MLCK is activated by calcium+calmodulin and phosphorylates the 5,5'-di-thiobis-2-nitrobenzoic acid "regulatory" light chains in the myosin S1 head groups. This increases the inherent myosin Ca sensitivity and brings it into the physiological range, allowing contraction to proceed. This system also operates in striated muscle, where it seems to play a subordinate role. Phosphorylation of myosin light chains on a second site by protein kinase C interferes with this process and leads to smooth muscle relaxation.

Isolated vascular smooth muscle contracts in response to ACh, but this compound relaxes intact blood vessels as a result of NO generated by endothelial cells. The NO relaxes vascular smooth muscle via cyclic guanosine monophosphate. Both vascular and airway smooth muscles relax in response to beta-adrenergic agonists via cAMP. These effects are of considerable medical significance in the treatment of hypertension and asthma.

ADENOSINE TRIPHOSPHATE HYDROLYSIS FOR MUSCLE CONTRACTION

For muscle contraction, myosin as ATPase walks along the actin filaments:
- The energy for muscle contraction comes from ATP hydrolysis. Actin catalyzes the ATPase activity of myosin. The rate-limiting step is the release of products of ATP hydrolysis (ADP and Pi). These remain noncovalently bound to the myosin molecule and prevent further ATP binding and hydrolysis. The binding of myosin to actin causes a rapid release of ADP and Pi from the myosin molecule.

- It is the globular head of the myosin molecule that binds to actin and hydrolyzes ATP. Each actin molecule in the thin filaments can bind one myosin head. The heads bind with the same orientation to each actin subunit and thus point all in the same direction. The actin filament has a plus and a minus end. The latter points toward the center of the sarcomere. The thin filaments on either side of the sarcomere are of opposite polarity to accommodate the oriented myosin heads appropriately. The myosin heads point in opposite directions away from the sarcomere center.
- The myosin heads walk from the minus ends of the thin filaments in center of the sarcomere to the plus ends on the Z disks. During this movement, ATP is hydrolyzed and subsequent dissociation of the tightly bound products (ADP and Pi) produce an ordered series of changes in the conformation of myosin, moving the actin filaments along the thick filaments.
- Phosphorylation of myosin light chains initiates contraction of smooth muscle.
- The MLCK is activated by calmodulin Ca^{2+} and then it phosphorylates the light chains and the same smooth muscle relaxes when the concentration of Ca^{2+} falls below 10^{-7} mol/L.

MUSCLE DISEASES

Muscular Dystrophies

Together myosin, actin, tropomyosin, and troponin make up over three quarters of the protein in muscle fibers. Some two dozen other proteins make up the rest. These are attaching and organizing the filaments in the sarcomere, and connecting the sarcomeres to the plasma membrane and the extracellular matrix. Mutations in the genes encoding these proteins may produce defective proteins and resulting defects in the muscles.

Among the most common of the muscular dystrophies are those caused by mutations in the gene for dystrophin. The gene for dystrophin is huge, containing 79 exons spread out over 2.3 million base pairs of deoxyribonucleic acid. Thus this single gene represents about 0.1% of the entire human genome (3×10^9 base pairs) and is almost half the size of the entire genome of *Escherichia coli*:

- *Duchenne muscular dystrophy (DMD):* Deletions or nonsense mutations that cause a frameshift usually introduce premature termination codons in the resulting messenger RNA. Thus at best only a fragment of dystrophin is synthesized and DMD, a very severe form of the disease, results.
- *Becker muscular dystrophy (BMD):* If the deletion simply removes certain exons but preserves the correct reading frames, a slightly shortened protein results that produces BMD, a milder form of the disease.

The gene for dystrophin is on the X chromosome, so these two diseases strike males in a typical X-linked pattern of inheritance.

Myasthenia Gravis

Myasthenia gravis is an autoimmune disorder affecting the NMJ. Patients have smaller EPPs than normal. With repeated stimulation, the EPPs become too small to trigger further action potentials and the fiber ceases to contract. Administration of an inhibitor of acetylcholinesterase temporarily can restore contractility by allowing more ACh to remain at the site.

Patients with myasthenia gravis have only 20% or so of the number of ACh receptors found in normal NMJs. This loss appears to be caused by antibodies directed against the receptors. Newborns of mothers with myasthenia gravis often show mild signs of the disease for a short time after their birth. This is result of the transfer of the mother's antibodies across the placenta during gestation. The reason some people develop autoimmune antibodies against the ACh receptor is unknown.

Cardiac Myopathies

Cardiac muscle, such as skeletal muscle, contains many proteins in addition to actin and myosin. Mutations in the genes for these may cause the wall of the heart to become weakened and, in due course, enlarged. Among the genes that have been implicated in these diseases are those encoding:
- Actin
- Two types of myosin:
  1. Troponin
  2. Tropomyosin.
- Myosin-binding protein C (which links myosin to titin).

The severity of the disease varies with the particular mutation causing it (over 100 have been identified so far). Some mutations are sufficiently dangerous that they can lead to sudden heart failure.

The clinical importance of *troponin* estimation
- Troponins have been investigated as markers of acute cardiac ischemia.
- These are protein components of striated muscle.
- TnT is the myofibrilla protein of the striated muscle, which is the building block of the contractile apparatus.
- Troponin is a protein complex consisting of three subunits with different structure and function, namely:
  1. *TnT:* Tropomyosin-binding element
  2. *TnI:* Actinomyosin ATPase inhibitory element
  3. *TnC:* Calcium binding.
- *TnT* is normally measured because a small pool of it is not compartmentalized in the contractile apparatus and may be a precursor for synthesis of the troponin complex.
- It is released into the blood within about 4 hours after the onset of symptoms, peaks at 12–16 hours and remains, elevated for 5–9 days post infarction.
- Therefore cardiac troponin is very useful as a marker at any time interval after the heart attack which is its great advantage.
- A level > 1.5 µg/L is indicative of myocardial damage.
- TnT is the specific and sensitive test for the diagnosis of myocardial infarction as compared to CPK and LDH enzymes.
- TnT is a very useful indicator of myocardial ischemia in these cases

Indications
- Acute myocardial infarction
- Subacute myocardial infarction
- Microinfarction
- Size of infarction
- Monitoring the outcome of thrombolysis therapy.

Advantages
- Highly sensitive for detecting myocardial ischemia
- Levels may help to stratify risk afterward
- The 14/32 hour ratio of troponin is a reliable indicator of success and thrombolysis
- *TnI* elevation is useful for predicting in-hospital risk for unstable angina patients admitted to a community hospital.

A level >1.2 suggests myocardial infarction.

SUMMARY

Muscles in the human body have biochemical specialization, which makes them to perform many physiological functions. Three different kinds of muscles are heart muscle, smooth muscle, and skeletal muscle. Skeletal muscle is made up of thousands of cylindrical muscle fibers often running all the way from origin to insertion. Each muscle fiber contains an array of myofibrils that are staked lengthwise and run the entire length of the fiber. Each fiber is composed of myofibrils and each myofibril is made up of arrays of parallel filaments, which is a series of repeating structural units called sarcomeres. Sarcomeres are composed of thick (myosin) and thin (actin) filaments. The thick filaments have a diameter of about 15 nm and composed of numerous protein strands, which are called myosin filaments. Each myosin filament is composed of a two twisted strands called heavy chains and two other, but each different, pairs of twisted strands called light chains. These light chains are found in the myosin heads. The thin filaments have a diameter of about 5 nm. Actin exists as a polymer of repeating globular proteins called G-actin. Two actin filaments are twisted into a single-stranded filament. These strands are anchored at one end to the Z disk, lying in the groove formed by the actin filaments are a series of rod-shaped protein molecules called tropomyosin. Each tropomyosin molecule is six to seven G-actin molecules in length. Bound to the end of each tropomyosin is a third protein called troponin. Troponin consists as three small bound protein molecules—TnI, TnT, and TnC. One molecule is bound to the actin filament, one to the tropomyosin, and the third is available to bind with Ca^{2+}. The junction between the terminal of a motor neuron and a muscle fiber is called NMJ. Together myosin, actin, tropomyosin, and troponin make up over three quarters of the protein in muscle fibers. Mutations in the genes encoding these proteins may produce defective proteins and resulting defects in the muscles. Among the most common of the muscular dystrophies are those caused by mutations in the gene for dystrophin. Myasthenia gravis is an autoimmune disorder affecting the neuromuscular junction.

MULTIPLE-CHOICE QUESTIONS

1. **The two principal contractile proteins found in skeletal muscle are:**
   a. Actin and myosin
   b. Troponin and tropomyosin
   c. Myosin and tropomyosin
   d. Actin and tropomyosin

2. **The sarcoplasmic reticulum in muscle cells acts as a:**
   a. Store of digestive enzymes
   b. Store of Na^+
   c. Store of lipid
   d. Store of Ca^{2+}

3. **An action potential arriving at the motor end plate causes release of:**
   a. Sodium ions, which binds to sodium receptors on the muscle membrane
   b. Calcium ions, which initiate an action potential along the muscle fiber
   c. Acetylcholine, which traverses the neuromuscular junction
   d. Noradrenaline, which increases muscle metabolic activity

4. **Trigger to initiate the contractile process in skeletal muscle is:**
   a. Calcium binding to tropomyosin
   b. ATP binding to the myosin cross-bridges
   c. Calcium binding to troponin
   d. ATP breakdown by actin

5. **Once the Ca^{2+} has been released from the sarcoplasmic reticulum, they:**
   a. Cause sodium channels to open in the sarcolemmal membrane
   b. Bind to troponin
   c. Bind to actin
   d. Initiate an action potential

6. **A muscle fiber relaxes when:**
   a. The nerve stimulus is too forceful
   b. The actin-binding sites are uncovered

Biochemistry of Muscle Structure and Function

   c. The actin-binding sites are saturated
   d. The nerve stimulus is removed
7. **Fast-twitch fibers contain a relatively:**
   a. Small number of mitochondria and high ATPase activity
   b. Large number of mitochondria and low ATPase activity
   c. Small number of mitochondria and low ATPase activity
   d. Large number of mitochondria and high ATPase activity
8. **Type I muscle fibers have the following characteristics:**
   a. Red, oxidative, slow contracting
   b. White, glycolytic, slow contracting
   c. Red, oxidative, fast contracting
   d. Red, glycolytic, slow contracting
9. **Cardiac muscle:**
   a. T is striated
   b. F has myosin, but not actin filaments
   c. F has multinucleated cells
   d. F cells are connected to other cardiac muscle cells at gap junctions
10. **Concerning Duchenne muscular dystrophy:**
    a. It is caused by partial deletion of the gene for dystrophin
    b. It is indicated by lowered serum creatine kinase of skeletal muscle fibers
    c. Females are not affected
    d. The disease is nonprogressive in its course
11. **Concerning malignant hyperthermia:**
    a. It can be induced by the administration of the drug dantrolene
    b. There is a high level of cytosolic Ca^{2+} in skeletal muscle
    c. There is decreased oxidative metabolism in skeletal muscle
    d. It is characterized by decrease in core body temperature
12. **Myosin:**
    a. Forms thin filaments in solutions of physiological ionic strength and pH
    b. Is composed of eight polypeptide chains
    c. Has a conserved sequence similar to that found in the active site of other ATPases
    d. Has two α-helical strands that point in opposite directions
13. **Concerning enzymatic cleavage of myosin:**
    a. Trypsin cleaves myosin into light and heavy meromyosin
    b. LMM has ATPase activity in the presence of Ca^{2+}
    c. HMM has kinase activity
    d. The S2 fragment has only one binding site for ATP
14. **Concerning the types of muscle fibers:**
    a. Type I fibers (slow oxidative) have high ATPase activity
    b. Type II fibers (fast oxidative) succumb to fatigue
    c. Type III fibers (fast glycolytic) are susceptible to fatigue
    d. Type III fibers are red because they contain myoglobin
15. **Cardiac muscle fibers:**
    a. Are susceptible to fatigue
    b. Are longer than those of skeletal muscle
    c. Can undergo tetanic contraction
    d. Are electrically coupled to each other
16. **Smooth muscle cells have:**
    a. Aligned sarcomeres
    b. Rudimentary sarcoplasmic reticulum
    c. Well-developed Z lines
    d. Identical myosin light chains
17. **Concerning the steps in excitation–contraction coupling:**
    a. The Ca^{2+}-calmodulin complex deactivates the enzyme myosin light chain kinase (MLCK)
    b. MLCK phosphorylates the 17 kDa light chains of the myosin heads
    c. Myosin phosphorylation exposes a binding site for actinin
    d. Myosin ATPase is activated when myosin binds to actin
18. **Concerning myosin and the power stroke:**
    a. ATP is hydrolyzed by the S2 head of myosin
    b. The myosin–ATP complex has no affinity for actin
    c. The myosin–ADP–Pi complex is at a low energy state
    d. Binding of actin to the myosin–ADP–Pi complex releases Pi
19. **Concerning skeletal muscle, which of the following is false?**
    a. Contraction is initiated by a nerve impulse
    b. It exhibits very rapid cycling of cross-bridges
    c. The plasmalemma lacks many hormone receptors
    d. T tubules are more developed compared to cardiac muscle

20. **Caldesmon:**
    a. Is not a ubiquitous protein
    b. Is a cofactor of MLCK
    c. Binds to actin and tropomyosin at low Ca^{2+}
    d. Binds to the Ca^{2+}–calmodulin complex at low Ca^{2+}

21. **Duchenne-type muscular dystrophy is:**
    a. Found only in males
    b. Caused by the deletion of a gene on the Y chromosome
    c. Usually observed to occur initially in the pelvis and legs
    d. Characterized by progressive necrosis and phagocytosis of cardiomyocytes

22. **Concerning malignant hyperthermia, all of the following are true, *except*:**
    a. It exhibits genetic heterogeneity in humans
    b. Elevated cytoplasmic Ca^{2+} is due to a mutation in the structural gene for the Ca^{2+} release channel
    c. Dantrolene inhibits the release of Ca^{2+} from the SR
    d. It is due to abnormal accumulation of Ca^{2+} in the cytoplasm of cardiac muscle cells

23. **Concerning muscle fiber types:**
    a. Long distance runners rely on mainly type II fibers
    b. Type I are also called fast-twitch fibers
    c. Lactic acid accumulates more readily in type IIB than IIA fibers
    d. Sprinters rely mainly on type I fibers

24. **Contraction of skeletal muscle depends on the:**
    a. Allosteric control of Ca^{2+}
    b. Enzymatic cleavage of myosin
    c. Binding of ATP to the S2 subunit of myosin
    d. Activation of myosin by MLCK

25. **Concerning thick and thin filaments in skeletal and cardiac muscles, all of the following are true, *except*:**
    a. Thick and thin filaments interact by cross-bridges
    b. Each thick filament is surrounded by six thin filaments
    c. Each thin filament has four neighboring thick filaments
    d. Overlapping filaments in the A band exhibit a hexagonal array in cross-section

26. **Concerning the mechanism of smooth muscle contraction:**
    a. Calmodulin binds to L-myosin
    b. MLCK phosphorylates L-myosin at serine 22
    c. Relaxation occurs by dephosphorylation of MLCK
    d. At low Ca^{2+} caldesmon binds actin

27. **Creatine:**
    a. Is formed by the methylation of guanidinoacetate
    b. Requires cysteine as a cofactor
    c. Is made in only skeletal muscle
    d. Exists as three isozymes

28. **Concerning myosin, it:**
    a. Lacks intrinsic ATPase activity
    b. Has two heavy and six light polypeptide chains
    c. Forms a viscous solution with F-actin
    d. Forms thin filaments in solutions of physiological ionic strength and pH

29. **The myosin S1 head region binds all of the following, *except*:**
    a. ATP
    b. Actin
    c. Actinin
    d. Light chain

30. **Concerning rigor mortis, which of the following is incorrect?**
    a. Reversal of myosin cross-linking does not occur
    b. Actomyosin complexes are poorly cross-linked
    c. It is a rigid state of muscle contraction that develops
    d. Cisternal and intracellular Ca^{2+} leak into the cytoplasm

31. **Concerning the myofilaments of the sarcomere, all the following are true, *except*:**
    a. Both thick and thin filaments are present in the I band
    b. Each thin filament has three neighboring thick filaments
    c. Each thick filament is surrounded by six thin filaments
    d. Actin is anchored to the Z line by actinin

32. **Concerning the contractile apparatus of smooth muscle, all of the following are true, *except*:**
    a. The contraction of smooth muscle is regulated primarily by bound Ca^{2+} concentration
    b. The thick filament proteins are myosin heavy chain and myosin light chains

c. The thin filament proteins are caldesmon, tropomyosin, calponin, and actin/tropomyosin
d. The Ca^{2+} binds to calmodulin at high Ca^{2+} concentration to effect contraction

33. **Concerning smooth muscle contractions:**
    a. The Ca^{2+} can regulate both contraction and relaxation in the same cell
    b. Caldesmon blocks the actin-binding site in relaxed smooth muscle at low Ca^{2+} levels
    c. At high Ca^{2+} levels, the Ca^{2+}-calmodulin complex removes caldesmon from actin and promotes cycling
    d. At intermediate Ca^{2+} levels cycling cross-bridges are formed between myosin head, caldesmon, and actin

34. **Thin filaments of skeletal and cardiac muscles are composed of all of the following, except:**
    a. F-actin
    b. Tropomyosin
    c. Troponins
    d. Kinesin

35. **The Ca^{2+}–Na^+ exchanger:**
    a. Transports one Na^+ for every three Ca^{2+} leaving the cell
    b. Is the principal route of exit of Ca^{2+} from myocytes
    c. Uses the energy from the downhill movement of Na^+ into the cell for the uphill movement of Ca^{2+} out of the cell
    d. Causes the direct increase of intracellular Na^+ and the indirect increase of Ca^{2+}

Answers

1. a	2. d	3. c	4. c	5. b
6. d	7. a	8. a	9. a	10. a
11. b	12. c	13. a	14. c	15. d
16. b	17. d	18. d	19. d	20. c
21. c	22. c	23. d	24. a	25. c
26. d	27. a	28. c	29. c	30. b
31. d	32. a	33. d	34. d	35. a

CHAPTER 24

Water and Electrolyte Balance

OBJECTIVES

At the end of this topic the student should be able to:
- Understand the mechanisms involved in the water balance
- Know the causes and symptoms of hyper and hypovolemia
- Know about the different types of electrolytes and the mechanisms involved in their regulation
- Get the knowledge of causes and symptoms of hyper and hypo conditions of electrolytes.

WATER BALANCE

Introduction

Water balance is the concept of human homeostasis that the amount of fluid lost from the body is equal to the amount of fluid taken in. Humans can survive for 4-6 weeks without food, but for only a few days without water. The amount of water varies with the individual, as it depends on the condition of the subject, the amount of physical exercise, and on the environmental temperature and humidity

- Water constitutes 60% of the total body weight.
- The body's water is distributed between two compartments.
- That is extracellular fluid (ECF) and intracellular fluid (ICF).
- Fluid found within the cells is called ICF and that found outside cells is called ECF **(Fig. 24.1)**.
- The ECF is further divided into that which is found as blood plasma within blood vessels and that which is found in the microscopic spaces between cells called interstitial fluid.
- Approximately two thirds of body fluid are intracellular, and the remaining one third is extracellular **(Table 24.1)**.
- Of the ECF approximately 80% is interstitial fluid and 20% is blood plasma.
- Selectively permeable membranes separate body fluids into distinct compartments.
- Plasma membranes of individual cells separate ICF from ECF and blood vessel walls separate blood plasma from interstitial fluid.
- The major components of these fluids include water and solutes.
- The solute mostly comprises electrolytes—inorganic compounds that dissociate into two ions, namely cations and anions.
- The cations are positively charged atoms and examples are sodium, potassium, calcium, and magnesium.
- The anions are negatively charged atoms and examples are chloride, sulfide, phosphate, bicarbonate, and carbonate.
- The exchange of interstitial and ICF is controlled mainly by the presence of the electrolytes, sodium and potassium.

Potassium is the chief intracellular cation and sodium the chief extracellular cation **(Fig. 24.2)**.

The body water is maintained at a constant volume by a regulation between intake and output water as given above.

Water and Electrolyte Balance

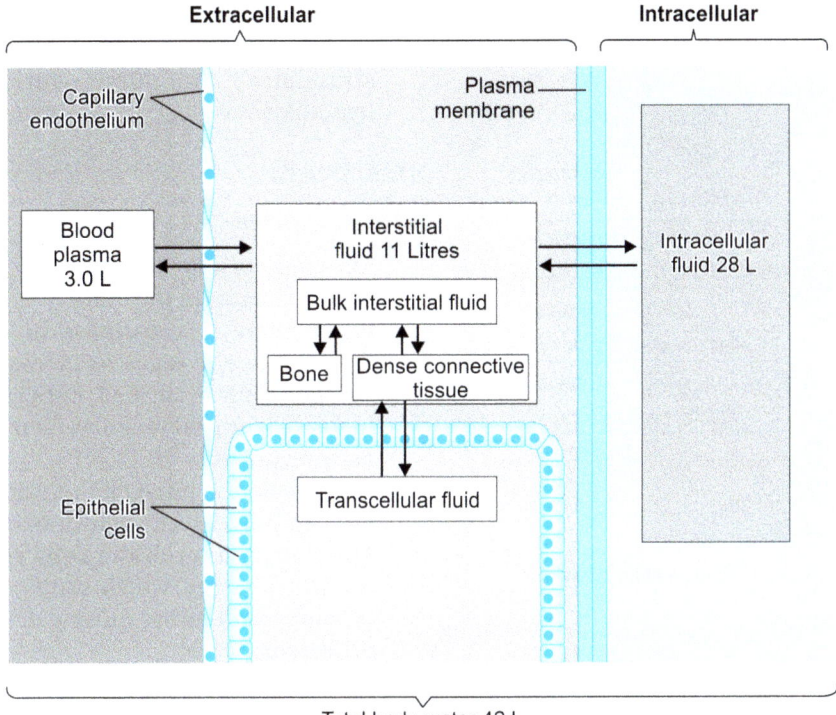

Fig. 24.1: Fluid distribution in different compartments.

Table 24.1: Fluid distribution in various compartments.

Fluid distribution	% of total body weight (70 kg)	Volume
Body water	60%	42 L
1. Intracellular	40%	28 L
2. Extracellular	20%	14 L
➢ Plasma (blood)	5%	3.0 L
➢ CSF		
➢ Interstitial fluid	15%	10.5 L
➢ Lymph		
➢ Synovial fluid		
➢ Ocular fluid		
➢ Pleural fluid		
➢ Pericardial fluid		

(CSF: cerebrospinal fluid)

Regulation of Fluid Balance

The term "fluid balance" defines the state where a body's required amount of water is

Fluid intake	(mL)
Ingested water	1,300
Ingested food	900
Metabolic oxidation	300
Total	2,500

Fluid output	(mL)
Kidneys	1,500
Skin	
Sweat	400
Lungs	400
Gastrointestinal	200
Total	2,500

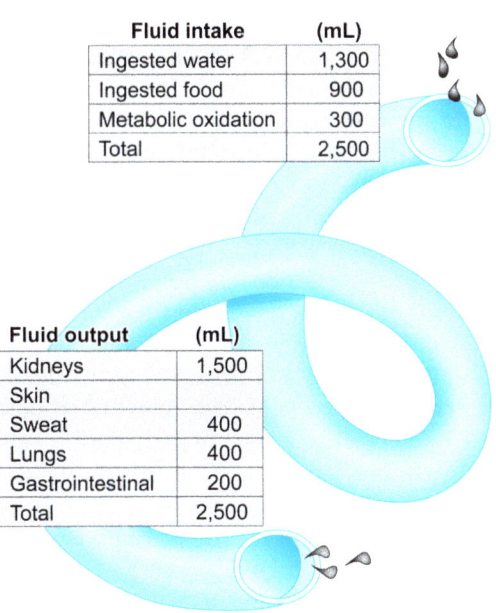

Fig. 24.2: Fluid input and output.

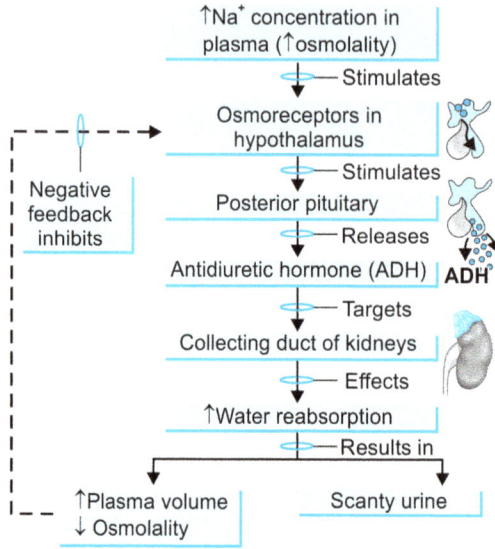

Fig. 24.3: Regulation of fluid balance.

present and proportioned normally among the various compartments **(Fig. 24.3)**.

Under normal conditions, water loss equals water gain and a body's water volume remains constant.

Water loss takes place through the kidneys, skin, lungs, feces, and menstruation.

Gain water mostly from dietary intake, this is called preformed water.

Metabolic processes such as cellular respiration and dehydration synthesis reactions generate a small component.

Water is not produced by the body to maintain homeostasis.

Metabolic water production is simply a by-product of cellular respiration.

The body regulates water intake via the thirst reflex which stimulates us to drink. When water loss is greater than water gain, the body reaches a state of dehydration, and dehydration stimulates the thirst reflex in three ways:
1. Saliva level drops resulting in a dry mucosa in the mouth and pharynx.
2. Increase in blood osmotic pressure, which stimulates osmoreceptors in the hypothalamus.
3. There is a drop in blood volume, which leads to the renin/angiotensin II pathway stimulating the thirst center in the hypothalamus.

Mechanism

Thirst Center

- The intake of water is regulated by the thirst center, situated in the brain.
- When there is a decrease in the body fluid volume, it leads to increase in the salt concentration; and hence, there is increased osmolality and an increase in the osmotic pressure the ECF.
- As a result, the intracellular water comes out and cells become dehydrated.
- The dehydration of the cells stimulates the thirst center, which sends messages to tongue and throat causing dryness and drink more water.
- Drinking inhibits the thirst center by stretching the stomach and intestines and reducing the osmotic pressure of the blood.

Antidiuretic Hormone

Antidiuretic hormone (ADH) helps in the reabsorption of water from renal tubules and thereby loss of water from the body is regulated.

Antidiuretic hormone is the hormone secreted by the posterior pituitary.

When there is a decrease in body fluid, osmotic pressure of ECF increases, which stimulates the cells of the hypothalamus, which then stimulates the posterior pituitary to secrete ADH.

Antidiuretic hormone acts on the kidney tubules and increases the reabsorption of water, thus conserving water. When the body fluid content is sufficient, the osmotic pressure of ECF is normal, or low. During this condition, there is no stimulation of the hypothalamic cells or posterior pituitary, so ADH is not secreted. As a result, there is a decrease in the reabsorption of water from the renal tubules and more water is lost in the urine.

CAUSES AND SYMPTOMS OF HYPOVOLEMIA AND HYPERVOLEMIA

Dehydration (Hypovolemia)

- Loss of water from the body in excess amounts leads to dehydration **(Table 24.2)**.
- First the plasma becomes concentrated followed by the ECF and then the ICF.
- When water comes out of the cells, it passes into ECF in exchange of K^+ and Na^+ passes into ICF from ECF.
- Loss of more than 20% of body water results in death.

Causes of Dehydration

The causes of dehydration are as follows:
- Severe diarrhea and vomiting
- Excessive heat
- Difficulty in swallowing and state of unconsciousness.
- Loss of fluid from skin in case of burns.
- Diabetes insipidus (ADH polyuria)
- Heart stroke
- Excitement
- Fever
- Excessive sweating.

Dehydration induces water to move from the reservoir inside cells into the blood. If dehydration progresses, body tissues begin to dry out and the cells start to shrivel and malfunction. The most susceptible cells to dehydration are the brain cells. Mental confusion, one of the most common signs of severe dehydration, may result and can lead to **coma**. Dehydration can occur when excessive water is lost with such diseases as **diabetes mellitus**, diabetes insipidus, and Addison's disease.

Dehydration is often accompanied by a deficiency of electrolytes, sodium and potassium in particular. Water does not move as rapidly from the reservoir inside of the cells into the blood when electrolyte concentration is decreased. Blood pressure can decline due to a lower volume of water circulating in the bloodstream. A drop in blood pressure can cause light headedness, or a feeling of impending blackout, especially upon standing (orthostatic hypotension). Continued fluid and electrolyte imbalance may further reduce blood pressure, causing **shock** and damage to many internal organs, including the brain, kidneys, and **liver**.

Features of Dehydration

The features of dehydration are as follows:
- Dryness of skin, tongue, and throat
- Changes in the values of packed cell volume, Hb, plasma protein, plasma electrolytes, urea, and decreased blood pressure.

Table 24.2: Observations related to fluid balance.

Observation	Fluid depletion	Fluid overload
Weight	Loss	Gain
Blood pressure	Lowered smaller pulse pressure	Normal or raised
Respirations	Rapid, shallow	Rapid, moist cough
Pulse	Rapid, weak	Rapid
Urine output	Reduced, concentrated	Increased or decreased if heart is failing
Skin	Dry, less elastic	Edematous
Saliva	Thick, viscous	Copious, frothy
Tongue	Dry, coated	Moist
Thirst	Present	No disturbance
Face	Sunken eyes	Periorbital edema
Temperature	May be raised	No disturbance

Treatment

Treatment for dehydration is as follows:
- Consuming plenty of plain water or water containing sugar and salt (depends upon the cause of dehydration).
- If the condition is very severe, intravenous infusion of fluids (normal saline) is required.

Water Excess (Hypervolemia)

It is a condition in which the body water content is excessive **(Table 24.2)**.

Causes

The causes of hypervolemia are as follows:
- Hypersecretion of ADH following the administration of anesthetics. This effect occurs for about 12–36 hours after the surgery.
- Renal failure.
- SIADH (syndrome of inappropriate ADH secretion).
   Here hypersecretion of ADH occurs.

Causes for SIADH: Some malignant conditions, disease of central nervous system, and side effects of certain drugs.

Overhydration can occur alone or in conjunction with excess blood volume. Distinguishing between the two conditions may be quite complicated. Overhydration induces water accumulation within and around the cells but does not typically show symptoms of fluid accumulation. On the other hand, with excess blood volume, there is an accumulation of sodium and the body cannot transfer water into the reservoir within cells. Conditions such as **heart failure** and liver cirrhosis may induce volume overload, whereby fluid accumulates around cells in the abdomen, chest, and lower legs.

Features

The features of hypervolemia are as follows:
- Mental confusion, incoordination, muscular weakness, nausea.
- Decreased packed cell volume.
- Decreased plasma electrolytes, plasma osmolality, increased urine osmolality, and increased blood pressure. When there is increased ADH secretion, more H_2O is absorbed from the renal tubules. As the volume of fluid increases, the salts get diluted. Hence, the plasma osmolality decreases.

Treatment

The treatment of hypervolemia is as follows:
- Withdrawal of fluids
- Administration of diuretics.

ELECTROLYTE BALANCE

Introduction

The electrolytes, anions or cations, which are present either in ECF or ICF should be maintained in balance otherwise the human body has to face several serious problems.

Electrolytes in Intracellular Fluid and Extracellular Fluid

Distribution of Electrolytes

Solutes plasma (mEq/L)	ECF	ICF
Cations		
Na^+	142	10
K^+	5	148
Ca^{2+}	5	2
Mg^{2+}	3	40
Anions		
Cl^-	103	
HCO_3^-	24	8
HPO_4^{2-}	2	136
SO_4^{2-}	1	
Protein	15	56
Organic ions	10	

- The sum of *cations* must be equal to the sum of *anions* to maintain electrical neutrality.

- Electrolyte composition of other ECF is similar to that of plasma except that of proteins. Protein concentration is higher in plasma than other ECF.
- *Sodium* is the major cation of plasma.
- *Chloride* and *bicarbonate* are the major anions of plasma.
- The total electrolyte concentration in ICF is higher than in ECF.
- The major cations in ICF are K^+ and Mg^{2+} and these are balanced mainly by the anions PO_4^{2-} and proteins.

Importance of Serum (Extracellular Fluid) and Urine Osmolality

Serum osmolality: Serum osmolality is a useful preliminary investigation for identifying the cause of hyponatremia. If a patient with significant hyponatremia (serum sodium <130 mmol/L) has a normal plasma osmolality, the patient may have pseudohyponatremia due to excess lipids or proteins, or the sample may have been collected from a drip arm containing dextrose. If the patient has an increased osmolality it is likely the patient has reactive hyponatremia due to an excess of solute pulling water out of cells. Examples of this include glucose in diabetes mellitus or hyperglycinemia after *trans*-urethral resection of the prostate.

Urine osmolality: Urine osmolality is an important test for the concentrating ability of the kidney. Interpretation of urine osmolality must always be made in the light of the appropriate physiological response to the state of hydration of the patient. The test is useful in the following areas:
- For determining the differential diagnosis of hyper- or hyponatremia.
- For identifying SIADH (urine osmolality >200 mmol/kg; urine sodium >20 mmol/L; low serum sodium; patient not dehydrated and no renal, adrenal, thyroid, cardiac, or liver disease or interfering drugs).
- For differentiating prerenal from renal kidney failure (high urine osmolality is consistent with prerenal impairment, in renal damage the urine osmolality is similar to plasma osmolality).
- For identifying and diagnosing diabetes insipidus.

Sodium Balance

- Kidney is the only organ involved in the excretion of sodium and helps to regulate the body Na^+ content.
- The filtered Na^+ in the glomerular filtrate is reabsorbed in the distal tubule.
- A hormone, namely *aldosterone* secreted by the adrenal cortex is involved in the regulation of sodium reabsorption in the renal tubules.
- Aldosterone increases the reabsorption of Na^+ whenever the plasma Na^+ is low.
- Along with Na^+, Cl^- is also reabsorbed.
- Absorption of Na^+ takes place in exchange for K^+.
- Aldosterone secretion is controlled by the volume of ECF and its Na^+ concentration.

Process of Balancing Sodium Maintained in the Human Body

- In addition to regulating total volume, the *osmolality* of body fluids is also highly regulated.
- Extreme variation in osmolality causes cells to shrink or swell, damaging or destroying cellular structure and disrupting normal cellular function.
- Regulation of osmolality is achieved by balancing the intake and excretion of sodium with that of water.
- Sodium is the major solute in ECFs, so it effectively determines the osmolality of ECFs.
- An important concept is that regulation of osmolality must be integrated with regulation of volume, because changes in water volume alone have diluting or concentrating effects on a bodily fluid.
- For example, when a person becomes dehydrated, they lose more water than

sodium. Then the osmolality of bodily fluids increases. In this situation, the body tries to conserve water but not sodium, thus stemming the rise in osmolality.
- When a person loses a large amount of blood from trauma or surgery, the losses of sodium and water are proportionate to the composition of bodily fluids. In this situation, the body should conserve both water and sodium.
- As discussed in the previous unit, ADH plays a role in lowering osmolality by increasing water reabsorption in the kidneys, thus helping to dilute bodily fluids. To prevent osmolality from decreasing below normal, the kidneys also have a regulated mechanism for reabsorbing sodium in the distal nephron. This mechanism is controlled by *aldosterone,* a steroid hormone produced by the adrenal cortex.
- Aldosterone secretion is controlled in two ways:
  1. When the osmolality increases above normal, aldosterone secretion is inhibited.
     - The lack of aldosterone causes less sodium to be reabsorbed in the distal tubule.
     - ADH secretion will increase to conserve water, thus complementing the effect of low aldosterone levels to decrease the osmolality of bodily fluids.
     - The net effect on urine excretion is a decrease in the amount of urine excreted, with an increase in the osmolality of the urine.
  2. The kidneys sense low blood pressure.
     - This triggers a complex response to raise blood pressure and *conserve volume*. Specialized cells in the afferent and efferent arterioles produce *renin*, a peptide hormone that initiates a hormonal cascade that ultimately produces *angiotensin II*.
     - Angiotensin II stimulates the adrenal cortex to produce aldosterone.

CAUSES AND SYMPTOMS OF DIFFERENT TYPES OF HYPONATREMIA AND HYPERNATREMIA

Hyponatremia

Hyponatremia refers to a lower-than-normal level of sodium in the blood.

Causes: Imbalance of water and sodium. Most frequently it occurs when excessive water dilutes the amount of sodium in the body or when not enough total sodium is present in the body. A common classification of hyponatremia is based on the amount of total body water that is present.

- Decrease in plasma sodium may be due to defect in kidneys or adrenal cortex.
- Sweating, burns, vomiting, or diarrhea which can cause loss of sodium containing fluids.
- In adrenocortical insufficiency (Addison's disease), decrease of serum sodium and increase in sodium excretion are seen.

Normal Volume (Euvolemic) Hyponatremia

The amount of water in the body is normal, but an ADH is being inappropriately secreted (SIADH) from the pituitary gland. This may be seen in patients with pneumonia, small cell lung cancer, bleeding in the brain, or brain tumors.

Excess Volume (Hypervolemic) Hyponatremia

Too much total body water dilutes the amount of sodium contained in the body. This can be seen in heart failure, kidney failure, and liver diseases like cirrhosis.

Inadequate Volume (Hypovolemic) Hyponatremia

The amount of water in the body is too low as can occur in dehydration. The ADH is stimulated, causing the kidneys to make very concentrated urine and hold onto water. This may be seen with excessive sweating and exercising in a hot environment. It can also occur in patients with excess fluid loss due to vomiting and diarrhea, pancreatitis, and burns.

Symptoms

The symptoms of hyponatremia are as follows:
- Confusion.
- Nausea and fatigue.
- Seizures.
- Some individuals do not show any symptoms.

Hypernatremia

Hypernatremia is an electrolyte disturbance with elevated sodium level in the blood.

It is generally not caused by an excess of sodium, but rather by a relative deficit of free water in the body. Water is lost from the body in a variety of ways, including perspiration, imperceptible losses from breathing, and in the feces and urine. If the amount of water ingested consistently falls below the amount of water lost, the serum sodium level will begin to rise, leading to hypernatremia. Rarely, hypernatremia can result from massive salt ingestion.

Even a small rise in the serum sodium concentration above the normal range results in a strong sensation of thirst, an increase in free water intake, and correction of the abnormality. Therefore hypernatremia most often occurs in people such as infants, those with impaired mental status, or the elderly, who may have an intact thirst mechanism but are unable to ask for or obtain water.

Common causes include:
- *Hypovolemic*
  - Inadequate intake of water typically in elderly or otherwise disabled (common cause)
  - Excessive losses of water from the urinary tract, which may be caused by glycosuria
  - Extreme sweating
  - Severe watery diarrhea.
- *Euvolemic:* Excessive excretion of water from the kidneys caused by diabetes insipidus, which involves either inadequate production of the hormone, vasopressin (ADH), from the pituitary gland or impaired responsiveness of the kidneys to vasopressin.

Hypervolemic
- Intake of a hypertonic fluid (a fluid with a higher concentration of solutes than the remainder of the body). This is relatively uncommon.
- Mineralocorticoid excess due to a disease state such as Conn's syndrome or Cushing's disease.

Signs and Symptoms

The signs and symptoms of hypernatremia are as follows:
- Lethargy
- Restlessness
- Spasticity
- Edema
- Seizures.

Treatment

Treatment option for hypernatremia is shown in **Figure 24.4**.

Potassium (K⁺)

- Potassium (K^+) is the most important cation of ICF.
- Average concentration in the ICF is 150 mEq/L.
- **Extracellular** potassium concentration is normally kept within a tight range of 3.5–5.0 mEq/L.
- **Extracellular** potassium is important for its controlling influence upon neuromuscular irritability, cardiac muscle (a proper balance between potassium and

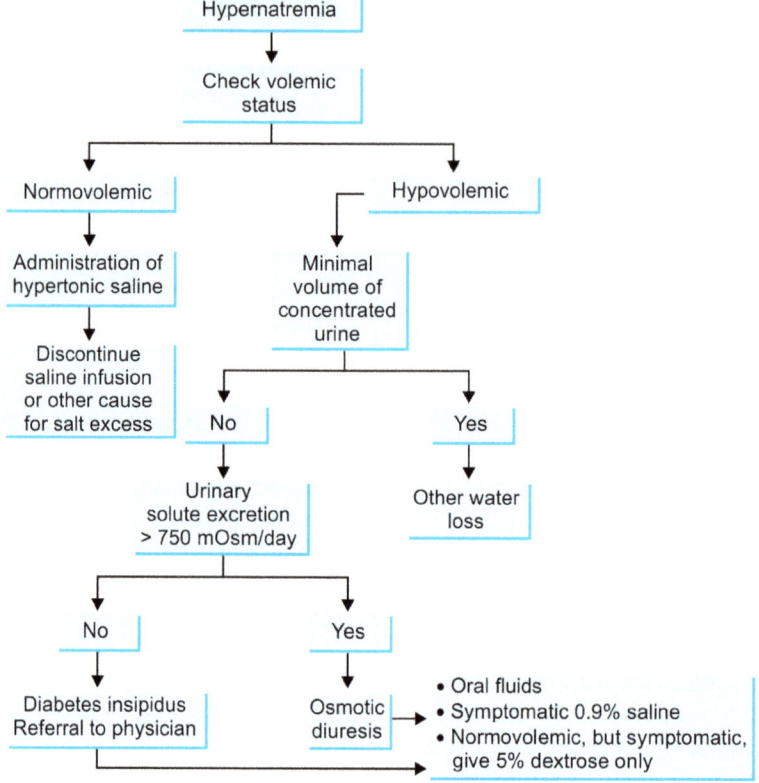

Fig. 24.4: Treatment option for hypernatremia.

calcium is essential for the contraction of heart muscle), and the operation of Na^+/K^+-ATPase (Na^+ pump) against the concentration gradient.

Hypokalemia

Hypokalemia is a metabolic disorder that occurs when potassium level in the blood drops too low.

It is the condition in which **serum potassium is reduced**.

This decreases the heartbeat and interferes with vital muscles such as those involved in respiration.

Possible causes of hypokalemia include:
- Antibiotics (penicillin, nafcillin, carbenicillin, gentamicin, amphotericin B, and foscarnet).
- Diarrhea.
  - *Gastrointestinal loss:* A more common cause is excessive loss of potassium, often associated with heavy fluid losses that "flush" potassium out of the body. Typically, this is a consequence of diarrhea, excessive perspiration, or losses associated with surgical procedures. Vomiting can also cause hypokalemia, although not much potassium is lost from the vomitus. Rather, there are heavy urinary losses of K^+ in the setting of postemetic bicarbonaturia that force urinary potassium excretion. Other GI causes include pancreatic fistulae and the presence of adenoma.
- Diseases that affect the kidneys' ability to retain potassium (Liddle syndrome,

Cushing's syndrome, hyperaldosteronism, Bartter syndrome, and Fanconi syndrome).
- Diuretic medications, which can cause excess urination.
- Eating disorders (such as bulimia).
- Magnesium deficiency.
  - Magnesium is required for adequate processing of potassium. This may become evident when hypokalemia persists despite potassium supplementation. Other electrolyte abnormalities may also be present
- Sweating.
- Vomiting.
- Aldosterone increases the excretion of potassium or administration of cortisone leads to hypokalemia.
- Certain diuretics increase the excretion of potassium. It is, therefore, important to supplement enough potassium when these diuretics are used.
- Reduced intake of potassium may cause hypokalemia but it is rare. Renal retention of potassium in response to reduced intake ensures that hypokalemia occurs only when intake is severely restricted.

Pseudohypokalemia

Pseudohypokalemia is a decrease in the amount of potassium that occurs due to excessive uptake of potassium by metabolically active cells in a blood sample after it has been drawn. It is a laboratory artifact that may occur when blood samples remain in warm conditions for several hours before processing.

Symptoms

A small drop in potassium usually doesn't cause symptoms; however, a big drop in the level can be life-threatening.
Symptoms of hypokalemia include:
- Abnormal heart rhythms (dysrhythmias), especially in people with heart disease
- Constipation
- Fatigue
- Muscle damage (rhabdomyolysis)
- Muscle weakness or spasms
- Paralysis (which can include the lungs).

Tests
- Serum potassium determination
- Arterial blood gas.

Treatment
Mild hypokalemia can be treated by taking potassium supplements by mouth. Persons with more severe cases may need to get potassium through a vein (intravenously).

Hyperkalemia
- Elevated plasma potassium concentration.
- It occurs in Addison's disease and in intravenous infusion of potassium at a rate excess of 25 mmol/h.
- Treatment using concentrated potassium solutions.

Causes
The causes of hyperkalemia are as follows:
- Renal insufficiency (renal failure).
- Medication that interferes with urinary excretion:
  - ACE inhibitors and angiotensin receptor blockers
  - Potassium-sparing diuretics (e.g. amiloride and spironolactone)
  - NSAIDs such as ibuprofen, naproxen, or celecoxib
  - The calcineurin inhibitor immunosuppressants ciclosporin and tacrolimus
  - The antibiotic trimethoprim
  - The antiparasitic drug pentamidine.
- Mineralocorticoid deficiency or resistance, such as:
  - Addison's disease
  - Aldosterone deficiency
  - Some forms of congenital adrenal hyperplasia

- Type IV renal tubular acidosis (resistance of renal tubules to aldosterone).
- Gordon's syndrome (pseudohypoaldosteronism type II), a rare genetic disorder caused by defective modulators of salt transporters, including the thiazide-sensitive Na–Cl cotransporter.
- Excessive release from cells.
  - Rhabdomyolysis, burns or any cause of rapid tissue necrosis, including tumor lysis syndrome
  - Massive blood transfusion or massive hemolysis
  - Shifts/transport out of cells caused by acidosis, low insulin levels, beta-blocker therapy, digoxin overdose, or the paralyzing agent succinylcholine.
- *Excessive intake:* Excess intake with salt-substitute, potassium-containing dietary supplements, or potassium chloride (KCl) infusion.
- *Pseudohyperkalemia:* Pseudohyperkalemia is a rise in the amount of potassium that occurs due to excessive leakage of potassium from cells, during or after blood is drawn. It is typically caused by hemolysis during venipuncture.
- Tissue trauma causing the cells to release potassium into the ECF includes burns, traumatic injury, and intestinal bleeding.

Signs and Symptoms

The signs and symptoms of hyperkalemia are as follows:
- Fatigue
- Weakness
- Tingling
- Numbness
- Paralysis
- Palpitations and difficulty in breathing.

Chloride (Cl⁻)

- Chloride (Cl⁻) is the major extracellular anion.
- Its average serum concentration is 105 mEq/L.

Functions

The functions of chloride are as follows:
- It is involved in maintaining osmotic pressure, proper body hydration, and electric neutrality.
- Dietary Cl^- is almost completely absorbed by the intestine.
- It is filtered out by the glomerulus and passively reabsorbed in conjunction with Na^+ by the proximal tubules.
- Excess Cl^- is excreted in urine and through sweating.
- Excessive sweating stimulates aldosterone secretion, which acts on the sweat glands to conserve Na^+ and Cl^-.

The normal level is between 94 and 111 mEq/L.

Hypochloremia

A low serum Cl^- is associated with loss of gastric HCl due to prolonged vomiting, salt-losing renal disease, in metabolic acidosis, etc.

Causes

The causes of hypochloremia are as follows:
- Diarrhea
- Congestive heart failure
- Pyloric obstruction
- Uremia
- Addison's disease
- Pulmonary emphysema
- Diabetic acidosis.

Hyperchloremia

High serum Cl^- is seen in dehydration and decreased renal blood flow.

Causes

The causes of hyperchloremia are as follows:
- Dehydration
- Acute renal failure.

SUMMARY

Water balance is the concept of human homeostasis that the amount of fluid lost from the body is equal to the amount of fluid taken in. Water constitutes 60% of the body weight. Thirst center and ADH mechanisms helps in the regulation of water balance in the body. Loss of water from the body leads to dehydration, which will become the cause for hypovolemia. Excess accumulation of water in the body leads to hypervolemia. Along with sodium water also has the effect on serum and urine osmolality. Serum osmolality is a useful preliminary investigation for identifying the cause of hyponatremia. Kidney is the only organ involved in the excretion of sodium and helps to regulate the body Na^+ content. The filtered Na^+ in the glomerular filtrate is reabsorbed in the distal tubule. A hormone, namely aldosterone secreted by the adrenal cortex is involved in the regulation of sodium reabsorption in the renal tubules. Aldosterone increases the reabsorption of Na^+ whenever the plasma Na^+ is low. Maintenance of electrolyte balance is equally important as water balance for the normal functioning of the body. Sodium is the major extracellular cation. Loss of sodium results in hyponatremia and more sodium level in the blood causes hypernatremia. Potassium is the major cation of intracellular fluid and its low level in the blood causes hypokalemia. High blood level of sodium causes hyperkalemia. Chloride is the extracellular anion. Low and high level of blood chloride results in hypo- and hyperchloremia, respectively.

SELF-ASSESSMENT QUESTIONS

1. Briefly discuss the regulation of fluid balance in the human body.
2. Give the causes and features of hypovolemia.
3. Write the causes of hypervolemia.
4. How does the thirst mechanism help to gain water?
5. Give the normal serum value of chloride.
6. What are the methods available to determine the concentration of sodium and potassium?
7. Name the method used to determine the cerebrospinal fluid chloride.
8. State the conditions in which serum calcium increases.
9. Explain the clinical significance of serum inorganic phosphorous estimation.

MULTIPLE-CHOICE QUESTIONS

1. The regulation of fluid balance is by:
    a. Antidiuretic hormone
    b. Thyroid hormone
    c. Insulin
    d. Oxytocin
2. All the following are the causes for hypervolemia, *except*:
    a. Renal failure
    b. SIADH syndrome
    c. Hypersecretion of ADH
    d. Diabetes insipidus
3. The concentration of sodium in the serum is
    a. 130–150 mEq/L   b. 135–140 mEq/L
    c. 100–120 mEq/L   d. 150–160 mEq/L
4. The major extracellular anion is
    a. Potassium   b. Chloride
    c. Sodium   d. Bicarbonate
5. Reduced calcium levels are seen in all the following conditions, *except*:
    a. Tetany
    b. Hypoparathyroidism
    c. Acidosis
    d. Childhood rickets
6. Elevated calcium levels are seen in all the following conditions, *except*:
    a. Primary hyperparathyroidism
    b. Vitamin D overdosage
    c. Bone tumors
    d. Liver disease
7. Elevated phosphorus levels are seen in:
    a. Renal failure
    b. Vitamin D overdosage
    c. Pancreatitis
    d. Liver disease

Answers

1. a 2. d 3. b 4. b 5. c
6. d 7. a

CHAPTER 25

Biochemistry of AIDS

OBJECTIVES
At the end of this chapter the learner should be able to:
- Understand the modes of transmission of HIV and the symptoms.

INTRODUCTION

Acquired immunodeficiency syndrome (AIDS) is a set of symptoms and infections resulting from the damage to the human immune system caused by the human immunodeficiency virus (HIV). This condition progressively reduces the effectiveness of the immune system and leaves individuals susceptible to infections and tumors.

FACTORS INFLUENCING TRANSMISSION OF AIDS

The AIDS is transmitted through direct contact of a mucous membrane or the bloodstream with a bodily fluid containing HIV, such as:
- Blood, semen
- Vaginal fluid
- Breast milk.

This transmission can involve:
- Anal
- Vaginal
- Oral sex
- Blood transfusion
- Contaminated needles
- Exchange between mother and baby during pregnancy
- Childbirth
- Breastfeeding.

There is currently no vaccine or cure. Antiretroviral treatment reduces both the mortality and the morbidity of HIV infection, but these drugs are expensive. Due to the difficulty in treating HIV infection, preventing infection is a key aim in controlling the AIDS epidemic, with health organizations promoting safe sex and needle-exchange programs in attempts to slow the spread of the virus.

SYMPTOMS OF HIV INFECTION

A generalized graph of the relationship between HIV copies and cluster of differentiation 4 (CD4) counts over the average course of untreated HIV infection; any particular individual's disease course may vary considerably. The symptoms of AIDS are primarily the result of conditions that do not normally develop in individuals with healthy immune systems. Most of these conditions are infections caused by bacteria, viruses, fungi, and parasites that are normally controlled by the elements of the immune system that HIV damages. Opportunistic infections are common in people with AIDS. HIV affects nearly every organ system. People with AIDS also have an increased risk of developing various cancers such as Kaposi's sarcoma (KS), cervical cancer, and cancers of the immune system known as lymphomas. Additionally, people with AIDS often have systemic symptoms of infection such as fevers, sweats, swollen glands, chills, weakness, and weight loss **(Fig. 25.1)**.

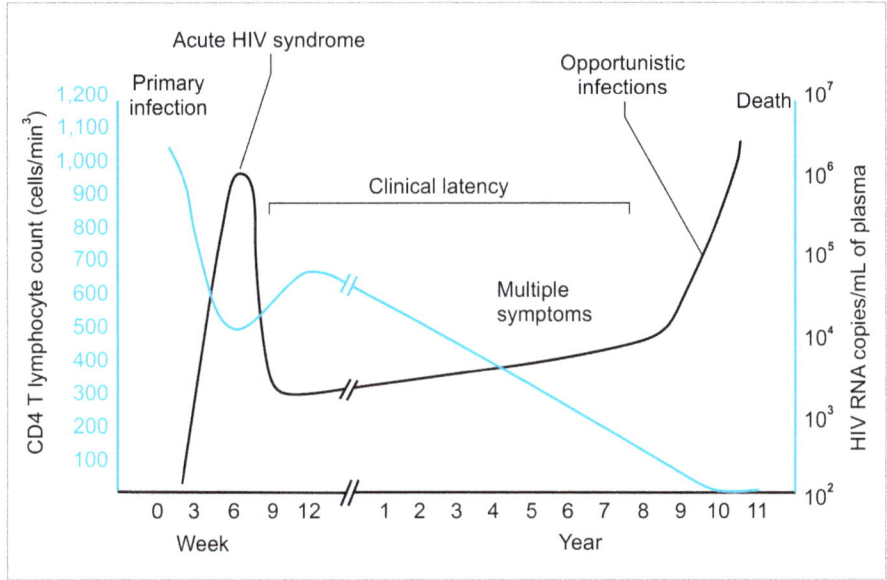

Fig. 25.1: Graph showing the symptoms of AIDS.
(RNA: ribonucleic acid; CD4: cluster of differentiation 4)

Lung Infections

Pneumocystis pneumonia is relatively rare in healthy, immunocompetent people, but common among HIV-infected individuals. It is caused by *Pneumocystis jirovecii*. Tuberculosis is unique among infections associated with HIV because it is transmissible to immunecompetent people via the respiratory route, is easily treatable once identified, may occur in early-stage HIV disease, and is preventable with drug therapy.

Gastrointestinal Infections

- Esophagitis is an inflammation of the lining of the lower end of the esophagus in HIV-infected individuals. This is normally due to fungal or viral infection in HIV-infected individuals.
- Unexplained chronic diarrhea in HIV infection is due to many possible causes, including common bacterial (*Salmonella, Shigella, Listeria,* or *Campylobacter*) and parasitic infections, uncommon opportunistic infections (cryptosporidiosis, microsporidiosis), mycobacterium avium complex, and viruses (astrovirus, adenovirus, rotavirus, and cytomegalovirus).

Neurological Symptoms

The HIV infection may lead to a variety of neuropsychiatric problems:
- Toxoplasmosis is a disease caused by the single-celled parasite called *Toxoplasma gondii*. It usually infects the brain causing toxoplasma encephalitis, but it can infect and cause disease in the eyes and lungs.
- Cryptococcal meningitis is an infection of the meninges by the fungus *Cryptococcus neoformans* and the symptoms are fever, headache, fatigue, nausea, and vomiting. Patients may also develop seizures and confusion.
- Progressive multifocal leukoencephalopathy is a demyelinating disease in which the gradual destruction of the myelin sheath covering the axons of nerve cells impairs the transmission of nerve impulses. It is caused by a virus called John

Cunningham virus, which occurs in 70% of the population in latent form, causing disease only when the immune system has been severely weakened, as is the case for AIDS patients. It progresses rapidly, usually causing death within months of diagnosis.
- The AIDS–dementia complex is a metabolic encephalopathy induced by HIV infection and fueled by immune activation of HIV-infected brain macrophages and microglia, which secrete neurotoxins of both host and viral origin.

Kaposi's Sarcoma

- Patients with HIV infection have substantially increased incidence of several malignant cancers. This is primarily due to coinfection with an oncogenic deoxyribonucleic acid (DNA) virus, especially Epstein–Barr virus (EBV), KS-associated herpesvirus (KSHV), and human papillomavirus (HPV).
- KS is the most common tumor in HIV-infected patients caused by a gamma herpesvirus called KSHV, it often appears as purplish nodules on the skin but can affect other organs as well, especially the mouth, gastrointestinal tract, and lungs.
- High-grade B-cell lymphomas such as Burkitt's lymphoma, Burkitt-like lymphoma, diffuse large B-cell lymphoma, and primary central nervous system (CNS) lymphoma present more often in HIV-infected patients. These particular cancers often foreshadow a poor prognosis. In some cases, these lymphomas are AIDS-defining. EBV or KSHV causes many of these lymphomas.
- Cervical cancer in HIV-infected women is considered as AIDS defining. It is caused by HPV.
- The AIDS is the most severe acceleration of infection with HIV. It is a retrovirus that primarily infects vital organs of the human immune system such as $CD4^+$ T cells (a subset of T cells), macrophages, and dendritic cells. It directly and indirectly destroys $CD4^+$ T cells. Once HIV has killed so many $CD4^+$ T cells that there are fewer than 200 of these cells per microliter of blood, cellular immunity is lost. Acute HIV infection progresses over time to clinical latent HIV infection and then to early symptomatic HIV infection and later to AIDS, which is identified either on the basis of the amount of $CD4^+$ T cells remaining in the blood and/or the presence of certain infections as mentioned above.

ROUTES OF TRANSMISSION

Sexual Transmission

Sexual transmission occurs due to the contact between sexual secretions of one person with the rectal, genital, or oral mucous membranes of another. Unprotected receptive sexual acts are riskier than unprotected insertive sexual acts and the risk for transmitting HIV through unprotected anal intercourse is greater than the risk from vaginal intercourse or oral sex. The risk of HIV transmission from exposure to saliva is considerably smaller than the risk from exposure to semen.

Exposure to Bloodborne Pathogens

This transmission route is particularly relevant to intravenous drug users, hemophiliacs, and recipients of blood transfusions and blood products. Sharing and reusing syringes contaminated with HIV-infected blood represent a major risk for infection with HIV. The risk of transmitting HIV to blood transfusion recipients is extremely low in developed countries, where improved donor selection and HIV screening are performed.

Perinatal Transmission

The transmission of the virus from the mother to the child can occur in utero during the last weeks of pregnancy and at childbirth. In the absence of treatment, the transmission rate between a mother and her child during pregnancy, labor, and delivery is 25%. However, when the mother takes antiretroviral therapy and gives birth by cesarean section, the rate of transmission is just 1%.

PATHOPHYSIOLOGY

The HIV causes AIDS by depleting CD4$^+$ T-helper lymphocytes. This weakens the immune system and allows opportunistic infections. T lymphocytes are essential to the immune response and without them; the body cannot fight infections or kill cancerous cells. During the acute phase, HIV-induced cell lysis and killing of infected cells by cytotoxic T cells account for CD4$^+$ T-cell depletion.

Although the symptoms of immune deficiency characteristic of AIDS do not appear for years after a person is infected, the bulk of CD4$^+$ T-cell loss occurs during the first weeks of infection, especially in the intestinal mucosa, which harbors the majority of the lymphocytes found in the body. The reason for the preferential loss of mucosal CD4$^+$ T cells is that a majority of mucosal CD4$^+$ T cells express the C–C chemokine receptor type five (CCR5) coreceptor, whereas a small fraction of CD4$^+$ T cells in the bloodstream do so. HIV seeks out and destroys CCR5 expressing CD4$^+$ cells during acute infection.

Continuous HIV replication results in a state of generalized immune activation persisting throughout the chronic phase. Immune activation, which is reflected by the increased activation state of immune cells and release of proinflammatory cytokines, results from the activity of several *HIV* gene products and the immune response to ongoing HIV replication. Another cause is the breakdown of the immune surveillance system of the mucosal barrier caused by the depletion of mucosal CD4$^+$ T cells during the acute phase of disease. This results in the systemic exposure of the immune system to microbial components of the gut's normal flora, which in a healthy person is kept in check by the mucosal immune system. The activation and proliferation of T cells that result from immune activation provide fresh targets for HIV infection. However, direct killing by HIV alone cannot account for the observed depletion of CD4$^+$ T cells since only 0.01–0.10% of CD4$^+$ T cells in the blood are infected. A major cause of CD4$^+$ T-cell loss appears to result from their heightened susceptibility to apoptosis when the immune system remains activated. Although new T cells are continuously produced by the thymus to replace the ones lost, the regenerative capacity of the thymus is slowly destroyed by direct infection of its thymocytes by HIV.

Cells Affected

The virus, entering through whichever route, acts primarily on the following cells.

Lymphoreticular System

- CD4$^+$ T-helper cells
- CD4$^+$ macrophages
- CD4$^+$ monocytes
- B lymphocytes
- Certain endothelial cells.

Central Nervous System

- Microglia of the nervous system
- Astrocytes
- Oligodendrocytes
- Neuron—indirectly by the action of cytokines and the glycoprotein 120 (gp120).

Effects

The virus has cytopathic effects, but how it does it is still not quite clear. It can remain inactive in these cells for long periods though.

This effect is hypothesized due to the CD4–gp120 interaction:
- The most prominent effect of the HIV virus is its T-helper cell suppression and lysis. The cell is simply killed off or deranged to the point of being functionless. The infected

B cells cannot produce enough antibodies either. Thus the immune system collapses leading to the familiar AIDS complications, such as infections and neoplasms.
- Infection of CNS cells causes acute aseptic meningitis, subacute encephalitis, vacuolar myelopathy, and peripheral neuropathy.
- The CD4–gp120 interaction (vide supra) is also permissive to other viruses such as cytomegalovirus, hepatitis virus, and herpes simplex virus. These viruses lead to further cell damage.

MOLECULAR BASIS OF HIV

Structure of HIV

- The HIV is different in structure from other retroviruses.
- It is around 120 nm in diameter and roughly spherical.
- The HIV-1 is composed of two copies of single-stranded ribonucleic acid (RNA) enclosed by a conical capsid comprising the viral protein p24, typical of lentiviruses. The RNA component is 9,749 nucleotides long. This is in turn surrounded by a plasma membrane of host cell origin. The single-stranded RNA is tightly bound to the nucleocapsid proteins p7 and enzymes that are indispensable for the development of the virion such as reverse transcriptase and integrase. The nucleocapsid (p7 and p6) associates with the genomic RNA and protects the RNA from digestion by nucleases. A matrix composed of an association of the viral protein p17 surrounds the capsid, ensuring the integrity of the virion particle. Also enclosed within the virion particle are Vif, Vpr, Nef, p7, and viral protease. The envelope is formed when the capsid buds from the host cell, taking some of the host cell membrane with it. The envelope includes the gp120 and gp41 (**Fig. 25.2**).

Genome Organization

The HIV has several major genes coding for structural proteins that are found in all retroviruses and several nonstructural genes that are unique to HIV. The *gag* gene provides the basic physical infrastructure of the virus and *pol* provides the basic mechanism by which retroviruses reproduce, while the others help HIV to enter the host cell and enhance its reproduction.

Though they may be altered by mutation, all of these genes except *tev* exist in all known variants of HIV:

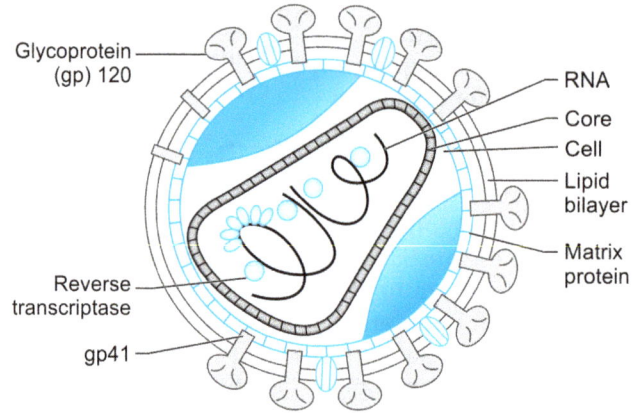

Fig. 25.2: Diagram of HIV.
(RNA: ribonucleic acid)

- *Group-specific antigen (Gag):* Codes for p24 (the viral capsid), p6 and p7 (the nucleocapsid proteins), and p17 (a matrix protein).
- *Pol:* Codes for viral enzymes, the most important of which are reverse transcriptase, integrase, and protease, which cleaves the proteins derived from gag and *pol* into functional proteins.
- *Envelope (env):* Codes for the precursor to gp120 and gp41, proteins embedded in the viral envelope, which enable the virus to attach to and fuse with target cells.
- *Tat, rev, nef, vif, vpr,* and *vpu:* Each of these genes codes for a single protein with the same name.
- *Tev:* This gene is only present in a few HIV-1 isolates. It is a fusion of parts of the *tat, env,* and *rev* genes, and codes for a protein with some of the properties of *tat,* but little or none of the properties of *rev.*

DIAGNOSIS OF AIDS

The diagnosis of AIDS in a person infected with HIV is based on the presence of certain signs or symptoms. In developing countries, the World Health Organization staging system for HIV infection and disease, using clinical and laboratory data, is used, and in developed countries, the Centers for Disease Control classification system is used.

Human Immunodeficiency Virus Test

- The donor blood and blood products used in medicine and medical research are screened for HIV.
- HIV tests are performed on venous blood.
- Many laboratories use screening tests, which detect anti-HIV antibody (IgG and IgM) and the HIV p24 antigen. The detection of HIV antibody or antigen in a patient previously known to be negative is evidence of HIV infection. Individuals whose first specimen indicates evidence of HIV infection will have a repeat test on a second blood sample to confirm the results.
- The window period (the time between initial infection and the development of detectable antibodies against the infection) can vary since it can take 3–6 months to seroconvert and to test positive.
- Detection of the virus using polymerase chain reaction (PCR) during the window period is possible, and evidence suggests that an infection may often be detected earlier, when using a fourth-generation enzyme immunoassays screening test.
- Routinely used HIV tests for infection in neonates born to HIV-positive mothers have no value because of the presence of maternal antibody to HIV in the child's blood. HIV infection can only be diagnosed by PCR testing for HIV proviral DNA in the child's lymphocytes.

PREVENTION OF AIDS

The three main transmission routes of HIV are sexual contact, exposure to infected body fluids or tissues, and from mother to fetus or child during perinatal period. It is possible to find HIV in the saliva, tears, and urine of infected individuals, but there are no recorded cases of infection by these secretions, and the risk of infection is negligible.

Sexual Contact

The majority of HIV infections are acquired through unprotected sexual relations between partners, one of whom has HIV. The primary mode of HIV infection worldwide is through sexual contact between members of the opposite sex. During a sexual act, only male or female condoms can reduce the chances of infection with HIV and other sexually transmitted diseases, and the chances of becoming pregnant. The male latex condom, if used correctly without oil-based lubricants, is the single most effective available technology to reduce the sexual transmission of HIV and other sexually transmitted infections. Manufacturers recommend that oil-based lubricants such as petroleum jelly, butter, and lard not be used with latex condoms, because they dissolve the latex, making the condoms porous. If necessary, manufacturers recommend using water-based lubricants.

The female condom is an alternative to the male condom and is made from polyurethane, which allows it to be used in the presence of oil-based lubricants. They are larger than male condoms and have a stiffened ring-shaped opening and are designed to be inserted into the vagina. The female condom contains an inner ring, which keeps the condom in place inside the vagina—inserting the female condom requires squeezing this ring. Prevention strategies are well known in developed countries.

Exposure to Infected Body Fluids

Health-care workers can reduce exposure to HIV by employing precautions to reduce the risk of exposure to contaminated blood. These precautions include barriers such as gloves, masks, protective eyewear or shields, and gowns or aprons, which prevent exposure of the skin or mucous membranes to blood borne pathogens. Frequent and thorough washing of the skin immediately after being contaminated with blood or other bodily fluids can reduce the chance of infection. Finally, sharp objects such as needles, scalpels, and glass are carefully disposed of to prevent needle stick injuries with contaminated items.

Mother-to-child Transmission

Current recommendations state that when replacement feeding is acceptable, feasible, affordable, sustainable, and safe, HIV-infected mothers should avoid breastfeeding their infant. However, if this is not the case, exclusive breastfeeding is recommended during the first months of life and discontinued as soon as possible.

TREATMENT OF AIDS

Abacavir is a nucleoside analog reverse transcriptase inhibitor (NARTI or NRTI). There is currently no vaccine or cure for HIV or AIDS. The only known methods of prevention are based on avoiding exposure to the virus or, failing that, an antiretroviral treatment directly after a highly significant exposure, called postexposure prophylaxis (PEP). PEP has a very demanding 4-week schedule of dosage.

Antiviral Therapy

Current treatment for HIV infection consists of highly active antiretroviral therapy (HAART). This has been highly beneficial to many HIV-infected individuals. Current optimal HAART options consist of combinations of at least three drugs belonging to at least two types, or "classes," of antiretroviral agents. Typical regimens consist of two NARTIs or NRTIs plus either a protease inhibitor or a nonnucleoside reverse transcriptase inhibitor. In developed countries where HAART is available, doctors assess the viral load, rapidity in CD4 decline, and patient readiness, while deciding when to recommend initiating treatment. HAART allows the stabilization of the patient's symptoms and viremia.

Alternative Medicine

- Various forms of alternative medicine have been used to treat symptoms or alter the course of the disease. Acupuncture has been used to alleviate some symptoms such as peripheral neuropathy, but it cannot cure the HIV infection.
- Some data suggest that multivitamin and mineral supplements might reduce HIV disease progression in adults, although there is no conclusive evidence on if they reduce mortality among people

with good nutritional status. Vitamin A supplementation in children probably has some benefits. Daily doses of selenium can suppress HIV viral burden with an associated improvement of the CD4 count. Selenium can be used as an adjunct therapy to standard antiviral treatments, but it cannot itself reduce mortality and morbidity.
- Current studies indicate that alternative medicine therapy has little effect on the mortality or morbidity of the disease, but it may improve the quality of life of individuals afflicted with AIDS.

SUMMARY

Acquired immunodeficiency syndrome is a set of symptoms and infections resulting from the damage to the human immune system caused by the HIV. It is transmitted through direct contact of a mucous membrane or the bloodstream with a bodily fluid containing HIV such as blood, semen, vaginal fluid, and breast milk. There is currently no vaccine or cure. Antiretroviral treatment reduces both the mortality and morbidity of HIV infection. Due to the difficulty in treating HIV infection, preventing infection is a key aim in controlling the AIDS epidemic, with health organizations promoting safe sex and needle-exchange programs in attempts to slow the spread of the virus.

CHAPTER 26

Biochemistry of Cancer

OBJECTIVES

At the end of this chapter, the student should be able to:
- Know about the development, genetics, causes and treatment of cancer
- Understand the cell cycle, its importance and regulation
- Know about abnormal cell growth, cell signaling and signal transduction
- Understand the mutagens and tumor suppressor genes
- Know about tumor markers and their importance.

INTRODUCTION

Cancer is a disease characterized by the development of a large number of abnormal cells that can divide rapidly and have the ability to infiltrate and destroy the normal body tissue. It can spread throughout our body. Once diagnosed as cancer it can be frightening, but we can understand what is going on inside our body and try to help us fell more in the control of the disease.

Development of Cancer

- In the body, when a normal cell dies, the body replaces it with another new normal cell.
- Cancer can occur when the cells grow in an uncontrolled manner.
- The cancerous cells do not die and start accumulating. As a result, large number of cells accumulates until a mass of cells called tumor is created.
- Not all tumors are cancerous and not all cancers form tumors (**Figs. 26.1 and 26.2**). For example, leukemia is a type of cancer that includes the bone marrow, blood, spleen, and the lymphatic system, but they do not form a single mass or a tumor.

Causes of Cancer

- Cancers are caused by abnormalities in the genetic material of the transformed cells. These abnormalities may be due to the effects of carcinogens such as tobacco smoke, radiation, chemicals, or infectious agents.

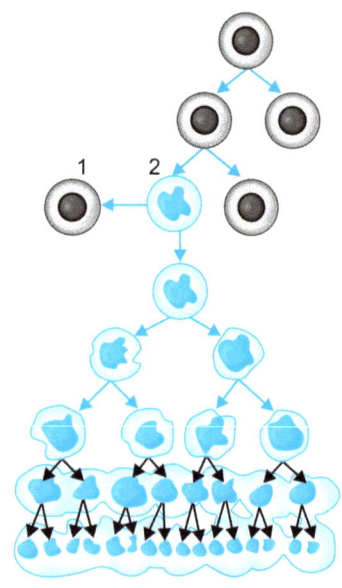

Fig. 26.1: Cancer cell production.

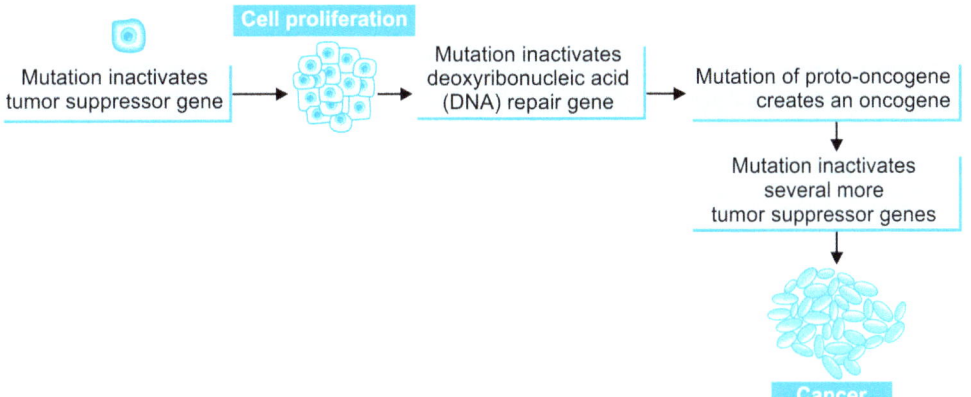

Fig. 26.2: Cell proliferation.

- Tobacco smoking is associated with lung cancer and bladder cancer.
- Prolonged exposure to asbestos fibers is associated with mesothelioma.
- Prolonged exposure to ultraviolet (UV) radiation from the sun can lead to melanoma and other skin malignancies.
- The main viruses associated with human cancers are human papilloma virus, hepatitis B and C virus, Epstein–Barr virus, and human T-lymphotropic virus.
- Some hormones can act in a similar manner to nonmutagenic carcinogens in that they may stimulate excessive cell growth. A well-established example is the role of hyperestrogenic states in promoting endometrial cancer.
- HIV is associated with a number of malignancies, including Kaposi's sarcoma, non-Hodgkin's lymphoma, and human papillomavirus (HPV)-associated malignancies such as anal cancer and cervical cancer.

Genetics of Cancer

- Most forms of cancer are "sporadic" and have no basis in heredity. There are, however, a number of recognized syndromes of cancer with a hereditary component, often a defective tumor suppressor allele.
- Certain inherited mutations in the genes *BRCA1* and *BRCA2* are associated with an elevated risk of breast cancer and ovarian cancer. Other cancer-promoting genetic abnormalities may be randomly acquired through errors in DNA replication (or are inherited) and thus be present in all cells from birth.
- New aspects of the genetics of cancer pathogenesis such as DNA methylation and microRNAs are increasingly being recognized as important.
- Genetic abnormalities found in cancer typically affect two general classes of genes. Cancer-promoting oncogenes are often activated in cancer cells, giving those cells new properties such as hyperactive growth and division, protection against programmed cell death (PCD), loss of respect for normal tissue boundaries, and the ability to become established in diverse tissue environments. Tumor suppressor genes are often inactivated in cancer cells, resulting in the loss of normal functions in those cells such as accurate DNA replication, control over the cell cycle, orientation and adhesion within tissues, and interaction with protective cells of the immune system.
- Cancer starts with damage or mutations in DNA. The normal cells of these develop

mutations in their DNA, but they do have the capacity to repair most of these mutations. Or, if they cannot make such repairs then the cells die. However, there are certain mutations, which are not repaired and cause the cells to grow and develop into cancerous cells.
- Mutations can also cause the cancer cells to live beyond a normal life span of cell. As a result cancerous cells begin to accumulate.

Risk Factors for Cancer

There are various factors known to increase the risk of cancer such as lifestyle, family history, health conditions, and environment. Studies have found that hereditary factor is one of the most common causes. Scientists believe that we need a number of changes within our cells to develop cancer, which include the following:
- There could be a genetic mutation caused by forces within our body such as hormones, viruses, and chronic inflammation. Genetic mutation can be caused by forces outside the body such as UV light from sun or carcinogens of our environment.
- A promoter to cause rapid cell growth; promoters cause cells to divide rapidly, which ultimately leads to a tumor. Promoters could either be inherited or could come from inside or outside the body. Promoters take advantage of the genetic mutations created by initiators.
- A progressor to cause cancer to become aggressive and spread; without a progressor a tumor can remain benign and localized. To make cancers more aggressive, there are progressors and they are more likely to spread. Progressors could also be inherited or they could come from environmental sources.
- The genetic makeup, lifestyle choice, forces within our body, and our environment can all set the stage for cancer or they could help the complete process once it is started. For example, smokers who work with asbestos are more likely to develop lung cancer than the smokers who do not, because the carcinogens play a role in cancer development.

Diagnosis

The only way to diagnose cancer is to examine the cells under the microscope. There are some imaging tests such as mammography or computerized tomography, which can indicate the possible presence of cancer and it looks like an abnormal mass, but cancer cells can be identified under a microscope.

Doctors use a surgical process called biopsy of the suspected tissue under the observation of the microscope. The normal cells look uniform with similar sizes and orderly organization. Cancer cells look less orderly, with different size and without apparent organization.

Treatment

There are anticancer agents that are used in the treatment of cancer. They are cytotoxic and when given in a proper dosage, they potentially kill the rapidly dividing cells such as cancer cells. The anticancer agents used are:
- Chronic lymphocytic leukemia—chlorambucil and cyclophosphamide (also used for the treatment of many types of cancer)
- Amethopterin
- 5′ fluorouracil
- Cytosine arabinoside and doxorubicin, etc.

CELL CYCLE

Definition

The **cell cycle**, or **cell division cycle**, is the series of events that take place in a **cell** leading to duplication of its DNA (DNA replication) and **division** of cytoplasm and organelles to produce two daughter **cells**. In bacteria, which lack a **cell** nucleus, the **cell cycle** is divided into the B, C, and D periods.

Purpose of the Cell Cycle

The most basic function of the **cell cycle** is to duplicate accurately the vast amount of DNA in the chromosomes and then segregate the copies precisely into two genetically identical daughter **cells**. These processes define the two major phases of the **cell cycle**.

Importance of the Cell Cycle

Cell cycle is important to organisms in different ways, but overall it allows them to survive. Zygotes also depend on the **cell cycle** to form its many **cells** in order to produce a baby organism at the end of its process. Plants require the **cell cycle** to grow and provide life for every other organism on earth.

The Four Stages of the Cell Cycle

Mitosis takes place in **four stages**: prophase (sometimes divided into early prophase and prometaphase), metaphase, anaphase, and telophase **(Fig. 26.3)**.

The Three Reasons for Cells Division

There are **three** main types of **cell** division exist: mitosis, meiosis, and binary fission. Mitosis creates two identical **cells** from one parent **cell**. The main goal of mitosis is growth and the replacement of worn out or old **cells**. Most of the **cells** in the human body go through mitosis.

The Consequence of Uncontrolled Procedure of the Cycle

Cells may grow and divide without performing their necessary functions, or without fully replicating their DNA, or without copying their organelles. Therefore the cell cycle needs to be highly regulated and tightly controlled.

The Consequence of Unregulated Cell Cycle

If the **cell cycle is not** carefully controlled, it can cause a disease called cancer, which causes **cell** division to **happen** too fast. A tumor can result from this kind of growth.

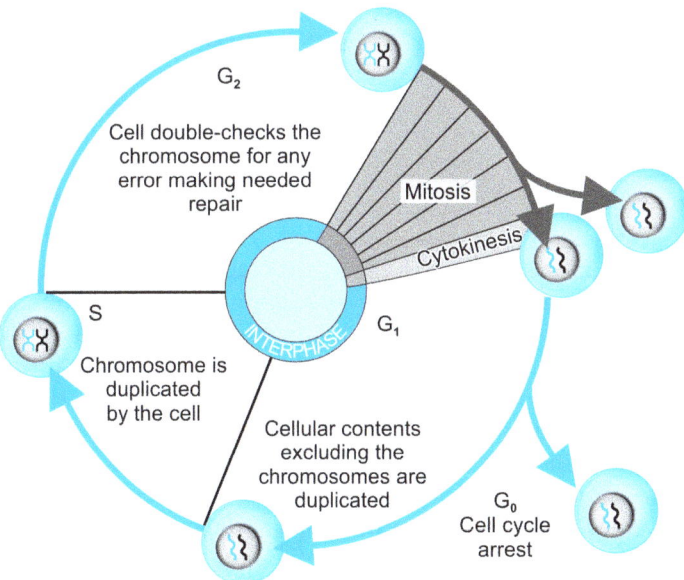

Fig. 26.3: Stages of cell cycle.

Control of the Cell Cycle

Control and Regulation of the Cell Cycle

Regulation of the cell cycle involves processes crucial to the survival of a cell. These include the detection and repair of damage to DNA, as well as the prevention of uncontrolled cell division. Uncontrolled cell division can be deadly to an organism and its prevention is critical for survival.

Cyclins and Kinases

The cell cycle is controlled by a number of protein-controlled feedback processes. Two types of proteins involved in the control of the cell cycle are **kinases** and **cyclins**. Cyclins activate kinases by binding to them, specifically they activate **cyclin-dependent kinases (CDKs)**. Cyclins comprise a group of proteins that are rapidly produced at key stages in the cell cycle. Once activated by a cyclin, CDKs are enzymes that activate or inactivate other target molecules through phosphorylation. It is this precise regulation of proteins that triggers advancement through the cell cycle (Leland H. Hartwell, R. Timothy Hunt, and Paul M. Nurse won the 2001 Nobel Prize in Physiology or Medicine for their discovery of these critical proteins).

Cyclin-dependent Kinases

Cyclin-dependent kinases are a family of protein kinases first discovered for their role in regulating the cell cycle. They are present in all eukaryotes and are small proteins with little more than the kinase domain. A CDK binds to a cyclin regulatory protein, activating the protein; without binding to cyclin, the CDK has little kinase activity. They phosphorylate their substrates on serines and threonines, so they are serine-threonine kinases. CDKs are also involved in regulating transcription, mRNA processing, and the differentiation of nerve cells.

Checkpoints

The cell cycle has key checkpoints. When the cell receives key signals or information via **feedback regulation**, the cell can begin the next phase of the cell cycle. The cell can also receive signals that delay passage to the next phase of the cell cycle. These signals allow the cell to complete the previous phase before moving forward. Three key checkpoints are the cell growth (G_1) checkpoint, the G_2 checkpoint, and the mitosis checkpoint. The DNA synthesis checkpoint is another checkpoint (**Fig. 26.3**).

The cell growth (G_1) checkpoint allows the cell to proceed into the S phase of the cell cycle and continue on to divide, or delay division, or enter a resting stage. The cell spends most of the cycle in the G_1 phase where the cell carries out its main functions. If the cell has performed its functions and has grown to significant size to be divided in half, key proteins will signal the cell to proceed to the S phase and stimulate DNA replication to begin. If the cells are not to divide, such as some muscle and nerve cells, the cell will stop at this checkpoint and move into a resting phase, G_0. Some cells may stay in this resting period permanently, without dividing.

The second checkpoint is located at the end of G_2 phase. Passing this checkpoint triggers the start of the mitosis. If this checkpoint is passed, the cell initiates the many molecular processes that signal the beginning of mitosis.

The mitosis checkpoint determines the end of one cycle and the beginning of the next. This checkpoint occurs at the point in metaphase where all the chromosomes should have aligned at the metaphase plate. This checkpoint signals the beginning of anaphase, allowing the cell to complete mitosis and prepare for the beginning of G_1 of the next cell cycle.

The DNA synthesis (S) checkpoint determines if the cell is ready for mitosis. DNA repair enzymes check the replicated DNA at this point. If the checkpoint is passed, the

Biochemistry of Cancer

many molecular mechanisms and processes needed for mitosis will begin.

Summary

- The cell cycle is controlled through feedback mechanisms involving cyclin and CDK proteins.
- Three important checkpoints are the G_1, G_2, and M phase checkpoints **(Table 26.1)**.

Abnormal Cell Growth

Abnormal regulation of the **cell** cycle can lead to the over **proliferation** of **cells** and an accumulation of **abnormal cell** numbers. Such uncontrolled, **abnormal growth** of **cells** is a defining characteristic of cancer.

Causes of Uncontrollable Cell Growth

Cancer is unchecked **cell growth**. Mutations in genes can **cause** cancer by accelerating **cell** division rates or inhibiting normal controls on the system, such as **cell** cycle arrest or PCD. As a mass of cancerous **cells** grows, it can develop into a tumor.

Causes of Abnormal Cell Growth

It describes the disease that results when **cellular** changes **cause** the uncontrolled **growth** and division of **cells**. Some types of cancer **cause** rapid **cell growth**, while others **cause cells** to grow and divide at a slower rate. Cancerous **cells** lack the components that instruct them to stop dividing and to die.

Common Causes of Cancer

- Smoking and tobacco
- Diet and physical activity
- Sun and other types of radiation
- Viruses and other infections

Programmed Cell Death

Programmed cell death or **apoptosis** is the **death** of a **cell** in any form, mediated by an intracellular program, and is also referred to as **cellular** suicide. Recently, a form of **programmed** necrosis, called necroptosis, has been recognized as an alternative form of PCD.

Cell commits suicide by apoptosis. Cellular homicide is necrosis **(Figs. 26.4A and B)**. Apoptosis is a process of PCD that occurs in multicellular organisms. Biochemical events lead to characteristic cell changes (morphology) and death.

Physiologic causes:

- The programmed destruction of cell during embryogenesis. It is programmed because it is death of specific cell types at defined times during development.

Table 26.1: Cell cycle regulation.

Regulation summary			
State	**Name**	**Abbreviation**	**Checkpoint**
• Quiescent • Senescent	Resting phase	G_0 phase	
Interphase	• First growth phase	G_1	• The G_1 checkpoint ensures that the cell has completed its homeostatic functions and is ready for DNA synthesis
	• Synthesis phase	S	• The S phase checkpoint ensures that DNA replication is complete
	• Second growth phase	G_2	• The G_2 checkpoint ensures that the cell is ready to enter the M (mitosis) phase and divide
Cell division	Mitosis	M	A checkpoint in the middle of mitosis (at metaphase) ensures that the cell is ready to complete cell division

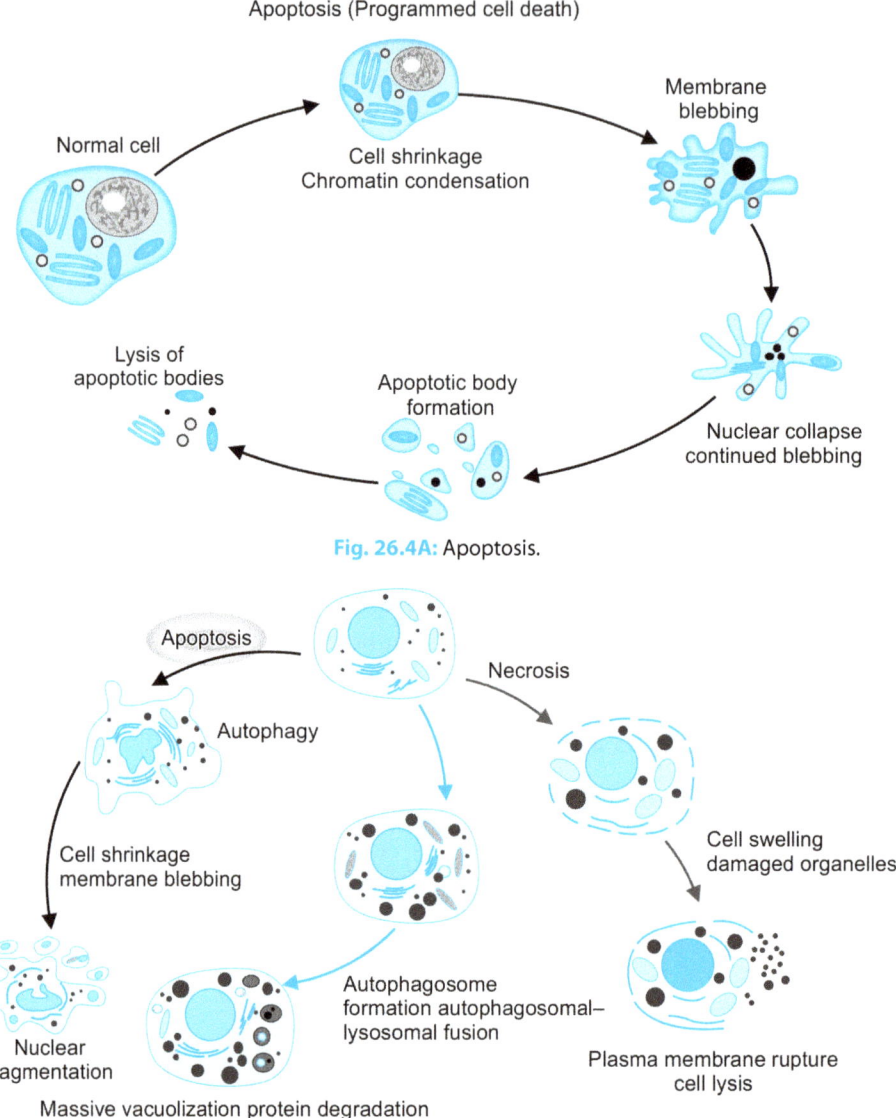

Fig. 26.4A: Apoptosis.

Fig. 26.4B: Apoptosis.

- Hormone-dependent physiologic involution, such as involution of the endometrium during the menstrual cycle.
- Cell deletion in proliferating cell population, such as intestinal crypt epithelium.
- Death of cells that have served their useful purpose, such as neutrophils in an acute inflammatory response.
- Elimination of potentially harmful self-reactive lymphocytes.

Pathological causes:
- Cell death produced by a variety of mild injurious stimuli such as heat, radiation, and cytotoxic cancer drugs that cause irreparable DNA damage that in turn triggers cell suicide pathways

- Cell injury in certain viral diseases such as viral hepatitis
- Cell death in tumors.

Cell Signaling

Cell signaling is a part of any communication process that governs basic activities of cells and coordinates multiple-cell actions. The ability of cells to perceive and correctly respond to their microenvironment is the basis of development, tissue repair, and immunity, as well as normal tissue homeostasis. Errors in signaling interactions and cellular information processing may cause diseases such as cancer, autoimmunity, and diabetes. With the knowledge of cell signaling, clinicians may treat diseases more effectively, and, theoretically, researchers may develop artificial tissues.

All cells receive and respond to signal from their surroundings. This is accomplished by a variety of signal molecules that are secreted or expressed on the surface of one cell and bind to receptor expressed by the other cells, thereby integrating and coordinating the function of the many individual cells that make up organisms. Each cell is programmed to respond to specific extracellular signal molecules. Extracellularly signaling usually involves the following steps:

- Synthesis and release of the signaling molecule by the signaling cell
- Transport of the signaling to the target cell
- Binding of the signal by a specific receptor leading to its activation
- Initiation of signal-transduction pathways.

Cell signaling can be classified as either mechanical or biochemical based on the type of the signal. Mechanical signals are the forces exerted on the cell and the forces produced by the cell. These forces can both be sensed and responded to by the cells. Biochemical signals are the biochemical molecules such as proteins, lipids, ions, and gases. These signals can be categorized based on the distance between signaling and responder cells. Signaling within, between, and amongst cells is subdivided into the following classifications:

- **Intracrine signals** are produced by the target cell that stay within the target cell.
- **Autocrine signals** are produced by the target cell, are secreted, and affect the target cell itself via receptors. Sometimes autocrine cells can target cells close by if they are the same type of cell as the emitting cell. An example of this is immune cells.
- **Juxtacrine signals** target adjacent cells. These signals are transmitted along cell membranes via protein or lipid components integral to the membrane and are capable of affecting either the emitting cell or cells immediately adjacent.
- **Paracrine signals** target cells in the vicinity of the emitting cell. Neurotransmitters represent an example.
- **Endocrine signals** target distant cells. Endocrine cells produce hormones that travel through the blood to reach all parts of the body.

Cells communicate with each other via direct contact (juxtacrine signaling), over short distances (paracrine signaling), or over large distances and/or scales (endocrine signaling).

The **endocrine system** is a chemical messenger system comprising feedback loops of hormones released by internal glands of an organism directly into the circulatory system, regulating distant target organs. In humans, the major endocrine glands are the thyroid gland and the adrenal glands. In vertebrates, the hypothalamus is the neural control center for all endocrine systems. The study of the endocrine system and its disorders is known as endocrinology. Endocrinology is a branch of internal medicine.

Signal Transduction

- Signal transduction is defined as the ability of a cell to change behavior in response to a receptor-ligand interaction.
- The ligand is the primary messenger.

- As the result of binding the receptor, other molecules or second messengers are produced within the target cell.
- Second messengers relay the signal from one location to another (such as from plasma membrane to nucleus).
- Often a cascade of changes occurs within the cell which results in a change in the cells function or identity.

Growth Factors

Growth factors act as messengers. In addition to nutrients, cell often need growth factors, which are listed in **Table 26.2**.

Disruption of growth factor signaling through receptor tyrosine kinases can have dramatic effects on embryonic development.
- The fibroblast growth factors (FGFs) and FGF receptors (FGFRs) function in both embryonic and adult signaling.
- FGFRs are important in the development of mesoderm, the embryonic tissue that eventually becomes muscle, cartilage, bone, and blood cells.
- A mutant receptor that, due to dimerization with normal versions of FGFR, has a dominant inhibitory effect upon the normal activity is a dominant negative mutation.

Hormones

Chemical signals known as hormones are secreted by one tissue to regulate another tissue. Hormones control many physiological functions, including growth and development, rates of physiological processes, concentrations of sugars and minerals, and responses to stress. Hormones can be proteins, peptides, steroids, and other molecules.

Hormonal signals can be classified by the distance that they travel to reach their target cells. An endocrine hormone travels through the circulatory system and a paracrine hormone acts only upon nearby cells. A paracrine hormone is roughly equal to a growth factor. Endocrine tissues secrete directly into the bloodstream and exocrine tissues into ducts for transport of the secretions to other parts of the body. The pancreas has both endocrine (insulin and glucagon) and paracrine (digestive enzymes) functions. Once in the circulatory system, the endocrine hormones will eventually reach their target tissue(s) such as heart and liver (epinephrine) or liver and skeletal muscles (insulin). In the target tissue, intracellular effects, such as the activation of the cyclic adenosine monophosphate (cAMP) pathway can control

Table 26.2: Growth factors with their function.

Growth factor	Abbreviation	Function
Epidermal growth factor	EGF	Stimulates epidermal and epithelial cells
Transforming growth factor-α	TGF-α	Same as above
Transforming growth factor-β	TGF-β	Inhibition of fibroblasts
Platelet derived growth factor	PDGF	Accelerates wound healing
Nerve growth factor	NGF	Growth of sensory neurons
Insulin-like growth factor-1	IGF-1	Sulfation into cartilage
Erythropoietin	EP	Stimulates erythropoiesis
Granulocyte macrophage colony-stimulating factor	GMCSF	Stimulates granulocytes, monocytes
Granulocyte colony-stimulating factor	GCSF	Stimulates granulocytes
Monocyte colony-stimulating factor	MCSF	Stimulates monocytes
Tumor necrosis factor-alpha	TNF-α	Necrosis of tumor cells

a number of cell functions. One example is by epinephrine binding to the beta-adrenergic receptor, activation of protein kinase A to cause the stimulation of glycogen breakdown.

Insulin activates a wide range of intracellular effects by the phosphorylation by the insulin receptor complex of its substrate insulin receptor substrate (IRS).

Cell Surface Receptors

Cell surface receptors (**membrane receptors**, **transmembrane receptors**) are receptors that are embedded in the plasma membrane of cells. They act in cell signaling by receiving (binding to) extracellular molecules. They are specialized integral membrane proteins that allow communication between the cell and the extracellular space. The extracellular molecules may be hormones, neurotransmitters, cytokines, growth factors, cell adhesion molecules, or nutrients; they react with the receptor to induce changes in the metabolism and activity of a cell. In the process of signal transduction, ligand binding affects a cascading chemical change through the cell membrane.

G Protein–coupled Receptor

G protein–coupled receptor (GPCR) (**seven-transmembrane receptor** or **heptahelical receptor**): Protein located in the cell membrane that binds extracellular substances and transmits signals from these substances to an intracellular molecule is called a G protein (guanine nucleotide-binding protein). GPCRs are found in the cell membranes of a wide range of organisms, including mammals, plants, microorganisms, and invertebrates (**Fig. 26.5**).

There are numerous different types of GPCRs—some 1,000 types are encoded by the human genome alone—and as a group they respond to a diverse range of substances, including light, hormones, amines, neurotransmitters, and lipids.

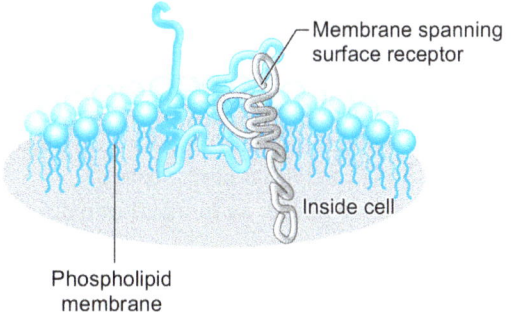

Fig. 26.5: Picture showing G-protein receptor.

Some examples of GPCRs include:
- Beta-adrenergic receptors, which bind epinephrine
- Prostaglandin E_2 receptors, which bind inflammatory substances called prostaglandins
- Rhodopsin, which contains a photoreactive chemical called retinal that responds to light signals received by rod cells in the eye.

GPCRs mediate the majority of cellular responses to external stimuli. Upon **activation** by a ligand, the **receptor** binds to a partner heterotrimeric **G protein** and promotes exchange of guanosine triphosphate (GTP) for guanosine diphosphate (GDP), leading to dissociation of the **G protein** into α and βγ subunits that mediate downstream signals.

An enzyme-linked **receptor**, also known as a **catalytic receptor**, is a transmembrane **receptor**, where the binding of an extracellular ligand causes enzymatic activity on the intracellular side. Hence, a **catalytic receptor** is an integral membrane protein possessing both enzymatic **catalytic** and **receptor** functions.

They have two important domains, an extracellular ligand-binding domain and an intracellular domain, which has a catalytic function, and a single transmembrane helix. The signaling molecule binds to the receptor on the outside of the cell and causes a conformational change on the catalytic function located on the receptor inside the cell.

Examples of the enzymatic activity include:
- Receptor tyrosine kinase, as in FGFR. Most enzyme-linked receptors are of this type (**Fig. 26.6**).
- Serine/threonine-specific protein kinase, as in bone morphogenetic protein.
- Guanylate cyclase, as in atrial natriuretic factor receptor.

Steroid Receptor Signaling

Steroid hormone **receptors** are found in the nucleus, cytosol, and also on the plasma membrane of target cells. They are generally intracellular **receptors** (typically cytoplasmic or nuclear) and initiate **signal** transduction for **steroid** hormones, which lead to changes in gene expression over a time period of hours to days.

Nuclear receptor (NR), in the absence of ligand, is located in the cytosol. Hormone binding to the NR triggers dissociation of heat shock proteins, dimerization, and translocation to the nucleus, where the NR binds to a specific sequence of DNA known as a hormone response element. The NR DNA complex in turn recruits other proteins that are responsible for transcription of downstream DNA into mRNA, which is eventually translated into protein, which results in a change in cell function (**Figs. 26.7A and B**).

Mutagens and Carcinogens

Mutagen

A mutagen is an agent, either a chemical substance or radiation, which can cause mutations. Mutations cause changes in the genetic information of an organism. Most mutagens are carcinogens.

Mutations may also arise by the errors in DNA replication. These types of mutations are called spontaneous mutations. Many of the mutations harm cells, causing diseases and cancers. Since mutagens modify the DNA sequence, they may cause nucleotide substitutions, insertions, deletions as well as chromosomal instability such as translocations and inversions. The mutagens that cause chromosomal instability are called

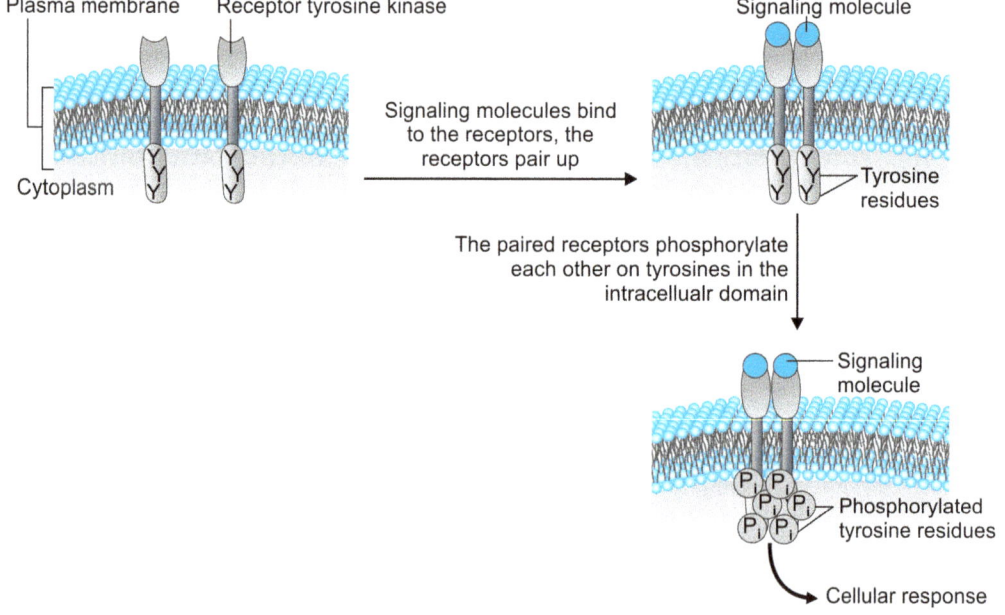

Fig. 26.6: Receptor tyrosine kinase.

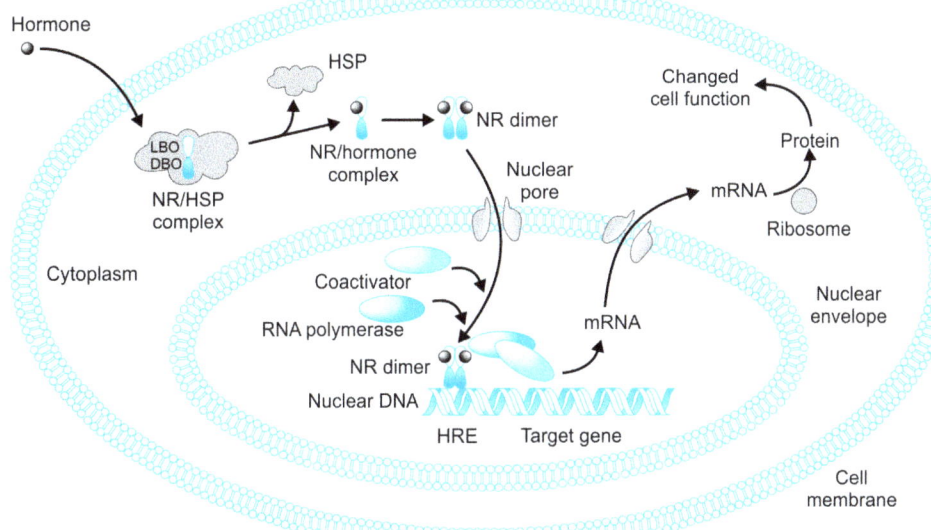

Fig. 26.7A: Steroid receptor signaling.

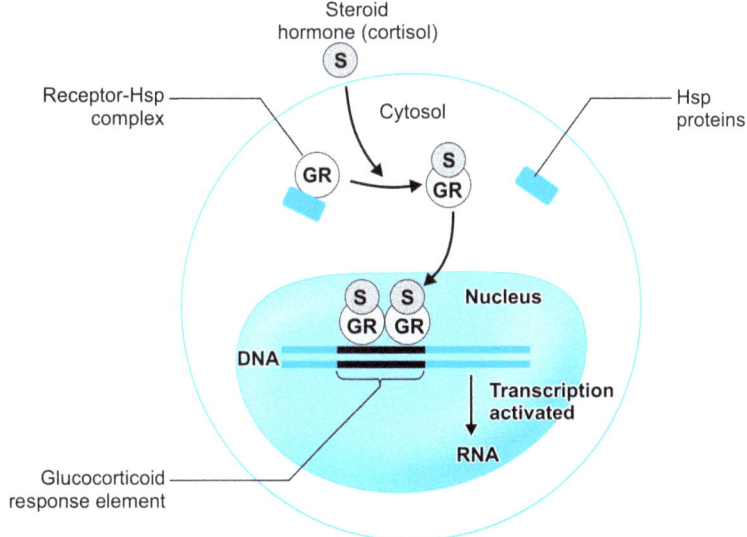

Fig. 26.7B: Steroid receptor signaling.

clastogens. Some mutagens can change the number of chromosomes in a cell.

Factors causing mutagens: Physical substances such as radioactive elements, X-rays, and UV radiation can cause mutations. The chemicals that interact with DNA such as reactive oxygen species, deaminating agents, sodium azide, and benzene also cause mutations. Intercalating agents such as ethidium bromide and metals such as nickel, arsenic, cadmium, and chromium are also mutagenic. Biological agents such as transposon, virus, and bacteria also cause mutations.

Carcinogen

Any physical, chemical, or biological substance, which can cause or promote cancer is referred to as a carcinogen.

Cancer-forming agents (carcinogens): Tobacco smoke, pathogens, radiation, environmental hazard, and the diet. Smokers and victim of secondhand smoke can easily be subjected to cancers. Smoking directly causes cancers in lungs, respiratory tract, and the esophagus and indirectly in the stomach, kidney, and the liver. Air, water, and soil pollution also cause cancers in bladder and lungs.

Proto-oncogenes and their Activation

A **proto-oncogene** is a normal gene that could become an oncogene due to mutations or increased expression. Proto-oncogenes code for proteins that help to regulate the cell growth and differentiation **(Fig. 26.8)**. Proto-oncogenes are often involved in signal transduction and execution of mitogenic signals, usually through their protein products. Upon acquiring an activating mutation, a proto-oncogene becomes a tumor-inducing agent, an oncogene.

Examples are *RAS, WNT, MYC, ERK,* and *TRK.* The *MYC* gene is implicated in Burkitt's lymphoma, which starts when a chromosomal translocation moves an enhancer sequence within the vicinity of the *MYC* gene.

Activation of Proto-oncogenes

The proto-oncogene can become an oncogene by a relatively small modification of its original function. There are three basic methods of activation:
1. A mutation within a proto-oncogene, or within a regulatory region, can cause a change in the protein structure, causing an increase in protein (enzyme) activity and a loss of regulation.
2. An increase in the amount of a certain protein (protein concentration), caused by:
   – An increase of protein expression (through misregulation)

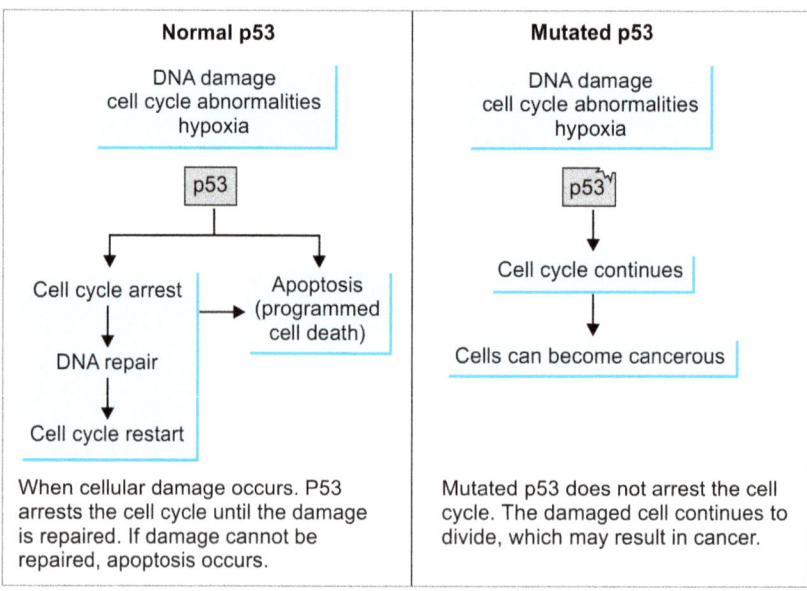

Fig. 26.8: Normal and mutated p53.

Biochemistry of Cancer

- An increase of protein (mRNA) stability, prolonging its existence and thus its activity in the cell
- G (one type of chromosome abnormality), resulting in an increased amount of protein in the cell.

3. A chromosomal translocation:
   - Translocation events that relocate a proto-oncogene to a new chromosomal site that leads to higher expression.
   - Translocation events that lead to a fusion between a proto-oncogene and a second gene (this creates a fusion protein with increased cancerous/oncogenic activity).
     - The expression of a constitutively active *hybrid protein*. This type of mutation in a dividing stem cell in the bone marrow leads to adult leukemia.
     - Philadelphia chromosome is an example of this type of translocation event.

Oncogene

An **oncogene** is a gene that has the potential to cause cancer. In tumor cells, these genes are often mutated, or expressed at high levels.

Tumor Suppressor Genes

A **tumor suppressor gene**, or antioncogene, is a **gene** that protects a cell from one step on the path to cancer. When this **gene** mutates to cause a loss or reduction in its function, the cell can progress to cancer, usually in combination with other **genetic** changes.

Tumor suppressor genes are normal **genes** that slow down cell division, repair DNA mistakes, or tell cells when to die (a process known as apoptosis or PCD). When **tumor suppressor genes** don't work properly, cells can grow out of control, which can lead to **cancer**.

Familial aggregation of human **cancers** is partly attributable to inherited **genetic** defects. Up to the **present**, more than 10 **tumor suppressor genes** have been identified as being responsible for autosomal dominant hereditary **cancer** syndromes.

Oncogenic Viruses

A number of **viruses** are suspected of causing cancer in animals, including humans, and are frequently referred to as **oncogenic viruses**.

Examples include HPVs. This can **cause** cervical and several other **cancers**. And hepatitis C can lead to liver **cancer** and non-Hodgkin's lymphoma.

The Epstein-Barr **virus**, and the hepatitis B **virus**, all of which have genomes made up of DNA.

Growth Factors and their Receptors

Growth factors are important for regulating a variety of **cellular** processes. **Growth factors** typically act as signaling molecules between **cells**. Examples are cytokines and hormones that bind to specific receptors on the surface of their target **cells**.

Growth factor receptors are present in the plasma membrane of resting cells as monomers or (pre)dimers. Ligand binding results in higher order oligomerization of ligand **receptor** complexes.

Growth factors are proteins that **function** as **growth** stimulators (mitogens) and/or **growth** inhibitors, stimulate **cell** migration, act as chemotactic agents, inhibit **cell** migration and invasion of tumor **cells**, and modulate differentiated **functions** of **cells**, involved in apoptosis and angiogenesis.

TUMOR MARKERS

Introduction

- A tumor marker is a substance produced by a tumor or by the tissue containing the tumor. Measurement of such substances in the tissue or in the body fluids is helpful to detect the presence of cancer.
- These substances can be found in the blood, urine, stool, tumor tissue, or other

tissues or bodily fluids of some patients with cancer.
- These are present in higher quantities in cancer tissue or in the blood of cancer patients.
- Normally its concentration is low.
- The goal is to be able to screen for and diagnose cancer early, when it is the most treatable and before it has had a chance to grow and spread.

The detection of tumor markers is clinically useful to:
- *Screen*
  - Most markers are not suited for general screening, but some may be used in those with a strong family history of a particular cancer.
  - In the case of genetic markers, they may be used to help predict risk in family members; prostatic specific antigen (PSA) testing for prostate cancer is an example.
  - These help to diagnose.
  - In a patient who has symptoms, tumor markers may be used to help identify the source of the cancer, such as CA-125 for ovarian cancer and to help differentiate it from other conditions.
  - Tumor markers cannot diagnose cancer themselves but aid in this process.
- *Stage*
  - If a patient does have cancer, tumor marker elevations can be used to help determine how far the cancer has spread into other tissues and organs.
  - Determine prognosis.
  - Some tumor markers can be used to help doctors determine how aggressive a cancer is likely to be.

Guide Treatment

Some tumor markers will give doctors information about what treatments their patients may respond to.

Monitor Treatment

- Tumor markers can be used to monitor the effectiveness of treatment, especially in advanced cancers.
- If the marker level drops, the treatment is working; if it stays elevated, adjustments are needed.
- The information must be used with care, however.
- Carcinoembryonic antigen (CEA), for instance, is used to monitor colorectal cancer but not every colorectal cancer patient will have elevated levels of CEA.
- If the marker level is not initially elevated with the cancer, it cannot be used later as a monitoring tool.

Determine Recurrence

- Currently, one of the biggest uses for tumor markers is to monitor for cancer recurrence.
- If a tumor marker is elevated before treatment, low after treatment, and then begins to rise over time, then it is likely that the cancer is returning (if it remains elevated after surgery, then chances is that not all of the cancer was removed).

The important tumor markers are shown in **Fig. 26.1** and **Table 26 3**.

Prostate-specific Antigen

- The major site of PSA production is the glandular epithelium of the prostate.
- A major function of PSA is the proteolytic cleavage of gel forming proteins and increases sperm motility.
- It is used as a marker for prostate cancer.
- Certain procedures involving prostate gland like transrectal biopsy, prostatectomy, and conditions like prostatitis and acute urinary retention, benign prostatic hyperplasia (BPH), and cancer of prostate will cause an increased PSA.

Table 26 3: Common tumor markers **(Fig. 26.9)**.

Name	Serum level increased in
AFP	Hepatoma, germ cell cancers
CEA	Colorectal, gastrointestinal, and lung cancer
Carbohydrate antigens CA-125	Ovarian cancer of epithelial origin
CA 15-3/CA-27.29 CA 72-4	Breast cancer
CA-19.9	Pancreatic and biliary tract cancers
ALP	Bone secondaries
Placental type ALP (Regan)	Lung, seminoma
PAP	Prostate cancer
PSA	Prostate cancer
Beta-hCG	Choriocarcinoma
Calcitonin	Medullary thyroid carcinoma
VMA	Pheochromocytoma and neuroblastoma
Hydroxy indole acetic acid	Carcinoid syndrome
Ig	Multiple myeloma, macroglobulinemia
Bence–Jones proteins (in urine)	Multiple myeloma

(AFP: alpha-fetoprotein; ALP: alkaline phosphatase; CEA: carcinoembryonic antigen; hCG: human chorionic gonadotropin; Ig: immunoglobulins; PAP: prostatic acid phosphatase; PSA: prostatic specific antigen; VMA: vanillyl-mandelic acid)

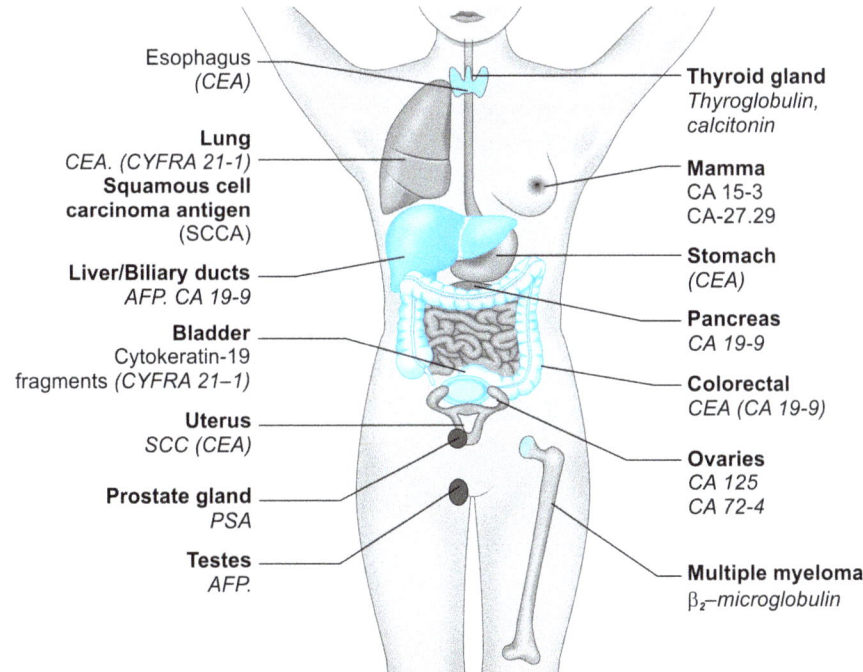

Fig. 26.9: Figure showing tumor markers for various organs.

Clinical Application

- Early detection of cancer:
  - PSA is specific for prostatic tissue but not for prostate cancer.
  - PSA level alone will not detect cancer in early stages.
  - PSA level is highest even in BPH. Serum PSA value together with digital rectal examination, transrectal ultrasonography is useful in the early detection of prostatic cancer.
  - Early detection is important because prostatic cancer can be detected in the early stage.
- Staging of prostatic cancer:
  - PSA level is found to be correlated well with the clinical stages of prostatic cancer.
  - Elevation of PSA level is seen in advanced stages of cancer.
- Monitoring treatment:
  - PSA level is useful in monitoring the definitive treatment of prostatic cancer.
  - After radial prostatectomy or radiation therapy, PSA level should decrease or should fall below the detection limit of the assay. High PSA levels even after prostate removal indicates the presence of residual tumor.

Normal range: 0–4 ng/mL.

Human Chorionic Gonadotropin

It is secreted by syncytiotrophoblast cells of the normal placenta.

It increases normally in pregnancy and also in trophoblastic disease and germ cell tumors.

Clinical Applications

- Human chorionic gonadotropin (hCG) is an excellent marker for early conformation and monitoring of pregnancy.
- Aiding in the detection of ectopic pregnancy.
- hCG is useful in identifying patients with trophoblastic tumors.
- Along with alpha-fetoprotein (AFP) it is useful in the detection of nonseminiferous testicular tumor where hCG levels correlate well with tumor volume of prognosis.
- High levels of hCG even in colony stimulating factor indicate brain metastasis. hCG is used to monitor the therapy of patients with central nervous system metastasis.
- Its level is useful in monitoring treatment and progression of trophoblastic disease.
- During chemotherapy and after remission, periodic levels are measured to detect the relapse.

Normal value: <5.0 mIU/mL.

Cancer Antigen 15-3/27.29 and 72-4

Primary tumor: Breast cancer.

Benign conditions: Breast, liver, kidney disorders, and ovarian cysts.

Normal value: 38 U/mL.

Level above which benign is >100 U/mL.

Cancer Antigen 19.9

Primary tumor(s): Pancreatic and biliary tract cancers.

Benign conditions:
- Pancreatitis
- Biliary disease and cirrhosis.

Normal value: 37 U/mL.

Level above which benign is more than 1,000 U/mL.

Cancer Antigen 125

CA 125 is a glycoprotein normally expressed in coelomic epithelium during fetal development.

This epithelium lines body cavities and envelopes the ovaries.

Normal values: <35 U/mL.

Primary tumor(s): Ovarian cancer.

Benign conditions:
- Menstruation
- Pregnancy
- Fibroids
- Ovarian cysts
- Pelvic inflammation

- Cirrhosis
- Pleural pericardial effusions
- Endometriosis.

Level above which benign: >200 U/mL.

Calcitonin: Thyroid medullary carcinoma.

Normal ranges:
- ≤0.155 ng/mL for men
- ≤0.105 ng/mL for women.

ONCOFETAL ANTIGENS

Oncofetal antigens are proteins produced during fetal life. These proteins are present in high concentration in the sera of fetuses and decrease to low levels or disappear after birth. These proteins reappear in cancer patients. The production of these proteins demonstrates that certain genes are reactivated as the result of the malignant transformation of cells. There are several examples for oncofetal antigens; AFP, CEA, beta-oncofetal antigens, and pancreatic oncofetal antigen.

Alpha-fetoprotein

- AFP is the best example for oncofetal antigen.
- It is a marker for hepatocellular and germ cell carcinoma.

Clinical Application

- For detecting fetuses with neural tube defect.
- Screening of hepatocellular carcinoma.
- Prognosis and monitoring the therapy of the patients.
- Along with hCG, it is used in classifying and staging germ cell tumors into a single type or a mixture.

Normal levels: 0–15 ng/mL.

Carcinoembryonic Antigen

Carcinoembryonic antigen is a marker for:
- Colorectal cancer
- Gastrointestinal cancer.

Clinical Applications

- CEA is elevated in the benign conditions such as cirrhosis, pulmonary emphysema, rectal polyps, benign breast diseases, and ulcerative colitis.
- It also increases in colorectal, lung, gastric, breast, pancreatic, ovarian, and uterine cancers. Moreover CEA is not a marker in these cases because of the elevations associated with benign disease of the number of tumors that do not produce CEA.
- It is used as an adjuvant in clinical staging. If CEA increases 5–10 times than the normal, it may be a colon cancer or may be associated with other cancers.
- If 28% increased than the normal, it may be a colorectal cancer of stage A. If it is 45% more, it is colorectal cancer of stage B.
- In the prognosis of the development of the metastasis.
- Monitoring the therapy of colorectal cancer.
- Monitoring breast, lung, gastric, and pancreatic carcinomas.
- Monitoring metastatic colon cancers.

Normal level: 0–4 ng/mL.

For smoker: 0–5 ng/mL.

Estrogen Receptor

Estrogen receptor (ER) is a protein found in the nucleus of breast and uterine tissues. The level of ER in the tissue is used to determine whether a person with breast cancer is likely to respond to therapy with tamoxifen, which binds to the receptors blocking the action of estrogen. Women who are ER-negative have a greater risk of recurrence than women who are ER-positive.

Progesterone Receptor

Tissue that does not express the progesterone receptors (PRs) is less likely to bind estrogen analogs used to treat the tumor. Persons who test negative for both ER and PR have less than a 5% chance of responding to endocrine therapy. Those who test positive for both markers have greater than a 60% chance of tumor shrinkage when treated with hormone therapy.

BIOCHEMICAL BASIS OF CANCER THERAPY

Chemotherapy

- Use of one or more type of anticancer drug **(Figs. 26.10 and 26.11)**
- Given with either curative intent, symptom reduction or with the aim to prolong life
- *Administered in many ways:* Oral, intravenous, injection, intra-arterial, topical.

Cancer still imposes a global threat to public health. After decades of research on cancer biology and enormous efforts in developing anticancer therapies, we now understand that the majority of cancers can be prevented. Bioactive phytochemicals present in edible plants have been shown to reduce the risk of various types of cancer.

Effect on Cancer Cells

Kills cancer cells by damaging DNA and preventing cell division. If the cell cannot divide, it dies.

Some types of chemo used:
- DNA-damaging agents, also called alkylating agents: These agents stop cells from dividing by changing the cell's DNA through the addition of hydrogen and carbon (alkyl groups), so it can't be copied. Because cancer cells grow and divide quickly, they end up dying because they don't have time to repair the damaged DNA.
- Antimetabolites act like the building blocks of DNA or RNA that cancer cells need to grow and survive. When a cancer cell uses the antimetabolite chemotherapy drug instead of their own substances, the DNA is damaged and the cell dies.
- Antimitotic agents block the process of cell division (mitosis) so cells can't divide and multiply.
- Antitumor antibiotics bind to DNA so it can't work properly, resulting in cell death. These drugs are different than antibiotics used to treat infection.

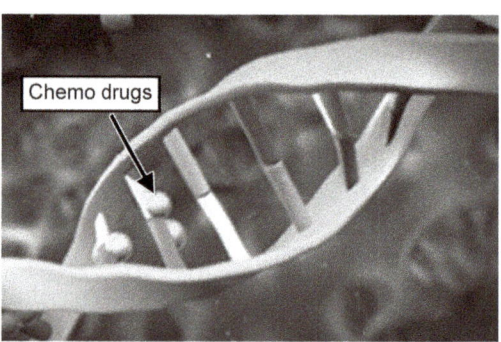

Fig. 26.10: Action of chemo drugs.

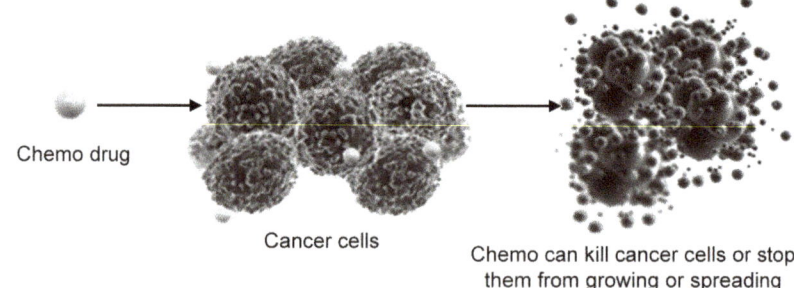

Fig. 26.11: Action of chemo drugs.

- DNA-repair enzyme inhibitors prevent the normal repair of DNA damage inside the cell. These chemotherapy drugs attack the enzymes that normally repair damage to DNA. If a cancer cell can't repair damage to DNA, it dies.
- Some chemo drugs kill cancer cells only when they are dividing and are called cell-cycle specific.
- Some kill cancer cells when they are at rest and are called cell-cycle nonspecific.
- A combo of chemo drugs are typically used, which target the cell at different stages of division thus making it overall more effective in killing cancer cells.

Effects on Normal Cells

- Because chemo drugs cannot distinguish between cancer cells and normal cells, normal cells are also targeted as they divide.
- Blood cells are most commonly affected as well as the mouth, hair follicles, stomach, and bowels as these cells tend to grow and divide quicker than others.
- These cells tend to grow back healthily, and thus damage does not usually last after treatment.
- However, side effects such as hair loss, low blood counts, diarrhea, nausea, and mouth sores occur in the interim.

Alkylating agents work by reacting with the proteins that bond together to form the very delicate double helix structure of a DNA molecule, adding an alkyl group to some or all of them. This prevents the proteins from linking up as they should, causing breakage of the DNA strands and, eventually, the death of the cell.

An **alkylating** antineoplastic **agent** is an **alkylating agent** used in cancer treatment that attaches an alkyl group (C_nH_{2n+1}) to DNA. The alkyl group is attached to the guanine base of DNA, at the number 7 nitrogen atom of the purine ring.

Examples of alkylating agents include:
- Altretamine
- Busulfan
- Carboplatin
- Carmustine
- Chlorambucil
- Cisplatin
- Cyclophosphamide
- Dacarbazine.

Anticancer Drugs

Surgery and radiotherapy are most effective to reduce the initial tumor load. These are the prime modalities of treatment in solid tumors. Chemotherapy is the sheet anchor of therapy in leukemias, advanced lymphomas, choriocarcinoma, and other widely disseminated malignancies. The effectiveness of cytotoxic drugs is directly proportional to the doubling time of the tumors and is inversely proportional to the number of cancer cells. Cytotoxic drugs affect all the cells that are in the dividing phase. Rapidly dividing normal cells (gastrointestinal tract, hematopoietic system, hair follicles, and gonads) are also affected by chemotherapeutic drugs, leading to toxicity.

Antimetabolites

Antimetabolites are drugs that interfere with one or more enzymes or their reactions that are necessary for DNA synthesis. They affect DNA synthesis by acting as a substitute to the actual metabolites that would be used in the normal metabolism (e.g. antifolates interfere with the use of folic acid).

Antimetabolites are drugs used in cancer chemotherapy. Cancer cells divide more rapidly compared to normal cells so antimetabolites affect cancer cell replication more than they affect normal cell replication **(Table 26.4)**.

Receptor Blockers

Angiotensin II **receptor blockers** (ARBs) are a class of drugs prescribed to control blood pressure, treat heart failure, and prevent

Table 26.4: Common anticancer drugs.

Name	Type	Mode of action
Methotrexate	Folic acid analog	Competitive inhibitor of dihydrofolate reductase. THFA is required for nucleotide synthesis
6-Mercapto purine	Purine analog	Inhibits the conversion of IMP to AMP
6-Thioguanine	Purine analog	Inhibits the conversion of IMP to AMP
Cyclophosphamide	Alkylating agent	Cross-linking of bases of DNA; inhibition of strand separation
Mitomycin C	Antibiotic	Cross bridges are formed between DNA base pairs
Actinomycin D	Antibiotic	Intercalates with guanine bases of DNA; prevents transcription
Vincristine and vinblastine	Alkaloids from *Vinca rosea*	Interferes with assembly of cytoskeleton and inhibits stathmokinesis (spindle movement)
Adriamycin	Anthracyclines	Topoisomerase-mediated breaks in DNA
Etoposide	Podophyllotoxin	Stabilizes topoisomerase-II-DNA cleavage complexes
Cisplatin	Platinum compound	Forms intrastrand DNA adducts
Imatinib	Monoclonal antibody	Tyrosine kinase inhibitor
FU	Pyrimidine analog	Inhibits thymidylate synthase

(FU: fluorouracil; DNA: deoxyribonucleic acid; THFA: tetrahydro folic acid; IMP: inosine monophosphate; AMP: adenosine monophosphate)

kidney failure in people with diabetes or high blood pressure.

Examples of ARBs include:
- Azilsartan (Edarbi)
- Candesartan (Atacand)
- Eprosartan
- Irbesartan (Avapro)
- Losartan (Cozaar)
- Olmesartan (Benicar)
- Telmisartan (Micardis)
- Valsartan (Diovan).

Monoclonal Antibody (Table 26.5)

These drugs are a relatively new innovation in cancer treatment. The mechanism of action of monoclonals against cancer may be:
- The antibody marks the cancer cell and makes it easier for the immune system to attack. The drug rituximab attaches to CD20 found only on B cells, which makes the cells more visible to the immune system to attack.

Table 26.5: Action of monoclonals.

Name	Target	Used against the cancer
Rituximab	CD20 on B cells	NHL, CLL, B-cell leukemia
Trastuzumab (Herceptin)	HER-2/neu (EGFR2, Erb-B2)	Breast cancer
Bevacizumab	VEGF	Colorectal, solid tumors of kidney, and breast
Alemtuzumab	CD52 on B cells	CLL
Cetuximab	KRas	Colorectal, head, and neck
Panitumumab	EGFR	Colorectal
Imatinib	Tyrosine kinase	CML

(EGFR: epidermal growth factor receptor; VEGF: vascular endothelial growth factor; HER: ??; NHL: ??; CLL: ??; CML: ??)

- Block growth factors. Certain cancer cells make extra copies of the growth factor receptor. This makes them grow faster than the normal cells. Monoclonal antibodies can block these receptors and prevent the growth signal. For example, cetuximab attaches to epidermal growth factor receptors on cancer cells. Blocking this signal from reaching its target on the cancer cells may slow or stop the cancer from growing.
- Stop new blood vessels from forming. To attract blood vessels, cancer cells send out growth signals. Monoclonal antibodies that block these growth signals may help prevent a tumor from developing a blood supply, so that it remains small. The monoclonal antibody bevacizumab intercepts vascular endothelial growth factor and stops them from connecting with their targets.

Radiotherapy

Radiotherapy is a treatment where radiation is used to kill cancer cells. It damages cancer cells and stops them from growing or spreading in the body. It uses high energy rays such as X-rays to destroy cancer cells in the area it is given.

There are many different ways of **radiotherapy**, but they all work in a similar way.

- *External beam radiotherapy:* Given outside the body by a radiotherapy machine.
- *Internal radiotherapy:* When a radioactive material is placed inside the body.

Radiation therapy damages the DNA of cancer cells. Ionizing radiation (X-ray and gamma) forms ions in the cells of the tissue it passes through. These ions can change the genes within DNA thus damaging it.

SUMMARY

Cancer is a disease characterized by the development of a large number of abnormal cells that can divide rapidly and have the ability to infiltrate and destroy the normal body tissue. It can spread throughout our body. Cancers are caused by abnormalities in the genetic material of the transformed cells. These abnormalities may be due to the effects of carcinogens such as tobacco smoke, radiation, chemicals, or infectious agents. Anticancer agents such as amethopterin, 5'-fluorouracil, cytosine arabinoside, and doxorubicin are used to treat cancer.

SELF-TEST ASSESSMENT

1. Define tumor markers.
2. State the clinical importance of tumor marker estimation in the laboratory.
3. Name any four tumor markers.
4. Which marker is used to find out the tumor of the prostate gland?
5. Write the clinical significances of PSA estimation.
6. Write the normal value for the following:
   a. PSA
   b. AFP
   c. CEA.
7. Write the clinical applications of β-hCG estimation.
8. What are oncofetal antigens? Give an example.
9. In which tumor the CA-125 increases?
10. Mention the other associated benign conditions in which CA-125 increases.
11. State the conditions associated with AFP increase.
12. Write the clinical applications of CA-27.29 estimation in the laboratory.

MULTIPLE-CHOICE QUESTIONS

1. **The specific tumor marker for prostate is:**
   a. Prostatic acid phosphatase
   b. Prostate-specific antigen
   c. Carcinoembryonic antigen
   d. Lactate dehydrogenase

2. The β-hCG is secreted from:
   a. Adrenal medulla
   b. Syncytiotrophoblastic cells of placenta
   c. Prostate gland
   d. Ovarian follicles
3. The following are the examples for oncofetal antigens, *except*:
   a. hCG
   b. CEA
   c. AFP
   d. α-Oncofetal antigens
4. CEA is not a marker for:
   a. Colorectal cancer
   b. Gastrointestinal cancer
   c. Lung cancer
   d. Liver cancer
5. Which of the following does not have AFP as a marker for?
   a. Detecting fetuses with neural tube defect
   b. Screening of hepatocellular carcinoma
   c. Yolk sac tumor
   d. Colon cancer

Answers

1. b   2. b   3. a   4. d   5. d

CHAPTER 27

Radioisotopes in Medicine

OBJECTIVES
At the end of this topic the students should be able to:
- Know about different types of radiation hazards and application of radioisotopes
- Understand the radioimmunoassay and enzyme linked immunoassay techniques.

INTRODUCTION

Radioisotope: A version of a chemical element that has an unstable nucleus and emits radiation during its decay to a stable form. Radioisotopes have important uses in medical diagnosis, treatment, and research.

Each molecule in our body is made up of atoms having a nucleus with particles revolving around it. A lot of facts about our body and disease are still unknown. But it is certain that in any disease, the problem starts at the level of a molecule in our body and the knowledge of this helps us to know more facts about health and disease. This chapter talks about how the knowledge of molecules can be exploited to our benefit for research, diagnosis, and treatment of disease.

The entire concept explained here and its application was developed by Henri Becquerel, who discovered a phenomenon called radioactivity in 1896.

Atom **(Fig. 27.1):** Its structure contains a nucleus in the center having positively charged protons and uncharged neutrons, and surrounded by electrons in the periphery.

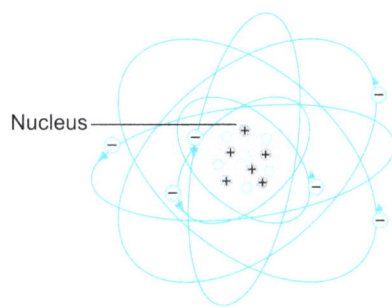

Fig. 27.1: Structure of an atom.

Nuclide: An atomic species with a given atomic number and a given mass number.

Isotope: Definition and Properties

- Nuclides have same atomic number (left subscript to the chemical symbol), but different mass number (left superscript to the chemical symbol).
- Behave similarly in chemical reactions.
- May be stable (nuclear composition does not change with time) or unstable (undergoes spontaneous decay).

Examples of isotopes:

Stable	Unstable
$_2H_1$ (deuterium)	$_1H_1$, $_3H_1$ (tritium)
$_{12}C_6$, $_{13}C_6$ (isotopes of carbon)	$_{14}C_6$, $_{127}I_{53}$ (isotope of iodine) $_{125}I_{53}$, $_{131}I_{53}$

Radioactivity

Radioactivity is a property of unstable isotopes to undergo spontaneous degradation of nucleus with emission of particles or rays to attain a stable conformation.

Units of Radioactivity

- International system unit of radioactivity is becquerel (Bq). It is defined as the activity of a quantity of radioactive material in which one nucleus decays per second.
- Older unit of radioactivity is curie.

Radioactive Decay

An unstable (radioactive) nucleus can become stable by spontaneously emitting particles and energy by a process called "decay." These particles or energy (in the form of electromagnetic waves) are collectively called radiation. The radiation emitted can either be alpha particles, beta particles, or gamma rays. This process is called radioactivity.

Half-life

During the decay process of a radioactive isotope, the radioactivity decreases with time. The time taken for an isotope to reach half of its original radioactivity is called half-life. Each radionuclide (radioactive isotope) has a characteristic half-life. The half-lives of radionuclides may vary from millionth of a second to millions of years **(Table 27.1)**.

Table 27.1: Half-life period of radioactive isotopes.

Radionuclides	Half-life
Radon-219	4 seconds
Potassium-38	7.6 minutes
Selenium-73	7.2 hours
Iodine-131	8 days
Cobalt-60	5.26 years
Cesium-137	30 years
Carbon-14	5,730 years
Iodine-129	15,700,000 years
Uranium-235	703,800,000 years
Potassium-40	1,277,000,000 years

TYPES OF RADIATION

Nonionizing Radiation

- Contains low-energy electromagnetic waves, e.g. ultraviolet, visible light, infrared, microwave, and radio wave **(Fig. 27.2)**
- Causes molecules to vibrate and induces heating effects
- Ultraviolet radiation: Although it is nonionizing, exposure to it could cause harmful sunburn.

Ionizing Radiation

- Ionizing radiation includes high-speed particles and high-energy electromagnetic waves.

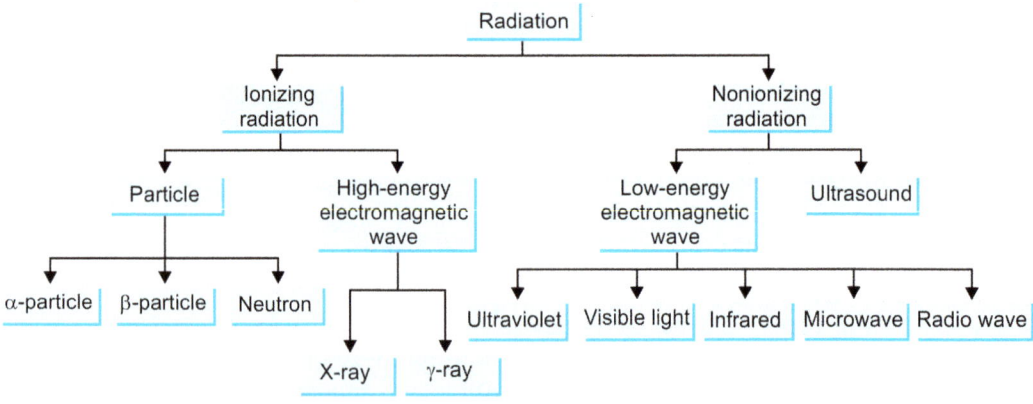

Fig. 27.2: Types of radiation.

- Their energy is high enough to remove orbital electrons from atoms.
- They can cause deoxyribonucleic acid (DNA) damage, mutation, and cancer.
- Their ability to destroy DNA has been exploited to kill cancer cells.

Types of Ionizing Radiations

Alpha (α) radiation
- Consist of two protons and two neutrons. After emission, they decrease atomic number by two and mass number by four (helium nucleus). For example:
  $_{88}^{226}Radium \rightarrow {_{88}^{222}}Radon \rightarrow {_{84}^{218}}Polonium \rightarrow {_{82}^{214}}Lead$
- Have maximum ionization.
- *Stopped by sheet of paper:* Minimum penetration.
- Not useful in clinical medicine because they cannot penetrate deep tissues.

Beta (β) radiation
- When neutron splits, it forms proton$^{(+)}$, β$^{(-)}$ particle (electron), and neutrino.
  For example:
  $_{6}^{14}C \rightarrow {^{14}N} + Neutrino + \beta(-)$
- So, they increase atomic number by one and have no effect on mass number.
- Negatively charged with negligible mass.
- Have more penetration than α-radiation.
- Used widely in clinical medicine for diagnosis and treatment.

Gamma (γ) radiation and X-rays
- γ-rays are emitted when neutron is converted to proton after emission of a particle or during electron capture by proton to form neutron. For example:
  $_{53}^{131}I \rightarrow {_{54}^{131}}Xenon \rightarrow {_{54}^{131}}Xenon + Gamma$
- γ-rays are electromagnetic waves, have no charge or mass. They are emitted from the nuclei of unstable atoms during radioactive decay. They are similar to visible light, except that they have higher frequency and energy.
- X-ray is also an electromagnetic radiation without charge or mass, but it is less powerful than γ-rays.
- γ-rays and X-rays have great penetrating power and can pass through human body.
- γ-rays and X-rays are similar; the major difference is their origin. X-rays are from the electron cloud as a result of electron excitation.
- These are widely used in treatment of cancers.

HANDLING RADIOACTIVE MATERIAL

Before knowing the applications, every student should know some precautions in handling radioactive material.

Radiation Hazard Symbol

If you see this symbol on any container/bottle/reagents, etc., you should be aware that the material inside is radioactive (**Fig. 27.3**).

Radioprotective Enclosure

Everyone who is standing as a bystander when taking X-ray, computed tomography scan or near an instrument, while giving radiation treatment for cancer patients, should wear a suitable enclosure so that radiation does not affect him/her. It is usually a thick and heavy coat made up of lead as shown in **Fig. 27.4**.

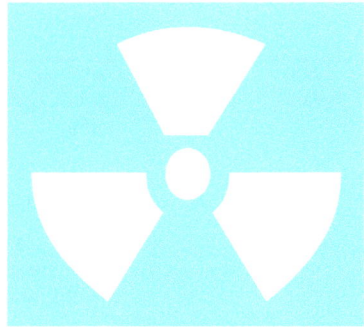

Fig. 27.3: Radiation hazard symbol.

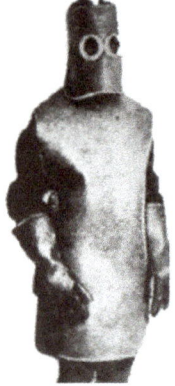

Fig. 27.4: Radioprotective enclosure.

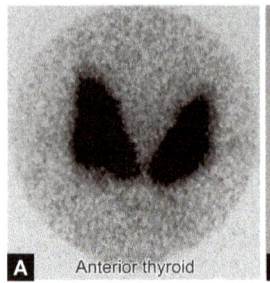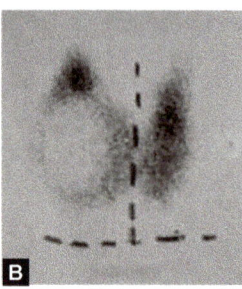

Figs. 27.5A and B: *Diagnosis:* (A) normal thyroid scan and (B) cold nodule in thyroid cancer (left side).

APPLICATIONS OF RADIOACTIVE ISOTOPES

Research

Tracer technique:
- ^{14}C: Study metabolic pathways **(Table 27.2)**
- ^{131}I: Study half-life of immunoglobulin
- ^{131}I-labeled albumin: Total body content, e.g. blood volume.

Diagnosis

- ^{51}Cr (chromium): Red blood cell life span, intravascular hemolysis **(Figs. 27.5A and B)**.
- ^{131}I: Thyroid uptake in normal/hyperthyroidism/hypothyroidism.
- ^{131}I: Thyroid scan, "cold nodule" (less/no uptake of radioactive isotope).
- ^{90}Sr (strontium): Osteoblastoma can be detected even before radiological changes have occurred.
- ^{125}I-labeled antigen: In radioimmunoassay (RIA) to quantitate hormones, tumor markers, etc. that are present in small amounts.

Radioimmunoassay

- Microgram or picogram of substances can be analyzed **(Fig. 27.6)**.
- Only microcuries of radioactivity are used and radiation hazard is minimal.
- Half-life of ^{125}I is 60 days.
- *Stringent laws:* Only approved laboratory can use.
- Expensive.

Uses: To quantify biological materials such as hormones, tumor markers, and antigens.

Note: As the number of drug molecules added increases from blank (0) to drug (12), the number of labeled drug particles getting displaced and appearing in the supernatant increases.

Enzyme-linked Immunosorbent Assay

- No radiation hazard **(Fig. 27.7)**
- Simple and less time-consuming than RIA
- Cheap
- No special detectors required.

Uses: Same as RIA.

Note: If sample contains antigen, it gets bound to antibody on plate and a second enzyme-labeled antibody helps in its detection.

Table 27.2: Examples for applications of radioactive isotopes.

Isotopes	Half-life	Radiation	Uses
^{14}C	5,600 years	α	Metabolism studies, carbon dating
^{32}P	14 days	α	Nucleic acid study
^{51}Cr	28 days	α	RBC kinetics
^{131}I	8 days	α	Thyroid scan, treatment of thyroid cancer
^{137}Cs	30 years	α	Teletherapy

(RBC: red blood cell)

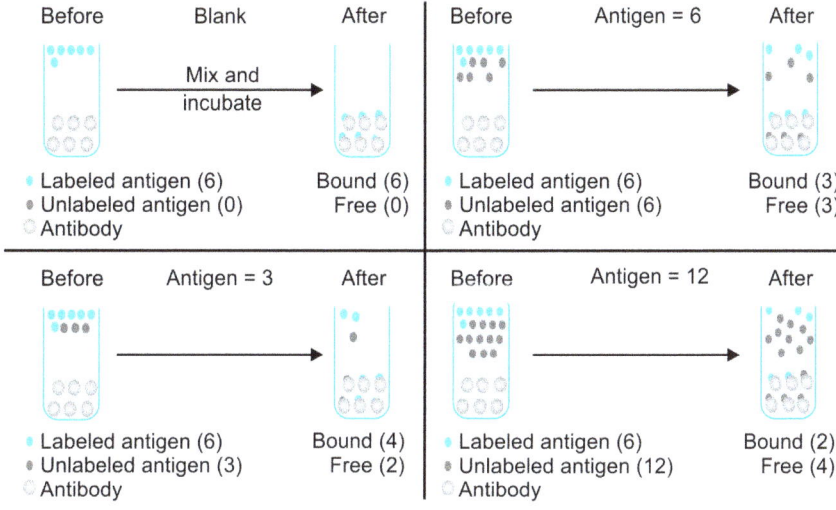

Fig. 27.6: Radioimmunoassay.

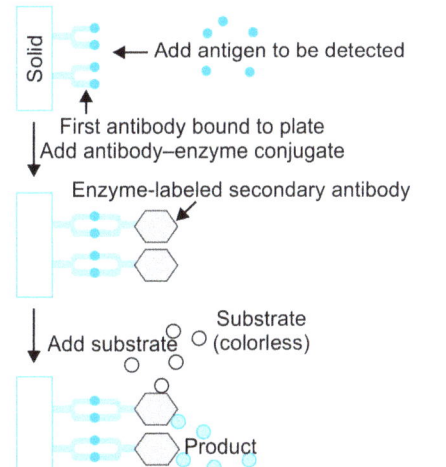

Fig. 27.7: Enzyme-linked immunosorbent assay.

Treatment

Radiotherapy

Three types of radiotherapy are as follows:
1. Unsealed.
2. Sealed
3. Teletherapy.

Unsealed

- Mainly β-rays: Liquid form of the isotope injected—selectively stored in cancer tissue
- ^{131}I: Treatment of thyroid cancer and secondaries
- ^{32}P (phosphorus): Treatment of polycythemia vera.

Sealed

- Utilize γ, which has good penetration
- Source applied on cancer tissue or as needle (brachytherapy)
- Radium/cesium needle for uterine, cervix, intestine, and buccal cancer.

Teletherapy

- Source kept at a distance in a thick-walled metal container with small aperture and focused on cancer tissue.
- γ-rays are used, e.g. ^{60}Co (cobalt)/^{137}Cs in deep-seated cancers.

Radiosensitivity

Success of treatment depends upon how much the tumor is sensitive to radiation:
- Lymphoma, Hodgkin's disease, and neuroblastoma are highly sensitive.
- Oral, cervical, and breast cancer are moderately sensitive.
- Osteoblastoma and malignant melanoma are poorly sensitive.

RADIATION EFFECTS

Radiotherapy can cause some unwanted effects on the body. This depends on the system or organ exposed to radiation:
- *Skin:* Epilation, dermatitis, hypopigmentation, and loss of elasticity
- *Mucous membrane:* Nausea, vomiting, ulceration, bleeding, adhesion, and fibrosis
- *Blood cells:* Thrombocytopenia and leukopenia
- *Reproductive organs:* Sterility and genetic alterations in offspring
- Can produce cancer.

SUMMARY

Isotopes are nuclides having same atomic number but different mass number. They may be stable (nuclear composition does not change with time) or unstable (undergoes spontaneous decay). Radioactivity is a property of unstable isotopes to undergo spontaneous degradation of nucleus with emission of particles or rays to attain a stable conformation. There are nonionizing and ionizing radiations. Types of ionizing radiations are α-radiation (having maximum ionization), β-radiation, γ-radiation, and X-rays. The γ-rays and X-rays have great penetrating power and can pass through human body. Radioisotopes are used to study metabolic pathways, half-life of immunoglobulin, thyroid scan, RIA, and enzyme-linked immunosorbent assay.

SELF-ASSESSMENT QUESTIONS

1. What are radioisotopes? Name any three radioisotopes and their clinical applications.
2. Define stable isotopes and radioisotopes. Give an example for each. Write the principle of RIA.
3. Write briefly on hazards of radioactivity.
4. Define half-life of a radioisotope. Give example.
5. Write isotopes of medical significance.
6. What are radioisotopes? Give three different uses of radioisotopes in biochemistry.
7. Briefly explain RIA and ELISA.

MULTIPLE-CHOICE QUESTIONS

1. Isotope of an element is defined as element having:
   a. Same atomic and mass number
   b. Same atomic, but different mass number
   c. Different mass, but same atomic number
   d. Different mass and different atomic number
2. The correct statement about property of ionizing radiation is:
   a. Can get ionized in solution
   b. Low-energy radiations
   c. Can remove orbital electrons from atoms
   d. Will never carry any positive or negative charge
3. The ideal type of radiation used for treatment should have the following properties, *except*:
   a. High energy and high frequency
   b. High mass and high charge
   c. Maximum penetration
   d. Maximum ionization
4. One of the statements concerning γ-radiation is true, they:
   a. Have high energy and frequency
   b. Are positively charged particles
   c. Are negatively charged particles
   d. Have maximum ionizing power

Answers

1. b   2. c   3. c   4. a

CHAPTER 28

Metabolism of Xenobiotics (Detoxification)

OBJECTIVES

At the end of this chapter, students should be able to:
- Understand detoxification of unwanted products from the body
- Explain the two phases of detoxification.

INTRODUCTION

Human body is exposed to a number of xenobiotics during the course of the lifetime, including a variety of pharmaceuticals and food components. Many of these compounds show little relationship to previously encountered compounds or metabolites and yet our bodies are capable of managing environmental exposure by detoxifying them. The enzyme systems generally function adequately to minimize the potential of damage from xenobiotics. However, much literature suggests an association between impaired detoxification and disease such as cancer, Parkinson's disease, and chronic immune dysfunction syndrome.

A number of biochemical pathways and sequences of chemical changes are involved in liver biotransformation. These are grouped into oxidation, reduction, or hydrolysis reactions (phase I) and conjugation reactions (phase II). Phase I reactions are catalyzed by a group of liver enzymes scientifically known as cytochrome P450 oxidases (P450 oxidases or cytochrome P450s). These enzymes introduce oxygen into the chemical structure of toxins or metabolites. Typically, by this process, the toxins are converted into intermediate substances such as alcohols and aldehydes and then into acids, which are water soluble and can be excreted via the urine.

PHASE I DETOXIFICATION

- The intermediate substances created during phase I detoxification (reactive oxygen species like free radicals) can be extremely toxic and therefore their harmful effects are primarily controlled by antioxidant enzymes of our body.
- Apart from free radicals, there are other intermediate metabolites (chloral hydrate, epoxides, and endogenous benzodiazepines).
- Excess toxic intermediates in the body induce more P450 enzymes in the liver. These are also induced by caffeine, alcohol, dioxin and other pollutants, exhaust fumes, high-protein diets, oranges, organophosphorus pesticides, paint fumes, steroid hormones, and a variety of drugs, including paracetamol, diazepam tranquilizers, sleeping pills, contraceptive pills, and cortisone.

Aldehydes

- Substances that can inhibit the action of P450 enzymes include:
    - Carbon tetrachloride (CCl_4)
    - Carbon monoxide (CO)
    - Barbiturates and quercetin.

Oxidation reaction can also be blocked by an excess of toxic chemicals, a lack of enzymes, lack of nutrients, and/or loss of oxygen.

- The blocking results in a buildup of more toxic substances such as formaldehyde and other aldehydes in tissue. This can lead to a spreading phenomenon with increasing sensitivity to more chemicals such as ketones and alcohols, and eventually even to natural chemicals occurring in foods, pollen, and mold. A buildup of aldehydes can in severe cases lead to tissue cross-linking causing vasculitis with possible seizures and brain damage.
- Although most aldehydes in the body are thought to occur as intermediate metabolites, external sources include exposure to formaldehyde gas and breakdown products of ethylene glycol and methanol.
- Two known sources of aldehydes are intestinal overgrowth with *Candida albicans*, as well as the peroxidation of polyunsaturated fats.

Amines

Cytochrome P450 and other oxidizing enzymes also oxidize amines such as phenylethylamine found in chocolate, tyramine found in cheese, and adrenaline, noradrenaline, and dopamine. These are oxidized into aldehydes by the enzyme mitochondrial monoamine oxidase.

Chemical Reactions in Phase I

The main chemical reactions involved in phase I detoxification are as follows:
- Oxidation
- Reduction
- Hydrolysis.

Examples of Detoxification by Oxidation

Ethanol + NAD$^+$ $\xrightarrow{\text{Alcohol dehydrogenase}}$ Acetaldehyde + NADH + H$^+$

- Methanol is oxidized to formaldehyde.

Acetaldehyde + NAD$^+$ $\xrightarrow{\text{Alcohol dehydrogenase}}$ Acetic acid + NADH + H$^+$

- Indole is oxidized to indoxyl.
- Skatole is oxidized to skatoxyl.

Serotonin $\xrightarrow{\text{Amine oxidase}}$ 5-hydroxyindole acetic acid + NH$_3$

Histamine $\xrightarrow{\text{Amine oxidase}}$ Imidazole acetic acid + NH$_3$

- Epinephrine and norepinephrine are converted to 4-hydroxy-3-methoxy-mandelic acid (vanillylmandelic acid) by amine oxidase.
- Benzene is oxidized to phenol or muconic acid.

Examples for Oxidation Involving Microsomal Hydroxylase System

Phenobarbital is oxidized to p-OH-phenobarbital. The enzyme system is inducible and activity depends on P450, reduced form of nicotinamide adenine dinucleotide phosphate, flavoprotein. Phenobarbital has been used in the treatment of hyperbilirubinemia in infants. This drug causes the synthesis of uridine 5′-diphospho (UDP)-glucuronyltransferase, which converts the bilirubin to bilirubin diglucuronide.

Oxidation of following compounds occurs:
- Acetanilide to paracetamol
- Morphine to its *N*-oxide
- Deamination of amphetamine to phenylacetone and ammonia (NH$_3$)
- Hydroxylation of steroid hormones.

Detoxification by Reduction

- Chloral is reduced to trichloroethyl alcohol.
- Picric acid is reduced to picramic acid.
- Nitro group of chloramphenicol is reduced to amino group.

Detoxification by Hydrolysis

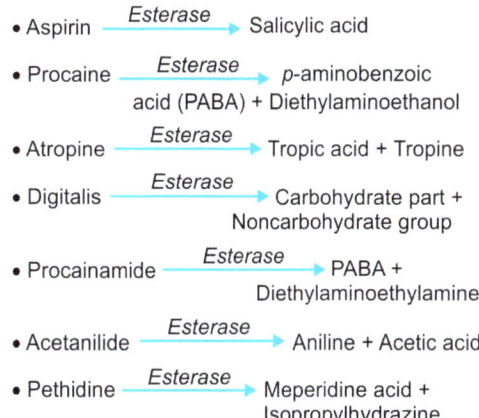

PHASE II DETOXIFICATION (CONJUGATION)

- Majority of the products formed in phase I mechanisms undergo conjugation.
- There are five main conjugation categories:
  a. Acetylation
  b. Acylation
  c. Sulfur conjugations
  d. Methylation
  e. Conjugation with glucuronic acid.
  Some substances enter phase II detoxification directly and others via phase I pathways.
- Conjugation involves the combining of a metabolite or toxin with another substance, which adds a hydrophilic (or water reactive), converting lipophilic (fat reactive) substances to water-soluble forms for excretion and elimination. Individual xenobiotics and metabolites usually follow a specific path, so while caffeine is metabolized by P450 enzymes, aspirin-based medications are conjugated with glycine and paracetamol with sulfate.

Acetylation

Acetylation requires pantothenic acid to function. It is the chief degradation pathway for compounds containing aromatic amines such as histamine, serotonin, para-aminobenzoic acid, p-amino-salicylic acid, aniline, and procaine amide. It is also a pathway for sulfur amides, aliphatic amines, and complex hydrazines.

Conjugation with Acetyl-CoA

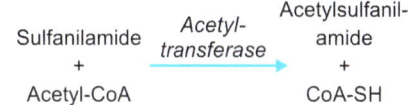

Acylation

- Acylation uses acyl-CoA with the amino acids glycine, glutamine, and taurine. Conjugation of bile acids in the liver with glycine or taurine is essential for the efficient removal of these toxic compounds. Disturbed acylation by pollutant overload decreases proper levels of bile in the gastrointestinal tract resulting in poor assimilation of lipids and fat-soluble vitamins, and disturbed cholesterol metabolism.
- Toluene, the most popular industrial organic solvent, is converted by the liver into benzoate, where aspirin must then be detoxified by conjugation with the amino acid glycine (glycination); large doses of glycine and N-glycylglycine are used in treating aspirin overdose. Benzoate itself is present in many food substances and is widely used as a food preservative.
- Glycine is a commonly available amino acid, but the capacity to synthesize taurine may be limited by low activity of the enzyme cysteine sulfinic acid decarboxylase. Damage can occur to this enzyme directly by pollutants or by overload/overuse resulting in depletion. Both taurine- and glycine-dependent reactions require an alkaline pH from 7.8 to 8.0.
- Glutathione conjugation, using the amino acid glutathione in its reduced form, is used for the transformation of xenobiotics such as aromatic disulfides, anthracene

and phenanthrene compounds, aliphatic disulfides, and the regeneration of endogenous thiols from disulfides. There is a cycle of replenishment for glutathione, allowing it to be reformed after conversion to glutathione reductase. Heavy metals can inhibit this process.

Conjugation with Glycine

Benzoic acid formed in the detoxification is converted to hippuric acid:

- Benzoic acid + CoA-SH + ATP $\xrightarrow{\text{Activation}}$ Benzoyl-CoA + ADP + Pi
- Benzoyl-CoA + Glycine ⟶ Hippuric acid

Conjugation with Glutamine

Indole acetic acid formed from tryptophan in Hartnup disease is converted to indoleacetyl glutamine.

Conjugation with N-acetylcysteine

Bromobenzene is conjugated with N-acetylcysteine to form p-bromophenylmercapturic acid.

Sulfation (Sulfur Conjugation)

- Neurotransmitters, steroid hormones, certain drugs, and many xenobiotic and phenolic compounds such as estrone, aliphatic alcohols, aryl amines, and alicyclic hydroxysteroids employ sulfation as their primary route of detoxification. Sulfate not only may be ingested from food but also is produced by the action of the enzyme cysteine dioxygenase on cysteine. This process is known as sulfoxidation.
- The body's ability to conjugate toxins with sulfate is "rate limited" by the amount of sulfate present; if there is inadequate sulfate present, toxins and metabolites can accumulate, perhaps building up to levels, which cause degeneration of nervous tissue after several decades.

Conjugation with Sulfate

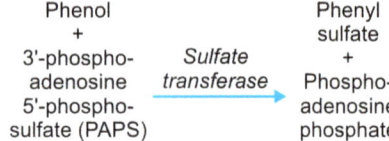

Phenol + 3'-phospho-adenosine 5'-phospho-sulfate (PAPS) $\xrightarrow{\text{Sulfate transferase}}$ Phenyl sulfate + Phospho-adenosine phosphate

Indoxyl, skatoxyl, steroid hormones, and paracetamol are conjugated by similar process.

Methylation

Methionine is the chief methyl donor to detoxify amines, phenols, thiols, noradrenaline, adrenaline, dopamine, melatonin, L-DOPA, histamine, serotonin, pyridine, sulfites, and hypochlorites into compounds excreted through the lungs. Methionine is required to detoxify the hypochlorite reaction. The methyltransferase enzyme activity is dependent on magnesium.

Conjugation with Transmethylation Reaction

Catechol-O-methyltransferase
  Adrenaline + S-adenosylmethionine (SAM) → Metanephrine + S-adenosylhomocysteine (SAH):
- Noradrenaline + SAM → Normetanephrine + SAH
- Histamine → N-methylhistamine.

Glucuronidation

The glucuronic acid, a metabolite of glucose, can conjugate with chemical and bacterial toxins such as alcohols, phenols, enols, carboxylic acid, amines, hydroxylamines, carbamides, sulfonamides, and thiols, as well as some normal metabolites in a process known as glucuronidation. This pathway is important if sulfation or glycination pathways are diminished or saturated. Damage to the capacity for oxidative phosphorylation in the mitochondria is likely to diminish the capacity for glucuronide conjugation.

Conjugation with Glucuronic Acid

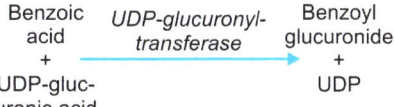

- Phenol + UDP-glucuronic acid → Phenyl glucuronide + UDP
- Chloramphenicol, morphine, paracetamol, salicylic acid, and menthol are conjugated by similar process.

SUMMARY

Human body is exposed to a number of xenobiotics during the course of lifetime, including a variety of pharmaceuticals and food components. The enzyme systems generally function adequately to minimize the potential of damage from xenobiotics. A number of biochemical pathways and sequences of chemical changes are involved in liver biotransformation. These are grouped into oxidation, reduction, or hydrolysis reactions (phase I) and conjugation reactions (phase II).

CHAPTER 29

Biochemistry of Free Radicals and Antioxidants

OBJECTIVES
At the end of this topic, the students should be able to:
- Understand the production and free radicals and their effects on the human body
- Know about the reactive oxygen species and different types of antioxidants
- Understand about the oxidative stress in diseases.

INTRODUCTION

Free radicals are chemical species possessing an unpaired electron that can be considered as fragments of molecules and are generally very reactive **(Fig. 29.1)**.

The free radicals are produced continuously in cells either as accidental by-products of metabolism or deliberately during phagocytosis.

The main danger from free radicals comes from the damage they can do when they react with important cellular components such as DNA or the cell membrane.

Reactive radicals formed within cells can oxidize biomolecules and lead to cell death and tissue injury.

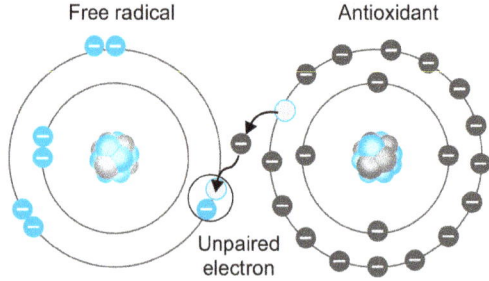

Fig. 29.1: Free radical and antioxidant.

To prevent free radical damage, the body has a defense system of **antioxidants**. These include enzymes to decompose peroxides, proteins to sequester transition metals, and a range of compounds to "scavenge" free radicals.

Formation of Free Radicals

- Normally, bonds do not split in a way that leaves a molecule with an odd, unpaired electron. But, when weak bonds split, free radicals are formed.
- Free radicals are very unstable and react quickly with other compounds, trying to capture the needed electron to gain stability. Generally, free radicals attack the nearest stable molecule, taking its electron. When the "attacked" molecule loses its electron, it becomes a free radical itself, beginning a chain reaction. Once the process is started, it can cascade, finally resulting in the disruption of a living cell.
- Some free radicals arise normally during metabolism and sometimes the cells of the immune system purposefully create them to neutralize viruses and bacteria. However, environmental factors such as pollution, radiation, cigarette smoke, and herbicides can also spawn free radicals.

REACTIVE OXYGEN SPECIES

There are many types of radicals, but those of most concern in biological systems are derived from oxygen, and known collectively as *reactive oxygen species (ROS)*. Oxygen has

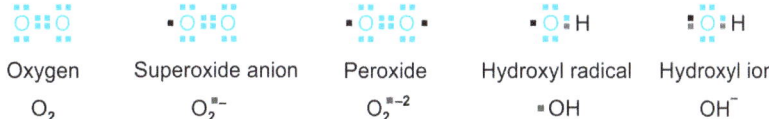

Fig. 29.2: Reactive oxygen species.

two unpaired electrons in separate orbitals in its outer shell. This electronic structure makes oxygen especially susceptible to radical formation.

Sequential reduction of molecular oxygen leads to formation of a group of ROS (**Fig. 29.2**):
- **Superoxide anion**
- **Peroxide** (hydrogen peroxide)
- **Hydroxyl radical**.

The structure of these radicals is shown in the figure above. One can observe the difference between hydroxyl radical and hydroxyl ion (not a radical).

Another radical derived from oxygen is **singlet oxygen**, designated as $^1O_2$. This is an excited form of oxygen in which one of the electrons jumps to a superior orbital following absorption of energy.

Formation of Reactive Oxygen Species

Oxygen-derived radicals are generated constantly as part of normal aerobic life. They are formed in mitochondria as oxygen is reduced along the electron transport chain. ROS are also formed as necessary intermediates in a variety of enzyme reactions. Examples of situations in which oxygen radicals are overproduced in cells include:
- **White blood cells** such as neutrophils specialize in producing oxygen radicals, which are used in host defense to kill invading pathogens.
- **Cells exposed to abnormal environments** such as hypoxia or hyperoxia generate abundant and often damaging ROS. There are many drugs that have oxidizing effects on cells and lead to production of oxygen radicals.
- **Ionizing radiation** is well known to generate oxygen radicals within biological systems. Interestingly, the damaging effects of radiation are higher in well-oxygenated tissues than in tissues deficient in oxygen.

Biological Effects of Reactive Oxygen

Free radicals are generated in a number of reactions essential to life and, as mentioned above, phagocytic cells generate radicals to kill invading pathogens.

Despite their beneficial activities, ROS clearly can be toxic to cells. By definition, radicals possess an unpaired electron, which makes them highly reactive and thereby able to damage all macromolecules, including lipids, proteins, and nucleic acids.

One of the known toxic effects of oxygen radicals is damage to cellular membranes (plasma, mitochondrial, and endomembrane systems), which is initiated by a process known as *lipid peroxidation*. A common target for peroxidation is unsaturated fatty acids present in membrane phospholipids. A peroxidation reaction involving a fatty acid is depicted in the **Figure 29.3**.

Reactions involving radicals occur in chain reactions. As shown in the **Figure 29.3**, the hydrogen is abstracted from the fatty acid by hydroxyl radical, leaving a carbon-centered radical as part of the fatty acid. The same radical then reacts with oxygen to yield the peroxy radical, which can then react with other fatty acids or proteins.

Peroxidation of membrane lipids can:
- Increase membrane rigidity

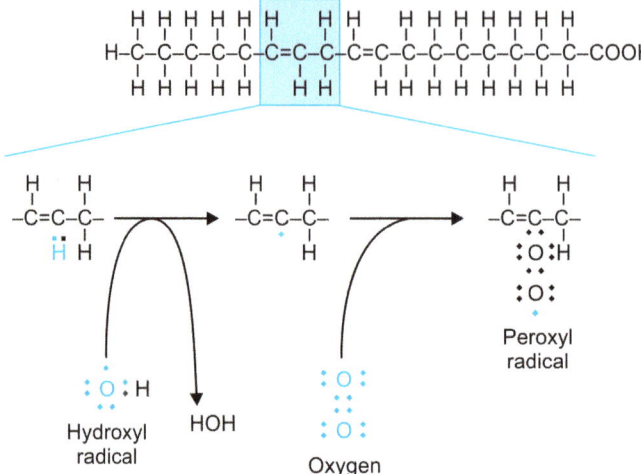

Fig. 29.3: Peroxidation reaction.

- Decrease activity of membrane-bound enzymes (e.g. sodium pumps)
- Alter activity of membrane receptors
- Alter permeability.

In addition to effects on phospholipids, radicals can also directly attack membrane proteins and induce lipid–lipid, lipid–protein, and protein–protein cross-linking, all of which obviously have effects on membrane function.

Mechanisms for Protection against Radicals

Life on Earth evolved in the presence of oxygen and necessarily adapted by evolution of a large battery of antioxidant systems. Some of these antioxidant molecules are present in all life forms examined, from bacteria to mammals, indicating their appearance early in the history of life.

Many antioxidants work by transiently becoming radicals themselves. These molecules are usually part of a larger network of cooperating antioxidants that end up regenerating the original antioxidant. For example, vitamin E becomes a radical, but it is regenerated through the activity of the antioxidants, vitamin C and glutathione.

ANTIOXIDANTS

- Antioxidants are involved in the prevention of cellular damage—the common pathway for cancer, aging, and a variety of diseases.
- An antioxidant is a molecule capable of slowing or preventing the oxidation of other molecules. Oxidation is a chemical reaction that transfers electrons from a substance to an oxidizing agent.
- Oxidation reactions can produce free radicals, which start chain reactions that damage cells. Antioxidants terminate these chain reactions by removing free radical intermediates and inhibit other oxidation reactions by being oxidized themselves.
- Plants and animals maintain complex systems of multiple types of antioxidants (e.g. glutathione, vitamin C, and vitamin E) as well as enzymes [e.g. catalase, superoxide dismutase (SOD)], and various peroxidases. Additionally, selenium is required for proper function of one of the body's antioxidant enzyme systems.
- The body cannot manufacture these micronutrients, so they must be supplied in the diet. Low levels of antioxidants, or inhibition of the antioxidant enzymes,

cause oxidative stress and may damage or kill cells.
- Antioxidants are also widely used as ingredients in dietary supplements in maintaining health and preventing diseases (cancer and coronary heart disease). In addition to uses of medicine, antioxidants have many industrial uses, such as preservatives in food and cosmetics.

Enzymatic Antioxidants

Enzyme Systems

$$O_2 \xrightarrow{\text{Superoxide dismutase}} O_2^{\cdot-} \xrightarrow{\text{Peroxidases catalase}} H_2O_2 \longrightarrow H_2O$$

Oxygen — Superoxide — Hydrogen peroxide — Water

The released superoxide is first converted to hydrogen peroxide and then further reduced to water. This detoxification pathway is the result of multiple enzymes, with SODs catalyzing the first step and then catalases and various peroxidases removing hydrogen peroxide.

Superoxide Dismutase

Superoxide dismutases are a class of closely related enzymes that catalyze the breakdown of the superoxide anion into oxygen and hydrogen peroxide. They are present in almost all aerobic cells and in extracellular fluids. SOD enzymes contain metal ion cofactors such as copper, zinc, manganese, or iron depending on the isoenzyme. In humans, the copper- or zinc-dependent SOD is present in the cytosol, while manganese-dependent SOD is present in the mitochondrion. There is third form of SOD in extracellular fluids, which has copper and zinc in its active sites.

Catalase

Catalases are enzymes that catalyze the conversion of hydrogen peroxide to water and oxygen, using either an iron or manganese cofactor. This protein is localized to peroxisomes in eukaryotic cells. It is an unusual enzyme; since hydrogen peroxide is its only substrate, it follows a ping-pong mechanism.

Peroxiredoxins

Peroxiredoxins are peroxidases that catalyze the reduction of hydrogen peroxide, organic hydroperoxides, as well as peroxynitrite. They are divided into three classes—(1) typical 2-cysteine peroxiredoxin, (2) atypical 2-cysteine peroxiredoxins, and (3) 1-cysteine peroxiredoxins. These enzymes share the same basic catalytic mechanism in which a redox-active cysteine (the peroxidatic cysteine) in the active site is oxidized to a sulfonic acid by the peroxide substrate.

Thioredoxin and Glutathione Systems

The thioredoxin system contains the 12-kDa protein thioredoxin and its companion thioredoxin reductase. Proteins related to thioredoxin are present in all sequenced organisms, with plants such as *Arabidopsis thaliana* having a particularly great diversity of isoforms. In its active state, thioredoxin acts as an efficient reducing agent, scavenging ROS and maintaining other proteins in their reduced state. After being oxidized, the active thioredoxin is regenerated by the action of thioredoxin reductase, using NADPH as an electron donor.

Glutathione

The glutathione system includes glutathione, glutathione reductase, glutathione peroxidases, and glutathione *S*-transferases. This system is found in animals, plants, and microorganisms. Glutathione peroxidase is an enzyme containing four selenium cofactors that catalyzes the breakdown of hydrogen peroxide and organic hydroperoxides. There are at least four different glutathione peroxidase isozymes in animals. Glutathione peroxidase 1 is the most abundant and is a very efficient scavenger of hydrogen peroxide, while glutathione peroxidase 4 is most active with lipid hydroperoxides.

Nonenzymatic Antioxidants

Melatonin

Melatonin is a powerful antioxidant that can easily cross cell membranes and the blood–brain barrier. Unlike other antioxidants, melatonin does not undergo redox cycling, which is the ability of a molecule to undergo repeated reduction and oxidation.

Vitamin E

- Vitamin E is the collective name for a set of eight related tocopherols and tocotrienols, with antioxidant properties.
- It is the abundant and efficient chain-breaking antioxidant available in the body (**Fig. 29.4**).
- It is the primary defender against oxidation and lipid peroxidation.

Vitamin C

- Vitamin C is the most abundant water-soluble chain-breaking antioxidant in the body.
- It acts primarily in cellular fluid and combating free radical formation caused by pollution and cigarette smoke.
- It also helps in returning the vitamin E to its active form.

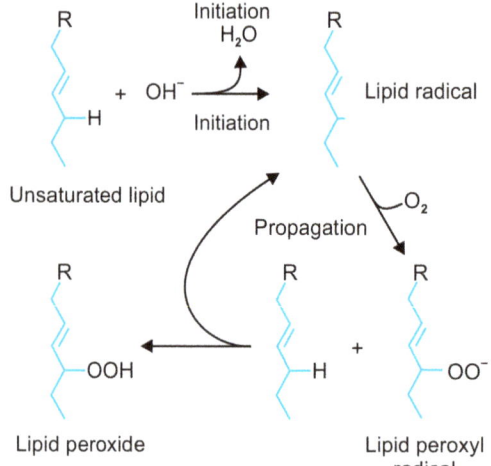

Fig. 29.4: Chain-breaking antioxidation.

β-Carotene (Carotenoids)

β-Carotene acts as a chain-breaking antioxidant by trapping peroxy radicals in tissues at low pressure of oxygen.

Selenium

Selenium is a trace element and is important constituent of various enzymes, such as glutathione peroxidase, which is an important scavenger for inorganic–organic peroxides. Deiodinase is an example.

Selenium deficiency results in the downregulation of glutathione peroxidase enzyme synthesis. Selenium and vitamin E reinforce each other in their action against lipid peroxides.

Transferrin and Ferritin

Transferrin and ferritin bind free Fe^{2+} and prevent it from initiating the formation of free radical.

Ceruloplasmin

Ceruloplasmin binds CU^{2+} and prevents it from initiating any oxidative damage.

Uric acid

Uric acid has the capacity of scavenging free electron (e^-) and thus prevents the progression of free radical damage in the blood. It has the sparing action on vitamin C. It prevents the initiation of free radical formation by transition elements ions by forming complex with them.

Ubiquitone

Ubiquitone is a lipid-soluble, radical-trapping antioxidant in membrane and plasma lipoproteins.

Bilirubin

Bilirubin also works as an antioxidant in plasma. A molecule of unconjugated bilirubin scavenges two hydroperoxy radicals and itself gets oxidized to bilirubin.

OXIDATIVE STRESS IN DISEASE

Oxidative stress can damage the cells, leading to a range of diseases and causes symptoms of aging, such as wrinkles.

Oxidative stress is thought to contribute to the development of a wide range of diseases, including Alzheimer's disease, Parkinson's disease, diabetes, rheumatoid arthritis, and neurodegenerative diseases. Low-density lipoprotein (LDL) oxidation appears to trigger the process of atherogenesis, which results in atherosclerosis and finally cardiovascular disease.

Impairment of Cognitive Function

Memory capabilities decline with age, evident in human degenerative diseases such as Alzheimer's disease, which is accompanied by an accumulation of oxidative damage.

Cause of Aging

Oxidative damage initiated by ROS is a major contributor to the functional decline that is characteristic of aging.

Male Infertility

Exposure of spermatozoa to oxidative stress is a major causative agent of male infertility. Sperm DNA fragmentation, caused by oxidative stress, appears to be an important factor in the etiology of male infertility.

Cancer

Reactive oxygen species are constantly generated and eliminated in the biological system and are required to drive regulatory pathways. Under normal physiological conditions, cells control ROS levels by balancing the generation of ROS with their elimination by scavenging system. But under oxidative stress conditions, excessive ROS can damage cellular proteins, lipids, and DNA, leading to fatal lesions in cell that contribute to carcinogenesis.

Cancer cells exhibit greater ROS stress than normal cells do, partly due to oncogenic stimulation, increased metabolic activity, and mitochondrial malfunction.

Reactive oxygen species at low level facilitate cancer cell survival since cell-cycle progression driven by growth factors and receptor tyrosine kinases requires ROS for activation, and chronic inflammation, a major mediator of cancer, is regulated by ROS. ROS at high level can suppress tumor growth through the sustained activation of cell-cycle inhibitor and induction of cell death as well as senescence by damaging macromolecules. In fact, most of the chemotherapeutic and radiotherapeutic agents kill cancer cells by augmenting ROS stress.

Carcinogenesis

Reactive oxygen species-related oxidation of DNA is one of the main causes of mutations, which can produce several types of DNA damage.

Cell Proliferation

Both exogenous and endogenous ROS have been shown to enhance proliferation of cancer cells.

Cell Death

A cancer cell can die in three ways—apoptosis, necrosis, and autophagy. Excessive ROS can induce apoptosis through both the extrinsic and intrinsic pathways.

Chronic Inflammation and Cancer

Reactive oxygen species induces chronic inflammation by the induction of COX-2, inflammatory cytokines [TNFα, interleukin 1 (IL-1), IL-6], chemokines (IL-8, CXCR4), and proinflammatory transcription factors (NF-κB).

Disease Treatment

Antioxidants are commonly used as medications to treat various forms of brain injury. SOD memetic, sodium thiopental, and propofol are used to treat reperfusion injury and traumatic brain injury. These compounds appear to prevent oxidative stress in neurons and prevent apoptosis and neurological damage. Antioxidants are also being investigated as possible treatments for neurodegenerative diseases such as Alzheimer's disease and Parkinson's disease.

Antioxidants and Disease Prevention

Heart Disease

Vitamin E may protect against cardiovascular disease by defending against LDL oxidation and artery-clogging plaque formation.

Cancer

Many studies have shown intake of high vitamin C reducing the rate of cancer, particularly cancers of the mouth and larynx.

SUMMARY

Free radicals are chemical species, possessing an unpaired electron, which can be considered as fragments of molecules. These are produced continuously in cells either accidental by-products of metabolism or during the processes of phagocytosis. Oxidation reactions can produce free radicals, which start chain reactions that damage cells. Antioxidants terminate these chain reactions by removing free radical intermediates and inhibit other oxidation reactions by being oxidized themselves. Antioxidants are also widely used as ingredients in dietary supplements in the hope of maintaining health and preventing diseases such as cancer and coronary heart disease. The important antioxidants are superoxide dismutase, catalase, and glutathione.

SELF-ASSESSMENT QUESTIONS

1. What are free radicals? Explain.
2. Why do they have damaging effect to human body?
3. How do vitamin E and the other antioxidant nutrients help to protect the body against free radical damage?
4. Explain the role of antioxidants in disease treatment and prevention.

CHAPTER 30

Immunology

OBJECTIVES

At the end of this chapter, students should be able to:
- Know about humoral and cellular immunity, antigen and vaccine development, types of vaccines, and the role of recombinant DNA technology in the development of vaccine
- Explain the structure, types, and functions of immunoglobulin (Ig)
- Describe the process of antibody production
- Explain multiple myeloma and human leukocyte antigen (HLA).

INTRODUCTION

Immunology is the study of the immune system and is a very important branch of the medical and biological sciences. The immune system protects us from infection through various lines of defense. If the immune system does not function as it should, it can result in disease, such as autoimmunity, allergy, and cancer. It is also now becoming clear that immune responses contribute to the development of many common disorders not traditionally viewed as immunologic, including metabolic, cardiovascular, and neurodegenerative conditions.

From Edward Jenner's pioneering work in the 18th century that would ultimately lead to vaccination in its modern form to the many scientific breakthroughs in the 19th and 20th centuries that would lead to safe organ transplantation, the identification of blood groups, and the now ubiquitous use of monoclonal antibodies throughout science and health care, immunology has changed the face of modern medicine. Immunological research continues to extend horizons in our understanding of how to treat significant health issues, with ongoing research efforts in immunotherapy, autoimmune diseases, and vaccines for emerging pathogens, such as Ebola.

Humoral and Cellular Immunity

There are two main mechanisms of immunity within the adaptive immune system:
1. **Humoral immunity** is also called antibody-mediated immunity. With assistance from helper T cells, B cells will differentiate into plasma B cells that can produce antibodies against a specific antigen. The humoral immune system deals with antigens from pathogens that are freely circulating, or outside the infected cells. Antibodies produced by the B cells will bind to antigens, neutralizing them, or causing lysis (dissolution or destruction of cells by a lysin) or phagocytosis.
2. **Cellular immunity** occurs inside infected cells and is mediated by T lymphocytes. The pathogen's antigens are expressed on the cell surface or on an antigen-presenting cell. Helper T cells release cytokines that help activated T cells bind to the infected cells' major histocompatibility complex (MHC)–antigen complex and differentiate the T cell into a cytotoxic T cell. The infected cell then undergoes lysis.

Cellular immunity is mediated by T lymphocytes, also called T cells. Their name refers to the organ from which they're produced: the thymus. This type of immunity promotes the destruction of microbes residing in phagocytes, or the killing of infected cells to eliminate reservoirs of infection. T cells do not produce antibody molecules. They have antigen receptors that are structurally related to antibodies. These structures help recognize antigens only in the form of peptides displayed on the surface of antigen-presenting cells.

T cells consist of functionally distinct populations. These include naive T cells that recognize antigens and are activated in peripheral lymphoid organs. This activation results in the expansion of the antigen-specific lymphocyte pool and the differentiation of these cells into effector and memory cells. Effector cells include helper T cells and cytolytic or cytotoxic T cells. In response to antigenic stimulation, helper T cells (characterized by the expression of CD4 marker on their surface) secrete proteins called cytokines, function of which is to stimulate the proliferation and differentiation of the T cells themselves, as well as other cells, including B cells, macrophages, and other leukocytes. Cytolytic or cytotoxic T cells (characterized by the expression of CD8 marker on their surface) kill cells that produce foreign antigens, such as cells infected by viruses and other intracellular microbes.

Vaccine development involves the process of taking a new **antigen** or immunogen identified in the research process and **developing** this substance into a final **vaccine** that can be evaluated through preclinical and clinical studies to determine the safety and efficacy of the resultant **vaccine**.

Vaccination

Vaccination is the administration of a **vaccine** to help the immune system develop protection from a disease. **Vaccines** contain a microorganism or virus in a weakened or killed state, or proteins or toxins from the organism.

There are four main types of vaccines:
1. Live-attenuated **vaccines**
2. Inactivated **vaccines**
3. Subunit, recombinant, polysaccharide, and conjugate **vaccines**
4. Toxoid **vaccines**.

A **recombinant vaccine** is a **vaccine** produced through **recombinant DNA technology**. This involves inserting the **DNA** encoding an antigen (such as a bacterial surface protein) that stimulates an immune response into bacterial or mammalian cells, expressing the antigen in these cells and then purifying it from them.

IMMUNOGLOBULINS

The defense strategies of the body are collectively known as immunity.

Two types of immunity identified:
1. *Cellular immunity:* This is mediated by T lymphocytes or T cells (thymic origin).
2. *Humoral immunity:* Mediated by a specialized group of proteins known as Igs or antibodies.
   - The B lymphocytes or B cells (mature in bone) are responsible for the production of Igs.
   - The Igs are also known as γ-globulins.
   - Protective in function.
   - Function as antibodies.
   - Synthesized in response to a foreign substance called antigen.
   - Provide immunity.
     - Five different types of Igs.
     - They are IgA, IgG, IgM, IgD, and IgE [remember it as Government (IgG) MADE] **(Table 30.1)**.

Structure of Immunoglobulin

- All the Ig molecules consist of two identical heavy (H) chains MW = 53,000 – 75,000 and

Immunology

Table 30.1: Different types of immunoglobulin and their properties.

Type	Heavy chains	Light chains	Serum conc. mg%	Placental transfer
IgG	γ	κ or λ	800–1,500	+
IgM	μ	κ or λ	50–200	–
IgA	α	κ or λ	150–400	–
IgD	δ	κ or λ	1–10	–
IgE	ε	κ or λ	0.02–0.05	–

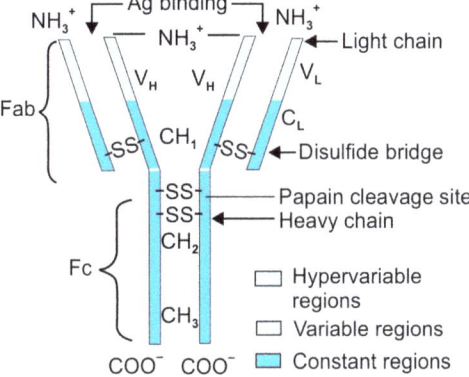

Fig. 30.1: Structure of immunoglobulin.

two identical light (L) chains MW = 23,000 (**Fig. 30.1**).
- They are held together by disulfide bridges.
- Heavy chains of Igs are linked to carbohydrates; hence, Igs are glycoproteins.
- Each chain (L or H) of Ig has two regions (domains), namely the constant and the variable.
- The amino terminal half of the light chain is the variable region (VL).
- The carboxy-terminal half is the constant region.
- There are five types of heavy chains: α, δ, ε, γ, and μ.
- Light chains are of two types: kappa (κ) and lambda (λ).
- One quarter of the amino terminal region of heavy chain is variable (VH). Remaining three quarters is constant (CH_1, CH_2, CH_3).

- The amino acid sequence of variable regions of light and heavy chains is responsible for the specific binding of Ig (antibody) with antigen.
- There are certain hypervariable regions within the variable regions of VL and VH.
- Light chains have three hypervariable regions.
- Heavy chains have four hypervariable regions.
- The hypervariable regions more specifically determine the antigen-binding site.

Functions of Immunoglobulin

The main function of Ig (antibodies) is to protect the body against infectious agents.

The Igs are able to provide resistance because they can neutralize viruses, opsonize microbes (the process by which antibodies make microorganisms more easily ingested by phagocytic cells) and activate complement, and prevent the attachment of microbes to mucosal surfaces.

Immunoglobulins act in direct and indirect way to protect the body against infections.

Direct Effect

Binding of antigen via antigen-binding fragment of antibody results in any one of the methods mentioned below:
- Precipitation of soluble antigens
- Agglutination by the cross-linking of particulate antigens (viruses or bacteria)
- *Neutralization:* By blocking of the attachment of viruses or bacterial toxins to membrane receptors, in which the antibodies cover the toxic sites of the antigenic substance
- Lysis of the cell membrane of the organisms to destroy them.

Indirect Effect

It is through the activation of the complement system, which is mediated through complement-binding site (Fc).

Indirect action is stronger when compared to direct effect.

The binding of one of the complement molecules to Fc portion results in any one of the following:
- *Opsonization and phagocytosis:* Activation of neutrophils and macrophages to engulf bacteria.
- Chemotaxis (movement of large number of phagocytes to the site of antigenic agent).
- Agglutination of foreign bodies.
- Neutralization.
- Activation of mast cells and basophils liberates histamine. This histamine dilates the blood vessels and increases capillary permeability. This results in the entry of plasma proteins from the blood to tissues to inactivate the antigenic products.

Different Types of Immunoglobulins

Immunoglobulin G

- Composed of a single unit (monomer).
- Major Ig of plasma (75–80%).
- Produced in response to various infections and protects the body against infections.
- IgG can cross the placenta from the mother's blood to the fetus and provide immunity to the fetus.
- Triggers foreign cell destruction mediated by complement system.

Immunoglobulin A

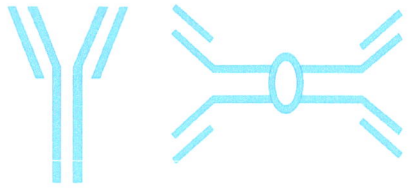

- Occurs as a single (monomer) or double unit (dimer) held together by J chain.
- Produced by the secretary cells of the respiratory tract, digestive tract, urinary tract, etc. and is present in the mucous secretions of these cells.
- It prevents the entry of bacteria into the body through these cells.

Immunoglobulin M

- Largest Ig composed of 5 Y-shaped units held together by a J polypeptide chain.
- Cannot traverse blood vessels, hence it is restricted to bloodstream.
- It is the first antibody to be produced whenever bacteria or virus attack the body.
- It is also produced in the fetal stage itself.

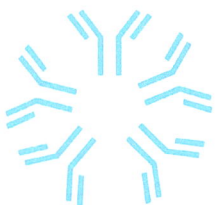

Immunoglobulin D

- It is composed of single Y-shaped unit.
- It is present in very small amount.
- IgD molecules are present on the surface of B cells.
- The synthesis and function of this are still unknown.

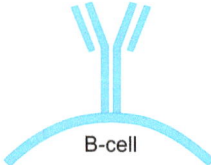

Immunoglobulin E

- Composed of single Y-shaped monomer.
- IgE molecules tightly bind with mast cells, which release histamine and cause allergy.
- It is produced by the plasma cells of the respiratory tract.
- Increases in allergic diseases.

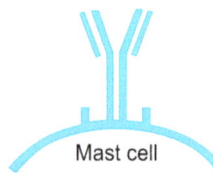

Mechanism of Antibody Production

The following animal model experiment explains the mechanism of antibody production **(Fig. 30.2)**.

A mouse is immunized by injection of an antigen X to stimulate the production of antibodies targeted against X. The antibody forming cells are isolated from the mouse's spleen.

Monoclonal antibodies are produced by fusing single antibody-forming cells to tumor cells grown in culture. The resulting cell is called a hybridoma.

Each hybridoma produces relatively large quantities of identical antibody molecules. By allowing the hybridoma to multiply in culture, it is possible to produce a population of cells, each of which produces identical antibody molecules. These antibodies are called "monoclonal antibodies" because they are produced by the identical offspring of a single, cloned antibody-producing cell.

Once a monoclonal antibody is made, it can be used as a specific probe to track down and purify the specific protein that induced its formation.

Quantitative Determination of Serum Immunoglobulins in Antibody-Agar Plates' Radial Immunodiffusion Method

The antibody in agar plate test has proved valuable for the quantitative measurement of individual serum Igs. With this technique, specific antiserum is mixed uniformly in an agar gel plate. Antigen-containing solutions are placed in small antigen wells cut in the agar. A concentric ring of antigen–antibody precipitate forms around the antigen well. By graphically comparing the ring diameters with those of appropriate standards, the protein concentration of the test sera can be determined. This procedure has been used to quantify protein concentrations as low as

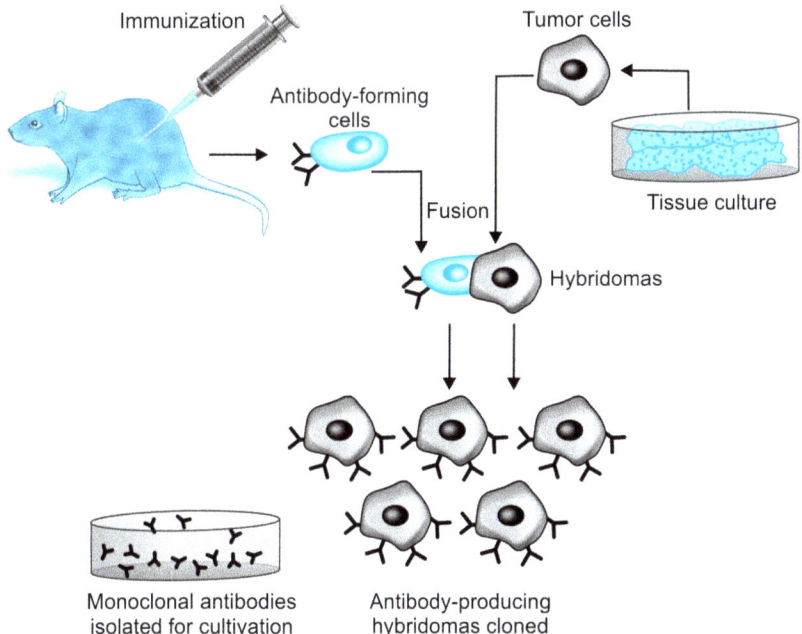

Fig. 30.2: Mechanism of antibody production.

0.003 mg/mL. Multiple samples can be easily tested.

A Sensitive Tube Method Developed by Eva and Peter

A sensitive and simple method for the quantitative determination of antibodies is reported. Tubes coated with antigen are incubated with antiserum followed by an enzyme-labeled preparation of anti-Ig. The enzyme remaining in the tubes after washing provides a measure of the amount of specific antibodies in the serum. Coating of polystyrene tubes with antigen is described, as well as the preparation of specifically purified antibodies against rabbit IgG, and their conjugation to alkaline phosphatase.

When rabbit antisera against human serum albumin or against the dinitrophenyl group were incubated in tubes coated with antigen, less than 1 ng/mL of specific antibody could be detected in both systems.

Antibodies in unknown sera could be quantitated by comparison with a standard antiserum.

Clinical Importance of Immunoglobulins

Quantitative determination of Igs will help to diagnose and treat the diseases. Abnormal amounts of certain Igs are found in plasma in several diseases.

HYPERGAMMAGLOBULINEMIA

Polyclonal Hypergammaglobulinemia

- Polyclonal (diffuse) hypergammaglobulinemia is due to increased production of a large number of different Ig types.
- Nonspecific increase in Ig levels in variety of infections and autoimmune diseases. This increased synthesis is from a number of cell lines, producing its own specific Ig and therefore is called polyclonal hypergammaglobulinemia.
- Liver diseases (hepatitis, cirrhosis) and recurrent or chronic infections such as rheumatoid arthritis and sarcoidosis stimulate B cells and an increased production of gammaglobulin takes place. This may affect all the types of Igs.
- This polyclonal hypergammaglobulinemia results in diffuse increase in protein mass throughout the gammaglobulin region on electrophoresis.

Monoclonal Hypergammaglobulinemia

Monoclonal (discrete) hypergammaglobulinemia is a group of disorders characterized by an abnormal benign or malignant proliferation of a single clone of B lymphocytes and/or plasma cells that produce homogeneous monoclonal Igs.

The discrete dense Ig bands seen with serum electrophoresis are known as paraprotein or monoclonal components.

This is due to the production of a single Ig fragment (light or heavy chain) by a single clone B cell.

Malignant proteinemia occurs in:
- Multiple myeloma
- Plasma cell leukemia
- Heavy chain disease
- Light chain disease
- Waldenström's macroglobulinemia
- Amyloidosis.

Multiple Myeloma

This is a malignant disease of the plasma cell.

In this case, one type of plasma cell multiplies abnormally and produces one type of Ig (IgG or IgA) in excess quantities.

The electrophoresis of such a serum shows a thick deeply stained protein band in the γ-globulin region. This band is called "M" band.

The Biochemical Findings

The biochemical findings of multiple myeloma are increased total proteins, decreased albumin, increased globulins and

Ca^{2+} levels in plasma. In some cases, multiple myeloma patients excrete light chains of Igs in the urine which are known as Bence–Jones proteins.

Bence–Jones Proteins

- Bence–Jones proteins are light chain fragments of Igs, which are excreted in urine, in some cases of multiple myeloma.
- These are discovered in the urine by its characteristic behavior on heating.
- These proteins precipitate between 40 and 60°C. But as the temperature increases above 60°C the protein redissolves. Again on cooling, the protein gets precipitated.

Waldenström's Macroglobulinemia

It is a malignant disease of the lymphoid elements, characterized by high serum level of IgM.

Amyloidosis

It is characterized by the deposition of insoluble fibrillar protein complexes in various tissues.

The deposition may contain fragments of light chains. This also occurs in multiple myeloma.

Cryoglobulinemia

Cryoglobulin is a serum IgM protein that precipitates at temperature lower than body temperature.

The patients with this disorder may develop thrombosis in cold environment.

Therefore the cryoglobulin examination maintenance of 37°C is very important during blood collection.

Benign Paraproteinemia

In this condition, paraproteins are found in patients, where there is no association of pathological features.

It may be transient occurs during acute infection and in autoimmune diseases due to antigen stimulation or it may be persistent due to a benign tumor of b cells.

Hypogammaglobulinemia

Plasma globulin levels are decreased in the following conditions:
- Congenital defect in the synthesis of γ-globulins (IgA and IgM will be low).
- Malnutrition particularly with protein deficiency.
- Malignancy (lymphoma, Hodgkin's disease).
- Infection (HIV, measles).
- Due to immunosuppressant drugs (cytotoxins, cyclosporine, and corticosteroids).
- Protein-losing diseases such as nephrotic syndrome and diabetes mellitus.

Human Leukocyte Antigen

The HLA region, located on the short arm of chromosome 6, is a highly polymorphic region containing about 200 genes. The HLA system is the name of the MHC in humans (Fig. 30.3).

The super locus contains a large number of genes related to immune system function

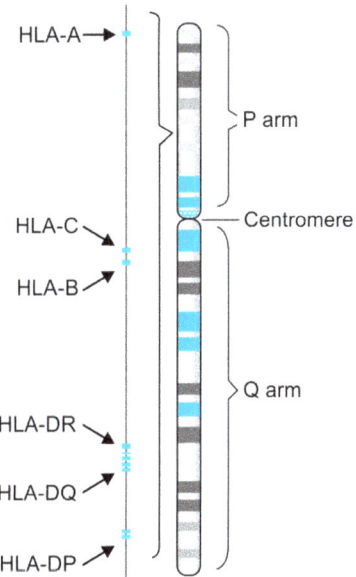

Fig. 30.3: HLA region of chromosome 6.
(HLA: human leukocyte antigen)

in humans. This group of genes resides on chromosome 6 and encodes cell-surface antigen-presenting proteins and many other genes. The proteins encoded by certain genes are also known as antigens.

The major HLA are essential elements in immune function.

Different classes have different functions. The Class I proteins, classically involved in presenting endogenous antigens to CD8+ T cells, are expressed by genes located in the HLA-A, -B, and -C loci. In contrast, the Class II proteins, which associate with and present exogenous antigens to CD4+ T cells, are expressed by the HLA-DR, -DQ, and -DP loci.

Human leukocyte antigens have other roles. They are sometimes involved in mate selection. They may protect against or allow cancer and may mediate autoimmune disease.

Human leukocyte antigen in human population is one aspect of disease defense, and, as a result, the chance of two unrelated individuals having identical HLA molecules on all loci is very low. Historically, HLA genes were identified as a result of the ability to successfully transplant organs between HLA similar individuals.

Leukocyte Antigen Typing

Human leukocyte antigen typing refers to the tissue type matching for transplant purposes.

Human leukocyte antigens are detected on the surface of white cells (leukocytes), from blood specimen, but they reside on the surface of all body cells.

These antigens regulate how the body can recognize and reject foreign tissues.

The phasing out of serological tissue typing and its replacement with DNA-based tissue typing has increased the accuracy and specificity of HLA typing, which allows for more precise HLA matching between donors and transplant patients.

Several large-scale studies have demonstrated that more precise HLA matching between donor and patient significantly:

- Improves overall transplant survival
- Reduces the incidence and severity of both acute and chronic graft-versus-host disease
- Improves rates of engraftment.

Studies on HLA and transplant outcome have also demonstrated HLA loci, which are critical to match in order to maximize the success of hematopoietic cell transplantation. Although matching at the three HLA loci traditionally associated with hematopoietic cell transplantation (HLA-A, -B, and -DR) can lead to successful transplantation outcomes, recent research has shown matching at HLA-C can also improve outcome.

Examining Leukocyte Antigen Types
Serotyping

In order to create a typing reagent, blood from animals or humans would be taken, the blood cells allowed to separate from the serum, and the serum diluted to its optimal sensitivity and used to type cells from other individuals or animals. Thus serotyping became a way of crudely identifying HLA receptors and receptor isoforms.

Gene Sequencing

Minor reactions to subregions that show similarity to other types can be observed to the gene products of alleles of a serotype group. The sequence of the antigens determines the antibody reactivates and so having a good sequencing capability (or sequence-based typing) obviates then need for serological reactions. Therefore different serotype reactions may indicate the need to sequence persons HLA to determine a new gene sequence.

Phenotyping

Gene typing is different from gene sequencing and serotyping. With this strategy, polymerase chain reaction (PCR) primers specific to a variant region of DNA are used (called sequence-specific primers-PCR), if a product of the right size is found, the assumption is that the HLA allele has been identified.

Immunology

Haplotypes

An HLA haplotype is a series of HLA "genes" (loci-alleles) by chromosome, one passed from the mother and father.

These haplotypes can be used to trace migrations in the human population because they are often much like a fingerprint of an event that has occurred in evolution.

Antibodies

Human leukocyte antigen antibodies are typically not naturally occurring, with few exceptions are formed as a result of an immunologic challenge of a foreign material containing nonself HLAs via blood transfusion, pregnancy (paternally inherited antigens), or organ or tissue transplant.

Antibodies against disease associated HLA haplotypes have been proposed as a treatment for severe autoimmune diseases.

Donor-specific HLA antibodies have been found to be associated with graft failure in kidney, heart, lung, and liver transplantation.

SUMMARY

Immunology is the study of the immune system and is a very important branch of the medical and biological sciences. There are two main mechanisms of immunity within the adaptive immune system:

Humoral and cellular immunity vaccination is the administration of a vaccine to help the immune system to develop protection from a disease. **There are four main types of vaccines:**
1. Live-attenuated **vaccines**
2. Inactivated **vaccines**
3. Subunit, recombinant, polysaccharide, and conjugate **vaccines**
4. Toxoid **vaccines**.

Immunoglobulin: The defense strategies of the body are collectively known as immunity. There are five different types of Igs, such as IgA, IgG, IgM, IgD, and IgE. There are two identical heavy and light chains they have.

CHAPTER 31

Biochemistry of Vision

OBJECTIVES

At the end of this chapter, students should be able to:
- Differentiate the rods and cones with their characteristic features
- Explain the process of transduction
- Describe the role of cone cells in color vision
- Explain the relationship of sorbitol pathway and diabetes.

INTRODUCTION

Visual phototransduction is a process by which light is converted into electrical signals in the rod cells, cone cells, and photosensitive ganglion cells of the retina of the eye.

Two types of photoreceptors distributed across the retina, i.e. rods and cones (**Fig. 31.1**). These photoreceptor cells absorb light and are sensitive to light of wavelength

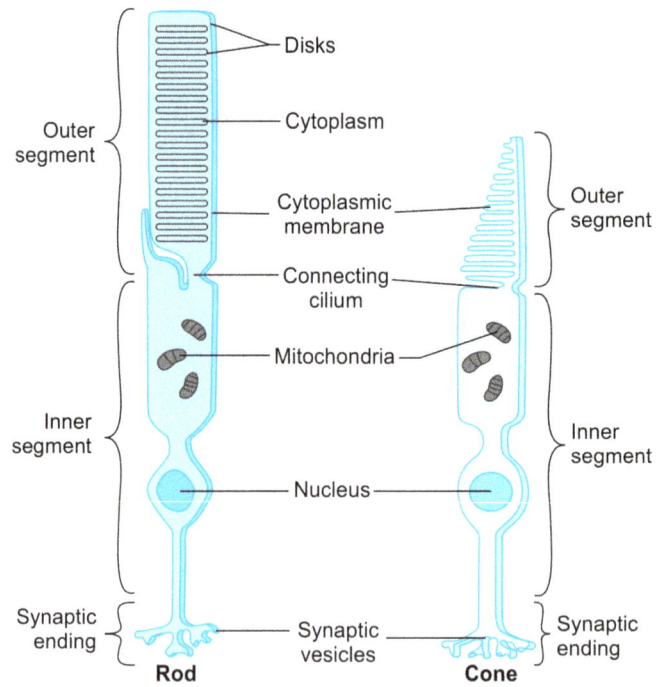

Fig. 31.1: Structure of rods and cones.

Table 31.1: Characteristics of rods and cones.

Rod cells	Cone cells
Function in dim light	Function in bright light
Do not distinguish color	Responsible for color vision
There are about 100 million in human retina	There are about 3 million in human retina
Require fewer than 10 photons produce flash of light	Require more photons for producing flash of light
Have high sensitivity to light	Have lower sensitivity to light
Specialized for night vision	Specialized for day vision
They have more photo pigment and capture more light	They have less photo pigment
Have high amplification, respond to single photon of light	Have lower amplification
Have low temporal resolution (slow response to light)	Have high temporal resolution (fast response to light)
More sensitive to scattered light	Most sensitive to direct axial rays
Have low visual acuity	Have high visual acuity with better spatial resolution
Not present in central fovea of the eye	Concentrated in fovea of the eye
Achromatic with one type of rod pigment	Chromatic with three types of pigment (red, green, and blue)
Absence of rods causing night blindness	Absence of cones causing legally blind

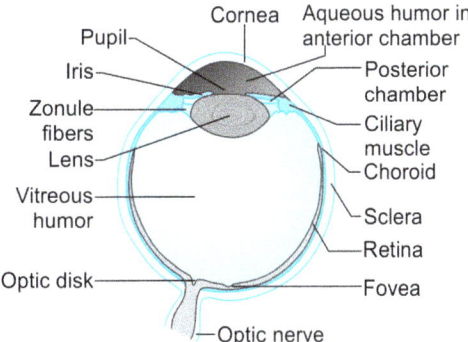

Fig. 31.2: Structure of eye.

300–850 nm. The rods and cones have different characteristics as shown in **Table 31.1**.

STRUCTURE OF THE EYE (FIG. 31.2)

Neuronal Cell Types in the Eye (Fig. 31.3)

Bipolar Cells

- When light hits a rod or cone cell, it hyperpolarizes and releases less glutamate.
- There are two types of bipolar cells reacting to this— (1) metabotropic (ON) cells (depolarize) and (2) inotropic (OFF) cells (hyperpolarize).

Amacrine Cells

- There are 40 different types.
- Most are inhibitory using either gamma-aminobutyric acid or glycine as neurotransmitters.
- Responsible for complex processing of retinal image, adjusting brightness, and detecting motion.

Horizontal Cells

- Help integrate and regulate the input from multiple photoreceptor cells.
- Allow eyes to adjust bright and dim conditions.

Ganglion Cells

- There are at least five main classes.
- Final output neurons of the retina.
- Information from bipolar and amacrine cells are transmitted directly to brain via axons.
- Only neuron cell type that transmits action potentials.

Retina Layers

- Multiple layers of interconnecting neurons in the retina of the eye.

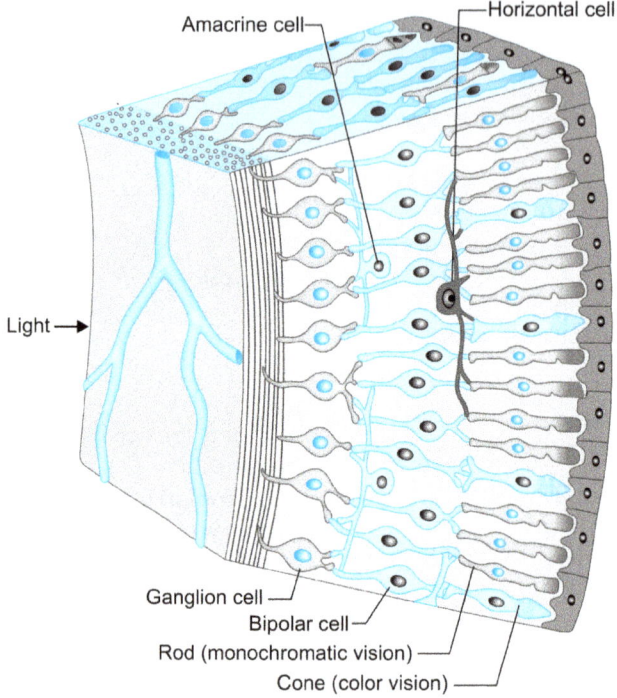

Fig. 31.3: Neuronal cell types in the eye.

- Cones and rods collect and transduce light.
- This relayed to bipolar cells in plexiform layer.
- Information processed further by amacrine cells.
- This passed to ganglion cells that send to brain.

PHOTOTRANSDUCTION

In the absence of light, the photoreceptors are depolarized to a membrane resting potential of –40 mV. Light will hyperpolarize the plasma membrane of the photoreceptor to –70 mV. This stimulus-induced hyperpolarization is a distinctive characteristic of the photoreceptor response, as many other neuronal types depolarize when stimulated:

- A key second messenger molecule responsible for maintaining a depolarized rest state in photoreceptors is the nucleotide cyclic guanosine 3'-5' monophosphate (cGMP) **(Fig. 31.4)**.
- High cGMP levels keep cGMP-gated ion channels in the open state and allow them to pass an inward Na^+ current.
- Light entering the eye activates the opsin molecules in the photoreceptors.
- Upon photon absorption, 11-*cis*-retinal undergoes an isomerization to the all-*trans*-form, causing a conformational change in the rhodopsin. The activated rhodopsin is called metarhodopsin II.
- The precursor for 11-*cis*-retinal is all-*trans*-retinol (vitamin A).

Retinal Synthesized from β-Carotene

- β-Carotene found in yellow, orange, and green leafy fruit, and vegetables.
- β-Carotenes oxidatively cleaved by the intestinal enzyme β-carotene dioxygenase.
- Retinal and retinol interconverted in the presence of nicotinamide adenine dinucleotide (NAD) or NAD phosphate (NADP) by dehydrogenases.

Biochemistry of Vision

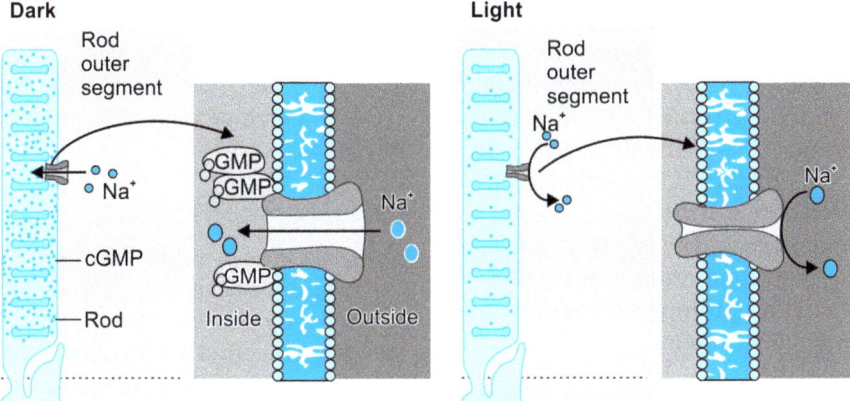

Fig. 31.4: Phototransduction.
(cGMP: cyclic guanosine 3′-5′ monophosphate)

Seeing the Light

Following are the absorption of light:
- Rhodopsin converts to bathorhodopsin:
  - Takes a few picoseconds.
  - 11-*cis*-retinal changes to all-*trans*.
  - Light energy converted into atomic motion.
  - Bathorhodopsin conformation is strained.
- Bathorhodopsin converts to metarhodopsin II:
  - Takes 1 millisecond.
  - Scotopsin undergoes significant reorganization.
  - Several intermediates between bathorhodopsin and metarhodopsin II.
- Metarhodopsin II activates transducin:
  - Metarhodopsin binds transducin and catalyzes exchange of bound guanosine diphosphate (GDP) for guanosine triphosphate (GTP).
  - GTP-α unit released.
  - Transducin is a trimeric G protein.
  - Alpha subunit has GDP and GTPase activity.
- Transducin activates cGMP phosphodiesterase (PDE):
  - GTP-α subunit of transducin binds to inhibitory unit of PDE and releases it.
  - Activated PDE potent enzyme that hydrolyzes cGMP.
- cGMP hydrolyzed to GMP by cGMP PDE.
- cGMP-gated channels close:
  - Reduction of cGMP causes cGMP-gated channels to close.
  - Results in reduction of entry of Na and Ca.
  - 1 A of Ca current for every 7 A of Na current.
- Hyperpolarization and reduction of glutamate release:
  - Closing of cGMP-gated ion channels stops Na and Ca entering cell.
  - As Na and Ca still being pumped out, net increase in negative charge inside cell.
  - Resting potential drops below resting value.
  - Diminished glutamate release.

Termination of Phototransduction Cascade

The light response is terminated by several mechanisms:
- Inactivation of rhodopsin occurs through phosphorylation by the opsin kinase, followed by the binding of arrestin to phosphorylated rhodopsin.
- Inactivation of transducin occurs through the hydrolysis of bound GTP to GDP via an

- intrinsic GTPase activity that is accelerated by the GTPase activating protein RGS9 (regulator of G-protein signaling).
- Inactivation of PDE is coupled to the inactivation of transducin. Inactivated transducin (Tα-GDP) dissociates from PDE, resulting in a cessation of PDE-mediated cGMP hydrolysis.
- Activation of guanylate cyclase by guanylate cyclase–activating protein restores cGMP levels and thus promotes the reopening of cGMP-gated channels.

VISUAL CYCLE

- This process occurs via G-protein-coupled receptors (GPCRs) (opsins), which contain the chromophore 11-*cis*-retinal.
- 11-*cis*-retinal is covalently linked to the opsin receptor via Schiff-base forming retinylidene protein.
- When struck by photon, 11-*cis*-retinal undergoes photoisomerization to all-*trans*-retinal, which changes the conformation of the opsin GPCR leading to signal transduction cascades, which causes closure of cyclic GMP-gated cation channel and hyperpolarization of the photoreceptor cell.
- Following isomerization and release from the opsin protein, all-*trans*-retinal is reduced to all-*trans*-retinol and travels back to the retinal pigment epithelium to be "recharged." It is esterified by lecithin–retinol acyltransferase and then converted to 11-*cis*-retinal by the isomerohydrolase RPE65.
- Finally it is oxidized to 11-*cis*-retinal before traveling back to the rod outer segment where it is again conjugated to an opsin to form new, functional visual pigment (rhodopsin).

COLOR VISION

Mediated by cone cells of which there are three types:

1. Blue pigment (the optimal absorption at 420 nm)
2. Green pigment (535 nm)
3. Red pigment (565 nm).

Mechanism of action is similar as seen in rod cells.

Visual Pigments for Color Vision

These are known as photopsins.

These are closely related to scotopsin.

Each pigment attached to 11-*cis*-retinal, which is converted to all-*trans*-retinal in light.

Amino acids close to the 11-*cis*-retinal impart different characteristics on the absorption spectrum.

HUMAN DISORDERS OF PHOTOTRANSDUCTION

- Bradyopsia (or slow vision) is a condition that results from mutations in genes encoding the transducin-inactivating protein RGS9 or the RGS9 anchor protein (R9AP).
- Retinitis pigmentosa is an inherited disorder characterized by degeneration of photoreceptor cells and accumulation of retinal pigments. This disorder often leads to blindness.
- Congenital stationary night blindness is an inherited disorder that affects rod photoreceptors and impairs vision under low-light conditions.

SORBITOL PATHWAY AND DIABETES MELLITUS

There are three metabolic fates of glucose:
1. Glycolysis
2. HMP shunt
3. Sorbitol pathway.

The sorbitol pathway is a minor bypass pathway that bypasses the regulatory steps of glycolysis. Mainly occurs in human lens:
- Activation of the polyol pathway results in a decrease of reduced NADPH and oxidized

NAD⁺; these are necessary cofactors in redox reactions throughout the body **(Fig. 31.5)**.
- The decreased concentration of these cofactors leads to decreased synthesis of reduced glutathione, nitric oxide, myoinositol, and taurine. Myoinositol is particularly required for the normal function of nerves.

- In uncontrolled diabetes, large amounts of glucose enter the cells, which are not dependent on insulin.
- Significant increase in intracellular glucose levels takes place in diabetes; the cells (lens, retina, nerve cells, and kidney) possess high activity of aldose reductase and sufficient supply of NADPH.
- This results in a rapid conversion of glucose to sorbitol.
- High level of galactose in blood is reduced by aldose reductase in the eye to galactitol, which accumulates causing cataract **(Fig. 31.6)**.

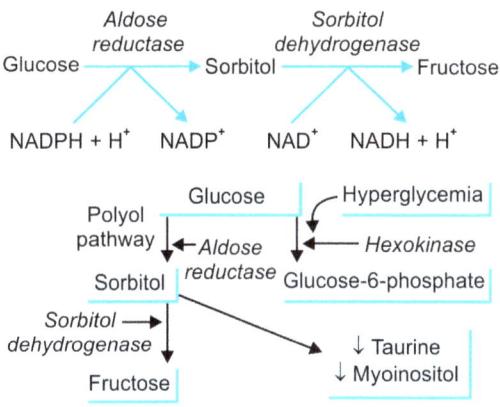

Fig. 31.5: Impact of hyperglycemia on polyol pathway.

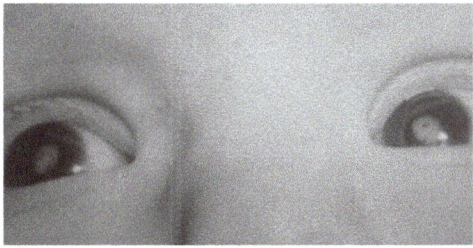

Fig. 31.6: Cataract.

SUMMARY

Phototransduction is a process by which light is converted into electrical signals in the retina of the eye. There are two types of photoreceptors distributed across the retina, i.e. rods and cones. The rods and cones function in dim and bright light, respectively. Rhodopsin is the pigment responsible for absorption of light.

MULTIPLE-CHOICE QUESTIONS

1. **The correct order of the visual cycle when light hits the retina of the eye (1 → 4) is:**
   1. 11-*cis* retinal changes to *all-trans* retinal
   2. Signal transduction cascade which causes the closure of cGMP-gated cation channel
   3. 11-*cis* retinol oxidized to 11-*cis* retinal
   4. All-*trans* retinal is reduced to all-*trans* retinol

   a. 1, 2, 3, 4   b. 1, 2, 4, 3
   c. 1, 4, 3, 2   d. 2, 1, 4, 3

2. **Concerning photoreceptor rod cells, they:**
   a. Are specialized for day vision
   b. Are chromatic with blue, green, and red pigment
   c. Are less sensitive to light than cone cells
   d. Have more photo pigments than cone cells and capture more light

3. **Which of the following enzyme deficiencies is responsible for diabetic cataract?**
   a. Aldose reductase
   b. Phosphofructokinase
   c. Sorbitol dehydrogenase
   d. Pyruvate kinase

4. **Cone cells:**
   a. Function in bright light
   b. Are more in number than rod cells
   c. Have high amplification and respond to a single photon of light
   d. Are absent in the fovea region of the eye

5. **Rod cells:**
   a. Function in bright light
   b. Are less in number than cone cells
   c. Have high amplification and respond to a single photon of light
   d. Are chromatic with more than two types of pigments
6. **The enzyme that converts cGMP to GMP is:**
   a. cGMP phosphodiesterase
   b. cGMP phosphorylase
   c. cGMP hydrolase
   d. cGMP lyase
7. **Concerning the absorption of light in the retinal layers of the eye, all of the following are true, *except*:**
   a. Rhodopsin changes to bathorhodopsin
   b. Bathorhodopsin converts to metarhodopsin II
   c. Scotopsin converts to metarhodopsin I
   d. Metarhodopsin II activates transducin
8. **During visual transduction, reduction in the concentration of cGMP:**
   a. Causes cGMP gated channels to open
   b. Reduces the entry of sodium into the cell
   c. Increases the entry of calcium into the cell
   d. Increases glutamate release in the presence of light

Answers

| 1. b | 2. d | 3. c | 4. a | 5. c |
| 6. a | 7. c | 8. b | | |

CHAPTER 32

Clinical Chemistry

OBJECTIVES
At the end of this chapter, students should be able to organize and manage their laboratory:
- Facilities and general laboratory design
- Designing and requirements of the various sections in the laboratory
- Laboratory operational flow
- Work force/staffing
- Equipment, instruments, and reagents used
- Laboratory safety
- Quality control (QC), quality assurance, and accreditation
- Reporting laboratory results and record keeping
- Financial considerations in laboratory planning
- Medicolegal concerns.

INTRODUCTION

Laboratory medicine is the base of the modern-day health-care system. The advance in technology, better understanding of the various disease processes, advancement of medical research, and the growing demand for reliable test results have greatly revolutionized the area of laboratory medicine.

Most of the present-day laboratories are now equipped with, to a varying degree, sophisticated automated instruments, with test results, which are accurate and reproducible. There is more emphasis on the QC programs.

Currently, in larger hospitals, major sections of the laboratory are specialized to the extent that they engage specialized staff and perform all the tests relating to their disciplines within sections. In smaller hospitals, the staff may be required to work in more than one section. It is not unusual for these smaller hospitals to establish and staff some sections and send the specimens to the other larger institutions.

Presently there is no prevailing legislation to check the labs, which do not satisfy the minimum standards, and hence do not provide quality results, which is a cause for great concern. The ministry has established an accreditation board to fix some rules and regulations for the small laboratories, which do not even have the recommended instruments and qualified persons.

In this changed scenario, organization and management of laboratory services is not only a complicated and complex process but also a great challenge.

PURPOSE OF THE LABORATORY MEDICINE

The laboratory results assist the clinician in
- Diagnosing the disease
- Providing guidelines in patient management
- Establishing prognosis
- Monitoring follow-up therapy.

Standard Operating Procedures

The preparation of test procedures comes under the broad heading of "Standard Operating Procedures" (SOPs). SOP is a clear, concise, and comprehensive written instruction of a method or procedure, which has been agreed upon and authorized as the operating policy of the department.

In general, SOPs, which mainly contain detailed descriptions of each analytical method, are essential for maintaining the same analytical quality over a long period of time. The procedures are a prerequisite to correct transfer of methods from one laboratory to another. The contents of SOP are as follows:
- Introduction
- Principle of method
- Specimen types, collection, and storage
- Reagents, standards, and control—preparation and storage
- Equipment, glassware, and other accessories
- Detailed procedure
- Calculations, calibration curve
- Analytical reliabilities (QC and statistical assessment)
- Hazardous reagents
- Reference range and clinical interpretation
- Limitations of method (e.g. interfering substances and troubleshooting)
- References
- Signature of authorization.

Quality Control and Quality Assurance

- All steps should be taken by laboratory to ensure reliability of lab results and the accuracy, reproducibility in and between other laboratories.
- The high quality and accuracy of the test results are achieved when the following points are taken into consideration:
  - Daily maintenance of the instrument
  - Use of specific and sensitive methods for the assay
  - The well-trained laboratory person.

Accuracy and Precision

See **Figure 32.1**.

Quality Control

- Set of measures useful in detecting errors.
- Errors can be minimized by exercising control on three factors.

Specimen Collection

Laboratory tests contribute vital information about a patient's health. Correct diagnostic and therapeutic decisions depend on the

ACCURACY VS. PRECISION
- Accuracy — how close a measurement is to the accepted value

(ACCURATE = CORRECT)

- Precision — how close a series of measurements are to each other

(PRECISE = CONSISTENT)

- Quality control is used to monitor both the precision and the accuracy of the assay in order to provide reliable results

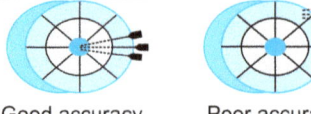
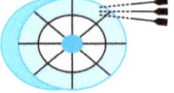
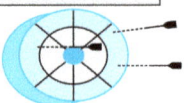

Good accuracy   Poor accuracy   Poor accuracy

Fig. 32.1: Accuracy and precision.

accuracy of test results. Adequate patient preparation, specimen collection, and specimen handling are essential prerequisites for accurate test results. The accuracy of test results is dependent on the integrity of specimens.

Safety and Disposal Considerations in Specimen Collection

In all settings in which specimens are collected and prepared for testing, laboratory and health-care personnel should follow current recommended sterile techniques, including precautions regarding the use of needles and other sterile equipment as well as guidelines for the responsible disposal of all biological material that is potentially hazardous as well as contaminated specimen collection supplies. There are four steps involved in obtaining a good-quality specimen for testing: (1) preparation of the patient, (2) collection of the specimen, (3) processing the specimen, and (4) storing and/or transporting the specimen.

Preparation

Prior to each collection, review the appropriate test description, including the specimen type indicated, the volume, the procedure, the collection materials, patient preparation, and storage and handling instructions.

Preparing the Patient

Provide the patient, in advance, with appropriate collection instructions and information on fasting, diet, and medication restrictions when indicated for the specific test.

Preparing the Specimen

Verify the patient's identification. Proper identification of specimens is extremely important. All primary specimen containers must be labeled with two identifiers at the time of collection. Process and store the specimen(s) as required. Appropriate storage and handling are necessary to maintain the integrity of the specimen and, consequently, the test results.

Avoiding Common Problems

Careful attention to routine procedures can eliminate most of the potential problems related to specimen collection.

General Specimen Collection

Some of the common considerations affecting all types of specimens are to:
- Make sure not to include **expired containers**
- Label a specimen correctly and provide all important information required on the test request form
- Submit a quantity of specimen sufficient to perform the test
- Use the container/tube indicated in the test requirements for appropriate specimen preservation
- Maintain the specimen at the temperature indicated in the test requirements.

Serum Preparation

The most common serum preparation considerations are to:
- Separate serum from red cells within 2 hours of venipuncture
- Mix specimen with additive immediately after collection
- Allow specimens collected in a clot tube (e.g. red-top or gel-barrier tube) to clot before centrifugation
- *Avoid hemolysis:* Red blood cells broken down and components spilled into serum
- *Avoid lipemia:* Cloudy or milky serum sometimes due to the patient's diet.

Plasma Preparation

The most common considerations in the preparation of plasma are to:
- Collect specimen in additive indicated in the test requirements

- Mix specimen with additive immediately after collection
- Avoid hemolysis or red blood cell breakdown
- Label transport tubes as "plasma"
- Indicate type of anticoagulant (e.g. ethylenediaminetetraacetic acid and "citrate").

Urine Collection

The most common urine collection considerations are to:
- Obtain a clean-catch, midstream specimen
- Store unpreserved specimens refrigerated or in a cool place until ready for transport
- Provide patients with instructions for 24-hour urine collection
- Add the preservative (as specified in the test requirements) to the urine collection container prior to collection of the specimen
- Carefully tighten specimen container lids to avoid leakage of specimen
- Divide specimen into separate containers for tests with such requirements
- Provide a complete 24-hour collection/aliquot or other timed specimen
- Provide a 24-hour urine volume when an aliquot from the 24-hour collection is submitted
- Preservatives vary for each test; refer to test information for the required preservative.

Preanalytical (Random) and Analytical (Systemic) Errors (Fig. 32.2)

There are two types of errors: Random or preanalytical errors and systemic or analytical errors.

1. *Random or preanalytical errors:* Errors that arise due to inadequate control on preanalytical variables, such as patient identification, test and patient correlation, labeling of samples, sample collection, handling and transport, and electric supply and equipment.
2. *Systemic or analytical errors:* Errors resulting from inadequate control on analytical variables. Systemic errors most often can be traced to faulty calibration, which includes use of impure calibration material, erroneous labeling of calibrators, use of wrong unstable or deteriorated calibrators, unstable reagent blanks, and inadequate use of sample blanks.

There are two types of QC programs available:
1. Internal QC program
2. External QC program.

Internal Quality Control Program

- Analysis of patient's serum
  - Clinical correlation of test results with the disease the patient is suspected to be suffered from.

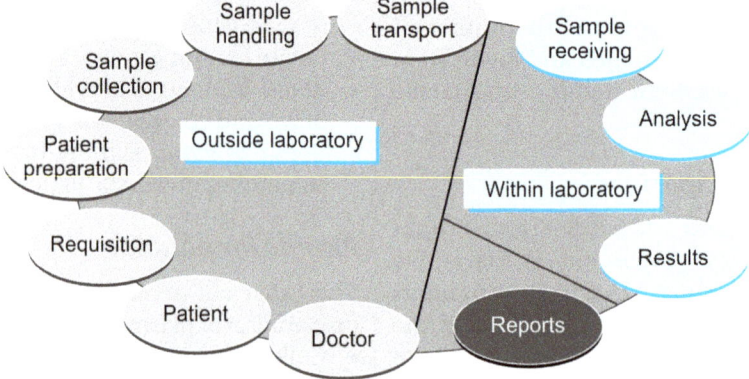

Fig. 32.2: Preanalytical and analytical variables.

- *Within-assay variation:* Analyze the same sample twice. Both the results should be identical. A large variation in results indicates the one or more errors.
- Correlation with other laboratory results. The results of a particular test must correlate with the results of other related tests. *Example:* In liver function tests, in a patient whose serum is visibly icteric, and alanine transaminase activity is high, total bilirubin concentration must be elevated proportional. If not, an error is indicated.
- *Intralab duplicates of 2 days:* A sample analyzed in duplicates for 2 days and the four values studied for reproducibility. Variations in the four values indicate one or more random or systemic errors.
- *Patient's daily and monthly average data:* The law of averages states that the average daily or monthly value for a particular parameter such as glucose must lie within a very small range. This can be calculated by the formula:

$$= \frac{\text{Sum of concentration of analyte in all samples}}{\text{No. of samples}}$$

If the average for a particular day or month varies greatly from the average for other 2 days or months, it is an indication of an error.
- Using pooled sera
Samples containing normal and abnormal levels of analytes may be pooled.
- Use of commercial assayed sera
An assayed control serum may be included in the assay and the result compared with the expected values provided with the control.

External Quality Control Program

Several external QC programs are available. The participating laboratory is sent vials of controls without reference values. The laboratory may analyze these samples as many times as they wish and send their best result to this reference laboratory.

Internal QC program is most useful in determining the reproducibility of results (precision).

External QC programs are useful in determining the closeness of a result to the true value (accuracy).

CRITICAL ALERTS

Critical values (panic or alert values) are laboratory test results that exceed established limit(s) (high or low) as defined by the laboratory for certain analytes as listed in the critical (panic) limits. Critical results are considered life threatening and require immediate notification of the physician, the physician's representative, the ordering entity, or other clinical personnel responsible for the patient's care.

A suggested approach for verbally reporting critical laboratory results is to:
- Place a call to report the critical results and identify yourself and the reason for calling
- State the patient's name, test name, time of draw, critical lab results, units of measure, and reference range
- Ask the recipient to repeat back the patient's name and the critical lab result
- Verbally correct any errors and repeat the request for a "read-back"
- Document the date, time, test results, and person to whom the test results were reported.

For example: Creatinine reference ranges from 0.7 to 1.5 mg/dL; less than 0.2 and more than 3.0 mg/dL is considered a critical result.

Glucose (fasting blood sugar, postprandial blood sugar, random blood sugar) ranges from 65 to 110 mg/dL; less than 40 and more than 500 is considered a critical result.

LEGAL AND ETHICAL REGULATIONS

Laws, guidelines, and recommendations on work in clinical laboratories: in particular, accident prevention and hygiene regulations, handling of isotopes, calibration, QC, education regulations, labor laws, and occupational diseases should be followed according to the laws and guidelines.

LABORATORY VALUES

Blood Tests

Tests	Normal values	To diagnose
Fasting glucose	60–100 mg/dL	Diabetes
Postprandial glucose	90–140 mg/dL	Diabetes
Random glucose	90–150 mg/dL	Diabetes
Urea (UN)	8–40 mg/dL	Prerenal and renal disorder
BUN	7–25 mg/dL	Prerenal and renal disorder
Creatinine	0.6–1.4 mg/dL	Renal disease and muscle degeneration
Sodium	130–143 mEq/L	Renal and cardiac disorder
Potassium	3.5–5.0 mEq/L	Renal disorder
Chloride	93–110 mEq/L	Renal disorder
Total CO_2	22–26 mEq/L	Renal and acid–base disorder
Anion gap	10–20 mEq/L	Acid–base disorder
Osmolality	270–285 mOsm/kg	Renal disorder
Uric acid	3–7 mg/dL	Renal disorder and gout
Calcium	8.5–10.6 mg/dL 8.5–10.3 mEq/dL	Renal and bone disorder
Phosphate	2.5–4.5 mg/dL	Renal disorder
Cholesterol	170–200 mg/dL	Atherosclerosis, diabetes, and hypothyroidism
Triglycerides	40–160 mg/dL	Atherosclerosis, hypothyroidism, liver disease, pancreatitis, myocardial infarction, and metabolic disorders
HDL cholesterol	45–70 mg/dL	High value indicates healthy metabolic system and low in liver disease

(BUN: blood urea nitrogen; HDL: high-density lipoprotein)

Tests	Normal values	To diagnose
LDL cholesterol	60–130 mg/dL	Atherosclerosis
Total bilirubin	0.2–1.2 mg/dL	Jaundice and liver disease
Direct bilirubin	0–0.2 mg/dL	Jaundice and liver disease
Total protein	6.0–8.0 g/dL	Liver disease, malabsorption lupus, chronic infections, and alcoholism
Albumin	3.5–5.0 g/dL	Liver disorder, shock, and multiple myeloma
Globulin	1.8–3.4 g/dL	Liver disease and chronic infections, multiple myeloma, and rheumatoid arthritis
A/G ratio	0.8–2.0 ng/mL	Liver disease, chronic infections, and multiple myeloma
Zinc turbidity	2–8 U	Liver disorder
SGOT (AST)	5–40 U/L	Liver and cardiac disease
SGPT (ALT)	5–40 U/L	Liver disease
ALP	35–125 U/L	Obstructive jaundice and bone disorder

Contd...

Contd...

Tests	Normal values	To diagnose
GGT	10–50 U/L	Liver disease, alcoholism, and obstructive jaundice
Amylase	80–240 unit	Pancreatitis
Acid phosphatase	Up to 11 U/L	Carcinoma prostate
LDH	0–250 U/L	MI and heart disease
LDH1	Up to 175 U/L	MI and heart disease
LDH1/LDH ratio	Less than 0.4	MI and heart disease
CK	10–80 U/L	MI and heart disease
T3	0.8–2.0 ng/mL	Thyroid disorder
T4	4.5–12.0 µg/dL	Thyroid disorder
TSH	0.3–5.0 mIU/mL	Thyroid disorder
Ferritin	27–300 ng/mL	Anemia
Cortisol: Morning	8–26 µg/dL	Cushing's syndrome
Cortisol: Evening	5–18 µg/dL	Addison's disease
β-hCG	0–5 mIU/mL	Choriocarcinoma
AFP	0–15 ng/mL	Carcinoma liver and neural tube defect
CEA	0–4 ng/mL	Colon cancer

(A/G: albumin/globulin; AFP: alpha-fetoprotein; ALP: alkaline phosphatase; CEA: carcinoembryonic antigen; GGT: gamma-glutamyl transpeptidase; LDH: lactate dehydrogenase; LDL: low-density lipoprotein; MI: myocardial infarction; SGOT: serum glutamic oxaloacetic transaminase; SGPT: serum glutamic pyruvic transaminase; TSH: thyroid-stimulating hormone; β-hCG: β-human chorionic gonadotropin; ALT: alanine transaminase; AST: aspartate transaminase; CK: creatine kinase)

Tests	Normal values	To diagnose
CA-125	0–35 U/mL	Ovarian cancer
PSA	0–4 ng/mL	Carcinoma prostate
FSH		
Men	1–12 mIU/mL	
Women: • Follicular • Midcycle • Luteal • Menopausal	• 3–20 mIU/mL • 9–26 mIU/mL • 1–12 mIU/mL • 18–153 mIU/mL	Fertility workup
LH		
Men	2.0 mIU/mL	
Women: • Follicular • Luteal • Menopausal	• 2–15 mIU/mL • 0.6–19.0 mIU/mL • 16–64 mIU/mL	Fertility workup
Prolactin		
Women: • Midcycle • Menopausal	• 5.4–22.5 ng/mL • 4.5–15 ng/mL	Fertility workup

Contd...

Contd...

Tests	Normal values	To diagnose
Testosterone		
Men	2.8–8.2 ng/mL	Fertility workup
Women: Progesterone	0.1–4.0 ng/mL or 1–20 ng/mL	Fertility workup
Estradiol		
Men	2–50 ng/mL	
Women: • Follicular • Midcycle • Luteal • Menopausal	• 23–145 ng/mL • 112–443 ng/mL • 48–241 ng/mL • 0–59 ng/mL	Fertility workup
IgG	1,200–1,480 mg/dL	Immune disorder
IgA	200–280 mg/dL	Immune disorder
IgM	110–136 mg/dL	Immune disorder
C3	90–150 mg/dL	Immune disorder
C4	15–50 mg/dL	Immune disorder
α-1-antitrypsin	90–150 U/dL	Acute-phase reactant
α-1-chymotrypsin	45–75 U/dL	Acute-phase reactant
C-reactive protein	Up to 6.0 mg/L	Immune disorder
Haptoglobin	70–240 mg/dL	Immune disorder
Glucose-6-phosphate dehydrogenase	8–18 U/g	Anemia
ANA	• <20 –ve • >160 +ve • 120–160 borderline	Autoimmune disorder
Anti-dsDNA antibodies	• <50 –ve • >65 +ve • 50–65 borderline	Autoimmune disorders
ACA, antiphospholipid	• <10 –ve • >15 +ve • 10–15 borderline	Autoimmune disorders
Hematology values	Normal	
Hb	12–16 g/dL	
HCT	37–47%	
MCH	27–33 pg	
MCV	80–100 fL	
MCHC	32–36%	
Red blood cell count (male)	4.2–5.6 mL/μL	
Red blood cell count (female)	3.9–5.2 mL/μL	
White blood cell count	3.8–10.8 thous/μL	

Contd...

Contd...

Tests	Normal values	To diagnose
Platelet count	130–400 thous/μL	
Neutrophil count		
Adult	48–73%	High in infection
Children	30–60%	
Lymphocyte count		
Adult	18–48%	High in viral infections
Children	25–50%	
Monocyte count	0–9%	High in chronic infections, leukemia, and carcinomas
Eosinophil count	0–5%	High in allergic reactions
Basophil count	0–2%	

(ACA: anticardiolipin antibodies; ANA: antinuclear antibodies; FSH: follicle-stimulating hormone; Hb: hemoglobin; HCT: hematocrit; IgG: immunoglobulin G; LH: luteinizing hormone; MCH: mean corpuscular hemoglobin; MCHC: mean corpuscular hemoglobin concentration; MCV: mean corpuscular volume; PSA: prostate-specific antigen)

Urine Tests

Tests	Normal values	To diagnose
Calcium	50–300 mg/24 h	
Phosphorus	400–1,300 mg/24 h	
Uric acid	200–500 mg/24 h	
Oxalate	17–53 mg/24 h	
Magnesium	60–120 mg/24 h	
Citrate	300–900 mg/24 h	
Cystine	Negative	
Xanthine	Negative	
Risk index	600–680	
pH	4.5–7.8	
Volume	600–2,000 mL/24 h	
Urea	10–35 g/24 h	
Creatinine	800–1,500 mg/24 h	
Creatinine clearance	60–120 mL/min	
Protein	24–180 mg/24 h	
Ammonia	140–1,500 mEq/24 h	
Sodium	40–220 mEq/24 h	
Potassium	35–90 mEq/24 h	
Chloride	60–125 mEq/24 h	
Osmolality	50–1,400 mOsm/kg	
Volume	1,000–2,000 mL/24 h	

Contd...

Contd...

Tests	Normal values	To diagnose
Estriol	4 mg/24 h	
17-ketosteroids: • Morning • Evening	 • 8–20 mg/24 h • 6–15 mg/24 h	
Catecholamines	Up to 150 µg/24 h	
VMA	2–8 mg/24 h	
HVA	3–28 mg/creatinine	
5-HIAA	1–10 mg/24 h	

(5-HIAA: 5-hydroxyindoleacetic acid; HVA: homovanillic acid; VMA: vanillylmandelic acid)

Cerebrospinal Fluid Tests

Tests	Normal values	To diagnose
CSF glucose	60 mg%	Meningitis
CSF protein	5–40 mg%	

(CSF: cerebrospinal fluid)

CHAPTER 33

Instrumentation and Techniques

OBJECTIVES

At the end of this topic, the students should be able to know about the:
- The principle and procedure involved with spectrophotometry
- Centrifugation, different types and their applications
- Electrophoresis, different types and their applications
- Chromatography, different types and their applications
- Radioimmunoassay and its applications
- Enzyme-linked immunosorbent assay and its applications

SPECTROPHOTOMETRY/COLORIMETRY

Introduction

Light: It is a form of energy.

Dual nature of light: Some of the properties of light can be explained by considering it as a stream of particles, whereas some other properties can be explained by considering it as a wave.

Wavelength of light: When light is considered as a wave the distance between two successive crests or troughs is called "wavelength" of that particular type of light. It is designated by "λ" (lambda) and expressed in terms of nm (nanometers) or Å (angstroms) **(Fig. 33.1)**.

Dispersion of light: When ordinary light (white light) is passed through a prism, it is split into seven different components (colors). This property is called "dispersion." The components from bottom to top will have the following order: violet (V), indigo (I), blue (B), green (G), yellow (Y), orange (O), and red (R). This visible light will cover a wavelength range from 400 to 700 nm **(Fig. 33.2)**.

Electromagnetic spectrum: It is constituted when all types of radiations are arranged in the increasing order of their wavelengths **(Fig. 33.3)**.

Principles of Spectrophotometry/Colorimetry

Both these techniques are based on the estimation of light-absorbing nature of the substances in solution. In colorimetry, only

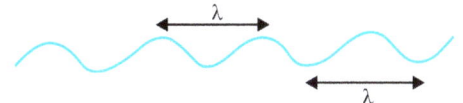

Fig. 33.1: Wavelength of time.

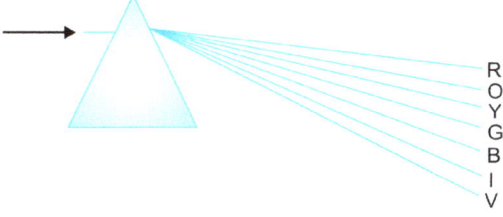

Fig. 33.2: Dispersion of light.

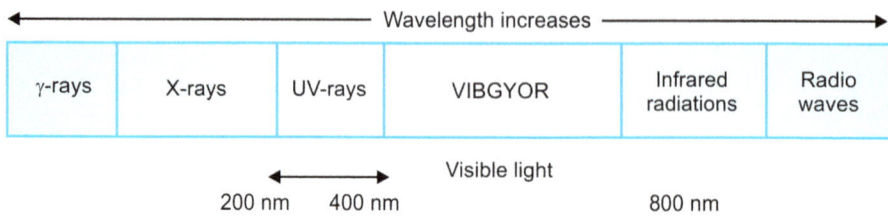

Fig. 33.3: Electromagnetic spectrum.

the colored compounds or the compounds capable of forming color complexes by reacting with reagents can be analyzed. In this the intensity of the color reflects the concentration of the substance, whereas in spectrophotometry not only colored but also colorless solution can be studied by means of ultraviolet (UV) spectral analysis. These techniques are based on two laws:

1. *Beer's law:* Absorbance of a solution is directly proportional to the concentration of the solution (i.e. $A \mu C$) or transmittance of a solution decreases exponentially with the increase in the concentration of the solution (i.e. $T = e - kC$).
2. *Lambert's law:* Absorbance of a solution is directly proportional to the thickness of the optical path (i.e. $A \mu t$) or transmittance of a solution decreases exponentially with the increase in the thickness of the optical light path (i.e. $T = e - kt$) **(Fig. 33.4)**.

Instrumentation

- Components of colorimeter or spectrophotometer **(Fig. 33.5)**

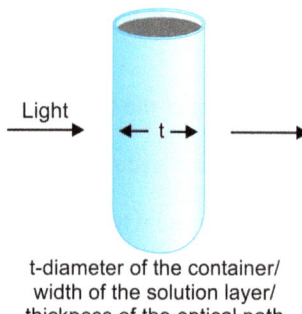

Fig. 33.4: Lambert's law.

- Spectrophotometer is more sophisticated compared to colorimeter. Instrumentation is almost similar except for certain differences.

Source of Light

In colorimeters, source of visible light is a tungsten lamp.

Spectrophotometers will have two sources of light—a tungsten lamp, which emits visible light (wavelength ranges from 400 to 700 nm) and a deuterium lamp, which emits

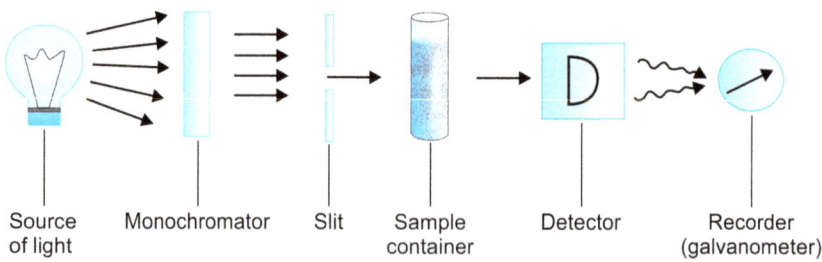

Fig. 33.5: Components of colorimeter or spectrophotometer.

UV radiations (wavelength range from 200 to 400 nm).

Monochromator

In colorimeters, replaceable colored glass filters are used to get the monochromatic light. The multiwavelength radiation from the source passes through the filter and the radiation of a narrow band width comes out. But in spectrophotometers, monochromators will not be the manually replaceable filters. Instead of this quartz prism or diffraction grating is used to obtain monochromatic light (diffraction grating is a glass slide like optical hardware consists of a series of ruled lines on a transparent or reflecting base).

Slit

Slit is to allow a narrow beam of selected monochromatic light to pass through the sample solution.

Cuvette

Cuvette is the glass container to keep the test solution, which has to be filled three fourth of its height. For UV analysis quartz cuvette is used.

Detector

Usually photomultiplier tubes (PMTs), which are based on "photoionic effect," are used as detectors. The light that comes out of the cuvette falls on this and gets converted into an electrical signal.

Photoionic effect: Light photons impinging on a metal surface in vacuum cause the emission of electrons in proportion to the intensity of the radiation.

Recorder

The electrical signal from the PMT is amplified and then recorded by the galvanometer. Usually the recorders are calibrated in such a way that they directly give the absorbance or transmittance values.

Applications

- In clinical diagnostic and research laboratories, these techniques are commonly used for the quantitative estimation of different compounds in various biological fluids, e.g. blood glucose, urea, cholesterol, creatinine, and cerebrospinal fluid protein.
- *Qualitative analysis:* Visible and UV spectra may be used to identify various compounds in both pure state and in biological preparations, e.g. proteins show a maximum light absorption at 280 nm, so we can observe a peak at 280 nm, when its absorption spectra is plotted.
  Similarly, nucleic acids show a absorption maximum at 260 nm. So these techniques can be used in the structural analysis of proteins and nucleic acids.
- Enzyme studies require these techniques.
- *Turbidimetry:* It is a form of spectrophotometry in which very dilute suspensions may be assayed by measuring the extent of turbidity.

CENTRIFUGATION

Introduction

Centrifugation is a separating technique commonly used in clinical and research laboratories. It is based on the behavior of particles in an applied centrifugal field.

Principle

If a solution of larger particles is allowed to stand, then the particles will tend to sediment under the influence of gravity. If the particles suspended in a liquid are so small or have a density so close to that of the liquid, then the force of gravity fails to sediment the particles into a separate layer. So the basis of centrifugation techniques is to exert a larger force than the gravitational force to enhance the effective sedimentation force for the separating such particles from the liquid.

In centrifugation, the particles are normally suspended in a specific liquid medium, held in tubes, which are located in a rotor. The rotor is positioned centrally on the drive shaft of the centrifuge. Particles, which differ in density, shape, or size, can be separated, since they sediment at different rates in the centrifugal field, each particle sedimentation at a rate, which is proportional to the applied centrifugal field.

The rate at which the sedimentation occurs in centrifugation is expressed in terms of sedimentation coefficient and is given by the formula:

$$S = \frac{V}{w2r}$$

where
V = migration (sedimentation) of the molecule
w = rotation of the rotor in radians/s (angular velocity)
r = distance in cm, from center of rotor.

The equipment used to perform centrifugation is called "centrifuge." The centrifuge should essentially have a rotor to keep the sample tube. The rotor can be of three types:
1. Fixed angle rotor
2. Vertical tube rotor
3. Swinging bucket rotor.

Types of Centrifuges

Centrifuges may be classified into four major groups:
1. Small bench centrifuges
2. Large-capacity refrigerated centrifuges
3. High-speed refrigerated centrifuges
4. Ultracentrifuges, which are of two types—preparative and analytical.

Applications of Centrifugation

Following are the applications of centrifugation:

- Separation of thick precipitates from solution:
  - Precipitating proteins from serum during colorimetric estimation of serum urea and creatinine. Trichloroacetic acid is added to serum sample, which denatures proteins and precipitates. The precipitate is separated by centrifugation. The protein free filtrate is used for further analysis.
  - Separation of serum from clotted blood.
  - Separation of erythrocytes from oxalated (or heparinized) blood.
- To determine packed cell volume (PCV) or hematocrit values. The oxalated blood is centrifuged in hematocrit tubes (110 mm long and 3 mm in bore diameter) at 3,000 revolutions per minute for 30 minutes. The proportionate volume of red blood cells (RBCs), settled in the bottom layer below the supernatant layer of clear plasma in the tube, is read from the graduations of the tube as PCV (normally it averages 45% in humans).
- *Isolation of subcellular organelles:* The cells are subjected to disruption by sonication or by osmotic shock or by the use of homogenizer. This is usually carried out in an isotonic (0.25 M) sucrose solution. The subcellular particles can be separated by differential centrifugation **(Fig. 33.6)**. The purity (or contamination) of the subcellular fraction can be checked by the use of marker enzymes. For example, deoxyribonucleic acid (DNA) polymerase is the marker for nucleus, glutamate dehydrogenase for mitochondrion, glucose-6-phosphatase for ribosome, and hexokinase for cytosolic fraction.
- Determination of molecular weight (in the fields of protein and nucleic acid chemistry) by studying their sedimentation characteristics.
- Estimation of purity of macromolecules, i.e. purity of DNA preparations, viruses, and proteins.

Instrumentation and Techniques

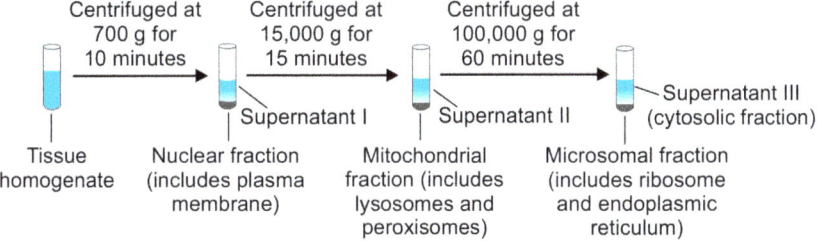

Fig. 33.6: Isolation of subcellular organelles.

6. Detection of conformational changes in macromolecules such as DNA and proteins.

ELECTROPHORESIS

Introduction

Electrophoresis and chromatography are the popular methods for the separation of closely related compounds such as mixture of proteins, amino acid, carbohydrates, steroid hormones, and drugs.

General Principle of Electrophoresis

Electrophoresis is a very common technique used in clinical and research laboratories. This technique is used for the separation of charged particles. Biological materials such as amino acids, peptides, proteins, and nucleic acids possess ionizable groups and hence exist as charged molecules in solutions, either as cations (positively charged) or anions (negatively charged) depending upon the pH of the medium (**Fig. 33.7**). Even typical nonpolar substances such as carbohydrates can be given charges by derivatization, e.g. as borate or phosphates.

These charged particles move (migrate) in an electric field, i.e. cations toward cathode (negatively charged electrode) and anions toward anode (positively charged electrode). So, it is obvious that the molecules having similar charges move in the same direction. But because of the difference in their molecular mass the extent to which they move differs; hence, the difference in charge occurs. Mass ratio (C/M) forms the basis for the differential migration of particles in an applied electric field and this forms the general principle of electrophoresis.

The following example of an amino acid shows how the extent of ionization and direction of migration is dependent on pH.

Types of Electrophoresis

Listed below are the types of electrophoresis:
- Depending upon the nature of supporting medium:
  - Agarose gel electrophoresis; agarose gel is used as the supporting medium
  - Polyacrylamide gel electrophoresis
  - Cellulose acetate electrophoresis (paper strip electrophoresis); cellulose acetate paper serves as the supporting medium.

$$H_3N^+-\underset{R}{CH}-COOH \underset{H^+}{\overset{OH^-}{\rightleftharpoons}} H_3N^+-\underset{R}{CH}-COO^- \underset{H^+}{\overset{OH^-}{\rightleftharpoons}} H_2N-\underset{R}{CH}-COO^-$$

pH:	Acidic	Isoionic point	Alkaline
Ionic form:	Cation	Zwitter ion	Anion
Migration:	toward cathode	Stationary	toward anode

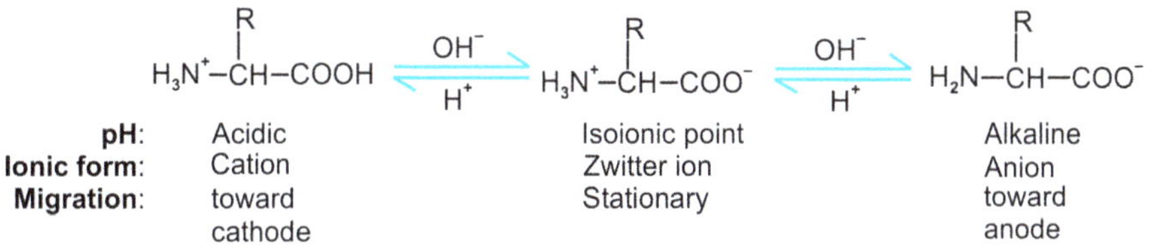

Fig. 33.7: Principle of electrophoresis (separation of charged particles).

- Depending upon the mode of technique:
  - Slide gel electrophoresis
  - Tube gel electrophoresis
  - Disk electrophoresis
  - Low- and high-voltage electrophoresis.

Applications

Applications of electrophoresis are given below:
- In separating serum proteins for diagnostic purposes
- Hemoglobin electrophoresis
- Lipoprotein electrophoresis
- Isozyme analysis
- Nucleic acid studies.

CHROMATOGRAPHY

Introduction

Chromatography is one of the most popular tools of biochemistry. This technique is used for the separation of a number of similar components in a mixture from each other so that these could be determined with a minimum of interference. These closely related compounds include proteins, peptides, amino acids, lipids, carbohydrates, vitamins, and drugs.

This technique is working on the principle of adsorption, partition, and ion exchange and exclusion properties.

General Principle of Chromatography

Chromatography usually consists of a mobile phase and a stationary phase. The mobile phase is a mixture of substance to be separated in a liquid or a gas. The stationary phase is a porous solid matrix through which the sample contained in the mobile phase percolates. The interaction between the stationary phase and the mobile phase causes the separation of compounds from the mixture. These interactions include adsorption, partition, ion exchange, and exclusion type of physicochemical properties.

Classification of Chromatography

The type of interaction medium used for stationary phase and mobile phase is the basis of classification of chromatography (**Fig. 33.8**).

Partition Chromatography

The molecules, which are to be separated, undergo continuous redistribution between a stationary phase and a mobile phase. The separation depends on the relative tendencies of the molecule in a mixture to associate more strongly with one or the other phases.

Since partitioning process is repeated hundreds or thousand times, small difference in partition ratio permits excellent separation.

In paper chromatography, paper serves as a solid support to hold the stationary phase. The solvent system provides both stationary phase and mobile phase. For amino acid chromatography, butanol, acetic acid, and water in the proportion of 4:1:5 v/v are used as solvent system. Butanol with a little acetic acid acts as the mobile phase and water–acetic acid forms the stationary phase, which will be held to the paper (**Fig. 33.9**).

Adsorption Chromatography

In this technique, separation of substances is based on the difference in adsorption on

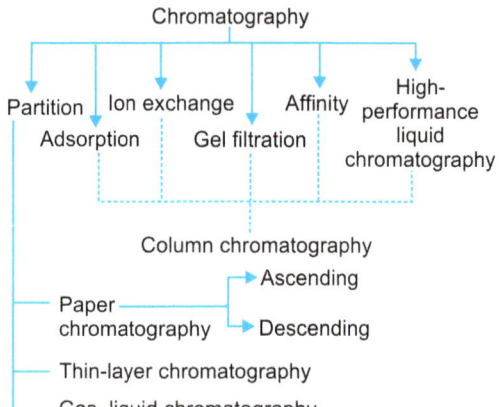

Fig. 33.8: Types of chromatography.

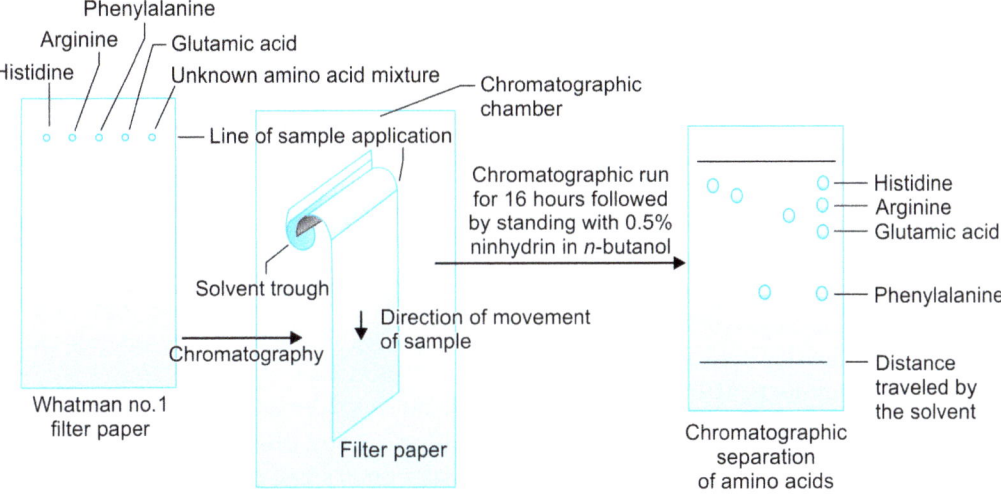

Fig. 33.9: Paper chromatography of amino acid.

the surface of a solid stationary medium such as silica gel or alumina. During the elution, weekly held substances move fast. Strongly held substances are eluted by changing pH and salt conditions **(Fig. 33.10)**.

Gas–liquid Chromatography

This is a method of choice for the separation of volatile substances such as lipids and drugs. Stationary phase is inert solid material, which is impregnated with a nonvolatile liquid such as polyethylene glycol. This is packed in a narrow column. Under proper condition, volatile material, which is to be separated, is passed through column with the help of an inert gas (argon). Separation of individual substance is based on partition of components.

Ion Exchange Chromatography

Here separation of molecules is based on their charges. Ion exchange resins used for this purpose are cation exchanger (e.g. carboxy-methylcellulose) and anion exchanger (e.g. diethylaminoethyl-cellulose) **(Fig. 33.11)**:
- Anion exchanger (R^+A^-): The R^+A^- exchanges its anion (A^-) with other anion,

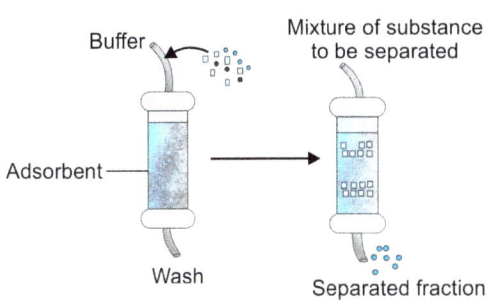

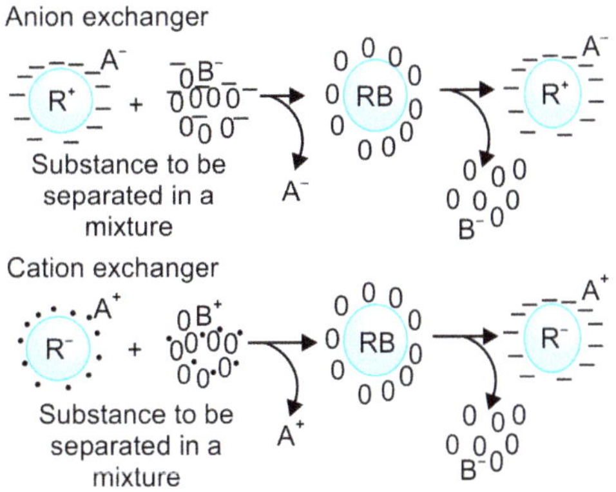

Fig. 33.10: Adsorption chromatography.

Fig. 33.11: Ion exchange chromatography.

i.e. the substance, which is to be separated (B⁻) in a solution.
- Cation exchanger: Similarly, the R⁺A⁻ exchanges its cation (A⁺) with other cation, i.e. the substance to be separated. This technique is highly pH dependent.

Gel Filtration Chromatography

Gel filtration chromatography separation is based on size, shape, and molecular weight of the substance to be separated. The gel serves as a molecular sieve for these substances. The larger particles cannot pass through the pores of the gel and therefore move faster. On the other hand, smaller particles enter the gel beads and are left behind, which comes out of the column very slowly, e.g. Sephadex G-100, Bio gel P-10 **(Fig. 33.12)**.

Affinity Chromatography

The principle of affinity chromatography is based on the specific and noncovalent binding of substances such as proteins and enzymes to a specific ligand (cofactor or substrates) attached to the gel matrix **(Fig. 33.13)**.

For example, separation of lactate dehydrogenase from RBC using NAD⁺ ligand linked to the affinity gel.

RADIOIMMUNOASSAY

- Radioimmunoassay (RIA) is an immunoassay technique that involves the reaction between an antigen and its specific antibody.
- It utilizes radioactive isotopes **(Table 33.1)**.

Antibody: It is a protective protein produced in an animal's body in response to a foreign substance and it is capable of binding with that of foreign substance.

Antigen: It is a foreign substance that stimulates the production of specific antibody molecules, when introduced into the animal's body.

Principle of Radioimmunoassay

This technique is based on the competition between unlabeled antigen and labeled antigen for a limited number of antibodies. At the end of the reaction time, the reaction

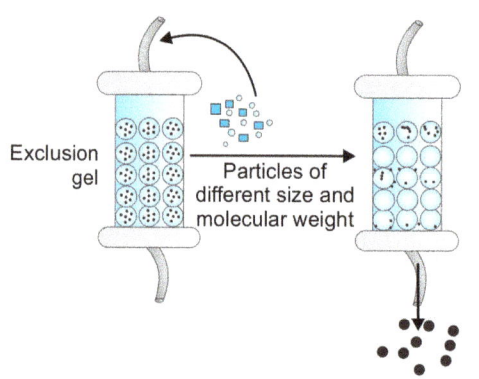

Fig. 33.12: Gel filtration chromatography.

Table 33.1: Radioimmunoassay techniques.

Isotope	Half-life (days)
3 H	>120
14 C	>120
125 I	60
131 I	8

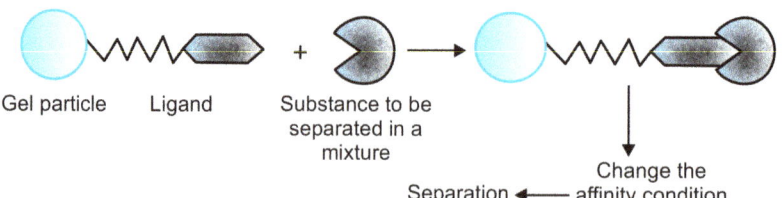

Fig. 33.13: Affinity chromatography.

tube would contain both antigen–antibody complex as well as free antigens (labeled and unlabeled). Under standard conditions, the amount of labeled antigen bound to the antibody will decrease as the amount of unlabeled antigen (antigen in the patient sample) increases. This is explained by the example given below:

$4 Ag^* + 4 Ab \rightarrow 4 Ag^* Ab$

$4 Ag + 4 Ag^* + 4 Ab \rightarrow 2Ag^*Ab + 2 Ag Ab + 2Ag^* + 2Ag$

$12 Ag + 4 Ag^* + 4 Ab \rightarrow Ag^*Ab + 3 AgAb + 3 Ag^* + 9 Ag$

where

Ab = antibody
Ag = antigen (unlabeled)
Ag* = labeled antigen
AgAb = antigen–antibody complex.

The radioactivity of the bound labeled antigen (Ag*–Ab) is measured. Hence, the radioactivity count is inversely proportional to the unlabeled antigen concentration.

Applications of Radioimmunoassay

A variety of compounds, which are present in serum or other biological fluids in very small amounts, can be estimated by this technique. For example:
- Hormones such as thyroxine, triiodothyronine, insulin, cortisol, renin, and aldosterone
- Tumor markers such as prostate-specific antigen (PSA), and alpha-fetoprotein (AFP)
- Vitamins
- Drugs such as digoxin.

ENZYME-LINKED IMMUNOSORBENT ASSAY

Introduction

In enzyme-linked immunosorbent assay (ELISA) technique, enzymes are used to label the antigens in place of radioactive isotopes in RIA.

Types and Principles

There are two types of methods in ELISA:
1. Single antibody method (competitive binding method) **(Fig. 33.14)**
2. Double antibody method **(Fig. 33.15)**.

Materials Used in Enzyme-linked Immunosorbent Assay

Following are the materials used in ELISA:
- Solid phase—plastic tubes or microtiter plates
- Enzymes:
  - Horse radish peroxidase for which substrate is hydrogen peroxide (H_2O_2)
  - Alkaline phosphatase, which substrate is p-nitrophenyl phosphate.

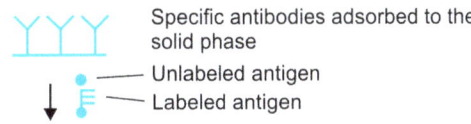
Specific antibodies adsorbed to the solid phase
— Unlabeled antigen
— Labeled antigen

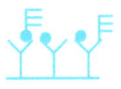
Labeled and unlabeled antigen bound to the antibody

Substrate for enzyme added and plates incubated

Enzyme activity measured

Fig. 33.14: Principle of single antibody method.

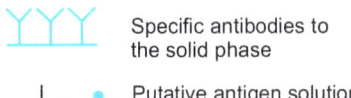
Specific antibodies to the solid phase

Putative antigen solution added; incubated and then washed

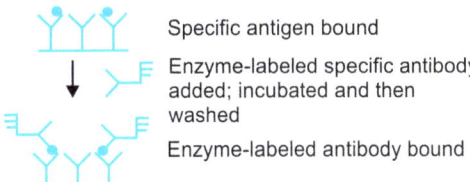
Specific antigen bound

Enzyme-labeled specific antibody added; incubated and then washed

Enzyme-labeled antibody bound

Enzyme substrate added

Enzyme activity measured

Fig. 33.15: Principle of double antibody method.

Applications of Enzyme-linked Immunosorbent Assay

Applications of ELISA are given below:
- The ELISA is used in the clinical biochemistry laboratories to measure hormones in the serum such as thyroid hormones, insulin, reproductive hormones, and pituitary hormones such as follicle-stimulating hormone, luteinizing hormone, and thyroid-stimulating hormone.
- It is used to measure the level of tumor markers in serum such as AFP, PSA, human chorionic gonadotropin, carcinoembryonic antigen, and cancer antigen 125.
- ELISA is used in the study of infectious diseases such as detection of bacterial toxins, viruses, and hepatitis B surface antigens.
- For the assay of antibodies in serum in infectious diseases, including antiviral antibodies. For example, Epstein-Barr virus, rubella virus, and antibacterial antibodies (*Brucella, Salmonella*).
- For the assay of autoantibodies, e.g. anti-DNA, antinuclear antibody, and antithyroglobulin.

SUMMARY

The spectrophotometry and colorimetry depends on the estimation of light-absorbing nature of the substances in solution. In colorimetry, the intensity of the color reflects the concentration of the substance, whereas in spectrophotometry, both colored and colorless solution can be studied by means of ultraviolet spectral analysis. These techniques are commonly used for the quantitative estimation of different compounds in various biological fluids, e.g. blood glucose, urea, cholesterol, creatinine, and cerebrospinal fluid protein. Also it is used for qualitative analysis and enzyme studies. Centrifugation is a separating technique commonly used in clinical and research laboratories. It is based on the behavior of particles in an applied centrifugal field. If a solution of larger particles is allowed to stand, then the particles will tend to sediment under the influence of gravity. Applications include separation of thick precipitates from solution, isolation of subcellular organelles, and determination of molecular weight. Electrophoresis is a very common technique used in clinical and research laboratories. This technique is used for the separation of charged particles. Biological materials such as amino acids, peptides, proteins, and nucleic acids possess ionizable groups and hence exist as charged molecules in solutions, either as cations (positively charged) or anions (negatively charged) depending upon the pH of the medium. Chromatography is one of the most popular tools of biochemistry. This technique is used for the separation of a number of similar components in a mixture from each other so that these could be determined with a minimum of interference. RIA technique is based on the competition between unlabeled antigen and labeled antigen for a limited number of antibodies. Applications include estimation of hormones, tumor markers, vitamins, and drugs such as digoxin. In enzyme-linked immunosorbent assay technique, enzymes are used to label the antigens. This technique has the similar applications as RIA, including the estimation of autoantibodies such as anti-DNA and antinuclear antibody.

SELF-ASSESSMENT QUESTIONS

1. Explain the different types of rotors used in centrifuges.
2. What are different types of centrifuges? Compare them.
3. Explain the process of subcellular fractionation.

4. Give some applications of centrifugation technique.

State Whether the Given Statements are True (T) or False (F)

1. Particles, which differ in their size and shape, can be separated by centrifugation.
2. One Svedberg unit means 10–15 seconds.
3. Analytical ultracentrifuges can be used to study the molecular structural changes of DNA.

Fill in the Blanks

1. The process by which white light is resolved into seven colors is called _____.
2. The wavelength range of visible light is _____ to _____ nm.
3. Source of UV light in a spectrophotometer is _____.
4. According to Lambert's law, absorbance of a solution is directly proportional to _____.
5. In a spectrophotometer the monochromator can be a prism or _____.
6. The photomultiplier tube in the spectrophotometer works on the principle of _____.
7. In UV spectral analysis, proteins show a maximum absorption at _____ nm.
8. In ELISA _____ are used as labels.
9. Labeled antigen and unlabeled antigen compete for the limited number of antibodies in _____ type of ELISA.
10. The enzyme activity measured is directly proportional to the antigen concentration in the test sample in _____ type of ELISA.
11. In RIA, labeled antigen and unlabeled antigen compete for the limited number of _____.
12. The radioactivity of _____ is measured at the end of radioimmunoassay procedure.
13. The radioactivity count is inversely proportional to the _____ concentration in the test sample.
14. Half-life of ^{125}I is _____.

Essay Questions

1. Write the general principle of electrophoresis.
2. Enumerate the application of electrophoretic techniques.
3. Define chromatography technique.
4. What are the different types of chromatography techniques?
5. Explain the principle of partition chromatography.
6. Write the steps involved in paper chromatography of amino acids.
7. Name the solvent system required for the paper chromatography of amino acids.

Short Essay Questions

1. Write the relation between absorbance and transmittance of a solution.
2. State Beer's law in terms of transmittance.
3. What is the function of photomultiplier tube (PMT) in a spectrophotometer?
4. Expand the term "ELISA."
5. Name any two enzymes used in ELISA.
6. Write the advantages of ELISA technique over RIA.
7. Name a few investigations, which can be done by ELISA.
8. What is an isotope? Give two examples.
9. What is the name of the instrument in which radioactivity is measured?
10. What is an antibody?

CHAPTER 34

Buffers and Biochemical Tests

OBJECTIVES

At the end of this topic, the students should be able to know about the:
- Preparation of buffers and the detection pH of various solutions

BUFFER

Buffer solutions are needed in some of the experiments which have to be carried out at a particular pH. This is possible because buffer solution resists the changes in pH upon addition of small portion of acid or alkali.

A buffer system consists of two chemicals in solution one of which is weak acid and the other Na or K salt of the same acid, e.g. acetate buffer is prepared by mixing sodium acetate and acetic acid. Buffer solutions are used in various enzymatic and other reactions. There are variety of buffer mixtures like phosphate buffer, citrate buffer, carbonate-bicarbonate buffer, etc.

A buffer solution is labelled with the strength and the pH it maintains like 0.2 M phosphate buffer, pH 7.8.

Phosphate Buffer

Solution *a*: 0.2 M KH_2PO_4 or 0.2 M NaH_2PO_4.
Solution *b*: 0.2 M Na_2HPO_4.

Mix solution '*a*' and solution '*b*' to get the required pH as shown in the example and adjust the pH with adding acid or base. If the mixed solution shows pH more than the required pH, use acid to decrease the pH, if it is less than the required one, then base is used to increase the pH.

Example 1: Preparation of 0.2 M phosphate buffer of pH 7.0 and 7.4.

Mix solution *a* of 61 mL and *b* of 30 mL and adjust the pH by adding solution *b* to get 0.2 M buffer, pH 7.0.

Example 2: Mix 80 mL 0.2 M monosodium dihydrogen phosphate and 20 mL of disodium hydrogen phosphate and check the pH if it is not 7.4 then adjust with acid or base prepared.

Volume of *a* and *b* to take to get a required pH:

pH	mL of *a*	mL of *b*
6.9	44.6	55.4
7.0	38.8	61.2
7.2	28.0	72.0
7.4	19.0	81.0
7.6	13.0	87.0

Acetate Buffer

pK 4.76
Solution *a*—0.2 M acetic acid.
Solution *b*—0.2 M sodium acetate.
Mix solution *a* with solution *b* in the volume given below.

Example 1: Preparation of 0.2 M acetate buffer of pH 4.0.

Mix 80 mL of 0.2 M acetic acid and 20 mL of sodium acetate and check the pH. If the pH is less than 4.0 add some more sodium acetate dropwise until pH 4.0 comes. If it is more than the required pH then add 0.2 M acetic acid to adjust the pH to 4.0.

Buffers and Biochemical Tests

Example 2: Preparation of 0.2 M acetate buffer of pH 5.0.

Mix 30 mL of 0.2 M acetic acid and 70 mL 0.2 M sodium acetate and check the pH.

pH	a (mL)	b (mL)
4.2	74.0	26.0
4.4	61.0	39.0
4.6	51.0	49.0
4.8	40.0	60.0
5.0	30	70

Tris-HCl Buffer

Solution a: Tris 0.2 M (hydroxymethyl) aminomethane is prepared.
Solution b: 0.2 M HCl.
Take 0.2 M tris in a beaker and adjust the pH with 0.2 M HCl.

Example 1: Preparation of 0.2 M Tris-HCl buffer, pH 7.6.
Take 100 mL of Tris and adjust the pH to 7.6 with 0.2 M HCl.

Example 2: Preparation of 0.2 M Tris-HCl buffer, pH 8.0.
Take 90 mL of tris in a beaker and adjust the pH to 8.0 with 0.2 M HCl.

Note: If the volume of the buffer required is more then proportionately take more acid and base solution before adjusting the pH.

ACIDS AND BASES

Acids liberate hydrogen ions (H^+) in solution. According to Bronsted theory, acids are proton donors and bases are proton acceptors. Acids change blue litmus paper to red and bases change red litmus to blue.

Strong and Weak Acids

Strong acids dissociate completely (complete ionization) in solution whereas weak acids dissociate partially.

Ionization is the phenomenon of splitting up of molecules into charged particles in solution, e.g. HCl ionizes as H^+ and Cl^-. This is reversible and written as

$$HCl \longleftrightarrow H^+ + Cl^-$$

Mineral acids like HCl, HNO_3 and H_2SO_4 ionize in solution to 90 to 95 percent so they are called as strong acids. Whereas organic acids like acetic acid and oxalic acid ionize to a less extent.

The same classification holds well with bases also. Sodium hydroxide is a strong base whereas disodium hydrogen phosphate (Na_2HPO_4) is a weak base.

Chemical Indicators

There are certain chemicals which are used as indicators in acid-base titration. These chemicals may be weak organic acids or bases or dye stuffs which change color as the hydrogen ion concentrations in solution increase or decrease. The reason for change of color is reversible ionization of these indicator molecules. The ionized particles will have one color and the unionized molecule of it have an entirely different color. Ionization of different indicators takes place at different pH ranges, e.g. Phenolphthalein is a colorless molecule; when it ionizes it is pink. This takes place between a pH of 8.3-10.00. So below pH 8.3 it is colorless. Beyond 8.3 and upto10 ionization goes on and different shades of pink color are obtained.

Beyond pH 10 no change in pink color is observed. Therefore, the pH 8.3-10.00 is called the effective pH range of phenolphthalein.

pH and pH Scale

Defined as the negative log of hydrogen ion concentration.

pH scale ranges from 0-14. pH 7.0 is considered as neutral, pH, below 7 is acidic and above 7 is alkaline.

Measurement of pH of Solution

Using the indicator papers, which are available in various pH ranges, the approximate pH of unknown solutions can be determined. For checking the pH of unknown solution a piece of indicator paper is immersed in it and the color change is compared with those given on the book of indicator paper.

List of indicators, their characteristics and preparation

Name	pH range	Color change	Preparation
Thymol blue	1.2 to 2.8	Red-yellow	0.1 g, in 4.3 mL of 0.05 N NaOH diluted to 250 mL with water
Topfer's reagent (p-Dimethyl-aminobenzene)	2.9 to 4.2	Red-yellow	0.5 g in 100 mL 95% alcohol
Methyl orange	3.0 to 4.4	Red-yellow	0.1 g in 100 mL water
Bromocresol green	3.8 to 5.4	Yellow-green	0.1 g, in 2.9 mL 0.05 N, NaOH diluted to 250 mL with water
Phenolphthalein	8.3 to 10.0	Colorless pink	0.1 g to 1% in 50% alcohol

The accurate pH of the prepared buffer or solution can be measured by using a pH meter. A pH meter consists of a glass electrode. The electrode is always kept immersed in water. The pH is displayed on the board when the electrode is immersed in a buffer and the pH mode button is pressed. The instrument is standardized with the standard buffer of pH nearer to that of unknown. For example, if prepared solution has pH around 4, the instrument is calibrated with the standard buffer of pH 4.0 or any buffer of nearer pH 4.0. If another is around 8, then the instrument is calibrated with standard buffer of pH 9.2 or any other standard buffer of near pH 8.

Procedure: Say, the pH of test solution is around needs modification 7. Put on the switch and wait for 5 minutes. Electrode is taken out from water by moving up the electrode, wash the of electrode with a jet of water. Dip the electrode into the standard buffer of pH 7 taken in a beaker. Press the button 'standardize' and then set it to '7' using the knob. Take out the electrode from the solution. Wash the electrode with a jet of water. Take test solution in a beaker. Dip the electrode into the test solution and press the button to read the pH. Remove the electrode from test solution. Wash the electrode with a jet of water. Keep it dipped in water.

Note:
- Handle the electrode carefully which is made of glass.
- Electrode is always dipped in water when not in use.

CHEMICAL COMPONENTS OF NORMAL URINE

Principles

- **Test for chlorides:** Chlorides present in urine react with silver nitrate to form a white ppt of silver chloride (AgCl).
- **Test for calcium:** Calcium present in the urine reacts with potassium oxalate to form a white ppt. of calcium oxalate.
- **Test for phosphates:** Phosphates present in the urine react with ammonium molybdate to form a canary yellow colored ppt. of ammonium phosphomolybdate.
- **Test for sulphates:** Sulphates present in the urine reacts with barium chloride to form white precipitate of barium sulphate.
- **Sodium hypobromite test:** The effervescence is due to liberation of nitrogen gas from the decomposition of urea into N_2 and CO_2 by the action of sodium hypobromite and CO_2 evolved reacts to form sodium carbonate.
- **Specific urease test:** The enzyme urease splits urea present in urine to form ammonium carbonate. The ammonium carbonate makes the urine alkaline. The change in

the pH is indicated by development of pink color by phenolphthalein indicator.
- **Test for ammonia:** In an alkaline medium the ammonium salts present in the urine decomposes to ammonia on boiling. The ammonia present in the vapours turns red litmus to blue color.
- **Benedict's uric acid reagent test:** Uric acid is a reducing agent. In an alkaline medium it reduces phosphotungstic acid to deep blue colored tungsten blue.
- **Schiff's test:** Uric acid reduces ammoniacal silver nitrate to metallic silver which is black in color.

- **Jaffe's test:** Creatinine present in urine reacts with picric acid in an alkaline medium to give orange red colored compound, creatinine picrate.
- **Sodium nitroprusside test:** The red colored complex is oxidized to give yellow color.

Physical Characteristics
- Volume
- Color
- Odor
- Reaction to litmus
- Specific gravity
- Deposits or turbidity.

Tests for Inorganic Constituents

Procedure	Observation	Inference
Tests for chlorides: 3 mL of urine in a test tube. Add 1 mL of conc.HNO_3 + 1 mL of silver nitrate and mix.	Formation of white ppt.	Shows the presence of chlorides
Tests for calcium: 3 mL of urine in a test tube. Make it alkaline by adding few drops of liquor ammonia. Then Add 1ml of potassium oxalate turbidity solution and mix.	Formation of white turbidity	Shows the presence of calcium
Tests for phosphates: 3 mL of urine in a test tube. Add 1 mL of conc.HNO_3 and 5 mL of ammonium molybdate solution. Then boil and cool and under tap water.	Formation of canary yellow ppt.	Shows the presence of phosphates
Tests for sulphates: 3 mL of urine in a test tube. Add 4 drops of conc.HCl and 2 mL of barium chloride solution and mix.	Formation of white ppt.	Shows the presence of Sulphates

Tests for Organic Constituents

Procedure	Observation	Inference
Tests for Urea:		
• **Sodium hypobromite test:** 3 mL of urine in a test tube. Add 1 mL of sodium hypobromite solution.	Effervescence is seen	Indicates the presence of urea
• **Specific urease test:** 3 mL of urine in a test tube. Add 4–6 drops of phenolphthalein indicator and 1 mL of urease solution. Mix the contents well and keep it for a few minutes.	Pink color develops	Confirms the presence of urea
Tests for uric acid:		
• **Benedict's uric acid reagent test:** 3 mL of urine in a test tube. Add 1 spoonful of sodium carbonate crystals and mix well. Then add 1 mL of benedict's blue colour. Add uric acid reagent and mix.	Formation of deep blue colour	Shows the presence of uric acid
• **Confirmatory test: Schiff's test:** Wet piece of filter paper with few drops of ammonical silver nitrate solution. Add 1 or 2 drops of urine sample on same paper.	Black color formed after sometime	Confirms presence of uric acid

Procedure	Observation	Inference
Test for ammonia: 3 mL of urine in a test tube. Add 2 mL of 10% NaOH solution. Boil and hold a red litmus paper to vapors at the mouth of the test tube.	Red litmus turns blue	Shows the presence of ammonia
Tests for creatinine:		
• **Jaffe's test:** Mix 5 mL of picric acid and 5 mL of 5% NaOH and divide into two parts—i) to one part add 5 mL urine, ii) another part add 5 mL of water.	Orange red color No color	Creatinine is present This is control test
• **Sodium nitroprusside test:** 5 mL of urine in a test tube + 5 drops of sodium nitroprusside solution. Then add 2 mL of 10% NaOH solution.	Red color changes to yellow	Shows the presence of creatinine

URINE ANALYSIS: ABNORMAL CONSTITUENTS OF URINE

Physical Characteristics

- **Volume**
- **Color**
- **Odor**
- **Reaction to litmus**
- **Specific gravity**
- **Deposits or turbidity.**

Tests for Abnormal Constituents

Principle

- **Sulphosalicylic acid test:** The protein present in the urine is precipitated by sulphosalicylic acid by neutralizing the charges on the protein.
- **Heat and acetic acid test:** Albumin is the major protein excreted in proteinuria. It is a heat coagulable protein and hence easily coagulated by heating the urine sample contaning it. Formation of turbidity is due to protein or phosphate present in the urine. Presence of turbity upon addition of dil. acetic acid indicates the presence of protein.

- **Benedicts test:** Refer carbohydrate chapter.
- **Rothera's test:** Sodium nitroprusside in alkaline medium reacts with ketone groups of acetone and acetic acid to form permanganate ring at the junction of the two liquids.
- **Gerhardt's test:** Acetoacetic acid gives red color with ferric chloride.
- **Benzidine glacial acetic acid test:** Heme part of hemoglobin has peroxidase like activity which acts on hydrogen peroxide to release nascent oxygen. This nascent oxygen oxidizes benzidine to give green color.
- **Hay's sulfur powder test:** Bile salts lower the surface tension of urine and hence the sulphur powder sinks to the bottom of the test tube.
- **Fouchet's test:** The bile pigment present in the urine gets adsorbed on to the precipitate of barium sulphate which is separated by filtration. The dried precipitate is then treated with Fouchet's reagent which contains ferric chloride. Ferric chloride is an oxidizing agent and it oxidizes bilirubin to biliverdin to give green color.

Experiment	Observation	Inference
Tests for proteins		
• **Sulfosalicyclic acid test:** 3 mL of urine in a test tube. Add 1 mL of sulfosalicyclic acid and mix.	Formation of white ppt	Proteins present
• **Heller's nitric acid test:** 3 mL of conc.HNO_3 in a test tube. Add 3 mL of urine by touching inside wall of test tube.	Formation of a white ring at the junction of two liquids	Proteins or phosphates present

Buffers and Biochemical Tests

Experiment	Observation	Inference
• **Heat and acetic acid test:** 10 mL of urine in a test tube and heat the upper column. Acidify the urine by adding few drops of dil.acetic acid.	Coagulum or ppt appears	Confirms the presence of proteins
Test for reducing sugars: • **Benedict's test :** 5 mL of Benedict's reagent in a test tube and boil. Then and 8 drop of given urine. Boil again and cool under tap water.	Formation of colored ppt. (green 0.5%, yellow 1%, orange 1.5%, red 2%)	Reducing sugar present
Test for ketone bodies • **Rothera's test** (for acetone and acetoacetic acid) 5 mL of urine in a test tube and saturate with ammonium sulfate. Then add 2–3 drops of sodium nitroprusside solution and 1 mL of liquor ammonia dropwise by the inside wall of test tube.	Appearance of permanganate ring at the junction of the two liquids	Ketone bodies present
• **Gerhardt's test:** 3 mL of urine in a test tube + few drops of 10% ferric chloride solution.	Red color is formed	Acetoacetic acid present
Test for blood: • **Benzidine glacial acetic acid test:** 2 mL benzidine glacial acetic acid and 2 mL of hydrogen peroxide solution and divide into two parts: ➢ One part add equal amount of urine ➢ Another part add equal amount of water	Formation of blue or green color. Stable only for few minutes then changes to brown	Blood present
Test for bile salts • **Hay's sulfur powder test:** 3 mL of urine in a test tube and sprinkle small quantity of sulfur powder without shaking.	Sulfur powder sinks to the bottom	Bile salts present
Tests for bile pigments • **Gmellin's test:** 3 mL conc. HNO_3 in a test tube. Add 2 mL of urine and just shake the test tube.	Play of colors are seen	Bile pigments present
• **Fouchet's test:** 10 mL of urine in a test tube and 3–4 mL of barium chloride solution+ 1–2 drops of ammonium sulfate. Filter and dry the ppt. between the folds of the filter paper. Then add 1–2 drops of fouchet's reagent on the ppt.	Formation of green color	Bile pigments present

DETERMINATION OF CREATININE CONTENT IN URINE, CALCULATION OF CREATININE CLEARANCE

Principle: Creatinine in urine is determined by its reaction with picric acid in alkaline medium to form orange colored tautomer of creatinine picrate. Since creatinine content of urine is high, it is suitable diluted. Equal volume of diluted urine, standard and blank is treated with picric acid and NaOH. The intensity of orange color is read using green filter (540 nm). The concentration of creatinine is calculated for 100 mL.

Procedure: Dilute 5 mL of urine in 50 mL volumetric flask. Label three test tubes as B, S, T. add 5 mL of distilled water into B and 5 mL standard into S. Pipette 5 mL of diluted urine into T. To each, add 2 mL of picric acid solution and 2 mL of 0.75 M NaOH. Mix and read optical density (OD) after 15 min;

Serum creatinine in mg/dL =
$$\frac{\text{OD of T} - \text{OD of B}}{\text{OD of S} - \text{OD of B}} \times 100$$

If the urine output per day is 1500 mL then creatinine is:

Serum creatinine in mg/dL =
$$\frac{OD \text{ of } T - OD \text{ of } B}{OD \text{ of } S - OD \text{ of } B} \times 100 \times \frac{15}{1000} \text{ g}$$

Clearance Test

Creatinine Clearance Test

It is the volume of plasma completely cleared off creatinine which is excreted in the urine.
Formula UV/P or UV/P × 173/A
U = Urine creatinine
P = Plasma
1.73 = generally accepted body surface area
A = Body surface area of the patient, under investigation.

The creatinine clearance is very convenient to measure GFR.

It fulfils all the requirement of the substance which is ideal for measuring GFR.

The amount of creatinine produced is relatively constant and also it is not affected by the dietary intake.

Normal values:
Males 105 ± 20 mL/min.
Female 95 ± 20 mL/min.
Abnormal results are lower than normal GFR measurements, and they indicate:
- Acute tubular necrosis
- Congestive heart failure
- Dehydration
- Glomerulonephritis
- Shock
- Acute nephrotic syndrome
- Acute and chronic renal failure.

ESTIMATION OF PLASMA PROTEINS

Determination of serum protein, albumin, globulin and their ratio by Biuret method:

Principle

Proteins react with the Biuret reagent to form a violet colored complex, which has a maximum absorbance at 540–560 nm. Biuret reagent consists of cupric ions (Cu^{2+}) which react with the N atoms of the peptide bonds of peptides and proteins, in an alkaline medium (presence of peptide bonds is the minimum requirement). The density of the purple color is directly proportional to the concentration of protein.

Biuret reagent consists of copper sulfate, sodium hydroxide, sodium potassium-tartrate and potassium iodide.
- The NaOH provides alkalinity to the solution
- Sodium potassium tartarate keeps the Cu^{2+} ions in solution.
- The conversion of Cu^{2+} to Cu^+ ions are prevented by potassium iodide.

Reagents

1. Sodium chloride, 0.9 percent.
   Dissolve 900 mg of sodium chloride in 80 mL of water and make up to 100 mL.
2. 0.2 N sodium hydroxide.
   Dissolve 8 g of sodium hydroxide in about 400 mL of water in a litre flask. Make up to one litre.
3. Biuret reagent: Dissolve 45 g of sodium potassium tartarate in 400 mL of 0.2 N sodium hydroxide (Reagent 2). Add 15 g of copper sulfate stirring continuously. Add 5 g of potassium iodide.
   Dissolve and make up to one litre with 0.2 N sodium hydroxide. This is the stock Biuret reagent. Store in a polythene bottle. It is stable for months.
4. 0.2 N sodium hydroxide containing 5 g of potassium iodide per litre. Add 5 g of potassium iodide per litre to Reagent 2 and dissolve.
5. Biuret reagent for use:
   Dilute 50 mL of stock Biuret reagent (Reagent 3) to 250 mL with 0.2 N sodium hydroxide containing 5 g potassium iodide per litre (Reagent 4).
6. Standard protein solution 6 mg/mL:
   Dissolve 714.3 mg of Bovine albumin and 100 mg of sodium azide used as preservative in 100 mL water. Store at 4°C.

7. **Sodium sulfite 28 percent:**
   Dissolve 28 gm of anhydrous sodium sulfite in about 70 mL of water. Make up to 100 mL.
8. Ether, AR grade.

Procedure

Reagents	B	S	A	Tp
Sodium sulfate, 28%	–	–	5.8 mL	–
Serum	–	–	0.2 mL	–
Ether	–	–	2.0 mL	–
Mix gently, centrifuge for 5 minutes. Aspirate and discard the ether layer. Pipette the lower layer for albumin estimation				
Supernatant	–	–	3.0 mL	–
Sodium chloride, 0.9%	3.0 mL	2.0 mL	–	2.9 mL
Serum (mL)	–	–	–	0.1
Standard protein solution	–	1.0 mL	–	–
Biuret reagent for use (mL)	3.0	3.0	3.0	3.0

Mix. Stand for 10 minutes
OD at 540 nm or green filter

Calculation

G of total proteins/100 mL =
$$\frac{T-B}{S-B} \times \frac{100}{Serum} \times \text{concentration of standard}$$

G of TP/100 mL taken = $\frac{T-B}{S-B} \times \frac{100}{0.1} \times 6 \times \frac{1}{1000}$

G of albumin /100 mL =
$$\frac{T-B}{S-B} \times \frac{\text{Total solution}}{\text{Taken solution}} \times \text{conc.} \frac{100}{\text{Serum taken}}$$

$$= \frac{T-B}{S-B} \times \frac{6}{3} \times 6 \times \frac{100}{0.2} \times \frac{1}{1000}$$

Globulins = Total proteins – Albumin.

A: G ratio is obtained by dividing albumin by globulin level.

For example, Say, Albumin = 4 g%, Globulin = 2 g%. Then, A:G Ratio = 4/2 = 2:1.

Note: When calculating for A: G ratio always globulin is always considered as one.

Clinical Significance

The change in the plasma protein value takes place either due to change in albumin or the globulin fraction. A reduced plasma protein level is mainly due to a decrease in albumin levels. Whereas, increased total protein is usually due to an increase in the globulin levels.

The conditions in which albumin are reduced are:

1. Nephrotic syndrome (more protein is excreted in urine).
2. Burns (dehydration).
3. Severe blood loss.
4. Reduced synthesis of proteins in liver diseases like cirrhosis of liver, hepatitis.
5. Impaired digestion and absorption of proteins as in peptic ulcer, carcinoma of stomach, cancer of pancreas and intestinal diseases, etc.
6. Increased breakdown of proteins as seen in fever, acute infections, untreated diabetes mellitus and hyperthyroidism.
7. Due to protein malnutrition (insufficient dietary protein intake).
8. In liver diseases like cirrhosis, albumin is decreased and globulin is increased.
9. Increased globulin levels are seen in few conditions like multiple myeloma, infections.

Index

Page numbers followed by *b* refer to box, *f* refer to figure, and *t* refer to table.

A

Acetaldehyde 177
Acetanilide 482
Acetate buffer 530
Acetazolamide 24
Acetic acid 146, 179
Acetoacetic acid 38
Acetylation 483
Acid
  base 531
    analysis, assessment of 254
    balance 246, 247, 250, 251*f*, 391
    disorders 251, 252, 254
    disturbances 252*t*
    homeostasis 246*s*
  phosphatase 27, 29, 515
  production of 251
Acidemia 250
Acidic amino acids 43
Acidic chyme 153
Acidosis
  chronic respiratory 254
  diabetic 442
Acquired immunodeficiency syndrome 444, 451
  biochemistry of 444
  diagnosis of 449
  factors influencing transmission of 444
  prevention of 449
  symptoms of 445*f*
  treatment for 450
Actinomycin D 472
Acyl carrier protein 163
Acylation 365, 483
Addison's disease 235, 400, 441, 435, 442
  diagnosis of 235

Adenine
  nucleotide of 330
  phosphoribosyltransferase 341
Adenoma 233
Adenosine
  deaminase, clinical significance of 344
  diphosphate 14, 15, 261, 262, 264, 270, 274, 331, 341, 344, 345, 423
  phosphorylation of 259
  monophosphate 14, 329, 331, 338, 340-342, 421, 472
  triphosphate 14, 15, 54, 93, 158, 194, 259, 261-264, 270, 274, 331, 341, 344, 345, 392, 416, 421, 423
  hydrolysis 425
  synthesis of 211, 261*f*
  structure of 13, 14, 14*f*, 331*f*
Adenovirus 445
Adipocytes 229
Adiponectin 201, 200, 325
  functions 200
  role of 201
Adipose tissue 155, 176, 196
  hormones 200
  fate of triacylglycerol in 155
Adrenal gland 399
  histology of 399*f*
  hormones 233
Adrenal insufficiency 235, 400
Adrenal medulla 237, 402
  functions 238
  secretes 237
  tumor of 238
Adrenaline 122, 238, 402

Adrenocorticotropic hormone 231, 234, 399, 400
  stimulation test 400
Adriamycin 363, 472
Aerobic glycolysis 96
  energetics of 100
  reactions of 96
Alanine 39, 169
  aminotransferase 387
  transaminase 218, 387, 390, 515
Albinism 75
Albumin 44, 268, 388, 514, 515
  estimation 388
  functions of 44
Alcohol 86, 142
  consumption 188
  effects of 179, 179*f*
  metabolism 177, 387
Aldehydes 481
Aldolase 118
Aldoses, oxidation of 85
Aldosterone 237, 401, 437, 438, 527
  deficiency 441
  function of 237
Alemtuzumab 472
Alkalemia 251
Alkali
  action of 85
  denaturation test 223*t*
Alkaline
  phosphatase 27, 28, 218, 387, 390, 467, 515
  urine, maintenance of 73
Alkalosis, chronic 250
Alkaptonuria 66, 67, 75
  causes of 67
  clinical symptoms of 67
Allopurinol 24, 343
Allosteric enzyme 26, 159

Alpha-fetoprotein 467-469, 515, 527
Alpha-helix structure 42*f*
Alpha-ketoglutarate dehydrogenase complex 294
Alpha-radiation 477
Amacrine cells 503
Amethopterin 24, 343, 454
  action of 24*f*
Amiloride 441
Amines 482
Amino acid 35, 37-39, 39*f*, 53, 54, 56, 59*t*, 74, 74*t*, 194, 220, 230, 268, 362, 393
  absorption of 54
  activation of 362
  carbon skeleton of 38, 59, 59*f*
  charge properties of 40
  chemical properties of 38
  classification of 38*f*
  decarboxylases 60
  degradation 194
  detection of 38
  essential 38, 65
  glucogenic 38, 39*t*, 59, 107*f*, 169
  ketogenic 39*t*
  metabolism of 53, 55, 59, 60, 71, 71*f*, 296
  nonessential 37, 58
  oxidative deamination of 387
  paper chromatography of 525*f*
  pool 55*f*
  proteins, chemistry of 35
  quantifying 38
  tyrosine 238
Amino alcohol sphingosine 143, 170
Amino group 35
  removal of 55
Amino sugars 87
Aminoaciduria 393
  primary 393
  secondary 393
Aminolevulinic acid synthase 296
Aminopterin 24, 343
  action of 24*f*

Ammonia 482, 517
  tests for 533, 534
Amphetamine 482
Amphotericin B 440
Amylase 29, 515
  clinical significance 29
Amyloidosis 498, 499
Amylopectin 81, 82*t*
Amylose 81, 82*t*
Anaerobic glycolysis 99
  energetics of 100
Anaplerotic reactions 105*f*
Anderson' disease 114
Anemia 292, 301, 393, 394
  hypochromic microcytic 279, 296
Anesthesia 255
Angiopathy 127
Anion gap 254, 514
Anomerism 83
Anorexia 294
Antagonists 297
Anthropometry 318
  advantages of 320
  disadvantages of 320
Antibiotic 440
  trimethoprim 441
Antibody 501, 526
  agar plates' radial immunodiffusion method 497
  anticardiolipin 517
  antinuclear 517
  antithyroglobulin 397
  primary 378*f*
  production, mechanism of 497, 497*f*
  secondary 379
Anticancer agents 454, 471, 472*t*
Antidiuretic hormone 231, 272, 434
Antigen 494, 526
Antimetabolites 471
Antioxidants 149, 486, 486*f*, 488, 492
  biochemistry of 486
  enzymatic 489
Antioxidation, chain-breaking 490*f*
Antithyroid peroxidase 397
Antitrypsin 45

Antiviral therapy 450
Apoenzyme 16
Apolipoprotein 172
Apoproteins 144, 174
Apoptosis 457, 458*f*
Appetite 202, 325
Arabidopsis thaliana 489
Arachidonic acid 146, 147, 180
Argentaffinoma 69
Arginase 57
Arginine 72
  catabolism of 64*f*
  fates of 64, 64*f*
  metabolism of 64
  synthesis of 64*f*
Argininosuccinase 57
Argininosuccinic acid synthetase 57
Ariboflavinosis 294
  signs of 294*f*
  symptoms of 294*f*
Arthritis 184
  rheumatoid 235
Ascorbic acid 291, 300
Asparagine 36, 54
  metabolism of 63
Aspartame 202
Aspartate
  aminotransferase 26, 204, 218, 387
  transaminase 56, 387, 390, 515
Aspartic acid 36, 63
  metabolism of 63
Asthma 235
Astrocytes 447
Astrovirus 445
Ataxia 293
  telangiectasia syndrome 355
Atherosclerosis 118, 127, 202, 203
  risk factors for 127, 203
Atom, structure of 475*f*
Atrial natriuretic peptide 272, 273
Autism 296
Autocrine signals 459
Autosomal recessive disorders 183
Azaserine 343
Azathioprine 333

Azidothymidine 334
Azilsartan 472

B

Barbiturates 481
Bartter syndrome 441
Basal metabolic rate 311-313
   calculation of 313
Basophil count 517
Becker muscular dystrophy 426
Beer's law 520
Bence-Jones proteins 47, 499
Benedict's test 87, 533-535
Benzidine glacial acetic acid test 534, 535
Benzoic acid, detoxification of 297
Beriberi
   cerebral 293
   dry 293
   infantile 293, 294
Beta-aminoisobutyricaciduria 346
Beta-carotene 490
Beta-human chorionic gonadotropin 515
Beta-oxidation, regulation of 158
Beta-radiation 477
Beta-thalassemia, types of 221
Bevacizumab 472
Bicarbonate 138, 437
Bicarbonate buffer system 248
   mechanism 248
Bile acid 147, 387
   synthesis 167
      clinical significance of 167
Bile duct
   cirrhosis of 388
   common 388
Bile pigments, tests for 535
Bile salts
   synthesis of 297
   tests for 535
Biliary tract
   cells 387f
   involvement 388
Bilirubin 387, 388, 490
   conjugated 218
   formation of 216f, 389, 389f
   indirect 217
   metabolism of 389
   transport 216
Biochemical pathways, number of 481
Biogenic amines 60
Biosynthesis 161
Biotin 17, 296, 301
Bipolar cells 503
   types of 503
Blood 218, 390, 444
   borne pathogens 446
   buffer system 247
   calcium 267
   cholesterol, high 186
   gas
      analyzer 255, 255f
      arterial 441
   glucose 123
      regulation of 101f, 106, 121, 124
   pH, regulation of 249
   pressure 271
      high 236, 401
      regulation of 181
      regulation of 122f
   sugar
      random 121
      regulation, fasting 121
   tests 514, 535
   transfusion 444
   urea nitrogen 514
   vessel disease 186
   volume of 271
Bloom syndrome 355
Blue pigment 506
B-lymphocytes 447
Body
   fluids 450
   surface area 312
   temperature 312
   water 433
Bohr effect 213f
Bone 233, 269
Bradyopsia 506
Brain 196, 197, 435
   cells of 307
   natriuretic peptide 273
Breast
   development of 240
   milk 239, 444
Breastfeeding 312, 444
Buffers 530
   and biochemical tests 530
   intracellular 250
   solutions 530
Bulimia 441
Bulk elements 267
Burkitt's lymphoma 446
Busulfan 471
Butyric acid 146

C

Calcitonin 268
   action of 269
Calcium 267, 368, 393, 514, 517
   complexes 268
   effect of 112
   element 267
   functions of 268
   ionized 268
   ions 53, 420, 424
   reabsorption of 288
   regulation 233f
   tests for 532, 533
Cancer 452, 457, 465, 473, 491, 492
   antigen 468
   biochemistry of 452
   causes of 452
   cell 470
      production 452f
   cervical 446
   colon 311
   colorectal 469
   common causes of 457
   control of 24
   development of 452
   early detection of 468
   endometrial 311
   forming agents 464
   gastrointestinal 469
   genetics of 453
   risk factors for 454
   therapy, biochemical basis of 470
Candesartan 472
Captopril 24
Carbaminohemoglobin 224
Carbamoyl phosphate
   synthetase 344

Carbenicillin 440
Carbohydrates 80, 87, 88, 91,
    305-307, 326, 387
  absorption of 91, 93f
  caloric value of 306, 306f
  chemistry of 80
  classification of 80
  complex 307
  dietary 94
  digestion of 91, 92f
  isomerism in 83
  metabolism 91, 94, 126, 196,
    197
    effects on 122
    hormonal regulation of
      197
    regulation of 198
  nutritional importance of
    307
  optical activity of 83
  reduction tests 87
  tests for 87
Carbon
  dioxide 155, 194, 210, 210f,
    247, 290
    volume of 306
  monoxide 481
  skeleton, part of 38
  tetrachloride 176, 481
Carbonic acid 212, 247
Carbonic anhydrase 249, 251
Carboplatin 471
Carboxyhemoglobin 223
Carboxypeptidase 54
Carcinoembryonic antigen 466,
    467, 469, 515
Carcinogenesis 491
Carcinogens 462, 464
Cardiac disease 230
Cardiac enzymes 204
  pattern of 28f
Cardiac glycosides 87
Cardiac muscle 416, 422, 424
  contraction 423f
  control of 423
Cardiolipin 142
Cardiomyopathy 187
Cardiovascular disease 203, 397
  risk of 185, 186
Cardiovascular disorders,
    development of 188
Carmustine 471

Carotenoids 490
Catabolism 55, 59, 63, 70
Catalase 277, 489
Catalytic receptor 461
Cataract 507f
Catecholamine 67, 518
  diagnosis of 68
  formation of 68f
  hormones 422
  synthesis of 67
  synthetic pathway, oxidase
    of 279
Cell 1, 454
  cycle 454, 455, 457
    control of 456
    purpose of 455
    regulation of 456, 457t
    stages of 455, 455f
  death of 458, 491
  deletion 458, 455
  division cycle 454
  fractionation 8
  growth 457
    abnormal 457
    causes of uncontrollable
      457
  membrane 1
  normal 1
  organelles 1, 2f, 9
  produce enzymes 26
  proliferation 453f, 457, 491
  signaling 459
  structure of 1f
  subcellular fractionation
    of 9f
  surface receptors 461
  types of 4
Cellular respiration 421
Cellulose 81
  acetate electrophoresis 222f
Central nervous system 68, 246,
    276, 446, 447
Centrifugation 521
  applications of 522
Centrioles 4
Ceramide 143
Cerebrosides 143
Cerebrospinal fluid 433, 518
  tests 518
Ceruloplasmin 45, 278, 490
Cetuximab 472
Chaulmoogric acid 147

Checkpoints 456
Cheilosis 295
Chemical
  coupling hypothesis 263
  indicators 531
  reaction 13, 482
Chemiluminescence method
    395
Chemiosmosis 263
Chemiosmotic hypothesis 263,
    263f, 264f
Chemo drugs, action of 470f
Chemotherapy 470
Chlorambucil 454, 471
Chloramphenicol 363
Chloride 267, 276, 437, 442, 514,
    517
  dietary 276
  functions of 276, 442
  high serum 276
  ions 276
  shift 214f, 249
  tests for 532, 533
Cholecalciferol 287, 288
Cholecystokinin 53, 91, 153
Cholestasis, intrahepatic 388
Cholesterol 147, 148, 164, 167,
    288, 310, 514
  biosynthesis, regulation of
    166
  estimation, clinical
    significance of 203
  functions of 148
  high-density level 186
  metabolic fate of 167
  metabolism 164
    hormonal regulation of
      200
  structure of 147f
  synthesis 165f
    regulation of 166, 166f
  transport, reverse 174f
Cholesteryl ester 174
  transfer protein 174
Cholinesterase 29
Chondroitin sulfate 82, 411
Chromatography 523, 524
  adsorption 524, 525f
  affinity 526, 526f
  classification of 524
  general principle of 524
  types of 524f

Chromium 282
  toxicity 282
Chylomicron 171, 174
  composition 171*f*
  remnant 172
  transport of 172*f*
Chymosin 53
Chymotrypsin 54
Cirrhosis 44, 388, 469, 498
Cisplatin 471, 472
Cistron 366
Citrate 268, 517
Citric acid 103
Cobalamin 299, 301
Cobalt 281
  toxicity 281
Cockayne syndrome 355
Coenzyme 17
  common 17*t*
  Q 261
  ubiquinone 262, 263
Cohn's syndrome 402
Collagen 44*f*, 407
  structure of 408*f*
  synthesis 291
  types of 407
Color vision 506
  visual pigments for 506
Colorimetry 519, 528
  principle of 519
Coma 435
Competitive inhibition
  technique 23, 23*f*
  therapeutic use of 23
Compound lipids 140, 141
Conjugation 483-485
Constipation 441
Convulsions 294
Copper 278
  deficiency 279*b*
  excess 279
Coproporphyria, hereditary 216
Cori cycle 108, 109*f*, 247
Corneal vascularization 295
Corticotropin-releasing
    hormone 234, 400
  stimulation test 401
Cortisol 121, 527
  release of 234*f*
  secretion, control of 234, 399
  synthesis of 400*f*
C-reactive protein 46

Creatine 74
  kinase 43, 204, 515
  phosphate 421
  phosphokinase 205
  synthesis of 74, 74*f*
Creatinine 392, 514, 517
  clearance test 391, 534, 536
Cretinism 232
Crigler-Najjar syndrome 215, 219
Crohn's syndrome 237
Cryoglobulinemia 499
Cryptococcus neoformans 445
Cunningham virus 446
Cushing's syndrome 236, 236*f*, 237, 400, 401, 441
Cyanmethemoglobin 224
Cyanocobalamin 17
Cyclic adenosine
    monophosphate 156, 228, 268, 330
Cyclic guanosine
    monophosphate 332, 505
Cyclophosphamide 454, 471, 472
Cystathionase deficiency 73
Cystathionine
  alpha-synthase 296
  gamma-lyase 296
Cystathioninuria 73
Cysteine 36, 39, 72
Cystinuria 72
Cystitis 394
Cytarabine 334
Cytidine monophosphate 171, 329, 338
Cytochrome 261, 262, 277
  oxidase 261, 279
Cytomegalovirus 445
Cytoplasm 228
Cytosine
  arabinoside 334, 454
  nucleotides 331
  triphosphate 331, 345

D

Dacarbazine 471
Dansyl chloride 39
Decarboxylases 296
  catalyze 60
Decarboxylation 60

Dehydration 392, 393, 435, 442
  causes of 435
  treatment for 436
Dehydrocholesterol 288
Dementia 185, 311
Deoxy sugar 87
Deoxyhemoglobin 223
  polymerization of 222*f*
Deoxypyridoxine 296
Deoxyribonucleic acid 228, 268, 288, 349, 352, 363, 382, 446, 472, 477
  amplification, artificial 370
  libraries 381
  repair 354
  structure of 335, 335*f*, 349*f*
Depression 296, 311
Dermatansulfate 82, 411
Dermatitis 301
Detoxification 297, 481-483
Dexamethasone 237
  suppression test 236, 237, 401
Dextrin 81
Diabetes insipidus 231, 435
Diabetes mellitus 124, 187, 435, 499, 506
  clinical complications of 126
  complications 202
  diagnosis of 126, 202
  gestational 126
  insulin-dependent 124
  metabolic changes 126, 202
  noninsulin-dependent 124
  signs 124
  symptoms 124
  types 124, 202
  uncontrolled 168
Diacylglycerol 142
Diamine oxidase 279
Diarrhea 94, 440, 442, 445
Diazo-norleucine 343
Dietary iron
  absorption of 278*f*
  transport of 278*f*
Dihydropyridine drugs 424
Dihydroxyacetone phosphate 96, 170
Diisopropylphosphofluoride 25
Dimercaptopropanol 262
Dipalmitoyl lecithin 140, 142

Dipalmitoyl
	phosphatidylcholine 143
Dipalmitoyl phosphatidyletha-
	nolamine 143
Dipalmitoyl phosphatidylserine
	143
Dipeptide 39
	formation 39
Disaccharides 81, 81*t*
Distal renal tubular acidosis 394
Disulfide linkages 42
Diverticulosis 310
Dopamine 279, 402
	synthesis of 67
Double antibody method 527
	principle of 527*f*
Down's syndrome, treatment
	of 296
Doxorubicin 454
Drug therapy 23
Dry beriberi 293
	symptoms of 293*f*
Dubin-Johnson syndrome 219
Duchenne muscular dystrophy
	359, 426
Dysrhythmias 441

E

Eating disorders 441
Ectopic adrenocorticotropic
	hormone syndrome 400
Edema 294, 439
Eicosanoids 180, 228
Elastase 54
Elastin 409
Electrolyte 436
	balance 432, 436
		regulation of 391
	distribution of 436
Electromagnetic spectrum 519,
	520*f*
Electron transport chain 179,
	260, 261*f*, 262*f*
	inhibitors of 261
	organization of 260
	reactions of 260
Electrophoresis 47, 523
	general principle of 523
	principle of 523*f*
	types of 523

Embden-Meyerhof-Parnas
	pathway 96
Emphysema 45
Enalapril 24
Endocrine
	glands location 229*f*
	signals 459
	system 459
Endocytosis 8, 173*f*
	process of 8*f*
Endometriosis 469
Endopeptidases 54
Endoplasmic reticulum 1, 2,
	2*f*, 9
Energy
	consumption 14
	expenditure 311
	releasing 14
Enkephalins 40
Enoic acid 145
Enterokinase 54
Enzyme 16, 26, 41, 55, 96
	activities of 14, 18
	catalysis, mechanism of 20
	catalyzed reaction 21
	chemical nature of 16
	classification of 19
	concentration, effect of 19,
		19*f*
	creatine kinase 204
	defect 412
	duplication of 358*f*
	extracellular 16
	extramitochondrial 165
	inhibition 23
	intracellular 16
	kinetics 21
	linked immunosorbent assay
		395, 478, 479*f*, 527
		applications of 528
	specificity 20
	synthesis, insulin-mediated
		124
	systems 489
		components of 267
Eosinophil count 517
Eosinophilia 236
Epidermal cells 460
Epidermal growth factor 460
	receptor 472
Epididymis, function of 240

Epimerism 84
Epinephrine 67, 198, 238, 402,
	421, 482
	synthesis of 67
Epithelial cells 460
Eprosartan 472
Epstein-Barr virus 446, 453, 465
Erythrocyte
	hemolysis of 289
	sedimentation rate 396
Erythroid cells 215
Erythromycin 363
Erythropoietic protoporphyria
	216
Erythropoietin 460
Escherichia coli 426, 368*f*
Esophagitis 445
Estradiol 516
Estriol 518
Estrogen 240
	receptor 469
Ethanolamine 142
Etoposide 472
Eukaryotic cell 4, 5, 5*f*, 368
	cytoplasm of 5
	gene regulation 369*f*
Excretory function test 393
Exocytosis 8
Exon 366
	gene 366
Exopeptidase 54
External beam radiotherapy 473
External quality control
	program 513
Extracellular matrix 407, 410
Eye, structure of 503, 503*f*

F

Fabry disease 182-184
Fanconianemia 355, 356
Fanconi syndrome 441
Farber's disease 182, 184
Farber's lipogranulomatosis 184
Fatigue 439, 441, 442
Fats 306, 308
	caloric value of 306, 306*f*
	cells 229
	metabolism 126
		hormonal regulation of
			198, 199, 199*f*

Fatty acid 142, 145-147, 157, 268
  alcohol sphingosine 143
  cis 147
  classification of 146
  de novo synthesis of 161
  essential 37, 140, 146, 147, 308
  functions of 147
  medium-chain 187
  metabolism, regulation of 159f
  nomenclature 145
  numbering of 146
  oxidation of 157, 194
  synthase 162
    enzyme complex 162f
  synthesis, steps of 163f
  trans 147
  unsaturated 146
Fatty liver 175, 175f, 176
  causes of 176
  prevent 147
  severe 176, 176f
  symptoms of 176
Favism 117
Ferritin 41, 277, 278, 490, 515
Fiber 307, 309, 310
Fibrillin 409
Fibrinogen 46
Fibroblasts, inhibition of 460
Fibroids 468
Fibronectin 410
Flavin
  adenine dinucleotide 102, 158, 260, 261, 262, 264, 294
  mononucleotide 260, 262, 263, 294
Flavoproteins 260
Floxuridine 334
Fludarabine 333
Fluid
  balance 433, 435t
    regulation of 391, 433, 434f
  depletion 435
  distribution 433
  extracellular 267, 423, 432, 436, 437
  input 433f
  intake 322

mosaic model 6
  output 433f
Fluoride 281
  excess 282
Fluorouracil 334, 472
Folacin 300
Folate
  deficiency of 321
  trap 299
Folic acid 17, 297, 300, 301, 321
Follicle-stimulating hormone 227, 230, 517
Food
  dairy technique 321
  products, digestion of 93
  stuffs, respiratory quotient of 306
Formamide 377
Formiminoglutamic acid 75, 298
  excretion test 298
Formylmethionine 71
Foscarnet 440
Fouchet's test 534, 535
Fragile blood vessels 292
Fragile X syndrome 359
Fredrickson's classification 174
Free fatty acid 144f
Free radicals 486, 486f, 492
  biochemistry of 486
  formation of 486
Fructosazone 86
Fructose
  intolerance 118
  metabolism 118, 119f
Fueling muscle contraction 420
Fumaric acid 57
Fungal rashes 311
Futile cycle 112

G

G protein 461
Gag linkage, structure of 413f
Galactose
  fates of 118
  metabolism 117, 118f
Galactosemia 117
  signs 117
  symptoms 117

Gallstones 311, 388
Gamma-aminobutyric acid 58
Gamma-glutamyl transferase 29, 218, 388, 390
  clinical significance 29
Gamma-glutamyl transpeptidase 390, 515
Gamma-radiation 477
Ganglion cells 503
Gangliosides 143
Gas 310
  liquid chromatography 525
Gastric
  acidity 268
  juice 92
  ulcer, prevention of 181
Gastrointestinal infections 445
Gastrointestinal loss 440
Gastrointestinal tract 233
  digestion in 92f
  enzymes of 92t
  proteins in 53
Gaucher's disease 143, 182
Gel filtration 46
  chromatography 526, 526f
Gemcitabine 334
Gene 366, 370, 465
  amplification 370
  expression of 366, 369
  rearrangement 371
  regulation 366, 368
  sequencing 500
Genetic code 362
Genome organization 448
Genomics 350, 351
Gentamicin 440
Gerhardt's test 534, 535
Ghrelin 325
Gilbert's syndrome 215, 219
Gland, enlarged 232
Globulin 45, 388, 514, 515
  estimation 388
  types of 45
Glomerular filtration rate 139, 391
Glomerulonephritis 392
  acute 392, 393
  chronic 393
Glossitis 295, 296, 299
Glucagon 121, 198, 200, 238
  action of 125f

functions 238
mechanism of action of 124
Glucocorticoid 177, 198, 122, 200, 234, 235, 240
  secretion, assessment of 399
Glucogenic lipid 109f
Glucokinase 99t, 197
Gluconeogenesis 94, 106, 106f, 387
  regulation of 107, 107f
  substrates for 108, 108f
Glucosazone 86
Glucose 94, 95f, 110, 110f
  6-phosphate 96, 110
    dehydrogenase 29, 116, 271, 516
  alanine cycle 108, 109f
  formation of 109f
  phenylhydrazine 86
  production, effect on 123
  starvation 368
  tolerance 129
    abnormal 129
    curve 129
    test 127, 128, 129, 129f, 129t
  transport, insulin-mediated 123
Glucuronic acid 85, 483, 485
  metabolism 120f
Glucuronidation 484
Glutamate 169
  compounds formed from 62
  dehydrogenase 56
  fates of 63f
  metabolic fate of 62
Glutamic acid 36, 58, 62, 221
Glutamine 36, 484
  formation of 58
Glutathione 39, 180, 489
  conjugation 483
  disulfide 180
  systems 489
Glycemic index 310
Glycerol 147
  phosphate, acylation of 170
Glycerophospholipids 140, 142
  dietary 154
  synthesis of 170, 170f
Glycine 36, 39, 169, 408, 483, 484
  detoxifies benzoic acid 62

fates of 62f
metabolic fate of 62
metabolism of 61
Glycinuria 62, 74
Glycogen 81, 110, 113, 307, 421, 422
  lysosomal degradation of 112
  metabolism 110, 198f
    compounds of 112
    regulation of 113f, 199f
  storage diseases 113
  synthesis 110f
Glycogenesis 94, 110, 113f, 387
  regulation of 112
Glycogenin 110
Glycogenolysis 96, 111, 111f, 112, 112f, 113f, 387
  regulation of 112
Glycolipids 143
Glycolysis 94, 96, 107, 194, 506
  enzymes of 16
  reactions of 97f, 98f
  regulation of 100, 100f
Glycoprotein 41, 87
  hormones 227
Glycosaminoglycan 410, 411, 413
  functions of 410
  location of 411t
  metabolism, disorders of 412t
Glycosides 87
Glycosidic bond 86
Glycosuria 439
Glyoxylate cycle 105
Gmellin's test 535
Goiter 232, 318f, 395
Golgi apparatus 3f
Golgi complex 3
  functions 3
Golgi membrane 9
Gordon's syndrome 442
Gout 311, 343
  acute 393
  causes of 343
  symptoms of 343
G-protein receptor 461f
Granulocyte colony-stimulating factor 460
Graves' disease 232, 240, 396, 397

Growth
  factor 460, 460t, 465
    receptors 465
  hormone 122, 227, 229
    deficiency symptoms 229
    effects of 229f
Guanine, nucleotide of 331
Guanosine
  diphosphate 341, 363, 364
  monophosphate 329, 331, 340-342
  nucleotides, structure of 332f
  triphosphate 270, 340, 341, 363, 364

H

Haplotypes 501
Haptoglobin 45, 516
Harris-Benedict formula 313
Hartnup's disease 69, 75
Hashimoto's thyroiditis 232, 397
Hay's sulfur powder test 534, 535
Head circumference 318
Heart
  beats, irregular 187
  disease 187, 309, 311, 441, 492
    coronary 185
    ischemic 203
  failure 436
    congestive 392, 442
  muscle 416
  rhythms, abnormal 441
Heat and acetic acid test 534, 535
Heavy chain disease 498
Height measurement 318
Heller's nitric acid test 534
Hematocrit 517
Hematuria 393
Heme biosynthesis, regulation of 215
Heme catabolism 216
Heme metabolism, clinical aspects of 215
Heme molecule 215
Heme proteins 210, 276
Heme synthesis 213

Index

Hemoglobin 43, 209, 210, 211, 211*f*, 212, 223, 249, 277, 517
   abnormal 220, 222, 222*f*
   buffer
      action of 249
      system 249*f*
   catabolism, disorders of 217
   compounds 223
   electrophoresis of 222, 524
   normal 222*f*
   quaternary structure of 43*f*
   role of 219
   structure of 209, 209*f*, 212*f*
   synthesis 213, 214*f*
   types of 210
Hemoglobinopathy 220
Hemosiderin 277, 278
Henderson-Hasselbalch equation 246
Heparan sulfate 82, 411
Heparin 82, 411
Hepatic cells 387*f*
Hepatitis 498
   A virus 391
   B virus 391, 453
   C virus 391, 453
   D 391
   E virus 391
Hepatobiliary tree 387*f*
Heptahelical receptor 461
Herceptin 472
Hers disease 114
Heteropolysaccharides 82
Hexokinase 26, 99*t*
Hexose monophosphate 29, 115
   pathway 196
   shunt 94, 114
      regulation of 117
High-density lipoprotein 144, 173, 174, 514
   cholesterol 514
   composition of 173*f*
High-energy compounds 14
Hip circumference 320
Histidine 36, 54
   catabolism of 70*f*
   metabolism 69
Hodgkin's disease 45, 499
Hodgkin's lymphoma 465
Holoenzymes 16
Homocysteinemia 73

Homocystinuria 73, 75
   types of 73*f*
Homogentisic acid 66
Homopolysaccharides 81, 81*t*
Hormones 41, 201, 227, 237, 268, 387, 527
   amine-derived 227
   chemical classes of 227
   hyperglycemic 124
   hypoglycemic 121
   hypophyseal 228
   regulation by 121
   role of 122*f*
   sensitive lipase 156, 156*f*
Human body 481, 485
Human chorionic gonadotropin 467, 468
Human immunodeficiency virus 444, 448*f*
   infection, symptoms of 444
   molecular basis of 448
   structure of 448
   test 449
Human leukocyte antigen 499, 500
Human papillomavirus 446, 453
Human T-lymphotropic virus 453
Hunger, control of 325*f*
Hunter's syndrome 411, 412
Huntington's disease 359
Hurler's syndrome 411, 412
Hurler-Scheie syndrome 412
Hutchinson-Gilford progeria syndrome 355
Hyaline membrane disease 142
Hyaluronic acid 82, 410, 411
Hybrid protein 465
Hydrochloric acid 53, 277
Hydrochloride 363
Hydrogen 210, 259
   bonds 42, 43
   ion 260
      balance 247
Hydrolysis 482, 483
Hydrophilic heads 6
Hydroxyl radical 487
Hyperaldosteronism 441
Hyperbilirubinemia 219
   acquired 218
   congenital 219

Hypercalcemia 233, 269, 270*t*
Hyperchloremia 276, 276*b*, 442
Hypercholesterolemia 164, 175, 203
Hypergammaglobulinemia 498
Hyperglycemia 230, 236, 401, 507*f*
Hyperglycemic hyperosmolar nonketotic coma 127
Hyperkalemia 274, 275*b*, 441
   causes of 441
   signs of 442
   symptoms of 442
Hyperlipidemia 127
Hyperlipoproteinemias 174
Hypernatremia 274, 438, 439, 440*f*
   signs of 439
   symptoms of 439
Hyperoxaluria 62
Hyperparathyroidism 233
Hyperphoshatemia 270, 271, 271*b*
Hyperplasia
   benign prostatic 466
   congenital adrenal 441
Hyperthyroid diseases 232
Hyperthyroidism 395, 396
Hypertriglyceridemia 202
Hyperuricemia 343
Hypervitaminosis 287
Hypervolemia 436
   causes of 435, 436
   features of 436
   symptoms of 435
Hypoalbuminemia 44
Hypocalcemia 269, 269*t*
Hypochloremia 276, 276*b*, 442
   causes of 442
Hypocholesterolemia 203
Hypogammaglobulinemia 499
Hypoglycemia 235, 236
Hypokalemia 236, 275, 275*b*, 440
   mild 441
   symptoms of 441
Hypolipidemic drugs, use of 166
Hyponatremia 236, 274, 276, 438, 439
Hypoparathyroidism 233

Hypophosphatemia 270, 271, 271*b*
Hypothalamus 394
Hypothyroid diseases 232
Hypothyroidism 395-397
   primary 397
   secondary 397
Hypoventilation 253
Hypovolemia 435
   causes of 435
   symptoms of 435
Hypoxanthine-guanine phosphoribosyltransferase 341

I

Ibuprofen 441
Imatinib 472
Immune system, human 444
Immunity 287
   cellular 493, 494
   humoral 494
   types of 494
Immunodeficiency disease, severe combined 343
Immunoglobulin 43, 467, 494, 501
   A 496
   clinical importance of 498
   D 496
   E 496
   functions of 495
   G 496, 517
   M 496
   structure of 494, 495*f*
   types of 496
Immunology 493
Inactivated vaccines 494, 501
Infarction, size of 427
Inflammation, chronic 491
Inhibition
   noncompetitive 25*f*
   uncompetitive 26*f*
Inosine monophosphate 472
   synthesis of 341*f*
Insomnia 311
Insulin 40, 121, 122, 238, 527
   action of 177
   deficiency
      signs of 125*f*
      symptoms of 125*f*
   dephosphorylates 164
   functions 238
   inhibits 198
   like growth factor-1 460
   mechanism of action of 123
   metabolic effects of 122
   promotes 164
   receptor 123
   secretion, factors inhibiting 122
   stimulates glycogenesis 197
Internal quality control program 512
Intestine, digestion in 53
Intoxication 252
Intracellular fluid 272, 432, 436
Intravenous glucose tolerance test 130
Introns 366
   reason for removal of 366
Inulin 81
Iodine 282, 318*f*
   deficiency 282*b*
   number 149
Iodoacetamide 25
Ion exchange chromatography 525, 525*f*
Ionic interactions 43
Ionizing radiation 476, 487
   types of 477
Irbesartan 472
Iron 276, 318*f*, 322
   absorption 277, 277*t*
      mechanism of 277
   deficiency 279*b*, 322
      anemia 322
   functions of 276
   sulfur protein 261, 277
Irritability 296
Irritable bowel syndrome 309
Isoenzymes 26
Isoleucine 36
Isomerases 19
Isonicotinic acid hydrazide 296
   treatment 25
Isotope 475, 480

J

Jaffe's test 533, 534
Jamaican vomiting sickness 159
Jaundice 217, 389
   abstractive 220
   hemolytic 218, 389
   hepatic 219, 389
   intrahepatic 220
   neonatal 219
   obstructive 203, 219, 389
   physiologic 219
   posthepatic 219
   prehepatic 218, 220
   types of 218*t*, 390*t*
Juxtacrine signals 459

K

Kaposi's sarcoma 444, 446, 453
Keratan sulfate 82, 411
Keratomalacia 287
Keratosis, follicular 287
Ketoacid 55
Ketoacidosis 252
   diabetic 127, 252
   mild 139
Ketogenic amino acids 38, 59
Ketogenic substances 169
Ketolysis 168, 169*f*
Ketone body
   formation 168
   metabolism 167
   synthesis of 167, 168*f*
   tests for 535
   utilization of 168
Kidney 233, 250, 269, 435
   disease 233
   function tests 391
   pathological conditions of 393
   role of 251*f*
Korsakoff's psychosis 293
Krabbe disease 182, 185
Krebs citric acid cycle 103
Krebs TCA cycle, aconitase of 277
Krebs-Henseleit cycle 56
Kussmaul breathing 252
Kwashiorkor 323, 324*t*, 326
   symptoms of 324*f*
Kynureninase 296

L

Laboratory medicine 509
Lacrimal glands, keratinization of 287

Lactate dehydrogenase 26, 43, 204, 515
Lactic acid 178, 247
Lactic acidosis 130, 252
Lactose 268
   intolerance 93, 94, 120, 121*f*
      cause 120
      signs 120
      symptoms 120
   operon 367
Lactosuria 94
Lambert's law 520, 520*f*
Laminin 410
Lecithin 148, 166
Lecithin-cholesterol
      acyltransferase 174, 187
   role of 166
Leptin 200, 201, 325
   deficiency 325
   functions 201
   role of 201
Lesch-Nyhan syndrome 343
Lethargy 439
Leucine 36, 54, 59
Leukemia 393
   chronic lymphocytic 454
Leukocyte antigen typing 500
Leukotrienes 147, 182, 188
Liddle syndrome 440
Ligase 19
   chain reaction 370
Light 519
   absorption of 505
   chain disease 498
   dispersion of 519, 519*f*
   dual nature of 519
   meromyosin 417
   source of 520
   wavelength of 519
Lignoceric acid 146
Lineweaver-Burk plot 22*f*
Linoleic acid 146
   sources 308
Lipase 29
Lipemia 511
Lipid 305, 387
   absorption of 155*f*
   amphipathic nature of 148
   biomedical importance of 140
   chemistry of 140

classification of 140
derived 145
digestion and absorption of 153
digestion of 154*f*
functions of 140
peroxidation 487
profile 202
properties of 148
simple 140, 141
storage disorders 182
synthesis of 179
Lipid metabolism 153, 157, 196, 197
   effects on 123
   regulation of 177
Lipolysis 160
Lipoprotein 143, 144*t*, 145, 176, 203
   characteristics of 143
   clinical importance of 145
   electrophoresis 524
   functions of 174
   intermediate-density 172
   metabolism 171
   separation of 144*f*
   structure and function 143, 171
   structure of 143*f*
Lipotropic factors 177
Lips, fissuring of 295
Live-attenuated vaccines 494, 501
Liver 176, 195, 435
   cell damage 388
   disease 387-389, 498
   enzymes 26
   failure 58
   in lipid metabolism, role of 177, 178*f*
   in starvation 196
   metabolic functions of 196
   synthesizes clotting factors 388
Liver function test 387
   indications of 387
Lobe, intermediate 228
Lock-and-key model 20, 20*f*
Loose teeth 292
Losartan 472
Louis-Bar syndrome 355

Lovastatin 24
Low phosphate level 268
Low plasma calcium 288
Low-density lipoprotein 144, 172, 194, 515
   cholesterol 309
   composition of 173*f*
Low-protein diet 58
Lung
   disease 311
   infections 445
Luteinizing hormone 227, 230, 517
   role of 230
Lyases 19
Lymphocyte count 517
Lymphocytosis 236
Lymphoma 499
   diffuse large B-cell 446
Lymphoreticular system 447
Lysine 36
   metabolism of 63
Lysophospholipase enzyme 154
Lysophospholipid 154
Lysosomes 3, 9
   nuclear envelope 2
Lysyl oxidase 279

M

Macroglobulins 45
Macrominerals 267
Macronutrients 267, 305
   caloric value of 306
Macrophages and granulocytes 8
Magnesium 267, 270, 271, 441, 517
   deficiency 441
Malabsorption 294
Male infertility 491
Malnutrition 58, 294
Manganese 280
   deficiency 280
   excess 280
Mannosazone 86
Maple syrup urine disease 71
Marasmus 323, 324, 324*t*, 326
   features of 324*f*
Marfan's syndrome 410
Maroteaux-Lamy syndrome 411

Massive blood transfusion 442
Massive hemolysis 442
McArdle's disease 114
Mean corpuscular hemoglobin 517
   concentration 517
Mean corpuscular volume 517
Megaloblastic anemia 298, 299, 321
Melanin 67
   synthetic pathway, tyrosinase of 279
Melatonin 490
Membrane
   active transport 7
   functioning, carrier proteins of 7f
   lipid
      bilayer of 148f
      synthesis of 170
   passive transport 6
   receptors 461
   transport mechanisms in 6
   uniport, symport and antiport 7
Menadione 290
Menaquinone 289
Menkes syndrome 279
Menopause 239
Menstruation 468
Mental confusion 436
Mental retardation 67
Mental stress 234
Mercaptopurine 333, 472
Messenger ribonucleic acid 268, 361
   molecule 361f
   stability 371
   synthesis of 361f
Metabolic acid-base disorders 251
Metabolic acidosis 138, 139, 251, 252
   and alkalosis 252f
Metabolic acids 247
Metabolic alkalosis 251
Metabolic blocks 73f
Metabolic disorder 62, 72
Metabolic fate 56, 59f
Metabolic rate 311
   measurement of 312
Metabolic water production 434

Metabolism 181, 195f
   after meal, integration of 201f
   hormonal regulation of 197, 198f, 200f
   inborn errors of 74, 74t
   integration of 194, 195f, 197f
   pathways of 194
Metalloenzymes 17
Methemoglobin 223
Methemoglobinemia
   causes of 223
   hereditary 224
   types of 224
Methionine 36, 54, 71, 363
   metabolism of 72f
Methotrexate 24
Methoxypyridoxine 296
Methyladenine 329
Methylation 365, 483, 484
Methylcobalamin 299
Methylguanine 329
Methylmalonic aciduria 299
Mevinolin 24
Michaelis-Menten equation 21, 21f, 22, 23, 25
Microinfarction 427
Micronutrients 267, 305
Microsomal hydroxylase system 482
Mid-upper arm circumference 318
Mineral 267, 283
   essential 306
   functions of 283, 283t
   metabolism 267
Mineralocorticoid 237, 401
   deficiency 441
Mitochondria 2-4, 9, 147, 159
   structure of 260
Mitochondrial membrane 157
Mitochondrion 4f
   sarcosome for 416
Mitomycin C 363, 472
Mixed acid-base disorders 253, 254
   types 254
Molecular biology 349
Molybdenum 280
Monoamine oxidase 279
Monoclonal antibodies 472, 497
Monoclonal hypergamma-globulinemia 498

Monocyte
   colony-stimulating factor 460
   count 517
Monosaccharides 80, 80t, 85
   absorption of 93
   chemical properties of 85
   oxidation of 85
Monounsaturated fats, sources of 308
Monounsaturated fatty acid 146
Moon face 401
Morquio's syndrome 411, 412
Mouth
   corners of 295
   inflammation of 299
Mucopolysaccharides 82, 82t
   biomedical of 82
Mucosal cells 154
Multicellular organisms 1, 10
Multiple myeloma 47, 220, 498
   biochemical findings 47
Muscle 416, 428
   contraction 425
      energy sources for 421f
   damage 441
   diseases 426
   fiber 416, 421t
   function, biochemistry of 416
   glycogen of 422
   glycogenolysis 112
   structure, biochemistry of 416
   types of 416
Muscular dystrophy 359, 393, 426
Muscular weakness 289, 441, 436
Mutagen 462
Mutarotation 83
Mutation 356
Myasthenia gravis 393, 426
Mycobacterium tuberculosis 344
Myocardial infarction 28, 28f, 205f, 515
   acute 427
   cardiac enzymes in 27
   laboratory tests in 204
   subacute 427
Myoglobin 210, 211, 211f, 277
   structure of 211

Index

Myosin light chain kinase 423
Myxedema 203, 232

N

N-acetyl
  cysteine 484
  glutamate 56
Nafcillin 440
Nails, spooning of 318*f*
Naproxen 441
Nausea 436, 439
Neomycin 363
Neotame 202
Nephritic syndrome 44
Nephritis, chronic 392
Nephron, structure of 391*f*
Nephropathy 127
  diabetic 393
Nephrosclerosis 392
Nephrotic syndrome 44, 203, 393, 394, 499
  acute 392
Nerve growth factor 460
Nervous system
  cells of 307
  microglia of 447
Neurological symptoms 183
Neuromuscular junction 29, 418
Neuron 447
Neuronal cell types 503
Neuropathy 127
Neutralization 496
Neutrophil count 517
Niacin 17, 295, 300, 301
Nicotinamide 295, 300
  adenine dinucleotide 68, 96, 259-262, 264, 287, 290, 341, 342, 344
  hydrogen 287
  phosphate 161, 290, 298, 345
  phosphate, role of 117*f*
Nicotinic acid 295, 300
Niemann-Pick disease 142, 182, 183
Nifedipine 424
Night blindness 287, 301
  congenital stationary 506
Ninhydrin 38
  reaction 38

Nitrobenzene 223
Nitrocellulose membrane 378
Nitrogen balance 55, 315
  expresses 55
Nonalcoholic fatty liver disease 176
Nonalcoholic steatohepatitis 176
Nonapeptide 40
Noncompetitive inhibition 25
Nonenzymatic antioxidants 490
Nonheme proteins 277
Non-Hodgkin's lymphoma 453
Nonionizing radiation 476
Nonoxidative deamination 56
Nonoxidative irreversible phase 116
Non-protein nitrogen 58
  substances
    elimination of 392
    excretion of 391
Noradrenaline 402
Norepinephrine 199, 402, 482
  synthesis of 67
Normal glucose tolerance test 129*f*
Northern blotting 377
Nuclear receptor 462
Nucleic acid 328, 338
  chemistry of 328
  metabolism 340
  studies 524
Nucleolus 4
Nucleoplasm 4
Nucleoside 328
  analog reverse transcriptase inhibitor 450
Nucleotide 328, 330
  function of 330
  repeat diseases 359
  structure of 330
Nucleus 4
Nuclide 475
Numbness 296, 442
Nutrition 305
Nutritional assessment,
  methods of 316
Nutritional deficiency
  clinical signs of 317*t*
  signs of 317
  symptoms of 317
Nutrition-related diseases 321

Nutritive function 44
Nystagmus 293

O

Obesity 311, 324, 325
  causes of 311
  central 401
Obstruction, types of 388
Ochronosis 67
Odd-chain fatty acids, oxidation of 158, 159*f*
Oic acid 145
Oleic acid 146
Oligodendrocytes 447
Oligomycin 265
Oligosaccharides 81
Oliguria 393
Olmesartan 472
Omega 146
  oxidation 161
Oncofetal antigens 469
Oncogene 465
Oncogenic viruses 465
One-carbon
  group 61*f*
  metabolism 61, 61*f*
Optical activity 83
Oral glucose tolerance test,
  performing 128
Organ function tests 387
Organic acids 247
Organic constituents, tests for 533
Organic solvents, recipitation by 47
Ornithine 72
  transcarbamylase transfers 57
Orotic aciduria 57, 346
  drug-induced 346
Osazone 86
  formation 86*f*
Osmolality 272, 514, 517
Osmotic function 44
Osteoarthritis 311
Osteomalacia 289
Osteoporosis 232
Ovarian cancer 468
Ovarian cysts 468
Ovarian hormones 228
Ovary 240

Oxalate 268, 517
Oxalosuccinate,
　　decarboxylation of 103
Oxidation 157, 160, 259, 264, 482
　biological 259
　reaction 481
　reduction reactions 259, 265
Oxidative deamination 56
Oxidative irreversible phase 115
Oxidative phosphorylation 261, 264f
Oxidative stress 491
Oxidoreductases 19
Oxygen 210, 212, 262
　binding, factors affecting 213
　dissociation curves 211
　to hemoglobin, binding of 212f
Oxyhemoglobin 223
　formation of 211
Oxytocin 142, 231
　production of 231

P

Pain and fever 181
Palmitic acid 146, 158
　β-oxidation of 158f
Pancreas
　carcinoma of 388
　Langerhans of 238
Pancreatic hormones 228, 238
Pancreatic juice 92
Pancreatic lipase 153
Pancreatic phospholipase 154
Pancreatitis 156
Panitumumab 472
Pantothenic acid 17, 297, 301
Paracetamol 482
Paracrine signals 459
Paralysis 441, 442
Paraproteinemia, benign 499
Parathyroid hormone 228, 233, 268, 269
　functions 233
Parathyroid secretes 240
Partition chromatography 524
Pellagra 295f, 296
Pelvic inflammation 468
Penicillin 440

Pentapeptide 40
Pentose phosphate pathway 114
Pepsinogen 17, 53
Peptide 39
　bond formation 39f
　hormones 227
Perinatal transmission 446
Periodic hyperlysinemia 63
Peripheral neuritis 293
Peroxidase 277
Peroxidation 149
　reaction 488f
Peroxide 487
Peroxiredoxins 489
Peroxisomal fatty acid oxidation 160
Peroxisomes 3, 9, 160
　detoxify 3
Persistent hyperlysinemia 63
pH
　effect of 18
　on enzyme activity, effect of 18f
　renal regulation of 250
Phagocytosis 8, 496
　process of 8f
Phenylacetone 482
Phenylalanine 37, 65
　and tyrosine, metabolism of 65
　catabolism of 59
　hydroxylase 65
Phenylhydrazine, action of 85, 86f
Phenylketonuria 65, 74
Pheochromocytomas 68
Phosphatases 28
Phosphate 252, 262, 514
　buffer 530
　　system 248
　inorganic 14
　reabsorption of 288
　tests for 532, 533
Phosphatidic acid 170
Phosphatidylcholine 141, 142
　metabolism of 171
Phosphatidylethanolamine 141, 142, 171
　metabolism of 171
Phosphatidylinositol 142
Phosphatidylserine 141, 142

Phosphocreatine 14
Phosphofructokinase 101
Phosphogluconate pathway 114
Phosphoglycerides 247
Phosphoguanidines 14
Phospholipid 148, 171
　metabolism 169
　nucleic acids 247
　types of 141
Phosphoribosyl pyrophosphate 341, 344
Phosphoric acid 142
Phosphorus 267, 270, 271, 393, 517
Phosphorylated nucleosides 330
Phosphorylation 264, 365
Photoionic effect 521
Photomultiplier tubes 521
Photopsins 506
Photoreceptors, types of 502
Phototransduction 504, 505f, 507
　cascade, termination of 505
　human disorders of 506
Phylloquinone 289
Pigmented scaly dermatitis 296
Pinocytosis 8
Pituitary adenoma 237, 401
Pituitary gland 394, 398
Pituitary hormones 228
　anterior 199, 229
Placenta 28
　developing 239
Plaque formation 204f
Plasma
　cell leukemia 498
　cholesterol, increased 167
　lipoprotein classes 143
　preparation 511
Plasma membrane 1, 6f, 9
　sarcolemma for 416
Plasma proteins 44, 46t
　estimation of 536
　separation of 46
　types of 46
Plasmalogen 142
　synthesis of 178f
Plasmid 379, 380f
　manipulation of 380
Plasmodium falciparum 222

Platelet
  aggregation and thrombosis 181
  count 517
  derived growth factor 460
Pleural pericardial effusions 469
Pneumocystis jirovecii 445
  pneumonia 445
Pneumonia 393
Polyamines 60
  clinical importance of 60
Polyclonal hypergammaglobulinemia 498
Polycystic kidney 392
Polycythemia vera 393
Polymerase chain reaction 370, 374, 375f, 500
Polyol pathway 118
Polypeptide 40, 42
  protein 53
Polysaccharides 81
Polyunsaturated fatty acid 146, 164
Porphobilinogen 216
Porphyria 215
  acute intermittent 216
  causes of 216t
  cutanea tarda 216
  hepatoerythropoietic 216
Positive nitrogen balance 55
Posterior pituitary hormones 231
Postexposure prophylaxis 450
Posthepatic jaundice 389
Postprandial blood sugar 121
Postprandial glucose 514
Post-renal causes 58
Potassium 267, 274, 439, 514, 517
  chloride 274
  depletion 253
  ion 260
  movement of 274f
Pregnancy 239, 312, 396, 468
Prehybridization 377
Premenstrual syndrome 296
Pre-renal causes 58
Primary aldosteronism 402
Proenzyme 17, 54

Progeria 355
Progesterone 239, 240
  receptor 469
Programmed cell death 453, 457
Progressive mental deterioration 185
Prokaryotic cell 4, 5, 5f
  gene regulation 367f
Prokaryotic gene regulation 367
Prokaryotic organisms 367, 369
Prolactin 231, 515
Proline 37, 39
  catabolism of 64f
  metabolism 64
    catabolism 64
    synthesis 64
  synthesis of 64f
Promoter 369
Prostacyclins 188
Prostaglandin 140, 147, 179, 180
  biochemical actions of 181
  synthesis 179, 180f
  inhibition of 180
Prostate gland, carcinoma of 29
Prostate-specific antigen 466, 467, 517, 527
Prostatic acid phosphatase 467
Prostatic cancer, staging of 468
Protein 8, 35, 40, 41, 268, 305, 307, 308, 326, 387, 517
  acute-phase 45
  after denaturation, modification of 44
  biological
    role of 41
    value of 315, 315f
  buffer system 249
  buffering 41
  caloric value of 306, 306f
  calorie malnutrition 323, 326
  catabolism, severe 401
  charge properties of 40
  chemistry of 35
  classification of 40
  complementary 308
  complete 307
  conjugated 41, 41t
  contractile 41
  degradation 55
  denaturation of 44
  derived 41

  digestion of 54f
  functions of 41
  general functions of 41
  immune 41
  incomplete 307
  intrinsic 5
  iron containing 276
  losing diseases 499
  metabolism 126, 197
    effects on 123
  modifications of 366
  post-translational modification of 364
  precipitation of 46
  primary structure of 42f
  receptor 41
  storage 41
  structural 41, 407
  synthesis 3, 387
    inhibitors of 363, 363t
    steps of 362
  tertiary structure of 43f
  tests for 534
  total 388
Proteinemia, malignant 498
Protein-energy malnutrition
  causes of 323
  signs of 323
  symptoms of 323
Proteinuria 393
Proteoglycan 87, 407, 411, 413f
  structure of 412f
Proteolytic enzymes 53
Proteome 350
Proteomics 350, 351
Proton gradient 263
Proto-oncogene 464
  activation of 464
Proximal renal tubular acidosis 394
Pseudohyperkalemia 442
Pseudohypoaldosteronism 442
Pseudohypokalemia 441
Pulmonary emphysema 442
Pulmonary shunt 258
Purine analogs 333
Purine metabolism 340
Purine nucleotide
  catabolism of 342, 342f
  phosphorylases 342
  salvage of 340

synthesis
  inhibitors of 343
  regulation of 340
Purine salvage pathway 340
Purine synthesis, clinical
  significance of 343
Puromycin 363
Putrescine 60
Pyelonephritis 393
  acute 138
Pyloric obstruction 442
Pyridoxal phosphate 296, 298
Pyridoxamine 300
Pyridoxine 17, 295, 296, 300
  active form of 296
Pyrimidine 345
  analogs 334
  catabolism of 345, 345f
  metabolism 344
    clinical significance of 346
  nucleotide
    biosynthesis of 344
    synthesis of 345f
  synthesis of 340
Pyruvate carboxylase 271
Pyruvate dehydrogenase
  complex 294
Pyruvic acid 178

R

Radiation
  effects 480
  hazard symbol 477, 477f
  therapy 473
  types of 476, 476f
Radioactive iodine uptake 397
Radioactive isotopes 478t
  applications of 478
  half-life period of 476t
Radioactivity 475
  units of 476
Radioimmunoassay 396, 478,
  479f, 526
  applications of 527
  principle of 526
  techniques 526t
Radioisotope 475
Radionuclides 476
Radioprotective enclosure 477,
  478f

Radiotherapy 473, 479, 480
  internal 473
Rancidity 149
Random glucose 514
Rapoport-Luebering cycle 101,
  101f
Reaction
  catalyzed and uncatalyzed
    18f
  reduction 85
Reactive oxygen
  biological effects of 487
  species 486, 487f
    formation of 487
Receptor tyrosine kinase 462f
Recombinant vaccine 494
Red blood cell 4, 214, 216, 289,
  394, 478, 522
  count
    female 516
    male 516
Redox reactions 259
  principle of 259
Refsum disease 160
Reichert-Meissl
  number 149
  value 149
Renal blood flow, reduced 393
Renal causes 58
Renal failure 393, 436, 441
  acute 392, 442
  chronic 268, 392
Renal function
  influence on 181
  test 70, 391
Renal insufficiency 441
Renal system 247
Renin 527
Rennin clots milk 53
Replication, types of 353f
Respiratory acid-base disorders
  253
Respiratory acidosis 251, 253,
  258
  and alkalosis 253f
Respiratory alkalosis 253, 258
Respiratory center 250
Respiratory distress syndrome
  142
Respiratory electron transport
  chain 260

Respiratory function, effects
  on 181
Respiratory system 247
Resting metabolic rate 312
Restriction enzymes 379
Restriction fragment length
  polymorphism 380
Retina layers 503
Retinitis pigmentosa 506
Retinoic acid 287, 291
Retinoids 286
Retinol 287, 291
Retinopathy 126
Rhabdomyolysis 441, 442
Rhodopsin 41, 287
Riboflavin 17, 294, 300
  active form of 294
Ribonucleic acid 352, 359, 363,
  371, 371f, 391, 445, 448
  functions of 336
  structure of 336, 336f, 359,
    360f
  types of 336
Richner-Hanhart syndrome 67
Rickets 318f
Rifampicin 363
Rituximab 472
Rod cells 287
Rods and cones, structure of
  502f
Rotavirus 445
Rothera's test 534, 535
Rothmund-Thomson syndrome
  355
Rotor's syndrome 219

S

Saccharin 202
S-adenosylmethionine 61, 71
Salivary amylase hydrolyzes 91
Sandhoff disease, treatment
  for 185
Sanfilippo's syndrome 411, 412
Saponification 148
Sarcolemma 416, 420
Sarcomere, structure of 417f
Sarcoplasmic reticulum 416
Sarcotubular system 420f
Satiety hormone 201
Saturated fats 308

Saturated fatty acids 146
Scheie's syndrome 412
Schiff's test 533
Scurvy, symptoms of 292f
Seborrheic dermatitis 295
Secretin 53
Seizures 439
   convulsive 296
   treatment of 296
Selenium 281, 490
Semen 444
Seminal vesicles 240
Sensory neurons, growth of 460
Sepsis 393
Serine 37, 39, 169
   catabolism of 74
   metabolism of 74
Serotonin 69
   physiological role of 69
   synthesis of 69, 69f
Serum
   calcium level, regulation of 268
   cholesterol 203
   electrophoresis 48f
   ferroxidase 278
   glutamic pyruvic transaminase 515
   immunoglobulins, quantitative determination of 497
   osmolality 272, 437
   preparation 511
   total protein estimation 388
   transaminases 390
Serum enzyme 27t, 218, 389, 390
   levels 205f
Serum glutamate
   oxaloacetate transaminase 56, 515
   pyruvate transaminase 55
Serum potassium 440
   determination 441
Serum protein 388
   electrophoresis 388
Sex hormones, female 238
Sexual maturation and fertility 227
Shock 392, 435
Shuttle pathways 100

Sialic acid 87
Sick euthyroid syndrome 397
Sickle cell
   anemia 221
   hemoglobin 221
   causes and symptoms 221
Sickle red blood cells 222f
Sickling test 222
Signal transduction 123f
Single antibody method 527
   principle of 527f
Singlet oxygen 487
Skeletal muscle 196, 416, 424
   activation of 418
   contraction of 418
   fibers 421
   in starvation 197
Skin 480
   folds 311, 318
Sleep apnea 311
Sliding filament model 419, 420f
Smooth muscle 416, 424, 425
   contraction of 425
Snoring 311
Sodium 267, 271, 437, 514, 517
   balance 437
   dodecyl sulfate 377
   hypobromite test 532, 533
   ion 260
   nitroprusside test 533, 534
Soft tissue swelling 230
Solitary thyroid nodules 395
Solubility test 223, 223t
Somatomammotropin 231
Somatotrophs, tumor of 230
Somatotropin 229
Sorbitol dehydrogenase 119
Sorbitol pathway 118, 119f, 506
Southern blotting 376, 377f
Spectrophotometry 519, 528
   components of 520f
   principle of 519
Spermidine 60
Spermine 60
Sphingomyelin 142, 143, 183
   deposition of 142
Sphingophospholipids 140, 142
Sphingosine 142
Spironolactone 441

Spongy gums 292
Sprinter, energy for 422
Starch, structure of 81f
Stearic acid 146
Steatorrhea 156
   causes 156
   treatment 157
Stereoisomerism 83
Steroid 147, 227
   hormone 147, 237, 401
     hydroxylation of 482
   receptors 462
   receptor signaling 462, 463f
Stevia 202
Stimulates erythropoiesis 460
Stimulates granulocytes 460
Stimulates monocytes 460
Stomach, digestion in 53
Streptomycin 363
Strong acids, action of 85
Stuart-Prower factor 24
Subcellular fractions, marker enzymes of 9t
Subcellular organelles, isolation of 522, 523f
Subclinical hyperthyroidism 397
Subclinical hypothyroidism 397
Substrate concentration, effect of 19, 19f
Succinate dehydrogenase 260, 294
Sucralose 202
Sugar alcohols 87
Sulfa drugs, treatment with 24
Sulfate 252, 484
Sulfhemoglobin 224
Sulfhydryl group 39
Sulfonamides 343
Sulfosalicyclic acid test 534
Sulfur conjugation 483, 484
Sulphates, tests for 532, 533
Sulphemoglobin 223
Superoxide anion 487
Superoxide dismutase 489
Suprarenal cortical hormones 228
Suprarenal medullary hormones 228
Sweating 441
Swollen lymph nodes 184

Synthesis 180
Synthetic nucleotide analogs 332

T

Tachycardia 294
Tandem enzyme 100
Tay-Sachs disease 182, 185
Teletherapy 479
Telmisartan 472
Temperature, effect of 19
Testes 240
Testicular hormones 228
Testosterone 516
Tetracycline 363
Tetrahydro folic acid 472
Tetrahydrofolate 61, 340, 341
　formation of 298f
Thalassemia 221
　minor 221
　types 221
Thiamine 17, 292, 300
　monophosphate 293
　pyrophosphate 292
　triphosphate 293
Thioguanine 333, 472
Thiokinase 271
Thiolase 157
Thioredoxin 489
Threonine 37, 39
　metabolism 63, 63f
Thromboembolic condition,
　dicumarol to 24
Thrombolysis therapy,
　　monitoring outcome of 427
Thromboxane 180, 188
Thymidine
　monophosphate 329, 344
　triphosphate 345
Thyroid
　autoantibodies 397
　binding globulin 398
　cancer 395, 478f
　cells 232, 394
　function, tests for 394, 395
　gland 232
　　function of 394
　hormone 228, 232, 240
　　role of 232

iodine uptake scan 398
peroxidase antibodies 397
scan 397, 399
Thyroiditis 395, 396
　chronic 397
Thyroid-releasing hormone 230, 394
　test 398
Thyroid-stimulating hormone 230, 394, 396t, 397t, 515
　pituitary production of 398
Thyrotropin 230
　releasing hormone 40, 227
Thyroxine 122, 199, 527
　induced hyperthyroidism 396
　therapy 398
Tissues
　development of 287
　growth of 287
Tocopherol 289
Total body weight 313
Toxic multinodulargoiter 396
Toxoid vaccines 494, 501
Toxoplasma
　encephalitis 445
　gondii 445
Trace elements 267, 276
Trans fat 309
　risks of 309
Transcarboxylation 61
Transcription 360, 361f
　factors 369
Transcription-mediated
　　amplification 370
Transfer ribonucleic acid 337, 360, 363
　structure of 337f, 360f
Transferases 19
Transferrin 277, 490
Transketolase transfers 116
Transmembrane receptors 461
Transmethylation 61
　reaction 484
Transport across membranes 5
Transport function 44
Transport protein 41
Trastuzumab 472

Triacylglycerol 153
　biosynthesis of 177
　composition of 141
　fate of 176
　synthesis 177f
Tricarboxylic acid 63, 104, 158, 195, 197, 259, 263
Tricarboxylic acid cycle 104
　amphibolic role of 105
　anapleurotic reactions of 105
　regulation of 104
Trichothiodystrophy 355
Triglycerides 140, 141, 148, 514
Trihydric alcohol 147
Triiodothyronine 527
Tripeptide 39
Tropomyosin 427
　filaments 418f
Troponin 205, 427
Trypsin 54
　hydrolyzes peptide 54
Trypsinogen 17
Tryptophan 37
　fate of 69f
　metabolic fate of 68
　metabolism of 68, 68f
Tuberculosis 25, 344, 445
Tubular disease 394
Tubular necrosis 392
　acute 392, 393
Tumor
　necrosis factor-alpha 460
　suppressor genes 465
Tumor cells
　necrosis of 460
　types of 63
Tumor markers 465, 467f, 527
　detection of 466
Typical buffalo hump 401
Tyrosine 37
　catabolism of 66f
　　metabolic block in 67f
　　phosphate hydroxy-
　　　phenylpyruvate
　　　hydroxylase of 279
　from phenylalanine,
　　synthesis of 65f
　metabolic fates of 66, 67f
　metabolism of 65
Tyrosinemia 67
　benign transient neonatal 67

U

Ubiquitone 490
Ulcerative colitis 235
Unsaturated fats 308
Uracil nucleotides 332
Urea 252, 392, 514, 517
    cycle 56, 57f
        inborn errors of 57, 57t
    synthesis 387
    tests for 533
Urease test, specific 532, 533
Uremia 442
Uric acid 393, 490, 514, 517
    tests for 533
Uridine diphosphate 332, 345
    glucose-glucuronate 119
Uridine monophosphate 329, 338, 344, 345
Uridine triphosphate 345
Urinalysis 138
Urinary ammonia 252
Urinary free cortisol level 236
    twenty-four-hour 401
Urinary tract
    infection 394
    obstruction 393
Urine 218, 390
    abnormal constituents of 534
    analysis 534
    collection 512
    formation 391
    osmolality 272, 437
    tests 517
Urobilinogen 218, 389
Uronic acid pathway 119
Uterine smooth muscles, contraction of 231

V

Vaccine 494
    development 494
    types of 494
Vaginal fluid 444
Valine 37, 39
Valsartan 472
Van den Bergh's reaction 389
Van den Bergh's test 217, 389
Vanillyl-mandelic acid 467
Variegate porphyria 216
Vas deferens 240
Vascular endothelial growth factor 472
Vasopressin 142, 231
Ventilation perfusion 258
Very low density lipoprotein 144, 171, 172, 174
    composition of 172f
    metabolism of 172f
Vinblastine 472
Vincristine 472
Viral hepatitis 388
    types of 391
Vision 287
    and hearing, loss of 183
    biochemistry of 502
    double 293
Visual cycle 506
Visual phototransduction 502
Vitamin 286, 291, 301, 387, 527
    A 140, 286, 291
        deficiency 301
        retinol form of 287
        role of 287
    B complex 292
    B1 300
    B12 299, 301
        deficiency of 321
    B2 300
    B3 300
    B5 301
    B6 300
    B7 301
    C 149, 291, 300, 322, 366, 490
        role of 292f
    D 140, 147, 268, 287, 288, 291
        action of 268
        deficiency of 289, 318f
    D3 148, 164, 288
        deficiency 289f
    E 140, 149, 286, 289, 291, 490, 492
    essential 306
    fats soluble 286, 291t, 301
    K 24, 140, 286, 289, 291
        cycle 290f
        dependent carboxylase enzyme requires oxygen 290
Vomiting 253, 294, 441
von Gierke's disease 114, 343

W

Waist circumference 319
Wald's visual cycle 287f
Waldenström's macroglobulinemia 498, 499
Water
    balance 432, 443
    depletion 392
    excess 436
Water-soluble vitamins 286, 291, 300t, 301
Watery diarrhea, severe 439
Weakness 442
Weight 312
    categories of 319f
    gain 308, 325
    loss 308
    measurement 318
Werner syndrome 355, 356
Wernicke-Korsakoff syndrome 293
Wet beriberi 293
White blood cell 487
Wilson's disease 279
Wound healing 460

X

Xanthine 517
    oxidase 294
Xanthochromatosis 203
Xenobiotics, metabolism of 481
Xeroderma pigmentosum 355, 356

Z

Zellweger syndrome 160
Zero-order kinetics 21
Zinc 279
    turbidity 514
Zona
    fasciculata 234, 399
    glomerulosa 234, 399
    reticularis 234, 399
Zygotes 455
Zymogens 17

EU GSPR Authorised Reprsentative
Logos Europe, 9 rue Nicolas Poussin
1700, La Rochelle, France
Phone: +33 (0) 6 67 93 73 78
E-mail: contact@logoseurope.eu

www.ingramcontent.com/pod-product-compliance
Ingram Content Group UK Ltd.
Pitfield, Milton Keynes, MK11 3LW, UK
UKHW050430150426
5217IPUK00019B/1319